RADIATION CARCINOGENESIS

CURRENT ONCOLOGY
Nathaniel I. Berlin, *Series Editor*

RADIATION CARCINOGENESIS

Edited by

ARTHUR C. UPTON, M.D.
Professor and Director, Institute of Environmental Medicine,
New York University Medical Center,
New York

ROY E. ALBERT, M.D.
Director, Institute of Environmental Health,
University of Cincinnati,
Cincinnati, Ohio

FREDRIC J. BURNS, Ph.D.
Professor, Institute of Environmental Medicine,
New York University Medical Center,
New York

ROY E. SHORE, Ph.D., D.P.H.
Associate Professor, Institute of Environmental Medicine,
New York University Medical Center,
New York

ELSEVIER
New York • Amsterdam • London

Elsevier Science Publishing Co., Inc.
52 Vanderbilt Avenue, New York, New York 10017

Distributors outside the United States and Canada
Elsevier Science Publishers B.V.
P.O. Box 211, 1000 AE Amsterdam, The Netherlands

Library of Congress Cataloging-in-Publication Data

Main entry under title:

Radiation carcinogenesis.

    (Current oncology, ISSN 0743-930X)
    1. Tumors, Radiation-induced. I. Upton, Arthur C., 1923-
    II. Series. [DNLM: 1. Neoplasms, Radiation-Induced. 2.
    Radiation Effects. QZ 200 R129]
RC268.55.R32 1986   616.99'4071   85-29243
ISBN 0-444-00859-4

Current printing (last digit)
10 9 8 7 6 5 4 3 2 1

Manufactured in the United States of America

CONTENTS

SECTION III. CARCINOGENESIS IN EXPERIMENTAL ANIMALS

EXPERIMENTAL CARCINOGENESIS IN THE SKELETON   **215**

Marvin Goldman

EXPERIMENTAL CARCINOGENESIS IN THE DIGESTIVE
AND GENITOURINARY TRACTS   **233**

Hiromitsu Watanabe, Akihiro Ito, and Fumio Hirose

SECTION IV. CARCINOGENIC EFFECTS IN HUMANS

LEUKEMIA, LYMPHOMA, AND MULTIPLE MYELOMA   **245**

Robert S. Miller and Gilbert W. Beebe

SECTION V. MODIFYING FACTORS AND RISK ASSESSMENT

PREFACE

Since the carcinogenic effects of ionizing radiation were first reported more than eighty years ago, they have been a subject of increasing epidemiological, clinical, and experimental study. Recently, however, serious credence has been given to the possibility that there might be no threshold for radiation carcinogenesis. Abandonment of the threshold hypothesis for purposes of radiological protection has prompted mounting debate about the shape of the dose–incidence curve in the low dose domain. As a result, rising public concern about the risks at low doses has led to growing numbers of congressional investigations, compensation claims, and law suits.

Attempts to predict the carcinogenic effects of low doses from effects observed at higher doses require assumptions about the shape of the dose–incidence relationship and, in turn, the mechanisms of carcinogenesis. Such risk assessments must thus seek to integrate all relevant epidemiological and experimental data. In order for the cogent information to appear together in a single volume, authoritative reviews on various aspects of radiation carcinogenesis have been compiled in the following chapters.

The editors are grateful to the many authors whose knowledge and perspectives are reflected in this compendium. We hope that the volume will be useful as a source book to those working in the field and will advance the understanding of the subject for readers in general.

CONTRIBUTORS

Editors
ARTHUR C. UPTON, M.D., ROY E. ALBERT, M.D., FREDRIC J. BURNS, Ph.D., and
ROY E. SHORE, Ph.D., D.P.H.

Chapter Authors
ROY E. ALBERT, M.D.
Institute of Environmental Health, University of Cincinnati, Cincinnati, Ohio

T. ASTIER, D.Sc.
Unité de Recherche de Radiobiologie Expérimentale et de Cancérologie, Bordeaux,
France

W. BAIR, Ph.D.
Environment, Health, and Safety Research Program, Battelle Pacific Northwest Laboratories, Richland, Washington

G. W. BARENDSEN, Ph.D.
Radiobiological Institute TNO, Rijswijk, and Laboratory for Radiobiology, Amsterdam,
The Netherlands

GILBERT W. BEEBE, Ph.D.
Clinical Epidemiology Branch, National Cancer Institute, National Institutes of Health,
Bethesda, Maryland

JOHN D. BOICE, Jr., Sc.D.
Clinical Epidemiology Branch, Environmental Epidemiology Branch, National Cancer
Institute, Bethesda, Maryland

V. P. BOND, M.D.
Brookhaven National Laboratory, Associated Universities, Inc., Upton, New York

FREDRIC J. BURNS, Ph.D.
Institute of Environmental Medicine, New York University Medical Center, New York

A. V. CARRANO, Ph.D.
Biomedical Sciences Division, Lawrence Livermore National Laboratory, Livermore,
California

GERALD L. CHAN, Ph.D.
Laboratory of Radiobiology, Harvard School of Public Health, Boston

JAMES E. CLEAVER, Ph.D.
Laboratory of Radiobiology and Environmental Health, University of California, San
Francisco

KELLY H. CLIFTON, Ph.D.
Departments of Human Oncology and Radiology, Wisconsin Clinical Cancer Center,
University of Wisconsin Medical School, Madison

J. F. DUPLAN, M.D.
Unité de Recherche de Radiobiologie Expérimentale et de Cancérologie, Bordeaux,
France

R. J. M. FRY, M.D.
Biology Division, Oak Ridge National Laboratory, Oak Ridge, Tennessee

MARVIN GOLDMAN, Ph.D.
Laboratory for Energy-Related Health Research, University of California, Davis

B. GUILLEMAIN, Ph.D.
Unité de Recherche de Radiobiologie Expérimentale et de Cancérologie, Bordeaux,
France

NAOMI H. HARLEY, Ph.D.
Institute of Environmental Medicine, New York University Medical Center, New York

LOUIS H. HEMPELMANN, M.D.
Department of Radiology, University of Rochester School of Medicine and Dentistry,
Rochester, New York

FUMIO HIROSE, M.D.
Research Institute for Nuclear Medicine and Biology, Hiroshima University, Hiroshima, Japan

S. HOLTZMAN, Ph.D.
Medical Department, Brookhaven National Laboratory, Upton, New York

AKIHIRO ITO, M.D.
Research Institute for Nuclear Medicine and Biology, Hiroshima University, Hiroshima, Japan

WOLFGANG JACOBI, M.D.
Gesellschaft für Strahlen und Umweltforschung, Institute for Radiation Protection,
Munich–Neuherberg, Federal Republic of Germany

ALFRED G. KNUDSON, Jr., M.D., Ph.D.
Fox Chase Cancer Center, Philadelphia

CHARLES E. LAND, Ph.D.
National Cancer Institute, National Institutes of Health, Bethesda, Maryland

JOHN B. LITTLE, M.D.
Laboratory of Radiobiology, Harvard School of Public Health, Boston

ROBERT W. MILLER, M.D.
Clinical Epidemiology Branch and the Environmental Epidemiology Branch, National
Cancer Institute, National Institutes of Health, Bethesda, Maryland

SURESH H. MOOLGAVKAR, M.D., Ph.D.
Fox Chase Cancer Center, Philadelphia

PHILIP E. SARTWELL, M.D.
Institute of Environmental Medicine, New York University Medical Center, New York

C. J. SHELLABARGER, Ph.D.
Medical Department, Brookhaven National Laboratory, Upton, New York

ROY E. SHORE, Ph.D., D.P.H.
Institute of Environmental Medicine, New York University Medical Center, New York

J. P. STONE, Ph.D.
Medical Department, Brookhaven National Laboratory, Upton, New York

JOHN B. STORER, M.D.
Biology Division, Oak Ridge National Laboratory, Oak Ridge, Tennessee

R. L. ULLRICH, Ph.D.
Biology Division, Oak Ridge National Laboratory, Oak Ridge, Tennessee

ARTHUR C. UPTON, M.D.
Institute of Environmental Medicine, New York University Medical Center, New York

JANET VAUGHAN, F.R.S., F.R.C.P., D.M.
Bone Research Laboratory, Nuffield Orthopaedic Centre, Oxford, England

HIROMITSU WATANABE, M.D.
Research Institute for Nuclear Medicine and Biology, Hiroshima University, Hiroshima, Japan

SHELDON WOLFF, Ph.D.
Laboratory of Radiobiology and Environmental Health and Department of Anatomy,
University of California, San Francisco

ELIZABETH D. WOODARD, M.D., M.P.H.
Department of Preventive, Family, and Rehabilitation Medicine, University of Rochester School of Medicine and Dentistry, Rochester, New York

KENJIRO YOKORO, Ph.D.
Department of Pathology, Research Institute for Nuclear Medicine and Biology, Hiroshima University, Hiroshima, Japan

SECTION I
INTRODUCTION AND OVERVIEW

HISTORICAL PERSPECTIVES ON RADIATION CARCINOGENESIS

ARTHUR C. UPTON, M.D.

Within weeks after Roentgen's discovery of the x-ray, in 1895, the first radiation injuries were reported (Table 1). These consisted predominantly of acute skin reactions involving the hands of those working with early radiation equipment (Brown, 1936). Within barely 1 year, 96 such cases were documented in a single report (Stone-Scott, 1897). During ensuing years, various other harmful effects of radiation were encountered, including the first case of cancer attributed to radiation (Frieben, 1902).

Since these early findings, study of the biological and carcinogenic effects of radiation has received continuing impetus from the expanding use of radiologic methods in medicine, science, and industry. Added impetus has come more recently from the military and peaceful applications of atomic energy.

Because of the long-standing professional and public interest in the carcinogenic effects of ionizing radiation, these effects have been investigated more thoroughly than those of any other environmental agent. The evolution of our knowledge of these effects and, in turn, the development of effective methods for radiation risk assessment and for radiologic protection, provide lessons of far-reaching scientific and practical importance.

EARLY OBSERVATIONS ON EXPOSED HUMAN POPULATION

Although it was evident early in the century, from carcinogenic effects in radiation workers, that cancer could result from excessive occupational exposure (Furth and Lorenz, 1954), it was not until decades later that epidemiologic studies of radiologists (Ulrich, 1946; March, 1950), patients irradiated therapeutically for ankylosing spondylitis (Court Brown and Doll, 1957) and other benign diseases (Simpson and Hempelmann, 1957), atomic bomb survivors

From the Institute of Environmental Medicine, New York University Medical Center, New York, New York.

TABLE 1. Early Reports of Radiation Injury Following Roentgen's Discovery of the X-Ray in 1895

Date	Type of injury	Reported by
1896	Dermatitis of hands	Grubbe
1896	Smarting of eyes	Edison
1896	Epilation	Daniel
1897	Constitutional symptoms	Walsh
1899	Degeneration of blood vessels	Gassman
1902	Cancer in x-ray ulcer	Frieben
1903	Inhibition of bone growth	Perthes
1903	Sterilization	Albers-Schonberg
1904	Blood changes	Milchner and Mosse
1906	Bone marrow changes	Warthin
1911	Leukemia in five radiation workers	Jagic
1912	Anemia in two x-ray workers	Belere

Source: Stone (1959)

(Moloney and Kastenbaum, 1955), and children exposed prenatally during radiographic examination of their mothers (Stewart et al, 1957) suggested the possibility that there might be no threshold for the carcinogenic effects of radiation (Lewis, 1957). The past 25 yr have produced a wealth of epidemiologic data bearing on this question (Table 2), which are reviewed in the chapters that follow. Although, in general, the data lend support to the hypothesis that the dose–incidence relationship may include no threshold for certain types of cancer, the data are imprecise enough, in most instances, to be compatible with any of several dose–incidence models. Hence, choice of the appropriate model for purposes of risk assessment is a matter of judgement, which must take into account all cogent information, including relevant data on the mechanisms of carcinogenesis.

EARLY OBSERVATIONS ON EXPERIMENTAL ANIMALS

Within several years after the first radiation-induced cases of cancer were observed in humans, the disease was produced experimentally in laboratory animals (Table 3). Since then, neoplasms of an increasing variety of histologic types have been associated with exposure to radiation (Lacassagne, 1945a&b; Brues, 1951; Furth and Lorenz, 1954; UNSCEAR, 1977). From the wealth of information that is now available, it may be concluded that

1. Neoplasms of almost any type can be induced by irradiation of an animal of suitable susceptibility, given appropriate conditions of exposure.
2. Not every type of neoplasm is increased in frequency by irradiation of animals of any one species or strain.
3. The carcinogenic effects of irradiation are mediated through a variety of mechanisms, depending on the type of tumor and the conditions of exposure.

4. Some mechanisms of carcinogenesis involve direct effects on the tumor-forming cells, themselves, but others may involve indirect (abscopal) effects on distant cells or organs.

5. Though the dose–incidence curve has not been defined precisely for any neoplasm over a wide range of doses, dose rates, and radiation qualities, the incidence generally rises more steeply as a function of dose and is less dependent on dose rates with radiations of high linear energy transfer (LET)—such as alpha particles or fast neutrons—than with radiations of low LET—such as x-rays and gamma rays.

6. The development of neoplasia appears to be a multicausal and multistage process, in which the effects of radiation may be modified by other physical or chemical agents.

7. At low to intermediate dose levels, the carcinogenic effects of radiation often remain unexpressed unless promoted by other agents.

8. At high dose levels, the expression of carcinogenic effects often tends to be suppressed by sterilization of the potentially transformed cells or by other forms of radiation injury, resulting in saturation of the dose–incidence curve.

9. The distribution in time of radiation-induced tumors characteristically varies with the type of tumor, the genetic background and age of the exposed animal, the conditions of irradiation, and other variables.

10. Because of the diversity of ways in which irradiation can influence the probability of neoplasia, the dose–incidence relationship may vary accordingly (Mole, 1975; UNSCEAR, 1977).

Owing to the complexity of neoplasia, attempts to elucidate the mechanisms of carcinogenesis have turned increasingly to model systems that enable the process to be analyzed at the cellular level. These approaches, among others, include the use of cell culture methods and transplantation of cells from irradiated donors into suitably conditioned recipients.

OBSERVATIONS AT THE CELLULAR LEVEL

For radiation carcinogenesis, there are strong grounds for questioning the assumption that the dose–response relationship must include a threshold (UNSCEAR, 1977; Whittemore and Keller, 1978; Brown et al, 1978; Crump, 1979; IRLG, 1979; NAS/BEIR, 1980). The evidence that many—if not most—cancers arise from a single cell (Fialkow, 1977), the putative role of DNA or chromosome damage in carcinogenesis (Cairns, 1981; Straus, 1981; Moolgavkar and Knudson, 1981; Bartsch et al, 1982; Yunis, 1983), the heritable nature of the neoplastic transformation in somatic cells, and the linear-nonthreshold nature of the dose–effect relationship for radiation-induced mutations and chromosome aberrations in the low-dose region (NAS/BEIR, 1980; UNSCEAR, 1982) imply that radiation-induced damage to the DNA or chromosomes of a single somatic cell, under certain conditions, may exert a potentially carcinogenic stimulus, even at low levels of exposure. In addition, unless other cancer-causing agents act through mechanisms unrelated to radiation carcinogenesis, the heterogeneity of the human population and its "background" incidence of

TABLE 2. Various Types of Cancer Associated with Radiation in Different Populations

Type of cancer	Atom bomb radiation			Medical radiation			
	Japanese atom bomb survivors	Marshall Islanders	Nuclear test participants	Ankylosing spondylitis (x-ray)	Ankylosing spondylitis (radium)	Benign pelvic disease	Benign breast disease
Leukemia	***		*	***		**	
Thyroid	***	**					
Female breast	***				*		***
Lung	***			***			
Bone				*	***		
Stomach	**			**			
Esophagus	**			**			
Bladder	**						
Lymphoma (including multiple myeloma)	**			**			
Brain							
Uterus						*	
Cervix	*						
Liver	*						
Skin							
Salivary gland	*						
Kidney				*	*		
Pancreas							
Colon	*					**	
Small intestine						*	
Rectum						**	

Source: Department of Health, Education and Welfare (1979)

*, Suggestive but unconfirmed associations; **, meaningful associations; ***, strong associations.

cancer are high enough so that any dose of radiation may be conceived to increase the risk of cancer in the most sensitive member of the population (Crump et al, 1979; Hall, 1980; Peto, 1978; Van Ryzin, 1982).

The inferences just mentioned are supported by observations on the kinetics of cell transformation in vitro. Although studies on the dose–effect relationship for transformation in vitro are few in number as yet, several important conclusions emerge from relevant experiments with Syrian hamster embryo (Borek, 1979a) and C3H 10T1/2 mouse embryo (Little et al, 1979; Elkind and Han, 1979; Lloyd et al, 1979) fibroblasts: 1) the percentage of cells transformed increases with increasing dose, reaching a plateau in the region of 150–400 rads of x-rays; 2) the transforming effectiveness of high LET radiation is greater than that of low LET radiation; 3) depending on the cell system used, transforming effects are detectable with doses as low as 0.1 rad of fast neutrons or

TABLE 2. (continued)

Medical radiation							Occupational radiation			
Multiple chest fluoroscopy	Tinea capitis (children)	Enlarged thymus (infants)	Thorotrast	Thyroid cancer (^{131}I)	In utero x-ray	Diagnostic x-ray	Radium dial painters	Radiologists	Uranium and other miners	Nuclear workers
		**	***	*	***	*	***			*
	**	***								
***										
			**						***	*
					***					
			*				**			*
	**			*			**			
			***							
	**	**					***	**		
	**	**	*							
										*
						*				

1.0 rad of x-rays; 4) the rate of transformation varies, depending on the cell system, radiation dose, and culture conditions used; 5) the rate of transformation may be modified by agents that promote or inhibit carcinogenesis in vivo; and 6) a dose of 50–300 rads of x-rays delivered in two or more fractions spread over an interval of hours can cause a higher rate of transformation than the same dose delivered in a single, brief exposure, depending on the culture conditions (Borek, 1979b; Elkind and Han, 1979).

Although research to date has not succeeded in defining the subcellular lesions involved in cell transformation, it has advanced our knowledge significantly. In the next few years, further understanding of the role of oncogenes (Duesberg, 1983; Weiss, 1983; Yunis, 1983, 1984; Rowley, 1984; Guerrero, et al. 1984), should provide important new insight into the mechanisms of radiation carcinogenesis at the molecular level.

TABLE 3. Early Experimental Radiation-Induced Cancers

Author (Date)	Radiation or isotope	Species	Type of tumor
Marie et al (1910)	X-ray	Rat	Sarcoma, spindle-celled
Marie et al (1912)	X-ray	Rat	Sarcoma, spindle-celled
Lazarus-Barlow (1918)	Ra	Mouse, rat	Carcinoma of skin
Bloch (1923)	X-ray	Rabbit	Carcinoma
Bloch (1924)	X-ray	Rabbit	Carcinoma
Goebel and Gerard (1925)	X-ray	Guinea pig	Sarcoma, polymorphous
Daels (1925)	Ra	Mouse, rat	Sarcoma, spindle-celled
Jonkhoff (1927)	X-ray	Mouse	Carcinoma-sarcoma
Lacassagne and Vinzent (1929)	X-ray	Rabbit	Fibrosarcoma, osteosarcoma, rhabdomyosarcoma
Schurch (1930)	X-ray	Rabbit	Carcinoma
Daels and Biltris (1931)	Ra	Rat	Sarcoma of cranium, kidney, spleen
Daels and Biltris (1931)	Ra	Guinea pig	Sarcoma of cranium, kidney, spleen
Daels and Biltris (1937)	Ra	Chicken	Carcinoma of biliary tract, osteosarcoma
Schurch and Uehlinger (1931)	Ra	Rabbit	Sarcoma of bone, liver, spleen
Uehlinger and Schurch (1935–47)	Ra,Ms-Th	Rabbit	Sarcoma of bone, liver, spleen
Sabin et al (1932)	Ra,Ms-Th	Rabbit	Osteosarcoma
Lacassagne (1933)	X-ray	Rabbit	Sarcoma, spindle-celled, myxosarcoma
Petrov and Krotkina (1933)	Ra	Guinea pig	Carcinoma of biliary tract
Sedginidse (1933)	X-ray	Mouse	Carcinoma, spindle-celled
Ludin (1934)	X-ray	Rabbit	Chondrosarcoma

Source: Lacassagne (1945a,b); Furth and Lorenz (1954); Upton (1968)

RISK ASSESSMENT AND RADIOLOGIC PROTECTION

In the early days, radiation safety standards were directed primarily toward the prevention of gross tissue damage, because protection against such effects was thought to be sufficient to eliminate all significant risk of harm. To achieve this objective, the Advisory Committee on X-ray and Radium Protection (later to become the National Council on Radiation Protection and Measurements) and the International Commission on Radiological Protection (ICRP) both recommended in the early 1930s that occupational exposure be limited to a maxium dose of 0.2 R/day (Table 4). Selection of this "tolerance" limit, as opposed to a higher or lower limit, was based on the observation that many radiation workers had been exposed at this level for years without apparent injury.

Later, as it was recognized that there might be no threshold for the genetic effects of radiation, and as the incidence of leukemia in radiologists was observed to be increased without other evidence of radiation injury, the exposure limit was reduced (Table 4) and the term "tolerance" dose was replaced by the term "maximum permissable" dose.

In the 1950s, large scale atmospheric testing of nuclear weapons led to growing concern about the genetic hazards to the world's population from mounting levels of radioactive fallout. As a consequence, dose limits to protect the population against such hazards were recommended (Table 4) (NAS, 1956). Since then, epidemiologic studies have suggested that the carcinogenic effects of low-level irradiation may be comparable in magnitude to the genetic effects (UNSCEAR, 1977, 1982; ICRP, 1977; NAS/BEIR, 1980). As a result, radiation protection standards for the individual have been strengthened accordingly (ICRP, 1977). Furthermore, to aid in assessing compensation claims, the U.S. Congress has mandated publication of a basis for estimating the likelihood that

TABLE 4. Historical Highlights in the Evolution of Radiation Protection Standards

1902	Rollins established photographic indication of "safe" intensity
1921	British X-ray and Radium Protection Committee considered "establishing a maximum tolerance dose"
1925	First attempt was made by Mutscheller to define a "tolerance dose"
1928	International Commission on Radiological Protection (ICRP) was established to develop radiation protection standards
1929	Advisory Committee on X-ray and Radium Protection was formed in the U.S. (later to become the National Council on Radiation Protection and Measurements)
1931	U.S. Advisory Committee on X-Ray and Radium Protection recommended a dose limit of 0.2 R/day for radiation workers (endorsed in 1934 by ICRP)
1936	U.S. Advisory Committee on X-Ray and Radium Protection reduced dose limit to 0.1 R/day
1950	International Commission on Radiological Protection reduced dose limit to 0.3 R/wk
1956	International Commission on Radiological Protection reduced dose limit to 5 R/yr
1956	National Academy of Sciences recommended a gonadal dose limit for general population of 10 R/30 yr
1960	Federal Radiation Council recommended 5 R/yr whole-body dose limit for radiation workers and 0.17 R/yr dose limit for general population, exclusive of natural background and medical radiation

Source: Stone (1959); Upton (1969)

TABLE 5. Comparative Estimates by the NAS/BEIR Committee and UNSCEAR of the Lifetime Risk of Fatal Cancer from Low-Level Low-LET Radiation

Source of estimate	Dose–response model[a]	Projection model	
		Absolute risk model	Relative risk model
		(Cancers per 10,000 person-Sv)	
BEIR (1980)	Linear, linear	167	501
BEIR (1980)	Linear-quadratic, linear	77	226
BEIR (1972)[b]	Linear, linear	117	621
UNSCEAR (1977)[c]	Linear, linear	75–175	—

Source: BEIR (1980).

[a] The first of each pair of models is used for leukemia, the second for other forms of cancer.

[b] Postnatal, age-specific risk factors applied to 1969–1971 life tables, with risk persisting throughout the lifetime remaining after irradiation (estimate b in the 1972 BEIR report). Because the average age of the 1969–1971 life table population exceeds that of the 1967 U.S. population used for the 1972 BEIR report, the numbers shown here for continuous exposure are larger, on a per-rad basis, than those obtainable from of the 1972 BEIR report.

[c] Range of estimates for low-dose, low LET radiation (p. 414, ¶ 318).

a cancer arising in a previously irradiated individual may have resulted from the radiation exposure (Rall et al, 1985).

Although there is strong concensus in the scientific community concerning the magnitude of the carcinogenic risks of low-level irradiation (Table 5), present estimates are fraught with considerable uncertainty. Hence, there has been ongoing scientific debate about them (NAS/BEIR, 1980; Darby and Reissland, 1981), leading to heightened public concern.

To refine existing risk estimates, greater understanding of dose–incidence relationships obviously will be necessary. For this purpose, further studies of irradiated human populations will be needed. Such studies cannot feasibly be large enough, however, to measure carcinogenic effects at the low radiation doses of interest, that is, in the range of 1–50 mSv (0.1–5.0 rem) (Land, 1980). Adequate clarification of dose–incidence relationships, thus, will require elucidation of the relevant mechanisms of carcinogenesis through appropriately designed experiments in laboratory animals and other model systems (UNSCEAR, 1977; Comptroller General, 1981). Future research, therefore, must seek to integrate knowledge of radiation carcinogenesis at all levels of biological organization.

REFERENCES

Bartsch H, Tomatis L, Malaveille C (1982) Qualitative and quantitative comparisons between mutagenic and carcinogenic activities of chemicals. In: Heddle JA (ed.), Mutagenicity: New Horizons in Genetic Toxicology. New York: Academic Press, pp 35–72.

Borek C (1979a) Malignant transformation in vitro: Criteria, biological markers, and application to environmental screenings of carcinogens. Radiat Res 70:209–232.

Borek C (1979b) Neoplastic transformation following split doses of x-rays. Br J Radiol 50:845–846.

Brown CC, Fears TR, Gail MH, Schneidermann MA, Torne RE, Mantel N (1978) Models for carcinogenic risk assessment. Science 202:1105.

Brown P (1936) American Martyrs to Science Through the Roentgen Rays. Springfield, IL: Charles C. Thomas.

Brues AM (1951) Carcinogenic effects of radiation. Adv Biol Med Phys 2:171–191.

Cairns J (1981) The origin of human cancers. Nature 289:353–357.

Comptroller General (1981) Problems in Assessing the Cancer Risks of Low-Level Ionizing Radiation Exposure. Report to the Congress of the United States. Gathersburg: U.S. General Accounting Office.

Court Brown WM, Doll R (1957) Leukemia and Aplastic Anemia in Patients Irradiated for Ankylosing Spondylitis. Medical Research Special Report Series, no. 295. London: H.M.S.O.

Crump KS (1979) Dose response problems in carcinogenesis. Biometrics 35:157–167.

Darby SC, Reissland JA (1981) Low levels of ionizing radiation and cancer—Are we underestimating the risk? J.R. Stat Soc 144.

Department of Health, Education and Welfare (1979) Interagency Task Force on the Health Effects of Ionizing Radiation. Report of the Working Group on Science. Washington: U.S. Government Printing Office.

Duesberg P (1983) Retroviral transforming genes in normal cells. Nature 304:219–226.

Elkind MM, Han A (1979) Neoplastic transformation and dose fractionation: Does repair of damage play a role? Radiat Res 79:233–240.

Fialkow PJ (1977) Clonal origin and stem cell evolution of human tumors. In: Mulvihill JJ, Miller RW, Fraumeni JF (eds.), Cancer Research and Therapy, Volume 3, Genetics of Human Cancer. New York: Raven Press, pp 439–453.

Frieben A (1902) Demonstration lines cancroids des rechten handruckens, das sich nach langdauernder einwirkung von rontgenstrahlen entwickelt hatte. Fortschr Geb Rontgestr 6:106.

Furth J, Lorenz E (1954) Carcinogenesis by ionizing radiations. In: Hollaender A (ed.), Radiation Biology, Vol. 1. New York: McGraw-Hill, pp 1145–1201.

Guerrero I, Calzada P, Mayer A, Pellicer A (1984) A molecular approach to leukemogenesis: Mouse activated c-ras oncogenes. Proc Natl Acad Sci (USA) 81:202–205.

Hoel DG (1980) Incorporation of background response in dose–response models. Fed Proc 39:73–75.

International Commission on Radiological Protection (1977) Recommendations of the International Commission on Radiological Protection. ICRP Publication 26. Annals of the ICRP, Vol. 1, No. 3. Oxford: Pergamon Press.

Interagency Regulatory Liaison Group (1979) Scientific bases for identification of potential carcinogens and estimation of risks. Natl Cancer Inst 63:241–268.

Lacassagne A (1945a) Les cancer produits par les rayonnements corpusculaires; mecanisme presumable de la cancerisation par les rayons. Actualites Scientifiques et Industriells No. 981, Paris: Hermann et Cie.

Lacassagne A (1945b) Les cancer produits par les rayonnements electromagnetiques. Actualites Scientifiques et Industrielles, No. 975, Paris: Hermann et Cie.

Land CE (1980) Estimating cancer risks from low doses of ionizing radiation. Science 290:1197–1203.

Lewis EB (1957) Leukemia and ionizing radiation. Science 125:965–975.

Little JB, Nagasawa H, Kennedy AR (1979) DNA repair and malignant transformation: Effect of x-irradiation, 12-0-tetradecanoyl-phorbol-13-acetate, and protease inhibitors on transformation and sister-chromatid exchanges in mouse 10T1/2 cells. Radiat Res 79:241–255.

Lloyd EL, Gemmell MA, Henning CB, Gemmell DS, Zabransky BJ (1979) Transformation of mammalian cells by alpha particles. Intl J Radiat Biol 36:467–478.

Mole RH (1975) Ionizing radiation as a carcinogen: Practical questions and academic pursuits. Br. J. Radiol. 48:157–169.

Moloney WC, Kastenbaum MR (1955) Leukemogenic effects of ionizing radiation on atomic bomb survivors in Hiroshima City. Science 121:308–309.

Moolgavkar SH, Knudson AG (1981) Mutation and cancer: A model for human carcinogenesis. J Natl Cancer Inst 66:1037–1052.

National Academy of Sciences–National Research Council (1956) The Biological Effects of Atomic Radiation: Summary Reports. Washington, DC: NAS/NRC.

National Academy of Sciences. Advisory Committee on the Biological Effects of Ionizing Radiation (BEIR) (1980) The Effects on Populations of Exposure to Low Levels of Ionizing Radiation. Washington, DC: National Academy of Sciences-National Research Council.

Peto R (1978) Carcinogenic effects of chronic exposure to very low levels of toxic substances. Envir Health Persp 22:155–159.

Rall JE, Beebe GW, Hoel DG, Jablon S, Land CE, Nygaard OF, Upton AC, Yalow RS, Zeve VH 1985. Report of the National Institutes of Health Ad Hoc Working Group to Develop Radioepidemiological Tables. Washington: NIH Publication No. 85–2748, U.S. Department of Health and Human Services.

Rowley JD (1984) Biological implications of consistent chromosome rearrangements in leukemia and lymphoma. Cancer Res 44:3159–3168.

Stone-Scott N (1897) X-ray injuries. Am X-Ray J 1:57–67.

Simpson CL, Hempelmann LH (1957) The association of tumors and roentgen-ray treatment of thorax in infancy. Cancer 10:42–56.

Stewart A, Webb J, Hewitt DA (1958) A survey of childhood malignancies. Br Med J 1:1495–1508.

Stone RS (1959) Maximum Permissible standards. In: Protection in Diagnostic Radiology. New Brunswick, NJ: Rutgers University Press.

Straus DS (1981) Somatic mutation, cellular differentiation, and cancer causation. J Natl Cancer Inst 67:233–241.

Ulrich H (1946) The incidence of leukemia in radiologists. N Engl J Med 234:45–46.

United Nations Scientific Committee on the Effects of Atomic Radiation (1977) Sources and Effects of Ionizing Radiation. Report to the General Assemby, with annexes. New York: United Nations.

United Nations Scientific Committee on the Effects of Atomic Radiation (1982) Ionizing Radiation: Sources and Biological Effects. Report to the General Assemby, with annexes. New York: United Nations.

Upton AC (1968) Radiation carcinogenesis. In: Busch H (ed.), Methods in Cancer Research, Vol. IV. New York: Academifc Press, pp. 53–82.

Upton AC (1969) Radiation Injury. Effects, Principles, and Perspectives. Chicago: University of Chicago Press.

Van Ryzin J (1982) The assessment of low-dose carcinogenicity. Biometrics Supplement: Current Topics in Biostatistics and Epidemiology pp. 130–139.

Vande Woude GF, Levine AJ, Topp WC, Watson JJ (eds.) (1984) Cancer Cells, Vol. 2, Oncogenes and Viral Genes. Cold Spring Harbor, NY: Cold Spring Harbor Laboratory.

Weiss R (1983) Oncogenes and growth factors. Nature 304:12–13.

Whittemore A, Keller JB (1978) Quantitative theories of carcinogenesis. SIAM Rev 20: 1–30.

Yunis JJ (1983) The chromosomal basis of human neoplasia. Science 221:227–236.

CARCINOGENIC EFFECTS: AN OVERVIEW

JOHN B. STORER, M.D.

Ionizing radiation should properly be classified as a weak carcinogen in man. If we accept the estimate of the UNSCEAR (1977) that 1 rad at a low dose rate carries a lifetime risk of 10^{-4} of developing fatal, radiation-induced cancer, then it follows that in the U.S. population where approximately 20% of deaths are from cancer, a dose of 2000 rads would be required to double the risk of death from cancer. This very large radiation dose is more than 10,000 times the average annual dose received from natural or background radiation sources, and millions of times larger than the lowest exposure levels that can be easily detected by routine monitoring devices.

Despite the fact that radiation is weakly carcinogenic, the quantitative risks from exposure are probably better known than those for any other environmental carcinogen. There are two reasons why this is so. First, there has been intense interest in radiation carcinogenesis over the past several decades and nearly every suitable population that has received radiation exposure for whatever reason has been or continues to be studied intensively. Secondly, because radiation exposures are easily measured, or can be reasonably well estimated retrospectively, and because record keeping on many populations (e.g., those exposed for medical purposes) has often been complete, it is possible to relate the observed effects to fairly accurate dose estimates. The good dosimetry contrasts sharply with the dosimetry of chemical carcinogens, where there are often major uncertainties in estimated exposure levels.

It should be noted at the outset that radiation differs from many chemical carcinogens, however, in that total-body exposure increases the cancer risk in a number of tissues or organs, whereas, many of the chemicals tend to be tissue- or organ-specific, presumably because of selective localization or metabolic activation. Radiation in high enough doses can increase the cancer risk for

From the Biology Division, Oak Ridge National Laboratory, Oak Ridge, Tennessee nearly all organs, although there are major differences in organ sensitivity, as will be shown.

Most of the topics covered in this brief overview are treated in more detail in other chapters. Here we have tried to identify what are considered to be major unresolved issues in radiation carcinogenesis. Some of the concepts are unorthodox and are presented to stimulate thought and discussion and ultimately, it is hoped, hypothesis testing.

RADIATION CARCINOGENESIS AS A STOCHASTIC PROCESS

In recent years there has been widespread acceptance of the concept that radiation carcinogenesis is a stochastic process. By this it is meant that the probability of the effect increases with increasing dose, but the severity of the effect is uninfluenced by dose. Implied in this terminology is the idea that the effect occurs at random in the irradiated population. If, in fact, the risk of radiation-induced cancer is independent of the natural incidence and there is no sensitive subset in the population, then it is reasonable to suppose that the process does occur at random and that excess cancers result. On the other hand, if the risk is a function of the natural incidence, then one can argue that there is interaction between the factors that make for proneness to cancer and the irradiation. In this event it is not at all clear that the process occurs entirely at random.

Additionally, it is our impression that in irradiated experimental animals there may be a dose-dependent effect on the grade of malignancy of certain tumors. This effect might be expected if the exposure depressed any host resistance factors that might slow the tumor growth rate or suppress metastasis. We have not been able to quantify our clinical impression, however.

Until such time as it is established whether or not radiation interacts with other factors making for cancer proneness, it is preferable to consider radiation carcinogenesis a quantal (all or none) response, rather than a stochastic (random) process.

PHYSICAL FACTORS

Dose and Dose Rate

The frequency of occurrence of radiation-induced cancer increases with increasing dose, although the precise mathematical function that describes the relationship is not known. In some cases, tumor frequency may pass through a maximum at some intermediate dose level and show a decline as the dose is further increased. This phenomenon is widely believed to result from cell killing, although there may be alternative explanations. (This will be discussed in greater detail later in this chapter.)

In general, with low-LET radiation, the effectiveness of the radiation in producing biological responses decreases significantly as the dose rate is lowered. Nearly all the dose rate information comes from experimental studies (NCRP, 1980), rather than from studies on human populations. About the only human populations that have shown an increase in cancer incidence as a result of protracted, relatively low-dose rate exposures are those patients who received thorotrast, workers who ingested or were injected with radium, uranium miners who inhaled radon and radon daughters, and the U.S. radiologists. The first three of these populations were exposed primarily to high-LET radiation (alpha particles from internal emitters), and it is known from experimental studies that high-LET radiations exert their effects relatively independently of dose rate. Exposure doses are not well known for radiologists who were exposed to low-LET radiations for protracted periods. If it is assumed that the total doses were high (1000 or more rads) then, by comparison with the Japanese survivors, it appears that the low-dose rate was perhaps 20% as effective as a high-dose rate. On the other hand, if the radiation dose to the radiologists was around 200 rads, then no dose rate effect is apparent (NCRP, 1980; Storer, 1982).

Multiple exposures at high dose rates but at low total doses per exposure may approximate the effects of low-dose rate exposures to the same total dose. In this case, the data on breast cancer in women exposed to multiple fluoroscopic examinations can be used to compare with the incidence seen in women given a single exposure or a limited number of fractionated exposures at high-dose rates. When this comparison is made there is no apparent decrease in the effectiveness of the multiple fractions (Land et al, 1980).

It is concluded that the data from human studies are inadequate to establish for most tumors whether or not there is a dose rate effect and certainly not its magnitude, if one exists. From experimental studies one would expect a dose rate effect, and NCRP (1980) has estimated that high dose rates are probably 2–10 times as effective as low-dose rates.

Radiation Quality

Radiation quality refers to the linear energy transfer (LET) characteristics of the various types and energies of ionizing radiations. High-LET radiations, such as alpha particles and the recoil protons produced in tissues by fission energy neutrons, are nearly always more effective (on a dose-for-dose basis) in producing biological effects than are low-LET radiations, such as x-rays or gamma rays. The ratio of doses required to produce equal levels of effect is defined as the relative biological effectiveness (RBE). Gamma rays or x-rays serve as the baseline radiation; thus, at an equal level of effect the RBE of neutrons, for example, is obtained from

RBE (neutrons) = dose of γ rays/dose of neutrons

An unusual characteristic of RBE is that for most effects, and particularly for delayed effects in experimental animals, RBE is not a constant over much of the usual range of dosages employed, but increases as the radiation dose decreases. This finding is a necessary consequence of differences in dose–effect curves. If, for example, the effect increases linearly for the high-LET radiation, but with the square of the dose for low-LET radiation, then the RBE will decrease with the square root of the dose of high-LET radiation. The biophysical basis and examples of the systematic variation have been described in detail by Kellerer and Rosi (1982).

As indicated earlier, most of the information on cancerogenic effects of high LET radiation in human populations comes from individuals exposed to alpha particles emitted by internally deposited radioisotopes, principally radium, thorium, radon, and its daughters. In these studies there are some uncertainties in dosimetry. Exposures are not well known in the case of uranium miners. For the radium cases, the dosimetry is much better, but knowledge of the relevant cell types at risk and the doses to these cells is not complete. Perhaps a greater problem in estimating the RBE arises from the fact there are no completely suitable populations comparably exposed to low-LET radiation. Thus, RBE values are not precisely known, but from the radium studies they appear to be high, perhaps on the order of 10–20. This estimate is in qualitative agreement with many experimental studies where, for most tumor types, the RBE for high-LET radiation is high.

Differences in the incidence of most cancers at equal dose levels have been consistently reported for the survivors in Hiroshima, as opposed to Nagasaki (Kato and Schull, 1982). In nearly all cases the incidence has been higher in Hiroshima. It has long been believed that there was a significant component of neutrons in the radiation at Hiroshima, whereas, the radiation at Nagasaki was considered to consist overwhelmingly of gamma rays. Differences in the weapon designs were believed to account for these differences in radiation fields. In the past there have been numerous attempts to estimate the RBE of the neutron component of the radiation. An RBE of greater than unity would, of course, account for the higher tumor incidence in Hiroshima.

Recently, the earlier tentative dosimetry (Auxier, 1977) was vigorously challenged, and it has been suggested that the neutron component was considerably overestimated, whereas the gamma ray component was underestimated at Hiroshima (Loewe and Mendelsohn, 1981). A number of groups are now actively reinvestigating the dosimetry, and at present the issue remains in doubt. If, in fact, there was not a significant neutron dose to the Hiroshima survivors, then we are left with little prospect of estimating RBE values for external exposure to high-LET radiation in human populations, and RBE values will necessarily be based primarily on experimental studies.

Fractionation

Both intuitively and on the basis of physical theory, one would expect a small number of high-dose fractionated exposures to low LET radiation to be more effective (on an equal total basis) than a large number of fractionated small doses. If the number of fractions is small and the dose per fraction is large, the effects should approximate those seen following a single large exposure to the same total dose. Conversely, a large number of small fractions should approximate continuous exposure at a low dose rate. Intermediate numbers of fractions and dose sizes should yield results intermediate between single high-dose rate exposures and protracted low-dose rate exposures. Although these questions have not been extensively investigated experimentally, the limited data available tend to confirm expectations mentioned.

Data from human studies are also consistent with some of these expectations. Many of the populations exposed for medical reasons, for example the patients irradiated for ankylosing spondylitis, received relatively large doses per fraction, and their cancer incidence agrees reasonably well with the data from the Japanese a-bomb survivor who received a single exposure. On the other hand, as discussed earlier, women exposed to multiple small doses from fluoroscopy procedures showed an excess incidence of breast cancer, which is consistent with that seen from single large exposures. Because of inadequacies in the data for many types of tumors in the human studies, we conclude that fractionation effects are not very well characterized for humans. In general, they probably follow the results seen experimentally with single high-dose rate exposures and continuous low-dose rate exposures, representing the extremes in biological effectiveness.

In experimental studies high-LET radiations, such as those resulting from fission energy neutron exposures, show much less of a fractionation effect than do low-LET exposures. In fact, fractionation may even enhance the carcinogenic effect in some cases. The reasons for this enhancement are not known, but may be related to changes in the number of sensitive cells at risk. Data from humans are inadequate to permit any conclusions about fractionation effects with high-LET radiation. On biophysical grounds one would expect that the effects should conform to those seen experimentally.

Total-Body Versus Partial-Body Exposure

The data from human studies indicate that in order for a tissue to be at risk for radiation-induced cancer it must be directly exposed to the radiation. It is conceivable that certain endocrine-associated tumors might be produced by indirect mechanisms (e.g., thyroid tumors might result from irradiation of the pituitary), but such an effect has not been established. In contrast to experimental studies, there are few cases in which humans have been exposed to uniform total-body irradiation. Those populations receiving exposures from internally deposited radioisotopes received most of the dose in the tissues in which the isotopes selectively localized. When patients were treated with radiation for medical purposes, the exposures were limited to specific tissues or organs, and only those tissues and the closely adjacent tissues received significant amounts of radiation. The Japanese survivors tended to receive more nearly total-body exposures but, even here, there were probably major inhomogeneities in dose, depending on shielding configurations. Despite these widely different patterns in dose distribution, it appears that the risk of radiation-induced cancer in a particular tissue primarily depends on the radiation dosage to the tissue, rather than on the extent to which the rest of the body is exposed. It should be noted, however, that this generalization contrasts sharply with findings in some experimental studies where the shielding of parts of the body, such as the mouse ovary or portions of the bone marrow, may significantly alter the expression of certain tumors. It may be that our risk estimates from human studies are not sufficiently precise to detect influences of dose inhomogeneities, and the possibility of such influences should not be dismissed.

TISSUE AND ORGAN SENSITIVITIES

There is general agreement that tissues and organs vary considerably in their sensitivity to the cancerogenic effects of ionizing radiation. A consensus is also emerging as to the rough ordering of sensitivities (UNSCEAR, 1977; BEIR-III, 1980). The tissues with the highest sensitivity are the thyroid, bone marrow, lung, and female breast. The exact ordering among these four is not precisely known, and the choice of risk model (see the section on relationship to spontaneous incidence) influences the ordering (Beebe, 1980). If the relative risk model is assumed, then the ordering is that given above. If the absolute risk model is used, then the ordering is female breast, thyroid, lung, and bone marrow. Cancers of three of the tissues carry a high risk of mortality. The fourth (cancer of the thyroid) is infrequently fatal and is often an incidental finding. Special procedures are frequently required to detect thyroid cancers clinically in the study populations, and for many studies questions can be raised about the adequacy of the control information. There is little doubt that there is positive association between radiation exposure and thyroid cancer, but, as pointed out by Boice and Land (1982) a controversy remains over the clinical importance of the cancers.

Other tissues and organs have a lower sensitivity to radiation carcinogenesis and, in fact, some do not appear to be sensitive at all. Tissues in this latter category would seem to include the prostate, testis, uterus, uterine cervix, rectum, and probably pancreas. Chronic lymphocytic leukemia and Hodgkin's disease are also refractory to induction. Most other tissues may be responsive, with low sensitivity, given appropriate circumstances. For many of these other tissues there are difficulties in reaching firm conclusions about sensitivity. In some cases, only one or very few studies have shown an association and other studies have been negative. There is a tendency on the part of investigators to report positive but not negative results. Finally, studies with low statistical power may frequently result in false-positive conclusions. These factors and others have been discussed extensively by Land (1980).

The evidence is convincing that cancers of bone and skin are associated with radiation exposure at high doses. There exists reasonably convincing evidence that the stomach and colon are also responsive. For many other tissues, such as the brain, salivary glands, esophagus, urinary tract, and liver, the evidence is not as consistent, though these tissues are probably susceptible under conditions of high radiation dosage.

DOSE–EFFECT RELATIONSHIPS

In order to estimate the cancer risk at low doses or low-dose rates it is necessary to choose not only a model for expressing the risk (e.g., absolute or relative risk), but to choose a model for the relationship between dose and effect. Historically, a linear, no-threshold, no dose-rate effect model has been used extensively (BEIR-I, 1972). This model offers some attractive features. First, it is believed to be conservative in that it is unlikely to underestimate the risks at low doses. Second, it offers great simplicity. Doses (or rem doses) can be added to arrive at an estimate of total risk, whereas, a more complicated model would require the adding of risks or of dose-equivalents, which are weighted for dose size and/or dose rate. Third, because data from human studies have large standard errors attached to most of the estimates, it has not been possible to reject this model rigorously, even though it conflicts with much of the literature on experimental radiation biology.

More recently, somewhat more complicated models have been accepted by expert committees that are concerned with risk estimation. UNSCEAR (1977) adopted the concept that low-LET radiation at low doses is less effective per rad than at high doses. The majority of the BEIR-III committee explicitly adopted a linear-quadratic equation to extrapolate cancer risk at high doses of low-LET radiation to low doses. The NCRP (1980) adopted a similar model and further assumed that at low dose rates the function would be linear, with the same coefficient as that of the first power term of the linear-quadratic model used for high-dose rate exposures. These recent changes in extrapolation models will complicate risk assessment to some extent, but they are likely to result in estimates that are more realistic.

Despite the likelihood that extrapolations are improved by the use of a linear-quadratic model for low-LET radiations delivered at high dose rates and the use of a linear model for high-LET radiations, there seems obvious room for further improvement. These two models and the linear model for low-LET radiation delivered at low dose rates come more from physical theory and microdosimetric considerations than from empirical observations of cancer incidence in irradiated human or experimental animal populations. In many cases, the models have been forced on the data even though the fit is not very good, particularly if a wide dosage range is considered. Again, these models cannot usually be rejected in favor of data from human studies because of uncertainties in the date; however, the models can often be rejected for animal studies.

In all fairness, it should be pointed out that for dose–effect curves in relatively simple biological systems, such as the production of chromosome aberrations and many effects studied in vitro, these models fit very well, indeed. The expression of cancer in animals and humans appears to be a complicated process, involving many host factors, and it is perhaps not surprising that models based on initial biophysical events may be too simplistic.

It is known from studies of irradiated experimental animals, and it is presumed to be the case in humans, that host factors may play an overriding role in determining tumor expression and, thus, the observed tumor incidence. Relatively minor manipulations of the endocrine status have been shown to profoundly affect the incidence of certain tumors in mice (Upton et al, 1958; Fry et al, 1980; Storer et al, 1982).

Factors other than the endocrine status have been less extensively studied, though it is known that manipulation of the immune system will affect the incidence of some tumors both in experimental animals and in humans (Holland et al, 1978; Melief and Schwartz, 1982). To date, the role of host factors has been explored to a limited extent. It is likely that there are many factors involved in tumor expression. Each may have its own distribution of radiation sensitivity. Some may exhibit radiation thresholds as, for example, if a critical number of cells must be killed before the host factor is compromised. Modelling of dose–effect curves based on effects on multiple host factors has not progressed, because of the lack of information about the detailed nature and radiation sensitivity of these postulated multiple factors. It may be that significant improvements in dose–effect modelling cannot be attained until we have a much more thorough understanding of the mechanisms of radiation carcinogenesis.

An unusual feature of the dose–effect curves for the incidence of most cancers in experimental animals and for some cancers in humans is that they do not contine to rise indefinitely as the dose is increased. A plateau or even a decline in corrected incidence is seen at very high doses. This effect is usually dismissed as representing cell killing, and mathematical models for dose–response curves have been altered by adding additional terms to account for this effect. There is little doubt that in some cases, such as skin carcinogenesis, indeed, the effect is due to cell killing; it appears less certain that this explanation applies in all (or even most) cases of radiation carcinogenesis. A possible alternative explanation that does not appear to have been widely considered is the following. Suppose, as we have suggested earlier in this chapter, the total incidence of a particular cancer is not increased by radiation, but the latent period for expression is decreased. (This reasoning probably does not appear to apply to radiation-induced leukemia.) Further, suppose that the decrease in latency is dose-dependent but that there is a limit to the acceleration of onset. This would also lead to a plateauing of incidence at high doses. It would not explain an actual decrease, but many of the reported decreases have been for uncorrected data. The well documented decreases occur only at very large radiation doses where cell killing may begin to play a role or where the general health of the animals is not conducive to tumor expression, in much the way that underfed mice show a decreased tumor incidence (Weindruch and Walford, 1982).

It is difficult to visualize how radiation would simply shorten the latent periods for tumors that would occur anyway in the absence of exposure, unless the radiation acts additively with some endogenous process that is responsible for the spontaneous incidence. Totter (1980) has suggested that the metabolism of oxygen, which must result in a significant production of reactive radicals, may represent the endogenous factor. Under some circumstances oxygen is a mutagen (Totter, 1981, and references therein), and apparently it may also be a carcinogen (Heston and Pratt, 1959).

Despite the issues just raised, there are certain conclusions that can be drawn about dose–effect curves for radiation-carcinogenesis. First, high-LET radiations tend to yield a more nearly linear relationship than do low-LET radiations. Second, high-LET effects tend to occur relatively independently of dose rate, whereas low-LET radiations usually (nearly always?) show a much lessened effectiveness at low-dose rates. Third, the dose–effect curves for low-LET radiation can be better approximated by a linear-quadratic model than a linear model when the radiation is delivered at a high dose rate. At low dose rates the effects tend to be more nearly a linear function of dose.

RELATIONSHIP TO SPONTANEOUS INCIDENCE

It is not known whether the incidence of radiation-induced cancer is a function of the spontaneous incidence or whether new cancers are produced independently of the natural frequency in the population. If the radiation risk of cancer induction is a function of the natural incidence, then the presumption is that the radiation acts to multiply the natural risk, and the corresponding model for risk assessment is the relative risk model. On the other hand, if there is no dependence on natural frequency and the number of radiation-induced tumors is simply added to the background incidence, then the appropriate model is the absolute risk model. The difference between these two models is of considerable importance in risk assessment but perhaps of even more importance is understanding the biology of radiation carcinogenesis.

It should be noted that for the population under study, either model necessarily describes precisely the excess risk. It is only when predictions are made for future risks in the study population or when extrapolations are made to other populations that the choice of models critically affects risk estimates. Risk estimates may vary by orders of magnitude depending on the model used. A good example of the variability is provided by BEIR-III (1980). Additionally, the ordering of sensitivity of different tissues and organs is influenced by the choice of model (Beebe, 1980). It is also of interest that sensitivity to subsequent tumor induction (all neoplasms except leukemia) in the Japanese survivors has shown a progressive decrease with age at the time of exposure, when the relative risk model has been used, but a progressive increase with age when the absolute risk model has been used (Kato and Schull, 1982). As previously indicated, it is not known at present which, if either, of these models is correct. It may turn out that for some types of cancer one model is correct and for others the alternative model applies. One would hope that this is not be the case, inasmuch as risk estimation is complicated enough without the additional problem of applying different models to different types of cancer.

If radiation produces a specific type of cancer independently of the tendency of the population to develop that cancer (either for genetic reasons or because of widespread exposure to some other environmental carcinogen), then one would not expect synergism between environmental carcinogens and radiation. The effects would be additive (independent action) under the absolute risk model. Synergism would be predicted under the relative risk model.

In human populations it has been suggested (Baum, 1973) that there is a subset that is extremely sensitive to radiation induction of cancer and that radiation standards should take into account this subset. The presumption being that the sensitivity is the result of the genetic constitution, it is difficult to believe that there is a single mutant gene or combination of genes that would result in sensitivity to the carcinogenic action of radiation only. It seems more plausible that the affected individuals would be more sensitive to an entire array of carcinogenic or cocarcinogenic agents. There is no doubt that there are individuals at high risk for specific types of cancer, and the genetic constitution leading to high risk has been extensively studied for many of these cancer types. (This problem is dealt with in a subsequent chapter.) Many, if not most, of these cancers known to be genetically controlled occur in childhood or early in adult life. Certain chromosome aberrations that result in a variety of constitutional diseases also result in a higher than normal risk for cancer. There also exist types of cancer that are inherited without evidence of chromosomal anomalies. These usually result from the expression of single dominant genes. It is not entirely clear if these high-risk individuals are also more sensitive to induction of cancer by radiation. One might expect that if the genetic effect were to alter host factors that normally might suppress cancer expression, then these individuals should be sensitive to radiation. On the other hand, if the defect is in the cellular regulatory mechanisms of a particular tissue (the tissue that is cancer prone), then it would not necessarily follow that radiation sensitivity would be increased. In any event, the proportion of the population carrying these genetic defects is likely to be small, and for many of the diseases the probability of developing cancer in the absence of radiation already approaches unity. Further, in many of these genetic diseases there are other overt constitutional abnormalities. More serious, at least numerically, is the possibility that a significant fraction of the population with normal phenotypes is unusually sensitive to carcinogens, including radiation. Albert and Altshuler (1976) have argued that, indeed, there is such a sensitive subset. This subset consists of those individuals who would develop the particular types of cancer induced by the carcinogen in the absence of any exposure to the carcinogen in question. By definition, thus, women who are sensitive to radiation-induced breast cancer, for example, are those who would develop the cancer anyway, whether they were irradiated or not. This reasoning, of course, is supportive of the relative risk concept and leads to some interesting inferences.

For those cancers that show a continuing increase in incidence or mortality rate with increasing age, it is impossible to distinguish between a higher total incidence and simply an earlier onset in an irradiated population. Many types of cancer associated with radiation exposure in human and animal populations fall into this category. Albert and Altschuler (1976) suggest that the principal effect of a carcinogen exposure may be to decrease the latent period for expression of a tumor in the subpopulation that would have developed the tumor later in the absence of exposure. According to this view, the "excess number of tumors" results from moving forward in time those tumors that otherwise would not have developed because the affected individuals would have died too soon from some competing risk. If we accept this view, then all exposed persons who develop a specific cancer may be presumed merely to develop it earlier than they would have if they had not been exposed; furthermore, the decrease in latency may be presumed to be dose-dependent. On the other hand, for cancers that do not show a progressive increase with age, such as some forms of leukemia, this reasoning does not apply.

Sponsored by the Office of Health and Environmental Research, U.S. Department of Energy, under contract W-7405-eng-26 with the Union Carbide Corporation.

REFERENCES

Albert RE, Altschuler B (1976) Assessment of environmental carcinogen risks in terms of life shortening. Environ Health Perspect 13:91–94.

Auxier JA (1977) Ichiban: Radiation Dosimetry for the Survivors of the Bombings of Hiroshima and Nagasaki. Technical Information Center, Energy Research and Development Administration. Available as TID-27080 from National Technical Information Service, U.S. Department of Commerce, Springfield, VA.

Baum JW (1973) Population heterogeneity hypotheses on radiation induced cancer. Health Phys 25:97–104.

Beebe GW (1980) Issue paper I. In: A Proposed Federal Radiation Research Agenda. Bethesda, MD: National Institutes of Health.

Beebe GW (1982) The estimation of risk from whole-body exposure to ionizing radiation. In: Critical Issues in Setting Radiation Dose Limits. Bethesda, MD: National Council on Radiation Protection and Measurements.

BEIR-I (1972) National Academy of Sciences/National Research Council. The effects on populations of exposure to low levels of ionizing radiation. Washington, DC: National Academy Press.

BEIR-III (1980) National Academy of Sciences/National Research Council. The effects on populations of exposure to low levels of ionizing radiations. Washington, DC: National Academy Press.

Boice JD, Jr, Land CE (1982) Ionizing radiation. In: Schottenfeld D, Fraumeni JF, Jr (eds.), Cancer Epidemiology and Prevention. Philadelphia: W. B. Saunders Co., pp 231–253.

Fry RJM et al (1980) Radiation toxicology: Carcinogenesis. In: Witschi H (ed.), The Scientific Basis of Toxicity Assessment. Amsterdam: Elsevier/North Holland Biomedical Press.

Heston WE, Pratt AW (1959) Effect of concentration of oxygen on occurrence of pulmonary tumors in strain A mice. J Natl Cancer Inst 22:707–717.

Holland JM et al (1978) Survival and cause of death in aging germfree athymic nude and normal inbred C3Hf/He mice. J Natl Cancer Inst 61:1357–1361.

Kato H, Schull WJ (1982) Studies of the mortality of A-bomb survivors. 7. Mortality 1950–1978. Part I. Cancer Mortality. Radiat Res 90:395–432.

Kellerer AM, Rosi HH (1982) Biophysical aspects of radiation carcinogenesis. In: Becker FF (ed.), Cancer. A Comprehensive Treatise, Vol. I. Etiology: Chemical and Physical Carcinogenesis, 2nd ed. New York: Plenum Press, pp 569–616.

Land CE (1980) Estimating cancer risks from low doses of ionizing radiation. Science 209:1197–1203.

Land CE et al (1980) Breast cancer risk from low-dose exposure to ionizing radiation: Results of parallel analysis of three exposed populations of women. J Natl Cancer Inst 65:353–376.

Loewe WE, Mendelsohn E (1981) Revised dose estimates at Hiroshima and Nagasaki. Health Physics 41:662–666.

Melief CJM, Schwartz RS (1982) Immunocompetence and malignancy. In: Becker FF (ed.), Cancer. A Comprehensive Treatise, Vol. I. Etiology: Chemical and Physical Carcinogenesis, 2nd ed. New York: Plenum Press, pp 161–199.

NCRP (1980) National Council on Radiation Protection and Measurements. The influence of dose and its distribution in time on dose effect relationships for low LET radiation. Report no. 64. Washington, DC: NCRP.

Storer JB (1982) Radiation carcinogenesis. In: Becker FF (ed.), Cancer. A Comprehensive Treatise, Vol. I. Etiology: Chemical and Physical Carcinogenesis, 2nd ed. New York: Plenum Press, pp 629–950.

Storer JB et al (1982) Causes of death and their contribution to radiation-induced life shortening in intact and ovariectomized mice. Radiat Res 89:618–643.

Totter JR (1980) Spontaneous cancer and its possible relationship to oxygen metabolism. Proc Natl Acad Sci 77:1763–1767.

Totter Jr (1981) The origins of cancer: A comparison of two hypotheses. Periodicum Biologorum 83:209–220.

UNSCEAR (1977) United Nations Scientific Committee on the Effects of Atomic Radiation. Sources and Effects of Ionizing Radiation. New York: United Nations.

Upton AC et al (1958) A comparison of the induction of myeloid and lymphoid leukemias in x-radiated RF mice. Cancer Res 18:842–848.

Weindruch R, Walford RL (1982) Dietary restriction in mice beginning at 1 year of age: Effect on life-span and spontaneous cancer incidence. Science 215:1415–1417.

SECTION II
BIOLOGICAL AND CELLULAR ASPECTS

PHYSICS: ENVIRONMENTAL SOURCES OF RADIOACTIVITY, LEVELS, AND INTERACTION WITH MATTER

NAOMI H. HARLEY, Ph.D.

Naturally occurring gamma rays, cosmic rays, and alpha- and beta-emitting radionuclides are present at varying levels in all environments. The specific cells that are targets for carcinogenesis are exposed constantly to radiation from these sources, and receive significant exposure from other sources, such as medical and dental x-rays.

Radiation exposure, absorbed dose, linear energy transfer (LET), and dose equivalent are described briefly in this chapter to define the concepts and terminology normally encountered. Recent data on sources and levels of environmental exposure to ionizing radiation are summarized, and the methods of calculating absorbed dose and dose equivalent are described.

The general levels of both external radiation and radiation from internal emitters are presented in tabular form so that estimates of environmental radiation from specific sources may be quickly assessed against this backdrop of existing information.

INTERACTION OF RADIATION WITH MATTER

The term "ionizing radiation" applies both to charged (alpha and beta) particles and photons (gamma rays and x-rays), which cause ionizations as they pass through matter. The unit used to describe radiation energy is the electron volt (eV) or multiples thereof (keV, MeV). Excitation, as well as ionization (in almost equal quantities) take place in the electrons of the absorbing atoms when alpha or beta particles pass through, whereas photons lose energy almost exclusively by ionization. Alpha and beta particles lose energy in quite similar ways through "collisions" (Coulomb interactions) with absorbing atoms. Beta particles, however, also lose a small fraction of their energy through a radiative

From the Institute of Environmental Medicine, New York University Medical Center, New York, New York.

loss process known as bremsstrahlung (braking rays), whereby a low-energy photon is released when beta particles are slowed down in matter. Bremsstrahlung is the mode of production of x-rays in x-ray tubes, for example.

Photons lose energy via three mechanisms: 1) photoelectric interaction, where all of the energy is lost to a single electron in an absorbing atom; 2) Compton interaction, where part of the energy is lost to a single electron of an absorbing atom, with the remainder being retained as the photon; 3) pair production, where energy is converted to the mass of a negative and positive electron pair. The latter process requires a minimum photon energy of 1.02 MeV (the mass equivalent of the two electrons), with any excess appearing as kinetic energy of the electrons.

Eventually, all of the energy from ionizing radiation is used up in producing excitation or ion pairs, where an ion pair consists of one electron and one positively charged residue atom. In dry air it requires about 34 eV (ICRU 1979) to produce one ion pair.

Ordinarily, alpha particles from any radionuclide have energies between 4 and 8 MeV. Beta particles from natural radionuclides have energies from almost 0 to 3 MeV, and photons have energies from about 0.04 to 3 MeV. Alpha and beta particle energy loss is characterized by a high ionization density (a relatively large number of ion pairs per unit path length) and, thus, the particles have a short range in absorbing material. In tissue, for example, the range of the 5.3 MeV alpha particle from ^{210}Po is 40 μm, and the range of the 1.16 MeV beta particle from ^{210}Bi is 0.5 cm. On the other hand, photons, are highly penetrating, and the 1.46 MeV gamma ray from ^{40}K, on an average, will travel 17 cm in tissue before interacting. Gamma-ray range is not a valid concept, and half-thickness is the more appropriate terminology. For example, a 1.0 MeV photon beam will lose half the initial number of photons in passing through 10 cm of tissue.

Linear Energy Transfer

The differential energy loss (dE) of a charged particle with energy (E) per unit distance travelled (dx) along its track is known as the total linear stopping power (S).

This energy loss includes both collision loss and the bremsstrahlung photons, which can escape from the site of origin, and although the loss is small, S does not quite describe the local energy deposition of the radiation. Linear energy transfer, L, describes the discrete local energy deposition or collision loss only.

L = S (collision) = − dE/dx (collision)

Greater biological damage results from radiation with a high energy deposition per μm micrometer than from radiation with a low deposition rate for a given total energy loss. To relate the biological effects of radiations with different values of LET, the quality factor (Q) is utilized. The quality factor gives an empirical scale of biological damage in relation to local energy deposition. Selected values of Q with respect to LET have been tabulated by ICRU (ICRU, 1971) and are given in Table 1. As a practical value, all photons and electrons (or beta particles) have a Q of 1, whereas, the heavy particles have larger Q values.

TABLE 1. Quality Factor (Q) as a Function of the Collision Stopping Power (LET) of Radiation

LET (keV/μmin Water)	Q
3.5	1
7.0	2
23.0	5
53.0	10
175.0	20

Exposure and Absorbed Dose

Exposure is defined uniquely for photons in air and does not usually apply to any other type of radiation. Exposure is the charge (dQ) produced per unit mass of air (dm), when electrons liberated by photons are completely stopped in air. The unit of exposure is the Roentgen (R) and is defined as exactly 2.58×10^{-4} Coulomb/kg air (ICRU, 1980).

Absorbed dose is the mean energy (de) imparted by ionizing radiation to a unit mass of any material (dm)

$$D = de/dm$$

The traditional unit for absorbed dose is the rad (1 rad = 100 erg/g) (ICRU, 1980). The unit for the absorbed dose in the International Standard (SI) system of units, which has been adopted by ICRP, but has not been adopted in the United States (as of writing) is the gray (Gy) and is equal to 1 joule (J)/kg (1 Gy = 100 rads).

The absorbed dose is generally calculated for the whole body, in the case of external gamma radiation, and for individual organs, in the case of internally deposited radionuclides. The dose to two cellular sites, basal cells in bronchial epithelium and bone stem cells close to bone surfaces, is also calculated for alpha irradiation of lung or bone, because these cells are thought to be the targets in radiation-induced cancer of these organs.

For a given gamma ray or x-ray exposure, the absorbed dose in air may be calculated by multiplying exposure in R by 0.87 to obtain the absorbed dose in rads.

Dose Equivalent

The dose equivalent is a quantity that attempts to provide additivity of radiation doses from different types of radiation. The dose equivalent (H) is the product of absorbed dose in rads times the quality factor (Q) selected from Table 1, times a factor N, which represents any other modifiers. The latter is presently taken as unity.

$$H = D\,Q\,N \text{ rem}$$

The traditional unit of dose equivalent is the rem. In the SI system of units, the dose equivalent is expressed in sieverts (Sv), where 1 Sv = 1 J/kg, and is the product of Gy and Q.

AVERAGE ENVIRONMENTAL EXPOSURE TO NATURAL RADIOACTIVITY

Individuals are exposed to alpha- and beta-emitters deposited internally from inhalation or dietary intake and to external radiation from terrestrial radionuclides and cosmic rays. The average dose from these sources is the basis of comparison for other environmental exposures.

Inhalation of Radon Daughters

Radon daughters deliver to people the highest dose of any natural background radioactivity. Radon-222 is the gaseous daughter of ^{226}Ra; which is found in all soils and rocks. The half-life of ^{222}Rn (3.82 days) allows its diffusion from the soil to the atmosphere, where the average surface wind speed of a few kilometers per hour allows radon to be transported for perhaps thousands of kilometers from its point of origin. The first short-lived alpha-emitting daughter of radon, ^{218}Po (RaA), with a half-life of 3.05 min, is formed as a free atom or ion. This decays to ^{214}Pb (RaB), a beta-emitter with a 26.8 min half-life, and then to ^{214}Bi (RaC), a beta-emitter with a half-life of 19.7 min. Polonium-214 (RaC'), an alpha-emitter with a half-life of only seconds, is always in equilibrium (equal activity) with its ^{214}Bi parent. The RaA, RaB, and RaC attach to the ambient aerosol particles [about 0.1 μm activity median diameter; George and Breslin (1980)]. When they are inhaled, about 5% of them deposit on the airway surfaces by diffusion deposition.

In environmental atmospheres, about 7% of the RaA activity persists as a free ion (small hydrated ion). This deposits with 100% efficiency on the upper airway surfaces and delivers about 25% of the total radon daughter dose, with 75% coming from the daughters attached to aerosol particles.

The short-lived alpha-emitting daughters deliver their primary radiation dose to the upper bronchial tree. The daughters must be supported in air by their parent ^{222}Rn, however, because they decay away in a few hours by themselves.

Radon concentrations are usually reported in activity units of pCi/L or pCi/m^3 (1 pCi$=10^{-12}$ Ci). Occupational exposures to radon daughters are conventionally reported in terms of the working level (WL), which describes the alpha energy released during complete decay of the short-lived daughters. One WL is numerically equal to 1.3 × 10^5 MeV/L and is equivalent to 100 pCi/L of ^{222}Rn in equilibrium with its daughters. Equilibrium is not a prerequisite, however, because any combination that yields the specified energy content is 1 WL. The WL is calculated from the expression

WL = 0.00105(pCi RaA/1) + 0.00517(pCi RaB/1) + 0.00378(pCi RaC/1)

In the IS system of units, the WL is equivalent to 2.08 × 10^{-5} J/m^3.

Cumulative exposure to radon daughters is expressed in units of the working level month (WLM). Although this unit was originally used for occupational exposure only (PHS, 1957), it is now common to report environmental exposure in this unit also. One working level month results from exposure to 1 WL for a work month of 170 hr. Environmental or occupational WLM may be calculated from the expression

WLM = [WL] [hours exposed]/170

Because indoor ^{222}Rn levels are considerably higher than outdoor levels, the average annual exposure in WLM is dependent on indoor radon, because most people spend 80% or more of their time indoors. Considerable effort is presently being spent to document exposures in the U.S., but only few long-term data are available. One study (George and Breslin, 1980) reported data for 18 homes in the New York–New Jersey area. The ^{222}Rn and radon daughter values were found to be log normally distributed, with a median outdoor concentration of 180 pCi of ^{222}Rn/L and a median indoor concentration of 830 pCi of ^{222}Rn/L. Both values had a geometric standard deviation (σ_g) of about 2.0. The measured values of WL were 0.0041 and 0.0016 for indoors and outdoors, respectively. The available data lead to an estimate of the average annual cumulative exposure of about 0.2 WLM (NCRP, 1984).

A considerable number of measurements have been reported in Canada. Fifteen thousand homes have been monitored in 19 Canadian cities (McGregor et al, 1980). The radon daughter concentration was found to be log normally distributed in these cities also. The medians ranged from 0.0009 WL for Vancouver to 0.0058 for Winnipeg, with an average value of σ_g of about 2.5. In this study it was reported that radon daughter levels could not be inferred from geological conditions and that measurements were necessary if accurate population exposures were desired.

Harley and Pasternack (1982) calculated the absorbed alpha dose to basal cells in bronchial epithelium in the upper bronchial tree using anatomically correct lung morphometry reported by Yeh and Schum (1980). The factors for individuals in the population are (NCRP, 1984a)

Men	0.52 rad/WLM
Women	0.50 rad/WLM
Children	1.20 rad/WLM
Infants	0.77 rad/WLM
Average	0.7 rad/WLM

It should be stressed that 90% of all lung cancer is bronchogenic, with its site of origin in the first few branching generations of the bronchial tree, and that the calculated absorbed alpha dose factors are highest in this region also (generations 2–4).

Table 2 indicates some of the average levels of radon daughters that have been measured in various parts of the world where levels are not thought to be unusually high (Harley, 1981).

The average absorbed alpha dose for all members of the population, assuming a cumulative environmental exposure of 0.2 WLM/yr, is 0.14 rad/yr or 2.8 rem/yr (Q=20).

TABLE 2. Summary of Indoor Measurements of ^{222}Ra Concentrations (pCi/m^3)

Location	Mean	Range	Duration[a]
Austria			
Innsbruck	1,200	<50–7,500	1 year
Salzburg	1,300	750–2,500	1 year
Canada			
13 Cities	410	140–880	
Finland			
Helsinki			
Bored wells	3,000 (median)		
City supply	1,000 (median)		
Hungary	2,600	700–5,800	
Norway	1,400	1,000–6,000	
Poland	330	80–2,100	
	230	20–5,300	
Sweden	1,500	30–16,000	
United Kingdom	200	5–1,200	
	1,300	60–6,900	19 months
USSR			
Tashkent	7,500	200–36,000	
	800	100–4,500	
US			
Grand Junction, CO			
Home on Tailings	35,000	200–240,000	
Background home	900	<400–2,300	
US			
Florida	1,300	30–3,600	
Polk County	4,500	1,500–7,700	
US			
Boston, MA	150	<5–940	
US			
New Jersey	2,000	80–7,400	Months
US			
New York	750	80–4,600	Months
New York City	100	60–170	1 year
	250	140–390	1 year
Howe Caverns, NY	17,000	13,000–32,000	3 months
Schenectady, NY	1,100		
US			
Canonsburg, PA	1,400	460–5,500	
US			
Tennessee	1,400	130–4,800	

Source: Adapted from Harley NH, Altman SM, Pasternack BS (1981) Genotoxic properties of radon and its daughters ENL/AUI conference on genotoxic effects of airborne agents. Conference Proceedings.

[a] When duration is not shown, measurements were short term.

Ingestion of ²²⁶Ra, ²¹⁰Pb, and Uranium

Radium. Radium-226 has been measured in 19 food categories in the diet in New York and San Francisco (Fisenne and Keller, 1970). The average daily intakes were found to be 1.7 and 0.8 pCi ²²⁶Ra/day, respectively. Radium-228 is also present in the diet, but few relevant data are available. Holtzman (1980) has summarized all of the existing ²²⁶Ra and ²²⁸Ra data, and these values are shown in Table 3. Samples of human bone ash from 26 countries in the world were measured for ²²⁶Ra, and the skeletal content was found to be distributed log normally. These data are shown in Figure 1, plotted as a fraction of the cumulative total of the population. These samples represent 1.4 billion persons, and the median value is 0.03 pCi ²²⁶Ra/g Ca, with a σ_g of 1.6. Since there are 1000 g of calcium in the skeleton, the median skeletal content is 30 PCi ²²⁶Ra. More than 95% of the body ²²⁶Ra is thought to reside in the skeleton (Schlenker et al, 1982).

The alpha dose factor is 84 mrad/yr for 1 pCi ²²⁶Ra/g wet bone to cells 10 μm from surfaces (Harley and Pasternack, 1976). This includes the dose from ²²⁶Ra and 33% of the alpha-emitting daughters of radon (the fraction remaining in bone through decay). A skeletal burden of 30 pCi in 5000 g of wet bone will yield an annual dose of 0.5 mrad (10 mrem/yr).

FIGURE 1. Cumulative population frequency distribution of measured ²²⁶Ra/g calcium in human bone ash. Reproduced from Health Physics 40:163–171 (1981) by permission of the Health Physics Society.

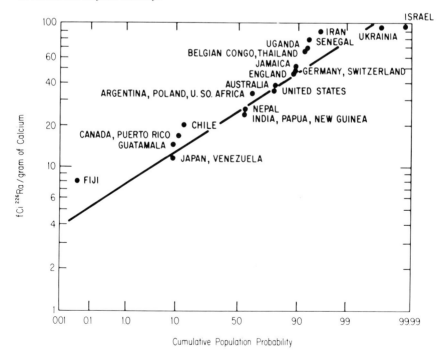

TABLE 3. Annual Absorbed Dose from Internal Alpha- and Beta-Emitting Nuclides in the Body

Nuclide	Average dietary intake (pCi/day)	Range (pCi/day)	Skeletal content (pCi or μg)	Alpha dose to cells 10 μm from bone surfaces for skeletal content indicated (mrem/yr)[a]
ALPHA EMITTERS				
^{226}Ra	1.4	0.7–2.4	30 pCi	10
^{228}Ra	1.1	1.0–1.2	—	—
^{210}Pb				
Nonsmokers	1.4	1.3–1.6	380 pCi	—
Smokers			780 pCi	—
^{210}Po				
Nonsmokers	1.6	1.3–1.6	240 pCi	32
Smokers			680 pCi	92
^{238,234}U	1.3 μ ^{238}U/day (0.82 pCi ^{238}U+^{234}U/day)	—[b]	6–70 μ ^{238}U	0.3–3
BETA EMITTERS				
^{40}K (Beta and Gamma)				15
^{14}C				1
^{3}H				0.001

[a] Q = 20

[b] 1 μ ^{238}U has an activity of 0.74 alpha disintegrations per minute. Since ^{238}U are reported to be in radioactivity equilibrium in samples of diet and skeletal ash the total radioactivity for 1 μg ^{238}U is 1.48 dpm or 0.67 pCi.

Lead-210. The bone dose from ^{210}Pb comes largely from the ^{210}Po daughter, which is an alpha emitter. Ingested ^{210}Po is found mostly in soft tissues, but that formed by decay of ^{210}Pb in bone tends to remain there. Spencer et al (1977) measured ^{210}Pb and ^{210}Po in the diet in a controlled metabolic study in Hines, Illinois. Their values were 1.3 pCi ^{210}Pb/day and 1.6 pCi ^{210}Po/day. Morse and Welford (1971) measured ^{210}Pb in 19 food categories in New York City and estimated a daily intake of 1.2 pCi. Holtzman (1980) summarized the ^{210}Pb/^{210}Po dietary intake in the United States and other countries, reporting mean values in the U.S. to be 1.4 pCi^{210}Pb/day and 1.6 pCi ^{210}Po/day. Holtzman (1966) also measured ^{210}Pb and ^{210}Po in skeletal ash of both smokers and non-smokers. He found 0.29 pCi ^{210}Pb/g ash and 0.14 pCi ^{210}Pb/g ash, with ^{210}Po/^{210}pb ratios of 0.87 and 0.62 for smokers and nonsmokers, respectively. The data indicate that much of the ^{210}Pb inhaled in tobacco smoke is translocated to the skeleton. The absorbed alpha dose from cigarette smoke is discussed in greater detail later in this chapter.

The dose factor is 34 mrad/yr for 1 pCi ^{210}Po/g wet bone. For the skeletal burdens reported by Holtzman, this yields an annual absorbed dose to critical cells at 10 μu from bone surfaces of 1.6 mrad for nonsmokers and 4.6 mrad for smokers (32 and 92 mrem/yr, respectively).

Uranium. There are few data on the naturally occurring isotopes ^{234}U and ^{238}U in diet and humans. Welford and Baird (1967) measured ^{238}U in 19 different food categories in New York City. They found the average daily intake to be 1.2 μg. Because there are 0.74 dpm/μg ^{238}U, this corresponds to a daily intake of 0.4 pCi ^{238}U. Uranium-234 is in near equilibrium with ^{238}U, and thus the total uranium intake is 0.8 pCi/day or about equal to the radium, lead, and polonium values.

Uranium has been measured in skeletal tissue, and the values appear to vary widely with geographic locations. Hamilton (1971, 1972) measured ^{238}U in the skeleton of persons living in the U.K. and estimated a total skeletal burden of 70 μg. Fisenne et al (1980, 1982) measured ^{234}U and ^{238}U in skeletal ash samples from Nepal, Australia, and Russia, and estimated skeletal contents of 43, 10, and 30 μg respectively. The ^{238}U and ^{234}U were found to be in equilibrium in these samples. Welford et al measured ^{238}U in bone from New York, and a skeletal content of 6.4 μg was calculated.

The alpha dose factors for cells 10 μm distant from bone surfaces for ^{238}U and ^{234}U are 13 and 20 mrad/yr per pCi/g wet bone, respectively. For the range of skeletal burdens indicated (6.4–70 μg) this corresponds to an annual alpha dose of 0.014–0.15 mrad (0.3–3.1 mrem/yr, respectively).

Body Potassium, Radiocarbon, and Tritium

A significant absorbed dose is received from ^{40}K, which is a naturally occurring radioactive isotope of potassium. Potassium is a necessary constituent of all body cells and is under homeostatic control. The average annual absorbed dose to the whole body from the beta and gamma rays emitted by ^{40}K is about 15 mrem.

Carbon-14 and tritium (^{3}H) are produced continuously in the upper atmosphere by cosmic radiation. Because carbon and hydrogen are major constituents of all organic materials, human tissue contains small amounts of ^{14}C and ^{3}H. The annual absorbed doses from their beta radiation are about 1 mrem and 0.001 mrem, respectively.

Terrestrial Gamma Ray and Cosmic Ray Exposure

Terrestrial radiation. The measurements of terrestrial gamma radiation in the U.S. are summarized by NCRP (1975). Aerial radiologic measuring surveys (ARMS) conducted by the U.S. Geological Service from 1958 to 1963 covered more than 26,000 km². In the Atlantic and Gulf coastal plains, the gamma ray dose in air averaged 23 mrad/yr, with the remainder of the U.S. averaging about 46 mrad/yr. Oakley (1972) estimated the overall population weighted outdoor dose rate in air to be 40 mrads/yr for the U.S., as a whole. Oakley (1972) derived a "housing factor" of 0.8 and defined it as the ratio of indoor to outdoor dose rates from terrestrial sources. Combining the housing factor with a body shielding factor of 0.8—which yields the gamma ray dose to gonads and bone marrow (Bennett, 1970)—and a quality factor of 1, he estimated a dose equivalent rate to gonads and bone marrow of $40 \times 0.8 \times 0.8 \times 1 = 26$ mrem/yr.

Cosmic Radiation. Cosmic rays at sea level are composed of energetic muons, electrons, protons, neutrons, and charged pions. Cosmic ray measurements in the U.S. are summarized by NCRP (1975). The cosmic ray intensity at sea level varies by about 2% with geomagnetic latitude over the U.S. and by about 10% over the 11-yr solar cycle (with a minimum during maximum solar activity). The average dose equivalent rate at sea level is 26 mrem/yr. The cosmic ray dose varies markedly with altitude, the atmosphere providing a significant shield at sea level. In Denver, Colorado (altitude 1600 m above sea level) the dose equivalent rate from cosmic rays is about 50 mrem/yr and in Leadville, Colorado (altitude 3200 m) the dose equivalent is 125 mrem/yr.

For persons travelling by air, the dose rate and dose equivalent rate vary by a factor of 20 between 4 and 12 km (14 μrad/hr–300 μrad/hr or 20 μrem/hr–450 μrem/hr, respectively; O'Brien, 1975). During a 7-hr flight at 11 km (New York to London) the observed dose from cosmic rays is estimated to be about 3 mrad (Wallace, 1975).

ELEVATED AND ENHANCED EXPOSURE TO NATURAL RADIOACTIVITY

Many locations in the world expose individuals to natural radionuclides in excess of levels that would be called average for the area. Either high concentrations of radionuclides are present naturally, because of the local geology (elevated areas), or commercial or individual activity has changed normal exposures by concentrating or uncovering radionuclides (enhanced areas). Uranium mill tailings under and around houses are an example of the latter.

The most significant exposure from either elevated or enhanced activity is from radon daughters. Radon daughter levels many times those considered average are found, for example, in the Florida phosphate region (an area with both elevated and enhanced activity) or near uranium mill tailings (Table 2). Uranium mill tailings are a clean, finely ground residue from uranium ore processing. They contain most of the radium from the ore, and poorly ventilated homes built on or with tailings can attain radon daughter levels that exceed those in uranium mines. The absorbed alpha dose to bronchial epithelium from enhanced or elevated radon daughter activity can exceed that allowed occupationally (4 WLM/yr in the U.S., which is equivalent to 2 rad/yr).

Elevated dietary intake of radionuclides in certain foods does not usually cause a significant increase in absorbed dose. Most individuals obtain food from a variety of sources, thus, a few items with high radionuclide content will not change the total daily intake substantially. For example, Hill (1965) measured 1400 pCi ^{210}Po/kg in crab meat, and reindeer and caribou meat are also known to contain high concentrations of ^{210}Pb and ^{210}Po (UNSCEAR, 1977). Turner et al (1958) reported up to 3000 pCi ^{226}Ra/kg in Brazil nuts.

Individual items such as these should not affect the total dietary intake; however, one possible exception is drinking water. Asikainen and Kahlos (1980) measured ^{226}Ra and uranium in drilled wells in Helsinki, Finland, and found 0.1–100 pCi ^{226}Ra/L and 1–3000 μg U/L. In areas where drinking water is elevated in radionuclide concentration, the average bone cell dose values in Table 3 possibly could be increased by an order of magnitude or more. Figure 1 shows the ^{226}Ra content in skeletal ash from 26 countries and indicates a range of about a factor of 10 in areas not known to be unusually elevated in dietary ^{226}Ra. This indicates that the variability from normal diets in elevated areas could probably add an additional order of magnitude to skeletal dose.

A few areas in the U.S. where there is elevated or enhanced exposure to radon daughters are described in greater detail later in this chapter.

Florida Phosphate Region

Phosphate rock is used extensively as a source of phosphorus for fertilizer. The countries supplying the majority of the phosphate rock are Morroco, U.S.S.R., and U.S. Sedimentary type phosphate ores, such as those found in Florida, tend to have high concentrations of ^{238}U and its daughters; 40 pCi ^{226}Ra/g is typical in central Florida (UNSCEAR, 1982).

About 600 km^2 of Florida land have been surface-mined for phosphate rock in the last 80 yr. In 1978, the Florida Department of Health and Rehabilitation Services (DHRS) adopted a control level of 0.029 WL (0.025 WL above an average indoor background of 0.004 WL) for existing structures in Florida (Roessler et al, 1980). The DHRS estimated that of the approximately 4000 structures built on reclaimed phosphate lands in west-central Florida (Roessler et al, 1980), about 6%–10% would require remedial action to attain the control level.

Guimond and Windham (1980) measured external gamma radiation in this same central Florida location and reported that in nonmineralized areas the average outdoor background gamma ray radiation was 6 μR/hr, on mineralized land 7 μR/hr, and on reclaimed land 11 μR/hr. The highest outdoor gamma ray exposure rate observed was 42 μR/hr. The average indoor-to-outdoor ratio was similar for all structures, at about 0.9.

Uranium Mill Tailings

Processing of uranium ore selectively removes the very small amount of uranium that is present (in the U.S. < 0.5%), and tailings, which make up the bulk of the ore brought to the surface, are stored in piles ranging from a few tenths to several square kilometers in area (Clements et al, 1980). In 1975, it was estimated that 10^{11} kg of uranium mill tailings were present in the U.S., and that they covered about 10 km². Predictions by the New Mexico Energy Institute indicate that about 2 × 10^{12} kg of tailings, requiring 200 km², will exist by the year 2000 (Clements et al, 1980).

Radon levels are highly variable on the tailing piles, themselves. Shearer and Sill (1969) measured 1–34 pCi ^{222}Rn/L, and their measurements indicate that levels are near normal background for distances greater than 1 km from the pile. Any off-pile levels above background are difficult to distinguish, because normal background in the area is quite variable (0.5–1.0 pCi/L).

Radon and radon daughter concentrations in homes built on uranium mill tailings are known to be high. In 1972, the Surgeon General issued guidelines for exposure in buildings built on, or with, uranium mill tailings and indicated that an indoor concentration greater than 0.05 WL required remedial action. The radon levels for a few homes built on tailings are shown in Table 2. The variation in ^{222}Rn concentration is considerable and depends primarily on ventilation.

Energy Conservation

As a cost-effective measure, many home owners in the northern heating zone in the U.S. have added insulating material and reduced leakage around doors and windows. The effect of this procedure on the ventilation rate is not known. Average ventilation rates are thought to be about 0.4 hr^{-1}, and even in a tightly sealed room ventilation rates of 0.1 hr^{-1} may be found. It seems probable that the ^{222}Rn concentration may be increased by a factor of 2–3 as a result of energy conservation measures.

MEDICAL EXPOSURE

Diagnostic X-Ray Dose

Medical exposure to x-rays are of interest because they deliver the highest man-made dose to individuals, short of accidental exposure (UNSCEAR, 1977). The reported trend with time has been an increase in the number of diagnostic x-rays in the population of many countries. Most studies of absorbed dose delivered during diagnostic radiation have reported gonad dose, mean marrow dose, or incident skin exposure. In one study in Sweden, information is given for whole body and mean marrow dose plus the absorbed x-ray dose to 5 organs. These values are shown in Table 4. In the U.S., the average annual genetically significant dose from diagnostic radiation is 20 mrad (USDHEW, 1973; NAS, 1980), and the corresponding dose to the bone marrow is 103 mrad (NAS, 1980).

Diagnostic Nuclear Medicine

UNSCEAR (1977) indicates that from about 1972 to present the number of diagnostic examinations using radiopharmaceuticals in developed countries is doubling approximately every 3 years. Roedler et al (1974) made a critical

TABLE 4. Average Organ Doses in Various Diagnostic X-Ray Examinations in Sweden (*mrad*)

Examination	Whole body[a]	Ovary	Testis	Active marrow	Thyroid	Breast	Lung
Hip and femur	170	370[b]	1,500[b]	250	<1[b]	<5[b]	<10[b]
Pelvis	125	190	310	190	<1[b]	<5[b]	<10[b]
Pelvimetry	440	460	—	680[b]	<10[b]	<10[b]	<50[b]
Lumbosacral region	150[b]	180[b]	100[b]	100[b]	<1[b]	<5[b]	<10[b]
Lumbar spine	590	620	180	410	16	120	<100
Urography	730	880	330	240	38	540	<100
Retrograde pyelography	1,000[b]	800[b]	1,300[b]	300[b]	50[b]	500[b]	<100[b]
Urethrocystography	600[b]	1,500[b]	2,000[b]	300[b]	5[b]	20[b]	20[b]
Stomach, upper GI tract	440	56	16	420	29	100	<50
Small intestine	300	180	100	250	3	11	<20
Colon	860	700	530	940	10	27	<20
Abdomen	300[b]	200[b]	200[b]	300[b]	3[b]	11[b]	<20[b]
Obstetrical abdomen	200[b]	150[b]	—	220[b]	2[b]	8[b]	<15[b]
Hysterosalpingography	130	590		170	<1[b]	<5[b]	<10
Cholecystography, cholangiography	130	24	6	150	3	15	<10
Dorsal spine	300	<100	<20	470	1,300	170	800
Lung, ribs	30	<3[b]	<3[b]	29	17	55	80
Lung (photofluorography)	105	<10[b]	<10[b]	90	100	200	350
Lung plus heart	57	<5[b]	<5[b]	54	24	61	120
Cervical spine	26	<1	1	38	140	<10	<10[b]
Shoulder, clavicle, sternum	60[b]	<1[b]	<1[b]	60[b]	50[b]	<50[b]	<10[b]
Head, sinus	97	<1	<1	122	790	<10[b]	<10[b]
Cerebral angiography	970	<10	<10	1,500	300	<10[b]	<10[b]
Femur (lower two thirds)	70[b]	50[b]	400[b]	1	<1[b]	<1[b]	<1[b]
Lower leg, knee	30[b]	<1	<1	1	<1	<1	<1
Arm	7[b]	<1	<1	1	<1	<1	<1
Dental (single exposure)	2.9	0.01	0.01	1	3	0.5	0.1

Source: Adapted from UNSCEAR, 1977.

[a] Assuming same mass as Reference Man (70 kg); not averaged over actual weight.
[b] Crude estimate.

review of the dose factors for the most frequently performed diagnostic tests. The doses to the examined or critical organs, the gonads and the skeleton, summarized from UNSCEAR (1977), are shown in Table 5.

Therapeutic Dose

High radiation doses have been used for treatment of both malignant and non-malignant skin lesions, with absorbed doses of 2000–3000 rad. Treatment of nonmalignant skin disease is now discouraged because of the long-term effects known to be induced by x-radiation. Many of the malignant skin lesions are treated with low-energy ($\sim$ 50 kvp) x-rays, which are sparing of the underlying organs and tissue because the radiation is not penetrating [half value layer (HVL) $\sim$ 0.8 mm Al].

Other neoplastic diseases treated with x-rays include all forms of cancer and invasive malignant disease. Radiation doses of 6000–7000 rad are given to localized tumors (UNSCEAR, 1977). UNSCEAR (1977) reports that about 50% of the new cancer cases arising each year are treated with radiotherapy, and that this proportion has not changed appreciably even with increased use of chemotherapy.

Although therapeutic doses to individuals are high, they do not contribute significantly to the average population dose.

MISCELLANEOUS SOURCES OF EXPOSURE

Fallout

Global fallout from nuclear weapons testing was most significant for atmospheric tests conducted prior to the moratorium in 1962 (NCRP, 1975). The major long-lived fission products or activation products that deliver a dose to the world's population are ^{90}Sr (^{90}Y; a beta-emitter), ^{137}Cs (^{137}Ba; a beta- and gamma-emitter), ^{3}H (a beta-emitter), and ^{14}C (a beta-emitter). The only short-lived internal emitter thought to have delivered a significant dose is ^{131}I, but no data are available to estimate the doses from this radionuclide during the high-fallout period. Direct measurements have been made on samples of skeletal ash and other tissue for both ^{90}Sr and ^{137}Cs (NCRP, 1975). Cesium–137 has been of high enough activity to be detected in vivo by whole body counting, during periods of high global fallout. During 1964, for example, the mean ^{137}Cs body content was estimated to be about 20 nCi, with a resultant dose of 2.4 mrad/yr (NCRP, 1975).

In order to evaluate absorbed dose per person for markedly varying annual doses, and with allowance for an absorbed dose to future populations from material deposited in the biosphere, UNSCEAR (1964) developed the concept of dose commitment which is defined as "the integral over infinite time of the average dose rates delivered to the world population as a result of a specific practice. The actual exposures may occur over many years after the explosions have taken place and may be received by individuals not yet born at the time of the explosions."

TABLE 5. Absorbed Dose per Examination in the Most Frequently Performed Radiopharmaceutical Examinations

Type of examination	Radio-nuclide	Chemical form	Average administered activity (μCi)	Examined and/or critical organ	Absorbed dose per examination (mrad)		
					Examined and/or critical organ	Gonads	Skeleton
Thyroid scan or function	^{131}I	Iodide	25	Thyroid	50,000	5	10
Thyroid scan	^{99m}Tc	Pertechnetate	1,000	Thyroid	600	20	20
Thyroid function	^{132}I	Iodide	25	Thyroid	750	2.5	2.5
Kidney function	^{131}I	o-Iodohippurate	20	Kidney	10	0.2	0.14
Bone scan	^{85}Sr	Nitrate/chloride	100	Skeleton	1,000	300	1,000
	^{87m}Sr	Nitrate/chloride	1,000	Skeleton	50	20	50
	^{99m}Tc	Polyphosphate	10,000	Skeleton	400	400	200
Kidney scan	^{203}Hg	BMHP	100	Kidney	50,000	1,000	1,000
	^{203}Hg	Chlormerodrine	150	Kidney	13,500	300	300
	^{99m}Tc	DTPA	3,000	Kidney	120	60	60
Brain scan	^{99m}Tc	Pertechnetate	10,000	Thyroid	6,000	200	200
Spleen scan	^{197}Hg	BMHP	300	Spleen	3,000	150	150
	^{99m}Tc	S-colloid	1,500	Spleen	150	7.5	15
Liver scan	^{198}Au	Colloid	150	Liver	6,000	45	75
	^{99m}Tc	S-colloid	1,500	Liver	600	7.5	15
	^{113m}In	Colloid	1,000	Liver	500	2	10
Pancreas scan	^{75}Se	Methionine	200	Pancreas	3,000	2,000	2,000
Blood (plasma) volume	^{131}I	HSA	10	Total body	20	20	20
	^{99m}Tc	HSA	100	Total body	2	2	2
Erythrocyte volume or survival time	^{51}Cr	Chromate	100	Total body	40	40	40
Lung scan	^{131}I	MAA	200	Lung	800	60	60
	^{99m}Tc	MAA	3,000	Lung	900	6	30
Iron kinetics	^{59}Fe	Citrate	15	Spleen	2,250	750	225

Adapted from UNSCEAR, 1977.

The mean dose commitments in the U.S. for all nuclear testing through 1970 are shown below (NCRP 1975).

External gamma radiation   80 mrad

Internal
^{137}Cs (whole body)   15 mrad
^{90}Sr (endosteal bone surfaces)   65 mrad
^{131}I   unknown
^{3}H (whole body)   2 mrad
^{12}C (whole body)   12 mrad

Consumer Products

There are many radioactive substances to which consumers are exposed. These are grouped into six categories: tobacco products; electronic devices that generate x-rays; static eliminators; smoke detectors; ceramics; and radioluminous products.

With the exception of tobacco products and dental porcelain, the absorbed dose to the individual is low from most of these items. The absorbed doses to individuals using these various devices are shown in Table 6.

Nuclear Power

The electricity generated by nuclear power reactors has approximately doubled from 1975 to 1979 (UNSCEAR, 1982). The total generating capacity in the world from 235 power reactors in 22 countries in 1979 was 120 GW(e).* The installed nuclear electricity generation capacity was 144 GW(e) in 1981, representing 261 nuclear power reactors. In the future, an additional 210 GW(e) will

TABLE 6. Absorbed Dose to Individuals from Various Consumer Products

Product		Reference
Airport baggage check	< 2 μR/inspection	NCRP, 1977
Ceramics		
Dental porcelain (0.044% uranium)	< 1 rem/yr	NCRP, 1977
Smoke detectors (^{241}Am 50 μCi/unit)	0.03 to 1.5 mrem	NCRP, 1977
Static Eliminators (^{210}Po ~ 0.5 mCi/unit)	< 1 μm/yr	
Tobacco products (^{210}Pb/^{210}Po dose to a few cells in bronchial epithelium)	≤ 10 rem/yr	Cohen et al, 1980 NCRP, 1975
Wrist watch		
^{226}Ra (1 μCi-gonad dose)	~ 3 mrem/yr	NCRP, 1977
^{3}H (1.3 mCi-from inhaled ^{3}H)	~ 0.6 mrem/yr	Moghissi, Carter
^{147}Pm (~ 0.05 mCi-gonad dose)	~ 0.25 mrem/yr	Moghissi, Carter

* 1 GW(e) = 109 watts of electric power.

be available from 227 power reactors presently under construction (UNSCEAR, 1982).

The radiation dose to people from nuclear power production stems from six sources: uranium mining and milling; fuel fabrication; reactor operation; fuel reprocessing; radioactive waste storage and disposal; and mill tailings.

The release of ^{222}Rn during mining is believed to yield the largest radiation exposure. Eight open pit mines in Wyoming are characterized by a ^{222}Rn emission rate of 5.4 mCi/1000 kg of ore mined (0.1%–0.2% uranium). Data reported from Canada and Australia also show the total radon released to be quite constant, at 27 mCi/1000 kg for each 1% of uranium in the ore.

Milling involves uranium extraction through crushing, grinding, leaching, and drying of the uranium concentrate. The process can release ^{222}Rn, uranium and its daughter products, and thorium.

Fuel fabrication releases some uranium and its daughter products to the atmosphere and effluent streams, but is a relatively small contributor. During reactor operation, radioactive gaseous fission products formed in the fuel, radioactive gases formed through neutron activation, tritium, radioactive iodine, and particulate fission products can be released.

The only commercial fuel reprocessing plants operating as of 1982 were in Windscale (U.K.) and La Hague and Marcoule (France). The effluents of concern from fuel reprocessing facilities are the long-lived radionuclides ^{3}H, ^{14}C, ^{85}Kr, ^{90}Sr, ^{106}Ru, ^{129}I, ^{134}Cs, and ^{137}Cs.

The absorbed dose from radioactive waste storage and disposal is not well known, because nuclides stored in geological repositories are expected to yield their maximum dose some millions of years after disposal.

Mill tailings are composed of uranium ore with most of the uranium removed. The principal radionuclide exposure from tailings is thought to result

TABLE 7. Summary of Collective Dose Equivalent Commitments to the Public from Nuclear Power Production

Local and regional contribution	Human-rem/GW(e)/year of operation
Mining	50
Milling	4.0
Fuel Fabrication	0.2
Reactor Releases	
Gases and particulates	410
Aquatic Releases	6
Fuel Reprocessing	
Atmospheric	30
Aquatic	70
Waste disposal (high level waste integrated to 10^6 yr)	3000
Mill Tailings	
Radon (integrated to 100 yr)	25

Source: Adapted from UNSCEAR, 1982.

from [222]Rn release. The collective dose equivalent commitments (the total dose equivalent in person-rem that will be delivered to the world's population) per year of operation of 1 GW(e) are summarized in Table 7 for each part of the nuclear power cycle.

SUMMARY

The sources and levels of radiation that affect people have been described. The major dose received from average exposure to natural radioactivity is from the short-lived daughter products of radon, which are always present in the atmosphere. The concentrations of radon daughters are not well documented in the United States. In areas in which radon levels are not thought to be elevated or enhanced, they deliver an alpha dose to the bronchial epithelium of about 3000 mrem/yr.

Natural potassium in the body gives an annual dose of about 15 mrem. Most of the other radionuclides ingested in the diet are bone seekers and normally deliver an annual alpha dose to cells on bone surfaces in the range of 10–30 mrem. Areas with elevated levels of naturally occurring radionuclides in the diet exist, but there are few data to estimate the resulting human dose. Factors of perhaps 10- to 100-times average may apply to a few individuals.

External gamma and cosmic radiations deliver an average annual dose of about 60 mrem. Small areas with elevated levels of gamma-emitting radionuclides, or elevated levels of cosmic radiation at higher altitudes, could increase this by a factor of two.

The annual doses to the bone marrow from diagnostic radiology and nuclear medicine showed average values of 103 and 0.5 mrem, respectively, for the U.S. in the 1970s. Therapeutic doses are high and variable, but apply to such a small number of individuals that their contribution to the population dose is not really comparable with the others.

Other miscellaneous sources, such as fallout, consumer products, and nuclear power, provide annual doses that are much smaller than those from the preceding sources. The average dose commitment from weapons test fallout, of about 100 mrem whole-body and 200 mrem to bone surfaces, is delivered over many years and cannot be expressed as an annual dose. Consumer product exposures are variable, depending on personal habits and use of various devices, but the average annual whole-body dose is only a few mrem. At the present time, nuclear power would deliver an annual dose of a few tenths of an mrem, based on U.S. nuclear capacity of about 50 GW(e).

The total doses to the whole body, thus, are somewhat more than 100 mrem/yr on the average, with small amounts of bone tissue receiving perhaps 50% more and the bronchial epithelium being exposed to about 3000 mrem/yr.

The author thanks Dr. John H. Harley for help in editing the text, Gordon B. Cook for the photographic reproduction, and Aimee Miranda for preparation and typing of the manuscript.

REFERENCES

Asikainen M, Kahlos H (1980) Natural Radioactivity of drinking water in finland. Health Physics 39:77–83.

Bengtsson G, (1976) Patient exposures in Swedish diagnostic radiology. Swedish National Institute of Radiation Protection Report 551:1976–2013.

Bennett BG (1970) Estimation of gonadal absorbed dose due to environmental gamma radiation. Health Physics 19:757.

Clements WE, Barr S, Marple ML (1980) Uranium mill tailings piles as sources of astmospheric radon-222. In: Gesell TF, Lowder WM (eds.), Natural radiation environmental III. National Technical Information Center USDOE, CONF 780422. Springfield, VA

Cohen BS, Eisenbud M, Harley NH (1980) Measurement of the alpha radioactivity on the mucosal surface of the human bronchial tree. Health Physics 39:619–632.

George AC, Breslin AJ (1980) The distribution of ambient radon and radon daughters in residential buildings in the New Jersey–New York area. In: Gesell TF, Lowder WM (eds.), Natural radiation environment III. Technical Information Center/USDOE, CONF 780422. Springfield, VA.

Guimond R, Windham ST (1980) Radiological evaluation of structures constructed on phosphate-related land. In: Gesell TF, Lowder WM (eds.), Natural radiation environment III, Vol. II. National Technical Information Center USDOE CONF Springfield, VA 780422, p 1457.

Fisenne IM, Keller HW (1970) Radium-226 in the diet in two U.S. cities. USAEC Report, HASL-224, Part I, National Technical Information Center, pp 1–8. Springfield, VA

Fisenne IM, Perry PM, Welford GA (1980) Determination of uranium in human bone ash. Anal Chem 52:777–779.

Fisenne IM, Keller HW, Harley NH (1981) Worldwide measurement of ^{226}Ra in human bone: Estimate of skeletal alpha dose. Health Physics 40:163–171.

Fisenne IM, Perry PM, Chu NY, Harley NH (1982) Measured ^{238,234}U and fallout ^{239,240}Pu in human bone ash from Nepal and Australia: Skeletal alpha dose. Health Physics 44:457–467.

Hamilton EI (1971) The concentration and distribution of uranium in human skeletal tissues. Calc Tiss Res 7:150–162.

Hamilton EI (1972) The concentration of uranium in man and his diet. Health Physics 22:149–153.

Harley NH, Pasternack BS (1976) A comparison of the dose to cells on trabecular bone surfaces from ^{239}Pu and ^{226}Ra based on experimental alpha absorption measurements. Health Physics 30:35–46.

Harley NH, Pasternack BS (1982) Environmental radon daughter alpha dose factors in a five-lobed human lung. Health Physics 42:789–799.

Harley JH (1981) Radioactive emissions and radon. Bull NY Acad Med 57:883–896.

Hill CR (1965) Polonium in man. Nature 208:423–428.

Holtzman RB, Ilcewicz FH (1966) Lead-210 and polonium-210 in tissues of cigarette smokers. Science 153:1259–1260.

Holtzman RB (1980) Normal dietary levels of ^{226}Ra, ^{228}Ra, ^{210}Pb and ^{210}Po for man. In: Gesell TF, Lowder WM (eds.), Natural radiation environment III. National Technical Information Center USDOE CONF 780422. Springfield, VA.

ICRU (1973) Supplement to Report 19. Dose equivalent. Washington, DC: International Commission Radiation Units and Measurements.

ICRU (1979) Report 31. Avergage energy required to produce an ion pair. Washington, DC: International Commission on Radiation Units and Measurements.

ICRU (1980) Report 33. Radiation quantities and units. Washington, DC: International Commission on Radiation Units and Measurements.

McGregor RG, Vasudev P, Letourneau EG, McCullough RS, Prantl FA, Taniguchi H (1980) Background concentration of radon and radon daughters in Canadian homes. Health Physics 39:285–289.

Moghissi AA, Carter MW (1975) Public health implications of radioluminous materials. Rockville, MD: US Department of Health, Education and Welfare Food and Drug Administration, DHEW Publication FDA 76-8001.

Morse RS, Welford GA (1971) Dietary intake of ^{210}Pb. Health Physics 21:53–55.

National Academy of Sciences Advisory Committee on the Biological Effects of Ionizing Radiation (BEIR) (1980) The effects on populations of exposure to low levels of ionizing radiation. National Academy of Sciences. Washington DC: National Research Council.

NCRP (1975) Report 45. Natural background radiation in the United States. Washington, DC: National Council on Radiation Protection and Measurements.

NCRP (1977) Report 56. Radiation exposure from Consumer Products and Miscellaneous Sources. Washington, DC: National Council on Radiation Protection and Measurements.

NCRP (1984) Report 77. Exposures from the uranium series with emphasis on radon and its daughters. Washington, DC: National Council on Radiation Protection and Measurements.

NCRP (1984) Report 78. Evaluation of occupational and environmental exposures to radon and radon daughters in the United States. Washington, DC: National Council on Radiation Protection and Measurements.

Oakley DT (1972) Natural radiation exposure in the United States. Report ORP/SID 72-1, U.S. Environmental Protection Agency, Washington, DC.

O'Brien K (1975) The cosmic ray field at ground level. In: Adams JHS, Lowder WM, Gesell TF (eds.), The natural radiation environment II. National Technical Information Center, CONF 720805. Springfield, VA.

PHS (1957) Publication 494. Control of radon and daughters in uranium mines and calculations on biologic effects. Washington, DC: Government Printing Office.

Roedler HD, Kaul A, Hinz G (1974) Genetically significant dose from the use of radiopharmaceuticals. In: Population dose evaluation and standards for man and his environment. Vienna: IAEA Publication STI/PUB/375, pp 377–393.

Roessler CE, Kautz R, Bolch WE, Jr. (1980) The effect of mining and land reclamation on the radiological characteristics of the terrestrial environment of Florida'a phosphate regions. In: Gesell TF, Lowder WM (eds.), Natural Radiation Environment III. National Technical Information Center, USDOE, CONF 780422. Springfield, VA.

Schlencker RA, Keane AT, Holtzman RB (1982) The retention of ^{226}Ra in human soft tissue and bone, implications for the ICRP 20 alkaline earth model. Health Physics 42:671–693.

Shearer SD, Sill CW (1969) Evaluation of atmospheric radon in the vicinity of uranium mill tailings. Health Physics 17:77–88.

Spencer H, Holtzman RB, Kramer L, Ilcewicz FH (1977) Metabolic balances of ^{210}Pb and ^{210}Po at natural levels. Radiat Res 69:166–184.

Turner RC, Radley JM, Mayneord WV (1958) The naturally occurring alpha ray activity of food. Health Physics 1:268–275.

UNSCEAR (1964) Report of The United Nations Scientific Committee on The Effects of Atomic Radiation. United Nations, NY: Official Records XVII Session (suppl 16) (A/5216).

UNSCEAR (1977) Sources and effects of ionizing radiation. United Nations, NY: UN Scientific Committee on The Effects of Atomic Radiation.

UNSCEAR (1982) Sources and effects of ionizing radiation. United Nations, NY: UN Scientific Committee on The Effects of Atomic Radiation.

USDHEW (1973) Population exposure to x rays, U.S. 1970. Washington, DC: US Department of Health Education and Welfare Publication, DHEW (FDA) 73-8047.

Wallace R (1975) Measurement of the cosmic radiation dose in subsonic commercial aircraft compared to the city pair dose calculations. University of California, Lawrence, Berkeley Laboratory, Report LBL-1505. Berkeley, CA.

Welford GA, Baird R (1967) Uranium, levels in human diet and biological materials. Health Physics 13:1321–1324.

Yeh HC, Schum M (1980) Models of human lung airways and their application to inhaled particle deposition. Bull Math Biol 42:461.

DNA DAMAGE AND REPAIR

JAMES E. CLEAVER, Ph.D.

The earliest approaches to understanding damage and repair were based on changes in the amount of tissue damage or of cell death resulting from varying regimens of irradiation. The clinical observation that a dose of x-rays caused less tissue damage when given in many fractions than in few, gave rise to the concept of the "sparing" effect of fractionation. Dose fractionation studies in cell culture gave rise to the concepts of "recovery from sublethal damage," and studies on relationships between growth demands on damaged cells, and their survival gave rise to concepts of "recovery from potentially lethal damage." The precise distinction between these concepts remains uncertain, but they are all related to repair of damage to DNA.

Biochemical approaches to DNA repair began with the identification of abnormal products and structures in irradiated DNA and analysis of their metabolism. Dimerized pyrimidine photoproducts formed by short wavelength ultraviolet (UV) light (260–280 nm) were among the first products found in DNA. Analysis of pyrimidine dimers led to the concept of excision-repair, which can be applied to repair of UV and many other kinds of damage.

These cellular and biochemical approaches have been complemented in recent times by discovery of various hereditary human diseases in which there are increases in the sensitivities of cells to radiation and chemical carcinogens in culture and in vivo. These diseases frequently exhibit an association of altered radiation sensitivities with increased carcinogenesis. In xeroderma pigmentosum (XP), ataxia telangiectasia (AT), and Cockayne's syndrome the increases in sensitivity are large and are an integral feature of the disease (Cleaver, 1980) (Figure 1, Table 1). Other diseases, such as retinoblastoma, Huntington's Chorea, and progeria, show increases in sensitivities that are of marginal biological significance, and may represent modulation of the radiation response by the altered cellular biochemistry (Figure 1, Table 1).

From the Laboratory of Radiobiology and Environmental Health, University of California, San Francisco, California.

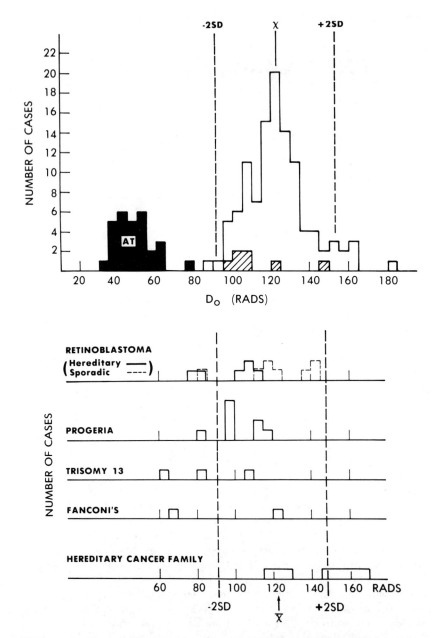

FIGURE 1. D_o (rads) of skin fibroblasts from normal individuals and those with various disorders. AT (solid histogram), ataxia telangiectasia; hatched histogram, ataxia telangiectasia heterozygotes. For some data, the D_o values were corrected so that the average D_o for normal cells corresponded to the value of Cox and Masson of 122 ± 17 rads. Dashed vertical lines indicate the range encompasing $\pm$ SD.

Data from Arlett and Harcourt, 1978; Cox and Masson, 1980; Little et al, 1980; Paterson et al, 1976, 1979; Weichselbaum et al, 1980.

TABLE 1. Human Diseases Showing Hypersensitivity to Radiations or Carcinogens

Disease	Agent	D_o ratio	Reference
Major Hypersensitivities[a]			
Xeroderma pigmentosum (A,C,D)	UV (chemical carcinogen)	5–10	Andrews et al, 1978
Xeroderma pigmentosum variant	UV light	1–6	Andrews et al, 1978
Ataxia telangiectasia	X-rays (gamma)	2.9–3.5	Paterson et al, 1979
Cockayne's syndrome	UV light	4.6	Wade and Chu, 1979
Fanconi's anemia	Mitomycin C	4–15	Fujiwara et al, 1977
Minor Sensitivities			
Ataxia telangiectasia heterozygotes	X-rays (gamma)	0.9–1.2	Paterson et al, 1979
Cockayne's heterozygote	UV light	1.8	Wade and Chu, 1979
Retinoblastoma	X-rays	1.2–1.5	Weichselbaum et al, 1980
Huntington's chorea	X-rays	1.25–2.0	Arlett, 1980
Huntington's chorea	MNNG[b]	2.1	Scudiero et al, 1981
Partial trisony 13	X-rays	1.6–2.0	Weichselbaum et al, 1980
Progeria	X-rays	1.1–1.6	Weichselbaum et al, 1980
Werner's syndrome	X-rays	1.1–1.6	Weichselbaum et al, 1980
Gardner's syndrome	UV light	2.3	Little et al, 1980
Gardner's syndrome	X-rays	1.4	Little et al, 1980
Chediak–Higashi syndrome	UV light	2.2	Kanaka and Oril, 1980

[a] The xeroderma pigmentosum variant is included in this category, because it has a major biochemical abnormality in DNA replication after UV, even though this does not cause large increases in sensitivity.

[b] N-methyl-N'-nitro-N-nitrosoguanidine.

These lines of investigation, cellular, biochemical and genetic, obviously overlap, but they provide useful categories to guide our thoughts. The term "recovery" will be used where changes in cell survival are measured with respect to alterations in dose fractions or growth conditions; the term "repair" will be confined to experiments that identify biochemical processes of removal of damaged sites from DNA. Although, historically, recovery experiments preceded the identification of repair processes, it is now possible to follow a more logical sequence from (1) damage, to (2) repair, to (3) recovery.

RADIATION DAMAGE TO DNA

The damage produced in DNA by ionizing and non-ionizing radiations is a welter of complex alterations to the reactive sites in DNA. X-rays produce direct X-ray–induced ionizations and indirect hydroxyl radical attack, all of which damage many sites in the purine and pyrimidine rings, destroy deoxyribose residues, break one or both strands of DNA, and produce DNA-protein crosslinks (Sonntag et al, 1982; Bernhard, 1981). In general, the damage from x-rays and other ionizing radiations is exclusively the result of ionizations in water and biological molecules; the energy deposited as excitations is of minor importance. Oxygen, which is a ubiquitous stable free radical, enters into the radiation-induced free radical reactions extensively and tends to exacerbate the biological effect. Ultraviolet light in the short wavelength range (260–280 nm), in contrast, is specifically absorbed in unsaturated chemical bonds in DNA, RNA, and proteins. Its biological effects are the consequence of chemical changes produced by specific excitations. Ultraviolet photoproducts in DNA consist mainly of cyclobutane and other kinds of pyrimidine dimers, with minor proportions involving water addition to pyrimidines (cytosine hydrates, thymine glycols) and DNA-protein adducts, but few strand breaks. Oxygen is of minor importance in the biological effects of UV light. One area of overlap has been observed recently with high-energy ionizing radiations that produce Cerenkov emission during passage though a liquid. Photoproducts characteristic of UV light can be detected as a result of these emissions (Morgan et al, 1982).

Damaged structures in DNA can be classified into general categories of singly modified bases, single-strand breaks, double-strand breaks, large structural modifications, and DNA-protein adducts. Single-strand breaks can be simple phosphodiester cleavage or more complex destruction or loss of bases and deoxyribose residues, and some sites may only produce breaks at high pH (alkali labile sites). Single-strand breaks and double-strand breaks are both produced as linear functions of x-ray dose, suggesting they are formed by single events; the breakage efficiencies seem to correspond to a single ionization cluster being the cause of a single-strand break (approximately 50 ev/break), whereas the ends of electron tracks are the cause of double-strand breaks (approximately 200 ev/break).

The termini of strand breaks produced in acqueous solution may consist of intact hydroxyl or more usually phosphate end groups on 3′ or 5′ sites. The break may involve a small gap from the loss of sugar and base, or there may be an altered sugar on the 3′ site and a 5′ phosphate end group. Modifications to sugar residues resulting in the loss of a base can be recognized as an alkaline-labile bond (Sonntag et al, 1981). Approximately 33% of the strand breaks are produced by direct action and the remainder from hydroxyl radical attack (Sonntag et al, 1981).

The D_o of about 100 rads of x-rays produces on the order of 1000 single-strand breaks (including alkaline-labile bonds), 1000 altered bases, and 40 double-strand breaks in a mammalian cell. The D_o of about 10 J/m^2 of UV light produces about 10^6 cyclobutane pyrimidine dimers. Clearly, the lethality of the average lesion from x-rays is far greater than for UV light, either because of differences in the structural devastation they cause to DNA or the relative efficiencies of their repair. Some of the DNA proton crosslinks may be the consequence of metabolic processes acting on damaged sites and, in the absence of repair, their frequency may increase slowly with time after irradiation (Fornace and Kohn, 1976).

DNA REPAIR SYSTEMS

The general scheme by which damaged DNA is repaired involves enzymatic pathways that convert damaged sites into suitable substrates for DNA polymerases and ligases, so that the damaged site can be replaced by a new, short stretch of nucleotides according to base-pairing requirements determined by the complementary strand. This scheme, excision repair, clearly will be most efficient for localized damage on individual strands; less efficient repair will be possible for damage in close proximity on both strands, such as that produced by densely ionizing tracks of heavy particles or crosslinks from some antibiotics (mitomycin C) or photoactive chemicals (the furocoumarins). Although the initial step of repair shows variation in enzymatic mechanisms, because of the large chemical variety of damaged sites, later steps are simpler and involve DNA polymerases and polynucleotide ligases that are also used for normal semiconservative replication.

Major branches for excision repair have been recognized on the basis of the initial mechanisms of action of excision enzymes: base excision-repair and nucleotide excision-repair, (Cleaver 1974) (Figure 2). Singly modified bases are

FIGURE 2. Pathways of nucleotide and base excision repair in mammalian cells. Single strand breaks are envisaged as involving an initial step in which damaged termini are modified, and subsequent steps would follow those depicted for base excision repair. Cleaver, 1978, used by permission.

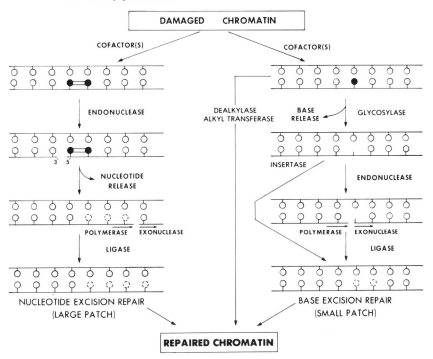

removed by cleavage of the glycosyl bond to release free damaged bases leaving apurinic or apyrimidinic sites (Lindahl, 1982). The glycosylases have narrow ranges of specificity, such as urea-DNA glycosylase, formamidopyrimidine-DNA glycosylase, 3-methyl adenine glycosylase, hypoxanthine-DNA glycosylase, uracil-DNA glycosylase, and thymidine glycol-DNA glycosylase (Lindahl, 1982). Many of these act quite rapidly in vivo, and the half-life of thymine glycols and other x-ray base damage is less than 15 min (Mattern et al, 1975; Paterson et al, 1975). Once the damaged base is removed, the remaining site is acted upon by apurinic/apyrimidinic endonucleases (Lindahl, 1982). The subsequent removal of the deoxyribose residues, their replacement by new bases and ligation produces a patch only a few bases long (Painter and Young, 1972).

Major chemical changes in DNA, such as UV-induced cyclobutane pyrimidine dimers, DNA-protein adducts, and chemical carcinogen adducts seem to

FIGURE 3. Excision repair of DNA damage including structural rearrangements required in relationship to the nucleosomal organization of eukaryotic DNA. The mended DNA is transiently in a state of looser DNA-protein association and can be easily digested by staphylococcal nuclease. Upon completion and ligation of the patch, the DNA returns to native chromatin structure with a half-time of about 15–20 min.
Cleaver, 1978, used by permission.

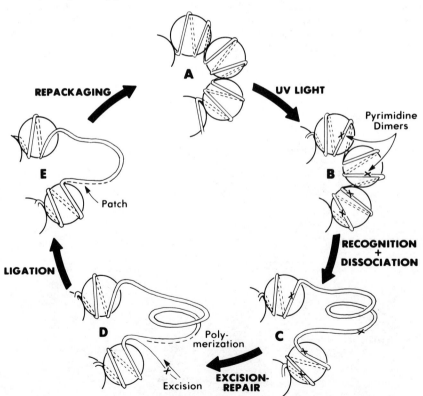

require extensive reconstruction of the damaged regions. The initial incision appears to be endonucleolytic, possibly removing a short oligonucleotide containing the lesion. The cleavage is indiscriminate with respect to the kind of chemical damage, but involves a large complex of proteins specified by numerous gene products (exemplified by the many complementation groups in the human disease XP; Cleaver and Bootsma, 1975). Following endonucleolytic cleavage, specific exonucleases remove the damaged strand, and a new polynucleotide strand is polymerized from the 3'OH terminus by DNA polymerase, α or β, according to cell type and the kind of damage (Ciarocchi et al, 1979; Seki and Oda, 1980), and then ligated. The patch eventually inserted into the DNA is large, up to 100 bases (Cleaver, 1974) and is apparently regulated at the nucleosomal level (Figure 3) by partial, temporary dissociation of chromatin during repair and subsequent reassembly (Cleaver, 1977; Smerdon and Lieberman, 1978; Bodell and Cleaver, 1981, 1982).

The initial step of repair of strand breaks must consist of enzymatic modification of the termini of the breaks, because these are rarely in a form suitable for immediate polymerization and ligation (Inoue et al, 1981). Single- and double-strand breaks are both rejoined efficiently and rapidly (Figure 4), although residual fractions of unrejoined breaks appear to be related to cell killing and to the high relative biological effectiveness of radiations of high linear energy transfer (LET) (Ritter, Tobias, and Cleaver, 1972).

FIGURE 4. (A) Rate of rejoining of single strand breaks in vivo, (●) and in vitro (○). Thymocytes were irradiated with 10 K rad and the number of breaks determined at various times by alkaline sucrose gradients (from Ono and Okada, 1974, used by permission). (B) Rate of repair of γ-radiation-induced double-stranded DNA breaks in normal human fibroblasts (HF-15) were exposed to 5000 rad (○) or 10,000 rad (●) and reincubated for various repair times. The number of double-stranded DNA breaks remaining after reincubation was determined based on the log of the relative retention of DNA on a filter after 4.5 hr of elution. Points represent the average ± SD of 3–5 separate experiments (from Woods, 1981, used by permission).

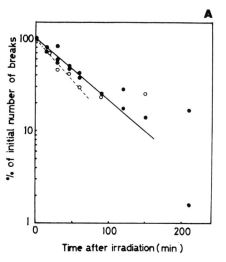

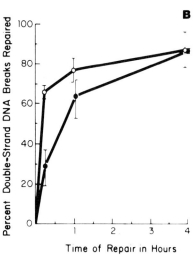

RECOVERY PROCESSES

Sublethal Damage

When doses of radiation are delivered in fractions separated by time intervals, the amount of cell killing observed is less than when the same total dose is delivered at once (Elkind and Sutton, 1959) (Figure 5). This implies that a certain amount of damage can be rapidly mended by cells, up to a certain limit (i.e., a sublethal amount). On single dose survival curves this limit corresponds approximately to the low dose shoulder of the curve (i.e., the quasi-threshold).

The rate and extent of recovery from sublethal damage varies considerably according to the kinds of radiation employed. After x-rays, for example, cells display an extremely rapid recovery within 30–60 min (Figure 5). After irradiation with densely ionizing radiations that commonly give exponential survival curves, very little recovery occurs. Recovery from non-ionizing radiations (i.e., short-wavelength UV light) is even more complicated. The extent of recovery after x-rays is independent of cell cycle and only modulated to a minor extent by progression of cells through more radiosensitive phases; after damage from

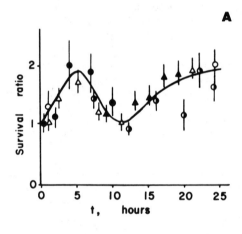

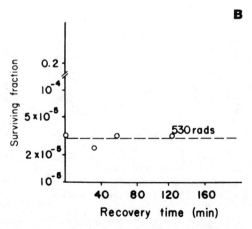

FIGURE 5. Relationship of the survival and the time interval between two fractionated doses of ionizing radiation.
(A) Colony-forming bone marrow cells in vivo (in mice). Cells were given two 200 rad doses separated by the interval t hours. Different symbols indicate separate experiments (from Till and McCulloch, 1963, used by permission).
(B) Chinese hamster H1 cells; dotted line with open circles: the cells received two fractionated neutron doses of 265 and 265 rads (from Schneider and Witmore, 1963, used by permission).

UV light the progression of cells around the cell cycle has a dominant effect. Most recovery between fractionated doses of UV light appears to occur within the S phase (Domon and Rauth, 1973; Todd, 1977).

Recovery from Potentially Lethal Damage

In many situations there seems to be a conflict between cells' recovery processes and their proliferative needs. A non-growing period after being damaged is generally beneficial, whereas DNA replication appears to fix damage in an irretrievable form with respect to survival, mutagenesis, and carcinogenesis. When confluent or non-growing cultures are maintained stationary for varying periods of time after irradiation before being forced to proliferate, the survival rate increases (Figure 6). Damage that would have been lethal in growing cells is apparently eliminated (i.e., the cells recover from "potentially lethal damage"). Xeroderma pigmentosum cell lines with differing abilities to remove damaged sites from DNA (Cleaver and Bootsma, 1975) show differing degrees of recovery (Figure 6). Over a 12- to 24-hr period, almost complete recovery from low UV doses is achievable by normal cells and XP cells with partial repair defects, but no recovery occurs in the XP cell lines with the most extreme defects (Maher et al, 1979).

Similarly, after irradiation with x-rays, recovery from potentially lethal

FIGURE 6. Rate of recovery of cells from potentially cytotoxic lesions induced by UV radiation. A series of confluent cultures was irradiated with the designated doses. Cells were released immediately or held in the confluent state for various lengths of time post-irradiation before being assayed for survival.
Maher et al, 1979, used by permission.

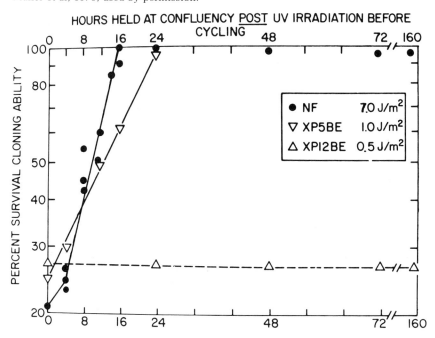

damage occurs in normal human cells and XP cells, but not in the x-ray–sensitive AT cell lines (Little et al, 1980; Weichenselbaum et al, 1979). This observation is more difficult to interpret for AT cells than for XP cells. AT cells have a complex abnormality (Painter and Young, 1980; Zampetti-Besseler and Scott, 1981; Murnane and Painter, 1982). Their failure to display recovery from potentially lethal damage may therefore be due to a complex interplay of repair and cycle progression effects.

Regulation of Recovery Processes

An intriguing and important question is to what extent cellular responses to radiation damage involve active, genetically controlled, repair systems in contrast to passive disturbances in normal processes. Cell cycle delays and mitotic delays that initially seemed to be passive disturbances now appear to have a strong genetically controlled aspect, from studies in AT (Painter and Young, 1980; Zampetti-Bosseler et al, 1981). Other features once associated with a postulated S phase repair process (postreplication repair) may reflect a more passive disturbance in the scheduling of DNA replication in UV-damaged cells (Park and Cleaver, 1979; Cleaver, 1978; Cleaver et al, 1980, 1983).

The association of radiation sensitivity with clinical disorders that often involve carcinogenesis (Table 1), provides insight into the biochemical mechanisms most closely connected with radiation carcinogenesis. Among four distinct disorders, exclision defective XP, XP variant, Cockayne syndrome, and AT, only the first has a clear defect in DNA repair, but all have abnormalities in DNA replication (Kaufmann and Cleaver, 1981; Cleaver et al, 1979, 1980; Lehmann et al, 1975, 1979; Painter and Young, 1980). This demonstrates clearly the crucial role that replication of damaged DNA has in relation to a wide spectrum of biological effects involving carcinogenesis, neurologic, immunologic and developmental abnormalities, and carcinogen sensitivity in general.

This research supported by the U.S. Department of Energy.

REFERENCES

Andrews AD, Barrett SF, Robbins JH (1978) Xeroderma pigmentosum neurological abnormalities correlate with colony-forming ability after ultraviolet irradiation. Proc Natl Acad Sci USA 75:1984–1988.

Arlett CF (1980) Survival and mutation in gamma-irradiated human cell strains from normal or cancer-prone individuals. In: Okada S, Imamura M, Terashima T, Yamaguchi H (eds.), Radiation research. Tokyo: Japanese Association of Radiation Research, pp 596–602.

Arlett CF, Harcourt SA (1978) A survey of radiosensitivity in a variety of human cell strains. Cancer Res 40:926–932.

Bernhard WA (1981) Solid state chemistry of DNA: The bases. In: Lett JT, Adler H (eds.), Advances in radiation biology, Vol. 9. New York: Academic Press, pp 199–280.

Bodell WJ, Cleaver JE (1981) Transient conformation changes in chromatin during excision repair of ultraviolet damage to DNA. Nucl Acids Res 19:203–213.

Bodell WJ, Kaufmann WK, Cleaver JE (1982) The structures of intermediates of excision repair in DNA and chromatin of human cells irradiated with ultraviolet light. Biochem. 21:6767–6772.

Ciarocchi G, Jose JA, Linn S (1979) Further characterization of a cell-free system for measuring replicative and repair DNA synthesis with cultured fibroblasts and evidence for the involvement of DNA polymerase-α in repair. Nucl Acids Res 7:1205–1219.

Cleaver JE (1974) Repair processes for photochemical damage in mammalian cells. In: Lett JT, Adler H, Zelle M (eds.), Advances in radiation biology, Vol. 4. New York: Academic Press, pp 1–75.

Cleaver JE (1977) Nucleosome structure controls rates of excision repair in DNA of human cells. Nature 270:451–454.

Cleaver JE (1978) DNA repair and its coupling to DNA replication in eukaryotic cells. Biochim Biochys Acta 516:489–516.

Cleaver JE (1980) DNA damage; repair systems and human hypersensitive diseases. J. Envir Pathol Toxicol 3:53–68.

Cleaver JE, Bootsma D (1975) Xeroderma pigmentosum: Biochemical and genetic characteristics. Ann Rev Genet 9:19–38.

Cleaver JE, Thomas GH, Park SD (1979) Xeroderma pigmentosm variants have a slow recovery of DNA synthesis after irradiation with ultraviolet light. Biochim Biophys Acta 564:122–131.

Cleaver JE, Arutyunyan R, Sarkisian T, Kaufmann WK, Greene AE, Corriel L (1980) Similar defects in DNA repair and replication in the pigmented xerodermoid and xeroderma pigmentosum variant. Carcinogenesis 1:647–655.

Cleaver JE, Kaufmann WK, Kapp LN, Park SD (1983) Replicon size and excision repair as factors in the inhibition and recovery of DNA synthesis from ultraviolet damage. Biochim Biophys Acta 739:207–215.

Cox R, Masson WK (1980) Radiosensitivity in cultured human fibroblasts. Intl J Rad Biol 38:575–576.

Domon M, Rauth AM (1973) Cell cycle specific recovery from fractionated exposures of ultraviolet light. Radiat Res 55:81–92.

Elkind MM, Sutton H (1959) X-ray damage and recovery in mammalian cells in culture. Nature 184:1293–1295.

Fornace AJ, Kohn KH (1976) DNA-protein cross-linking by ultraviolet radiation in normal human and xeroderma pigmentosum fibroblasts. Biochim Biophys Acta 435:95–103.

Fujiwara Y, Tatsumi M, Sasaki MS (1977) Crosslink repair in human cells and its possible defects in Fanconi'sanemia cells. J Molec Biol 113:635–650.

Inoue T, Yokoiyama A, Kada T (1981) DNA repair enzyme activity and in vitro complementation of the enzyme activity in cell-free extracts from ataxia telangiectasia fibroblasts. Biochim Biophys Acta 655:49–83.

Kanaka H, Orii T (1980) High sensitivity but normal DNA-repair activity after UV irradiation in Epstein–Barr virus-transformed lymphoblastoid cell lines from Chediak-Higoshi syndrome. Mutat Res 72:143–150.

Kaufmann WK, Cleaver JE (1981) Inhibition of replicon initiation and DNA chain elongation by ultraviolet light in normal human and xeroderma pigmentosum fibroblasts. J Molec Biol 149:171–187.

Lehmann AR, Kirk-Bell S, Arlett CF, Paterson MC, Lohman PHM, DeWeerd-Kastelein EA, Bootsma D (1975) Xeroderma pigmentosum cells with normal levels of excisio repair have a defect in DNA synthesis after UV-irradiation. Proc Natl Acad Sci USA 72:219–223.

Lehmann AR, Kirk-Bell S, Mayne L (1979) Abnormal kinetics of DNA synthesis in ultraviolet light irradiated cells from patients with Cockayne's syndrome. Cancer Res 39:4237–4241.

Lindahl T (1982) DNA repair enzymes. Ann Rev Biochem 51:59–85.

Little JB, Nove J, Weichselbaum RR (1980) Abnormal sensitivity of diploid skin fibroblasts from a family with Gardner's syndrome to the lethal effects of x-irradiation, ultraviolet light and mitomycin C. Mutat Res 70:241–250.

Maher VM, Dorney DJ, Mendrala AL, Konze-Thomas B, McCormick JJ (1979) DNA excision-repair processes in human cells can eliminate the cytotoxic and mutagenic consequences of ultraviolet irradiation. Mutat Res 62:311–323.

Mattern MR, Hariharan PV, Cerutti PA (1975) Selective excision of gamma ray induced thymine glycols from the DNA of cultured mammalian cells. Biochim Biophys Acta 395:48–55.

Mitchel DL, Clarkson JM (1981) The development of a radioimmune assay for the detection of photoproducts in mammalian cell DNA. Biochim Biophys Acta 655:54–60.

Morgan TL, Redpath JL, Ward JF (1982) Further studies on Cerenkov-induced photoreactivatable damage in E. coli. Radiat Res 89:217–226.

Murnane JP, Painter RB (1982) Complementation of the defects in DNA synthesis in irradiated and unirradiated ataxia telangiectasia fibroblasts. Proc Natl Acad Sci USA 79:1960–1963.

Ono T, Okada S (1974) Estimation in vivo of DNA strand breaks and their rejoining in thymus and liver of mouse. Intl J Radiat Biol 25:291–301.

Painter RB, Young B (1972) Repair replication in mammalian cells after X-irradiation. Mutat Res 14:225–235.

Painter RB, Young B (1980) Radiosensitivity in ataxia telangiectasia: A new explanation. Proc Natl Acad Sci USA 77:7315–7317.

Park SD, Cleaver JE (1979) Post-replication repair: Questions of its definition and possible alterations in xeroderma pigmentosum cell strains. Proc Natl Acad Sci USA 76:3927–3931.

Paterson MC, Smith BP, Lohman PHM, Anderson AK, Fishman L (1976) Defective excision repair of γ-ray-damaged DNA in human (ataxia telangiectasia) fibroblasts. Nature 260:444–447.

Paterson MC, Anderson AK, Smith BP, Smith PJ (1979) Radiosensitivity of cultured fibroblasts from ataxia telangiectasia heterozygotes: Defective colony forming ability and reduced repair replication after hypoxic irradiation. Cancer Res 39:3725–3734.

Ritter MA, Tobias CA, Cleaver JE (1977) High LET radiations induce a high proportion of non-rejoining DNA breaks in mammalian cells. Nature 266:653–656.

Schneider DO, Whitmore GF (1963) Comparative effects of neutrons and X rays on mammalian cells. Radiat Res 18:286–306.

Scudiero DA, Meyer SA, Clatterbuck BE, Tarone RE, Robbins JH (1981) Hypersensitivity to N-methyl-N'-nitro-N-nitroso-guanidine in fibroblasts from patients with Huntington's disease, familial disautonomia, and other primary neuronal degenerations. Proc Natl Acad Sci USA 78:6451–6455.

Seki S, Oda T (1980) Effects of 2',3' dideoxythymidine triphosphate on replicative DNA synthesis and unscheduled synthesis in permeable mouse sarcoma cells. Biochim Biophys Acta 606:246–250.

Smerdon MJ, Tlsty TD, Lieberman MW (1978) Distribution of ultraviolet-induced DNA repair synthesis in nuclease sensitive and resistant regions of human chromatin. Biochemistry 17:2377–2386.

Sonntag C, von Hagen U, Schon-Bopp A, Schulte-Frohlinde D (1981) Radiation-induced strand breaks in DNA: Chemical and enzymatic analysis of end groups and mechanistic aspects. In: Latt JT, Adler H (eds.), Advances in radiation biology, Vol. 9. New York: Academic Press, pp 109–142.

Till JE, McCulloch EA (1963) Early repair processes in marrow cells irradiated and proliferating in vivo. Radiat Res 18:96–105.

Todd P, Dalen H, Schroy CB (1977) Survival of synchronized cultured human liver cells following single and fractionated exposures to ultraviolet light. Radiat Res 69:573–582.

Wade MH, Chu EHY (1979) Effects of DNA damaging agents on cultured fibroblasts derived from patients with Cockayne's syndrome. Mutat Res 59:49–60.

Weichselbaum RR, Nove J, Little JB (1978) Deficient recovery from potentially lethal radiation damage in ataxia telangiectasia and xeroderma pigmentosum. Nature 271:261.

Weichselbaum RR, Nove J, Little JB (1980) X-ray sensitivity of 53 human diploid fibroblast cell strains from patients with characterized genetic disorders. Cancer Res 40:920–925.

Woods WG (1980) Quantitation of the repair of gamma-radiation induced double strand DNA breaks in human fibroblasts. Biochim Biophys Acta 655:342–348.

Zampetti-Besseler F, Scott D (1981) Cell death, chromosome damage and mitotic delay in normal human, ataxia telangiectasia and retinoblastoma fibroblasts after x-irradiation. Intl J Radiat Biol 39:547–558.

RADIATION-INDUCED CHROMOSOME ABERRATIONS AND CANCER

SHELDON WOLFF, Ph.D. AND A.V. CARRANO, Ph.D.

In exposed individuals, radiation can induce gene mutations or chromosomal abnormalities, as well as cancer. A possible connection between cancer and an abnormal chromosome constitution was proposed as early as 1914, by Boveri. More recently, the correlation between the mutagenicity and carcinogenicity of certain organic chemicals has refocused attention on models of carcinogenicity that relate the initiation of neoplastic growth to mutational events. Because the largest portion of radiation-induced mutational events take the form of chromosome aberrations, some of which are lethal to cells and some of which have genetic consequences, it has been particularly attractive to postulate that radiation-induced aberrations, themselves, can be a cause of cancer. This point of view is strengthened by the observation that chromosomes of tumor cells are often abnormal, and that patients with human diseases characterized by high levels of spontaneous chromosome aberrations are at increased risk of developing cancer.

RADIATION-INDUCED CHROMOSOME ABERRATIONS

When cells are exposed to ionizing radiation, one of the most readily noted effects is the production of aberrant chromosomes, particularly observable when the cells are in metaphase of mitosis (Evans, 1962; Lea, 1946; Wolff, 1961). These aberrations, which are the result of either simple breakage of the chromosomes or the interaction of the broken ends to form rearrangements, can be classified into two different types according to the stage of the cell cycle in which the exposure takes place. If cells are exposed in G_1 before the DNA is replicated, the chromosomes react as if they were single-stranded structures,

From the Laboratory of Radiobiology and Environmental Health, and Department of Anatomy, University of California, San Francisco, San Francisco, California (S.W.), and the Biomedical Sciences Division, Lawrence Livermore National Laboratory, Livermore, California (A.V.C.).

even though, as a minimum, a chromosome consists of a DNA double helix and its associated proteins. Thus, the unit of breakage and rejoining is the whole unreplicated chromosome, which doubles when the cell proceeds through the S phase, leading to full chromosome aberrations in which both chromatids are affected similarly. If, however, S or G_2 cells are irradiated, the individual chromatid is now the unit of breakage and rejoining, which leads to the formation of chromatid aberrations.

Most of the breaks produced by radiation restitute or become repaired (i.e., they rejoin in the original configuration and do not lead to observable aberrations). A small proportion, however, simply remain unrepaired, leading to the formation of fragmented chromosomes that can be seen and analyzed under the microscope. With sparsely ionizing radiations, such as x-rays, these simple breaks are found to increase approximately linearly with dose, indicating that radiation can break chromosomes with a probability that is directly proportional to the dose. Some broken ends, however, neither remain unrepaired to form terminal deletions nor undergo restitutional repair to reform the original chromosome. Rather, they undergo a form of misrepair in which broken ends from different breakpoints rejoin with one another to form two-break aberrations, such as dicentric or ring chromosomes, which are observable cytologically. Other configurations may also result, such as translocations, inversions, and interstitial deletions, which often can be observed cytologically only with specialized high-resolution banding techniques. Further, it should be noted that because deletions or rearrangements of the genome comprise a large class of mutational events, termed intergenic mutations, often apparently normal chromosomes can be shown to be abnormal if specialized genetic techniques are used. The two-break aberrations, whether detected cytologically or genetically, are found to increase approximately as the square of the dose after exposure to acute doses of x- or γ-rays. This is what might be expected, because these aberrations require the interaction of two independent breaks, each of which is produced in direct proportion to the dose. Therefore, the chance of obtaining two interacting breaks would be the product of the probabilities of getting each break individually.

The two breaks that interact to form these aberrations must be induced very close to one another in the cell nucleus. The first indication of this came from experiments showing that although single breaks were produced randomly within the nucleus, those aberrations requiring the interaction of two breaks were produced nonrandomly. (Sax, 1940). This distance factor was also found in experiments with densely ionizing particles, such as neutrons, which project protons within the cell. Under such densely ionizing conditions, both interacting breaks are produced by a single ionizing particle, so that the formation of two-break aberrations increases linearly, rather than as the square of the dose (Conger and Giles, 1950; Giles, 1940).

The formation of two-break aberrations produced by sparsely ionizing radiation is also subject to dose intensity or dose fractionation effects. If the radiation is administered over a long enough period of time, then breaks produced early during the exposure can undergo restitutional repair and, thus, not be present in the cell concurrently with breaks produced later during exposure. This precludes their interacting to produce two-break aberrations. It should be noted that with high linear energy transfer (LET) radiations, such as neutrons, where both breaks are produced by the same particle, no such intensity effects occur. Interestingly, the tracks of ionizations produced by x-rays contain not only portions in which the ionizations are well spaced, but also densely ioniz- ing tails in which the patterns of ionization resemble those found with neu- trons. Thus, as might be expected, the yield of two-break aberrations contains a linear component, in which the two interacting breaks are produced by the densely ionizing tails with one-hit kinetics, as well as a component produced by the interaction of the breaks produced independently by the sparsely ioniz- ing portions of the tracks. A more precise description of the kinetics of induc- tion, which takes into account both of these phenomena, is given by the equa- tion

$$Y = \alpha D + \beta D^2$$

where Y is the yield of two-break aberrations, D is the dose, α is the coefficient of aberration induction relating to the probability that both breaks will be produced by the densely ionizing tail of the radiation track, and β is related to the square of the probability that a break will be produced by a sparsely ioniz- ing portion of the track (Lea, 1946). Thus, the curve consists of a linear compo- nent and a two-hit component and, under acute conditions, the total yield increases as a linear-quadratic function of the dose. If the radiation is given under chronic conditions, however, the quadratic term becomes diminished because of restitutional repair. Under these conditions, even with sparsely ionizing radiations, the yield of two-break aberrations increases linearly with the dose. This is also true for acute radiation when the total dose is so low that the cell is not traversed by more than one track. Under these circumstances, only the linear term can contribute to the production of two-break aberrations.

In addition to there being a difference in the shapes of the dose–response curves for two-break aberrations induced by neutrons versus those induced induced by x- or γ-rays, densely ionizing radiations are more efficient at pro- ducing broken chromosomes (i.e., they have a high relative biological effective- ness [RBE]). The difference in the shapes of the curves, however, means that under acute conditions the RBE differs at each dose. The RBE is high at low doses but becomes progressively smaller as the dose increases because of the relatively larger contribution of two-track aberrations with x- or γ-rays. In fact, at high enough doses, more two-break aberrations are produced by sparsely ionizing radiations than by neutrons, leading to RBE of less than 1. This lack of a constant RBE over the dose–response curve has led some to select arbitrarily the dose at which 50% of cells are aberration-free as the dose at which to determine RBEs when making comparisons between various types of radia- tions (Conger et al, 1958). The difference in the shapes of the curves also leads to exceedingly high RBEs, or limiting RBEs, when the irradiation is carried out under chronic exposure conditions (Neary et al, 1963). When this is done with sparsely ionizing radiations, the two-track component of the dose no longer contributes to the production of two-break aberrations, leading to a comparison of the intensity-independent total dose of neutrons with the small intensity- independent portion of the x-ray dose that is contributed by the densely ioniz- ing tails of the tracks. Under these circumstances, comparisons are being made between the biological effect of the entire high-LET radiation dose and that caused by only a small portion of the dose of x- or γ-rays.

The kinetics of aberration induction are quite similar to those for radiation-induced cancer, which can be seen in the adoption of a linear-quadratic model for the induction of cancer by the National Academy of Sciences Advisory Committee on the Biological Effects of Ionizing Radiation (BEIR) (1980). As with chromosome aberrations, the limiting form of the equation, applicable at low doses and low intensities, would have only the linear term, whereas, at higher doses, the quadratic term would predominate. The equation the BEIR committee used has an additional exponential term representing a competing effect of cell killing that could lead to a decline in the dose-response at high doses. The same decline can be seen when mutational damage is measured by genetic means (Russell, Russell, and Kelly, 1958). In the usual study in which the damage is measured cytologically, however, aberrations are observed at the first mitosis after their induction, which is before cell division can lead to the genetic imbalance that causes death of the affected cell.

CHROMOSOME CHANGES IN CANCER

Over 100 yr ago, Arnold (1879) first described nuclear changes in human malignant tumors. Today, a preponderance of the evidence indicates that malignant cells often have abnormal chromosome constitutions (Sandberg, 1980). The mechanisms for such chromosome changes, however, are not yet resolved, and the hypothesis developed by Boveri (1914) relating malignant transformation to abnormal chromosome segregation is still debated. Although not every malignant cell possesses an abnormal karyotype, it has been argued that the apparently normal cells actually are karyotypically abnormal, but that the abnormalities are below the limit of detection by the light microscope. The critical unanswered question is whether the chromosome alterations observed in malignant cells are the cause of the malignancy or a by-product of the agent initiating the cancer.

The chromosomal alterations found in tumor cells can include numerical changes, structural changes, or both. The numerical abnormalities are deviations in chromosome number that can arise either by nondisjunction, involving only one or a few chromosomes, or by polyploidization as a consequence of cell fusion or defective karyokinesis. For cancer of the uterine cervix, the changes in chromosome number or structure have been observed to coincide with changes in the pathology of the tumor, as the disease progresses from mild dysplasia, to carcinoma in situ, to invasive carcinoma (Granberg, 1971; Ng and Atkin, 1973; Spriggs, 1974). Because within each patient multiple cells with the same structurally rearranged marker chromosomes can be found superimposed on a background of abnormal chromosome number, and because the frequency of cells with marker chromosomes tends to increase as the disease progresses, a clonal origin for the tumor cells has been suggested.

The structural chromosomal rearrangements observed in malignant cells include balanced as well as unbalanced translocations, inversions, duplications, and deletions. It is noteworthy that for some cancers the type of structural rearrangement is specific for the type of disease rather than unique to the

TABLE 1. Some Chromosome Changes Associated with Certain Human Malignancies

Malignancy	Chromosome rearrangement[a]	Percentage of patients with change
Leukemias		
Chronic myelogenous	t(9q;22q)	85
Acute promyelocytic	t(15q;17q)	40
Acute myelogenous	t(8q;21q)	15
Burkitt's lymphoma	t(8q;14q)	90
Meningioma	22q− or −22	68
Breast cancer	trisomy 1q	90
Retinoblastoma	13q−	—[b]
Wilms' tumor	11p−	—[b]

Source: Adapted from Rowley, 1980.

[a] Nomenclature: p, short arm; q, long arm; −, missing material; t, translocation involving chromosomes and arms indicated in parenthesis.
[b] Not adequately established.

individual. These findings alone provide the most provocative evidence that chromosomal changes may be involved in either the initiation or progression of malignancy. Table 1, derived from Rowley (1980), lists several malignancies in which a fairly specific chromosome change is found. It should be pointed out that not all cells within a given cancer contain the same aberration and that the specific aberrations are not necessarily the only chromosome changes that are present but are merely the most consistent.

In addition to being adjunctive diagnostic indicators of specific diseases, at least for certain leukemias, karyotypic rearrangements have been used to indicate prognosis and to evaluate patient response to therapy. Thus, for chronic myelogenous leukemia (CML) the translocation between chromosomes #9 and #22 produces a characteristic derivative chromosome called the Philadelphia (Ph) chromosome (Nowell and Hungerford, 1960; Rowley, 1973). A patient with CML who possesses the Ph chromosome is found to have a significantly better prognosis than a CML patient without a Ph chromosome; the mean survival times are 42 versus 15 mo, respectively (Whang-Peng et al, 1968). In addition, the clinical changes that occur between the chronic and acute phases of CML are accompanied by further chromosomal changes, the most common of which is the addition of another Ph chromosome. Other common changes include an extra chromosome #8 or an isochromosome #17 (Whang-Peng et al, 1968).

Some types of cancer are often linked to specific constitutional chromosomal changes. These include retinoblastoma which, in some patients, is associated with a deletion of a region on the long arm of chromosome #13 (Yunis and Ramsay, 1978), and Wilms' tumor, with a deletion on the short arm of chromosome #11 (Riccardi et al, 1978).

Both the numerical and the structural chromosome changes observed in cancers can be induced by radiation. For instance, irradiation of mammalian cells in vitro has been shown to induce polyploidy in a dose-dependent manner (Yu and Sinclair, 1972) and, as already discussed, structural rearrangements are induced with well-defined kinetics. Because initial radiation damage is a stochastic process, chromosomes should be involved in the rearrangements in proportion to their size. The presence of specific rearrangements in malignancies is therefore a likely consequence of selection of one rearrangement among many that are induced. The basis for this in vivo selection is unknown, although recent work in which oncogenes were moved next to active promoters suggests a possible mechanism for this selection (vide infra).

CHROMOSOMAL INSTABILITY AND SENSITIVITY SYNDROMES

If chromosomal alterations are associated with either the initiation or progression of cancer, then one might expect that individuals with an increased incidence of spontaneous aberrations would be at high risk for cancer. This, in fact, is the case for individuals with any of the three autosomal recessive diseases, Bloom's syndrome, Fanconi's anemia, and ataxia telangiectasia (AT). Similarly, people who are hypersensitive to the induction of chromosome damage by radiation or chemicals might also be expected to be at an elevated risk for cancer. Indeed, such is the case in individuals with the autosomal recessive disease xeroderma pigmentosum (XP) and individuals with Down's syndrome (trisomy for chromosome 21), who can be characterized by increased chromosomal sensitivity and a predisposition for cancer. The neoplasms associated with these disorders are shown in Table 2.

Bloom's syndrome is characterized by a high baseline frequency of sister chromatid exchange (SCE) (Chaganti, Schonberg, and German, 1974). In the lymphocytes, at least, there appear to be two populations of cells, one with a very high frequency of SCE and one with a normal frequency (German et al,

TABLE 2. Some Chromosomal Instability and Sensitivity Syndromes

Syndrome	Associated neoplasms	Cytogenetic defect
Bloom's	Leukemia, other cancers	High spontaneous frequency of quadriradials and SCE
Fanconi's anemia	Leukemia	High spontaneous frequency of chromosome breaks and gaps
Ataxia telangiectasia	Lymphoma, other cancers	High spontaneous frequency of chromosome breakage, especially translocations involving chromosome #14
Xeroderma pigmentosum	Skin cancers	Hypersensitivity to UV induction of SCE and aberrations
Down's	Acute leukemia	Hypersensitivity to x-ray induction of aberrations

1977). The high frequency of SCE is also observed in bone marrow cells from these patients (Shiraishi, Freeman, and Sandberg, 1976). Bloom's syndrome cells also contain a high frequency of chromosome breaks. As many as 15% of the lymphocytes from Bloom's syndrome patients characteristically possess quadriradial configurations resulting from translocations between the chromatids of homologous chromosomes. Such quadriradial configurations also have been observed in cultured fibroblasts from these patients. The frequency of chromosome and chromatid breaks, but not quadriradials, is also increased in bone marrow, suggesting that for aberrations, at least, the chromosome instability exists in vivo (Shiraishi, Freeman, and Sandberg, 1976). At the molecular level, the rate of DNA chain elongation is retarded in Bloom's syndrome cells (Hand and German, 1975). The relation between the malignant transformation and any of the stigmata associated with Bloom's syndrome cells is still unknown.

Cells from patients with Fanconi's anemia have an increased frequency of chromosome and chromatid gaps, breaks, and exchanges. The increase is generally greater than that observed for Bloom's syndrome patients, but quadriradial configurations are not commonly observed. The increased incidence of aberrations is more prevalent in lymphocytes than in bone marrow preparations (Hirschman et al, 1969). Unlike the situation in Bloom's syndrome patients, the spontaneous SCE frequency in Fanconi's anemia patients is normal (Chaganti, Schonberg, and German, 1974; Latt et al, 1975). A striking feature is the high susceptibility of Fanconi's anemia cells to killing and aberration induction after exposure to DNA crosslinking agents (Sasaki and Tonomura, 1973). This is postulated to be related to a defect in repair of the DNA damage produced by these agents (Fujiwara, Tatsumi, and Sasaki, 1977).

The autosomal recessive trait AT is also characterized by a high spontaneous frequency of chromosomal aberrations (Hecht and McCaw, 1977). In addition, lymphocytes from these patients often possess clones of cells carrying a specific translocation involving the long arm of chromosome #14 (Sandberg, 1980). The spontaneous SCE frequency in these patients is normal (Bartram, Roske-Westphal, and Passarge, 1976; Chaganti, Schonberg, and German, 1974; Calloway and Evans, 1975) but the cells are more sensitive to killing by ionizing radiation (Taylor et al, 1975).

Other disorders that demonstrate chromosomal instability are also associated with increased cancer risk (Sandberg, 1980; Sasaki and Ejima, 1981) but they are not as well characterized. These include incontinentia pigmenti (Hecht and McCaw, 1977), scleroderma (Emerit, 1976), porokeratosis of Mibelli (Goerttlerand and Jung, 1975; Taylor, Harnden and Fairburn, 1973), glutathione reductase deficiency anemia (Hampel et al, 1969) and basal cell nevus syndrome (Happle and Kupferschmid, 1972).

Unlike the chromsomal instability syndromes, the chromosomal sensitivity disorders, XP and Down's syndrome, do not demonstrate an increased spontaneous incidence of either chromosome aberrations or SCE. After exposure of cultured fibroblasts to ultraviolet (UV) light or certain chemicals, xeroderma pigmentosum cells, however, are hypersensitive to induction of aberrations (Parrington, Delhanty, and Baden, 1971), SCE (de Weerd-Kastelein et al, 1977; Wolff, Rodin, and Cleaver, 1977), and mutations (Maher et al, 1976). These cells, however, do not show an increased sensitivity to ionizing radiation, which is consistent with their known DNA repair defect (Cleaver, 1969; Setlow et al, 1969). Specifically, xeroderma pigmentosum cells lack a functional endonuclease that incises the DNA as one of the early steps in the excision repair process. Because ionizing radiation itself produces polynucleotide strand breaks, the loss of an endonuclease does not prevent the later steps of repair from occurring in irradiated XP cells.

A high incidence of acute leukemia in Down's syndrome is well documented (Miller, 1940; Wald et al, 1961), but the role of the additional chromosome #21 material in the causation of the leukemia is uncertain. Cells from Down's syndrome patients have been shown to be hypersensitive to the induction of chromosomal damage by ionizing radiation (Countryman, Heddle, and Cranford, 1977; Sasaki and Tonomura, 1969).

CHROMOSOME ABERRATIONS AND THE ETIOLOGY OF CANCER

The association of specific chromosomal rearrangements with certain cancers and the incidence of spontaneous or enhanced chromosomal breakage in individuals prone to malignancy suggest that chromosome abnormalities play a role in either the etiology or progression of cancer. Until we better understand the mechanisms by which chromosomal alterations occur as well as their biological consequences, however, this association can only remain suggestive and not an indication of cancer causation.

Two pieces of evidence, namely, the relatively consistent cytogenetic patterns is specific cancers and the uniformity of X-linked biochemical genetic markers (e.g., G6PD) observed in cells of a given tumor in a heterozygous individual indicate that tumors originate in single cells (Fialkow, 1977; Rowley, 1980). Evidence from cancer epidemiology in humans and from experimental cancer induction in animals indicates that at least two steps are needed for the conversion of cells to malignancy (Knudson, 1971; Mole, 1964; Moolgavkar and Knudson, 1981). It has been proposed that either or both of these steps could involve a heritable alteration at the molecular or chromosomal level (Strong, 1977). This idea is strengthened by the knowledge that radiation is a mutagen and that a close correlation exists between mutagens and carcinogens (Ames et al, 1973).

The types of radiation-induced genomic alterations that might induce a malignant transformation must be consistent with cellular viability. Therefore, unstable aberrations such as dicentrics, rings, and large deletions, which lead to cellular inviability, would not contribute directly to a developing tumor. On the other hand, the stable aberrations, such as balanced translocations, inversions, and small deletions, which are induced with similar frequency and similar dose kinetics as are unstable aberrations, could do so (Buckton et al, 1978). As indicated by Table 1, translocation-bearing cells often can have a selective advantage for growth as malignant cells. This is true for nonmalignant cells, as well (Carrano, Minkler, and Piluso, 1973; Hainden et al, 1976). Thus, stable aberrations (as well as any possible point mutations) could be candidates for either step in the transformation process, although the precise mechanisms by which the chromosomal mutations actually lead to cancer are still unknown.

Recently it has been postulated that oncogenes could be activated by having their positions in the genome translocated to regions where they would come under the influence of highly active promoters, which might lead to the over-production of some important regulator (Cairns, 1981; Klein, 1981; Radman, Jeggo, and Wagner, 1982). Alternatively, a promoter region could be moved closer to an oncogene. It has also been postulated that chromosome aberrations might lead to changes in gene dosage that would affect the signals responsible for the fine balance achieved in normal growth control (Klein, 1981).

Recent evidence at the molecular level suggests that stable rearrangements in somatic cells have a role in either the etiology or progression of cancer (Dalla-Favera et al, 1982; Dalla-Favera et al, 1983). For example, Burkitt's lym-phoma is associated with a specific translocation involving the long arm of chromosome #8 with the long arm of chromosome #14. Minor variants of this translocation involve chromosome #8 with either #2 or #22. An oncogene, c-myc, the homolog of the transforming gene of an avian myelocytomatosis virus, which produces a B-cell lymphoma in chickens, has been mapped distal to the breakpoint on chromosome #8 in patients with Burkitt's lymphoma and is translocated to chromosome #14 at a site within or very close to the genes coding for one of the heavy chain immunoglobulins. Because these Ig chains are overexpressed in the lymphoma cells, one hypothesis envisions the onco-gene to be translocated downstream from a promoter on chromosome #14, causing the abnormal production of the genes along the transcriptional path-way. Ig genes have also been mapped to chromosomes #2 and #22, which are involved in the variant translocations of Burkitt's lymphoma. These results have renewed interest in the potential biological consequences of stable chro-mosomal rearrangements in somatic cells as they relate to oncogenes (Marx, 1984).

The two-step model of carcinogenesis, in which either or both of the two events are chromosomal mutations, can accommodate many aspects of radia-tion-induced carcinogenesis, such as the latent period and the age dependency of cancer. That is, because mutation at the cellular level is a rare event, it should take time for most individuals to accumulate sufficient mutations from radiation exposure alone to put a somatic cell at risk for cancer from a second mutational event. The probability of two mutations being induced by radiation in the same cell at about the same time is approximately the probability of a single mutation squared. Therefore, there is likely to be a latent period before both mutations are present and the cancer is induced. Similarly, the age-related incidence of radiation-induced cancer can be interpreted as reflecting the accu-mulation of first mutational events in the aging individuals and the increased probability with time of acquiring the second mutation. Exposure to carcino-gens other than radiation would further increase the likelihood of a mutation. For those individuals at high risk for cancer induction, it might be imagined that they had acquired the first mutational event. This could explain the early onset of cancer and increased susceptibility of retinoblastoma patients to radia-tion-induced sarcomas (Sagerman et al, 1969; Strong, 1977).

Two observations must be reconciled before a generalized scheme of trans-formation based on cytogenetic damage can be derived: first, the apparent insufficiency of a single chromosomal event to produce cancer, and second, the uniqueness of the chromosomal alteration associated with some malignancies.

Certain cancers, such as retinoblastoma and Wilm's tumor, are inherited in an autosomal dominant fashion. In hereditary retinoblastoma, some of the affected individuals possess a deletion of a small region on the long arm of chromosome #13. For these individuals, the first step in carcinogenesis can be assumed to have been present in the zygote, so that the defect is constitutional. A second mutagenic event occurring in a somatic cell might trigger the carcinogenic process (Moolgavkar and Knudson, 1981). An argument in support of this two-step model lies in the fact that the chromosome #13 deletion does not appear to be sufficient by itself to induce the tumor; otherwise, all cells would be at the same risk and there would be a multicellular origin for this tumor, which is not consistent with the pathogenesis of the disease. It is attractive to speculate that the second mutational event occurs at loci homologous to those in the deleted region, thereby converting a hemizygous genotype to one that is homozygous recessive.

The concept of the recessive nature of cancer has sparked much debate and stimulated new thought on potential recombinational mechanisms for converting a heterozygous locus to homozygosity. One such mechanism involves mitotic recombination in a somatic cell (Kinsella and Radman, 1978). In the process of mitotic recombination a chromosome containing a mutant gene is postulated to exchange DNA with its normal homologue at a point of somatic pairing. If the reciprocal DNA exchange occurs proximal to the mutant gene, a homozygous mutant genotype will segregate in one of the daughter cells. Quadriradial formation among homologous chromosomes of Bloom's patients has been suggested to be a mechanism leading to homozygosity at a cancer gene locus in this disease (Festa, Meadows, and Boshes, 1979).

Whether or not the events leading to the induction of cancer are indeed chromosomal is unknown. The appearance in cancers of structural chromosomal alterations, often specific to particular malignancies, suggests, however, that they do play a role in carcinogenesis.

This work was performed under the auspices of the U.S. Department of Energy under contract numbers W-7405-ENG-48 and DE-AC03-3-76-SF01012.

REFERENCES

Ames BN, Durston WE, Yamasaki E, Lee FD (1973) Carcinogens are mutagens: A simple test system combining liver homogenates for activation and bacteria for detection. Proc Natl Acad Sci USA 70:2281–2285.

Arnold J (1879) Beobachtungen uber kernteilungen in dem zellen der geschwulste. Virch Arch Pathol Anat 78:279–301.

Bartram CR, Koske-Westphal T, Passarge E (1976) Chromatid exchanges in ataxia telangiectasia, Bloom syndrome, Werner syndrome, and xeroderma pigmentosum. Ann Hum Genet 40:79–86.

Boveri T (1914) Zur frage der enstehung maligner tumoren. Jena: Gustav Fisher.

Buckton KE, Hamilton GE, Paton L, Langlands AO (1978) Chromosome aberrations in irradiated ankylosing spondylitis patients. In: Evans HJ, Lloyd DC (eds.), Mutagen-induced chromosome damage in man. Edinburgh: Edinburgh University Press.

Cairns J (1981) The origin of human cancers. Nature 289:353–357.

Carrano AV, Minkler J, Piluso D (1975) On the fate of stable chromosomal aberrations. Mutat Res 30:153–156.

Chaganti RSK, Schonberg S, German J (1974) A manyfold increase in sister chromatid exchanges in Bloom's syndrome lymphocytes. Proc Natl Acad Sci USA 71:4508–4512.

Cleaver JE (1969) Xeroderma pigmentosum: A human disease in which an initial stage of DNA repair is defective. Proc Natl Acad Sci USA 63:428–435.

Committee on the Biological Effects of Ionizing Radiation, National Research Council (1980) The effects on populations of exposure to low levels of ionizing radiation. Washington, DC: National Academy Press.

Conger AD, Giles NH, Jr. (1950) The cytogenetic effect of slow neutrons. Genetics 35:397–419.

Conger AD, Randolph ML, Sheppard CW, Luippold HJ (1958) Quantitative relation of RBE in Tradescantia and average LET of gamma-rays, x-rays, and 1.3-, 2.5-, and 14.1-Mev fast neutrons. Radiat Res 9:525–547.

Countryman PI, Heddle JA, Crawford E (1977) The repair of x-ray-induced chromosomal damage in trisomy 21 and normal diploid lymphocytes. Cancer Res 37:52–58.

Dalla-Favera R, Bregni M, Erikson J, Patterson D, Gallo RC, Croce CM (1982) Human c-myc oncogene is located on the region of chromosome 8 that is translocated in Burkitt lymphoma cells. Proc Natl Acad Sci USA 79:7824–7827.

Dalla-Favera R, Martinotti S, Gallo RC, Erikson J, Croce CM (1983) Translocation and rearrangements of the c-myc oncogene locus in human undifferentiated B-cell lymphomas. Science 219:963–967.

de Weerd-Kastelein EA, Keijzer W, Rainaldi G, Bootsma D (1977) Induction of sister chromatid exchanges in xeroderma pigmentosum cells after exposure to ultraviolet light. Mutat Res 45:253–261.

Emerit I (1976) Chromosomal breakage in systemic sclerosis and related disorders. Dermatologica 153:145–156.

Evans HJ (1962) Chromosome aberrations induced by ionizing radiations. Intl Rev Cytol 13:221–321.

Festa RS, Meadows AT, Boshes RA (1979) Leukemia in a black child with Bloom's syndrome. Cancer 44:1507–1510.

Fialkow PJ (1977) Clonal origin and stem cell evolution of human tumors. In: Mulvihill JJ, Miller RW, Fraumeni JF, Jr. (eds.), Genetics of human cancer. New York: Raven Press.

Fujiwara Y, Tatsumi M, Sasaki MS (1977) Cross-link repair in human cells and its possible defect in Fanconi's anemia cells. J Molec Biol 113:635–649.

Galloway SM, Evans HJ (1975) Sister chromatid exchange in human chromosomes from normal individuals and patients with ataxia telangiectasia. Cytogenet Cell Genet 15:17–29.

German J, Schonberg S, Louie E, Chaganti RSK (1977) Bloom's syndrome. IV. Sister-chromatid exchanges in lymphocytes. Am J Hum Genet 29:248–255.

Giles NH, Jr. (1940) The effect of fast neutrons on the chromosomes of Tradescantia. Proc Natl Acad Sci USA 26:567–575.

Goerttler EA, Jung EG (1975) Parakeratosis Mibelli and skin carcinoma. A critical review. Humangenetik 26:291–296.

Granberg I (1971) Chromosomes in preinvasive, microinvasive and invasive cervical carcinoma. Hereditas 68:165–218.

Hampel KE, Lohr GW, Blume KG, Rudiger HW (1969) Spontane und chloramphenicolin-duzierte chromosomemutationen und biochemische Befunde bei zwei fallen mit glu-tathionreduktasemangel (NAD(P)H: Glutathione oxidoreductase, E.C. # 1.6.4.2.). Humangenetik 7:305–313.

Hand R, German J (1975) A retarded rate of DNA chain growth in Bloom's syndrome. Proc Natl Acad Sci USA 72:758–762.

Happle R, Kupferschmid A (1972) A further case of basal cell nevus syndrome and structural chromosome abnormalities. Humangenetik 15:287–288.

Harnden DG, Benn PA, Oxford JM, Taylor AMR, Webb TP (1976) Cytogenetically marked clones in human fibroblasts cultured from normal subjects. Somat Cell Genet 2:55–62.

Hecht F, McCaw BK (1977) Chromosome instability syndromes. In: Mulvihill JJ, Miller RW, Fraumeni JF, Jr. (eds.), Genetics of human cancer. New York: Raven Press.

Hirschman RJ, Shulman NR, Abuelo JG, Whang-Peng J (1969) Chromosomal aberrations in two cases of inherited aplastic anemia with unusual clinical features. Ann Intern Med 71:107–117.

Kinsella AR, Radman M (1978) Tumor promoter induces sister chromatid exchanges: Relevance to mechanisms of carcinogenesis. Proc Natl Acad Sci USA 75:6149–6153.

Klein G (1981) The role of gene dosage and genetic transpositions in carcinogenesis. Nature 294:313–318.

Knudson AG, Jr. (1971) Mutation and cancer: Statistical study of retinoblastoma. Proc Natl Acad Sci USA 68:820–823.

Latt SA, Stetten G, Juergens LA, Buchanan GR, Gerald PS (1975) Induction by alkylating agents of sister chromatid exchanges and chromatid breaks in Fanconi's anemia. Proc Natl Acad Sci USA 72:4066–4070.

Lea DE (1946) Actions of radiations on living cells. Cambridge: Cambridge University Press.

Maher VM, Ouellette LM, Curren RD, McCormick JJ (1976) Frequency of ultraviolet light-induced mutations is higher in xeroderma pigmentosum variant cells than in normal human cells. Nature 261:593–595.

Marx JL (1984) What do oncogenes do? Science 223:673–676.

Miller RW (1970) Neoplasia and Down's syndrome. Ann NY Acad Sci 171:637–644.

Mole RH (1964) Cancer production by chronic exposure to penetrating gamma radiation. In: Control of cell division and the induction of cancer. National Cancer Institute Monograph No. 14, Washington DC.

Moolgavkar SH, Knudson AG, Jr. (1981) Mutation and cancer: A model for human carcinogenesis. J Natl Cancer Inst 66:1037–1052.

Neary GJ, Savage JRK, Evans HJ, Whittle J (1963) Ultimate maximum values of the RBE of fast neutrons and gamma-rays for chromosome aberrations. Intl J Radiat Biol 6:127–136.

Ng ABP, Atkin NB (1973) Histological cell type and DNA value in the prognosis of squamous cell cancer of uterine cervix. Br J Cancer 28:322–331.

Nowell PC, Hungerford DA (1960) A minute chromosome in human chronic granulocytic leukemia. Science 132:1497.

Parrington JM, Delhanty JDA, Baden HP (1971) Unscheduled DNA synthesis, u.v.-induced chromosome aberrations and SV_{40} transformation in cultured cells from xeroderma pigmentosum. Ann Human Genet 35:149–160.

Radman M, Jeggo P, Wagner R (1982) Chromosomal rearrangement and carcinogenesis. Mutat Res 98:249–264.

Riccardi VM, Sujansky E, Smith AC, Francke U (1978) Chromosomal imbalance in the aniridia-Wilms' tumor association: 11p interstitial deletion. Pediatrics 61:604–610.

Rowley JD (1973) A new consistent chromosomal abnormality in chronic myelogenous leukemia identified by quinacrine fluorescence and Giemsa staining. Nature 243:290–293.

Rowley JD (1980) Chromosome abnormalities in cancer. Cancer Genet Cytogenet 2:175–198.

Russell WL, Russell LB, Kelly EM (1958) Radiation dose rate and mutation frequency. Science 128:1546–1550.

Sagerman RH, Cassady JR, Tretter P, Ellsworth RM (1969) Radiation induced neoplasia following external beam therapy for children with retinoblastoma. Am J Roentgenol Radium Ther Nucl Med 105:529–535.

Sandberg AA (1980) The chromosomes in human cancer and leukemia. New York: Elsevier North Holland.

Sasaki MS, Ejima Y (1981) Procancer class of genes and generation of chromosome mutation. In: Inui N, Kuroki T, Yamada M, Heidelberger C (eds.), Mutation, promotion and transformation in vitro. Tokyo: Japan Scientific Societies Press.

Sasaki MS, Tonomura A (1969) Chromosomal radiosensitivity in Down's syndrome. Jap J Hum Genet 14:81–92.

Sasaki MS, Tonomura A (1973) A high susceptibility of Fanconi's anemia to chromosome breakage by DNA cross-linking agents. Cancer Res 33:1829–1836.

Sax K (1940) An analysis of x-ray-induced chromosomal aberrations in Tradescantia. Genetics 25:41–68.

Setlow RB, Regan JD, German J, Carrier WL (1969) Evidence that xeroderma pigmentosum cells do not perform the first step in the repair of ultraviolet damage to their DNA. Proc Natl Acad Sci USA 64:1035–1041.

Shiraishi Y, Freeman AI, Sandberg AA (1976) Increased sister chromatid exchange in bone marrow and blood cells from Bloom's syndrome. Cytogenet Cell Genet 17:162–173.

Spriggs AI (1974) Cytogenetics of cancer and precancerous states of the cervix uteri. In: German J (ed.), Chromosomes and cancer. New York: John Wiley.

Strong LC (1977) Theories of pathogenesis: Mutation and cancer. In: Mulvihill JJ, Miller RW, Fraumeni JF, Jr. (eds.), Genetics of human cancer. New York: Raven Press.

Taylor AMR, Harnden DG, Fairburn EA (1973) Chromosomal instability associated with susceptibility to malignant disease in patients with porokeratosis of Mibelli. J Natl Cancer Inst 51:371–378.

Taylor AMR, Harnden DG, Arlett CF, Harcourt SA, Lehmann AR, Stevens S, Bridges BA (1975) Ataxia telangiectasia: A human mutation with abnormal radiation sensitivity. Nature 258:427–429.

Wald N, Borges WH, Li CC, Turner JH, Harnois MC (1961) Leukaemia associated with mongolism. Lancet i:1228.

Whang-Peng J, Canellos GP, Carbone PP, Tjio JH (1968) Clinical implications of cytogenetic variants in chronic myelocytic leukemia (CML). Blood 32:755–766.

Wolff S (1961) Radiation genetics. In: Errera M, Forssberg A (eds.), Mechanisms in radiobiology, Vol. 1. New York: Academic Press.

Wolff S, Rodin B, Cleaver JE (1977) Sister chromatid exchanges induced by mutagenic carcinogens in normal and xeroderma pigmentosum cells. Nature 265:347–349.

Yu CK, Sinclair WK (1972) Polyploidy induced by x-rays during the cell cycle of Chinese hamster cells in vitro. Radiat Res 52:509–519.

Yunis JJ, Ramsay N (1978) Retinoblastoma and subband deletion of chromosome 13. Am J Dis Child 132:161–163.

ROLE OF VIRUSES

J.F. DUPLAN, M D., B. GUILLEMAIN, Ph.D.,
AND T. ASTIER, D. Sc.

The purpose of this review is to report and evaluate a number of observations that indicate 1) oncogenic viruses can be derepressed as a consequence of radiation exposure, 2) some radiation-induced tumors contain such viruses, and 3) a causal relation between viral activation and radiocarcinogenesis can be envisaged. The notion that "latent" viruses might be "activated" by chemical or physical agents arose from the experiments on lysogeny. The induction of the development of prophage was first observed by Lwoff, Siminovich, and Kjeldgaard (1950) after ultraviolet (UV) irradiation. Latarjet (1951) described a similar effect after exposure of B-megatherium to x-radiation. It was soon discovered that besides UV and x-radiations, several chemicals displayed inductive activity that correlated with their mutagenic activity in bacteria. It was also noted that those agents which were both mutagenic and inductive were also carcinogenic (Lwoff, 1953). In retrospect, it seems difficult to assess what would have been the impact of lysogenic induction on cancer research if it had not coincided with the demonstration by Gross that spontaneous leukemia of AKR mice could be transfered by cell-free extracts (Gross, 1951), and also with several decisive improvements in cell culture techniques and in biochemistry.

In relation to the specific subject of this review (i.e., the role of viruses in radiocarcinogenesis) a decisive event was the work initiated in the early 1950s on radiation leukemogenesis by Kaplan et al (Kaplan, 1978). One highlight in this series of experiments was the demonstration that a nonirradiated thymus could become malignant when transplanted into a previously thymectomized irradiated recipient (Kaplan and Brown, 1954). Two hypotheses were successively formulated to account for this indirect carcinogenic effect: 1) the malignant transformation of the grafted thymus was the result of a proliferation of cells in the subcapsular thymic zone, elicited by the radiation-induced deple-

From the Unité de Recherche de Radiobiologie Expérimentale et de Cancérologie, INSERM, Fondation Bergonié, Bordeaux, France.

tion of the hemopoietic system (Kaplan and Brown, 1957), and 2) irradiation activated a thymotropic leukemogenic virus, which in turn induced the thymic lymphoma. The prevention of radioleukemias by a postirradiation injection of nonirradiated hemopoietic cells provided indirect evidence supporting the first assumption (Kaplan et al, 1953). The second possibility prevailed when Gross (1958) and Lieberman and Kaplan (1959) described the cell-free transmission of radiation-induced thymic lymphomas in C3H and C57BL mice, respectively. The virus suspected to be the leukemogenic agent was named the radiation leukemia virus (RadLV).

Ionizing radiation is a universal carcinogen that can induce a variety of neoplasms. A number of publications have reported the detection of viral particles by electronmicroscopy in radiation-induced tumors. In 1969, Timmermans et al described the presence of B viral particles in mammary tumors induced by the combined effects of x-radiation and urethane in mice of the strain 020 which were otherwise resistant to the mouse mammary tumor virus (MuMTV). A similar finding was reported by Goldfeder (1972) in mammary tumors developed in X/Gf mice exposed to x-rays. These were important findings because it had been generally suggested that chemical or physical agents could not potentiate a latent MuMTV. Another example of the participation of a virus in radiation-induced cancer involves the osteosarcomas produced by bone seeking radionuclides, such as ^{90}Sr or ^{224}Ra. Studies of this virus were initiated in 1971 by Reilly and Finkel and were developed further when an osteosarcoma-inducing virus (FBR) was recovered from ^{90}Sr-induced osteosarcomas in mice of the X/Gf strain (Finkel and Reilly, 1973).

Thus, three different viruses have been studied as possible causative agents of radiation-induced cancer, and all three belong to the retrovirus group (oncogenic RNA viruses). Radiation-induced osteosarcoma virus (FBR) is a murine sarcoma virus(MuSV). RadLV pertains to the murine leukemia virus group (MuLV). Both are C-type viruses, whereas, MuMTV is related to viruses of the B-type. There is no indication of the involvement of DNA viruses in radiocarcinogenesis, although radiation might conceivably favor the carcinogenic activity of oncogenic DNA viruses.

CHARACTERISTICS OF RETROVIRUSES

Retroviruses contain a 35S single-stranded RNA genome and an RNA-dependent DNA polymerase (reverse transcriptase), allowing synthesis of a double-stranded DNA provirus, which becomes integrated into the cellular DNA. Unlike DNA tumor viruses, retroviruses do not kill the cell to replicate.

The proviral DNA (8.8 Kb) is bounded by two sets of repetitive sequences (long terminal repeats, LTR), which play an important role in the integration and transcription of the proviral genome. Three proviral genes are found from the 5 prime to the 3 prime terminals of the RNA transcript: gag, pol, env. The gag gene codes for the internal structural proteins p15, p12, p30, and p10 for MuLV, or p10, p28, p23, and p14 for MuMTV. The pol gene codes for the reverse transcriptase. The env gene of the MuLV codes for the gp71 envelope glycoprotein and in addition for the p15E (immunosuppressive protein); the env gene of MuMTV gives the gp52 and gp36 envelope glycoproteins (Figure 1A) (Stephenson, 1980).

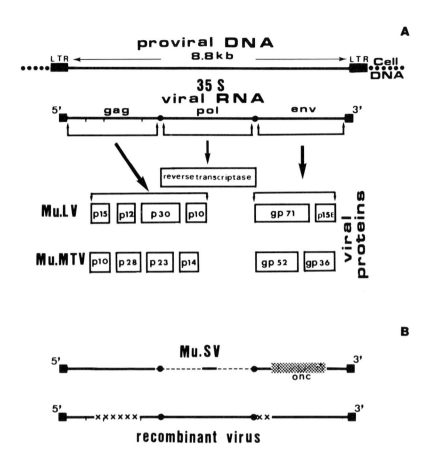

FIGURE 1. (A) Schematic representation of the retroviral genome and of its protein products. The proviral DNA, inserted into the DNA of the cell (dotted line), is transcribed into 35S viral RNA, which represents the viral genome and contains three genes: *gag, pol, env*. The *gag* proteins of MuLV and MuMTV, and the reverse transcriptase, are transcribed from the viral RNA—acting as an mRNA—through several intermediate precursor polypeptides that have been omitted in the figure. The *env* proteins gp71 and p15E (MuLV), or gp52 and gp36 (MuMTV), are translated from a specific env-mRNA, which does not appear in the figure and which results from the processing (splicing) of the 35S viral RNA. (B) Genomic structure of MuSV and recombinant viruses. MuSV are defective viruses that proceed from a genetic recombination between the genome of a deleted MuLV and cellular DNA sequences (oncogenes). Deleted sequences are represented by a broken line, the oncogene (dotted zone) substitutes for the deleted sequences of the *env* gene. Missing viral proteins—for instance, those replaced by the oncogene—are provided by the helper virus. Recombinant viruses are competent viruses that arise from recombination between the genomes of two different MuLV. The figure illustrates a B-tropic recombinant in which most of the viral proteins are encoded by an N-tropic MuLV (continuous line) except for the p30 and a fraction of the gp71, which are encoded by a xenotropic viurs (xxx).

MuLV

Most naturally occuring MuLV are endogenous viruses. They belong to two main types, depending on their ability to reinfect cells of their natural host (ecotropic virus) or cells of foreign species (xenotropic virus, X-tropic). The proviral information for both types of virus can exist simultaneously in the same host but at different loci. It must be stressed that 0.04%–0.3% of the mouse genome is formed of proviral sequences and that most of them are never expressed, at least in the form of infectious particles (Weinberg and Steffen, 1981).

All endogenous ecotropic MuLV studied so far are N-tropic and deprived of leukemogenic activity. B-tropic viruses, however, are frequently isolated from normal or malignant tissues, but they do not transform or convert fibroblastic cells, although many of them are leukemogenic after a long latent period. These B viruses arise from a genetic recombination between N and X endogenous viruses. This recombination always involves the part of the gag gene, which codes for the p30, but changes may also occur at the p15 and p12 levels. In addition, different types of env polytropic (amphotropic, dualtropic) recombinants that can infect both host and foreign cells may occur. All these recombinants are actual exogenous viruses; consequently, they may appear in the cellular DNA as new proviral copies. It must be made clear, however, that their presence in a tumor is not, in itself, definite proof that they are causative agents of the tumor (Figure 1B).

Acute Defective Retroviruses and Oncogenes

These defective viruses—which include MuSV—arise from recombination between a C-type virus (i.e., an MuLV), which has lost a large fraction of its genome by deletion and host cell genetic information (Figure 1B). The nature of the involved host cell gene sequences (onc genes) varies among viruses. The acquired host cell oncogenes are responsible for the high oncogenic potential of this group of viruses.

MuMTV

Schematically, two main types of MuMTV can be recognized: the endogenous type and the milk-born exogenous type (Hilgers and Bentvelzen, 1978). The expression of the endogenous MuMTV is 1) controlled by Mendelian loci of the host, which are strain-dependent, and 2) influenced by additional factors, such as disturbances in hormonal balance. Most inbred strains of mice contain genetic information for an MuMTV, but its exact role in mammary carcinogenesis remains controversial. There is some evidence, however, that the number of MuMTV–DNA copies in normal cellular DNA is increased in strains with a high incidence of mammary tumors, and that new virus-related RNA can be detected in mammary carcinomas (Marcus et al, 1981).

IN VITRO ACTIVATION OF ENDOGENOUS RETROVIRUSES

Unlike exogenous proviruses, endogenous proviruses are either not expressed or expressed at a very low level by non-target cells in animals of tumor-resistant strains. Proviruses, however, may be induced to replicate in vitro by a variety of chemicals, such as halogenated pyrimidines and protein synthesis inhibitors. So far, these agents have not been found to activate proviruses in vivo, nor have they displayed any oncogenic effects.

In spite of its potent carcinogenic activity, ionizing radiation is 100 times less efficient than the above-cited chemicals with respect to proviral activation in vitro (Rowe et al, 1971). Nevertheless, the possible role of retroviruses as causative agents in radiation carcinogenesis has prompted the study of the activation of endogenous viruses by ionizing radiation in vitro.

Experiments have been carried out on mouse embryo fibroblasts and established cell lines from mice of various strains, such as C57BL/Ka (Decleve et al, 1976), AKR (Tennant et al, 1977; Niwa and Sugahara, 1979), RFM (Otten et al, 1976), and BALB/c (Otten et al, 1976; Niwa and Sugahara, 1979). In most cases, the radiation dosage has ranged from 50 to 1000 rads, which are doses frequently used for exposures in vitro.

From these different reports, it can be concluded that x- and gamma-rays may activate endogenous viruses, with an induction rate of about $10^{-4}-10^{-5}$, as opposed to 10^{-1} for halogenated pyrimidines. It has been demonstrated by Otten et al (1976) that efficient virus induction requires cell division during irradiation, which was interpreted as an indication that irradiated cells are induced only if cellular DNA synthesis is initiated prior to repair of lesions in a virus-associated region of the DNA. The mechanism of induction and the types of activated viruses are different for x-rays and for IUdr or BrUdr, although both require at least transient transcription of cell DNA. After exposure to ionizing radiation, the viruses that are induced are those which are also subject to spontaneous expression (i.e., those that are less tightly restricted at the level of spontaneous activation).

IN VIVO ACTIVATION OF ENDOGENOUS VIRUSES

Activation of MuLV

With respect to radiation carcinogenesis, it is important to ascertain whether or not viral derepression occurs in irradiated animals previous to tumor development. The subject has been dealt with in the past by two different techniques: detection of viral particles by electron microscopy (Gross, 1970) and assay of cell-free extracts for carcinogenicity (Haran-Ghera, 1966; Haran-Ghera and Peled, 1967). Both methods have provided some positive results, but they are open to criticism, from a strictly virologic viewpoint. Actually, they suffer from weak sensitivity with respect to viral detection and also fail to characterize properly the induced viruses. These limitations are of special importance in the interpretation of the assay in vivo of cell-free extracts. Because the activated endogenous viruses are deprived of carcinogenicity, the test cannot be positive unless oncogenic recombinants either already exist in the extract or are formed secondarily in the recipient.

Several experiments have been carried out to detect viral activation subsequent to radiation exposure and prior to tumor development. The gross results of these experiments are reported in Table 1. It must be noted that the level of expression of N, B and X viruses remained very low and that, depending on the mouse strain, the percentage of positive mice varied from 25% to 64%,

TABLE 1. Detection of Ecotropic, Xenotropic, or Recombinant MuLv in Mice Prior to Tumor Development

Experiment number	Mouse strain	Dose (rad) and type of radiation	Time of appearance[a]	Type of virus[b]	Viral expression Organs tested[c] Spleen	Bone marrow	Thymus	Blood	Expected type and percentage of tumor[e]	Reference
1	C57BL/6	170 × 4 X-rays	8 days	B, X	—	+++	+	NT[d]	L 70%	Hass, 1977
2	ICR/JCL	170 × 4 X-rays	20 days	N, B	++	+++	+	NT	L 87%	Yokoro et al, 1977
3	NZB	630, [60]Co	4 wk	X	NT	NT	NT	+++	L 75%	Harvey et al, 1979
4	C57BL/Ka	175 × 4 X-rays	2 mo	N, B, X,	+++	+++	+++	NT	L 90%	Sankar-Mistry and Jolicoeur, 1980
5	(C3Hx101)F1	0.5 Ci [224]RA	1 mo[a]	N, B	NT	NT	NT	+++	O 100%	Erfle et al, 1980a and b
6	BALB/c	150 × 5 [137]Cs	4 mo[a]	N, B, NB	NT	NT	NT	+++	L 71%	Ellis et al, 1980a

[a] Time elapsed between the end of radiation exposure and the first detection of viruses. In Experiment 5, repeated injections of [224]Ra were carried out for 9 mo, and the mice were found positive 1 mo after the beginning of the treatment. In Experiments 3 and 6, the mice were not tested prior to the indicated time.

[b] Experiment 2: Xenotropic virus could not be detected for technical reasons. Experiment 3: NZB mice do not express ecotropic virus.

[c] Besides the listed organs, uterus and muscle were positive in Exp. 3, and bone in Exp. 5.

[d] NT, Not tested.

[e] L, lymphoma; O, Osteosarcoma.

whereas, the tumor incidence always exceeded 70%. Even at the individual cell level, the presence of MuLV antigen has not correlated with the expression of thymus leukemia (TL) antigen on the thymocytes of irradiated C57BL/6 mice (Stockert and Old, 1977).

In at least two cases (experiments 1 and 5), early viral expression was transient but viral production was resumed later at the outset of tumor development. The data in Table 1 (experiments 1, 2, and 4) are in agreement with those of Haran-Ghera (1976) and Lieberman et al (1977) obtained by detection tests in vivo, where it was found that the bone marrow is the primary site of viral production and also the organ in which viruses are most frequently expressed.

All the facts just mentioned demonstrate that, as with irradiation in vitro, whole-body exposure to ionizing radiation activates endogenous MuLV; however, none of the results provides evidence for a direct role of the derepressed viruses in carcinogenesis; indeed the N- and X-tropic viruses are devoid of leukemogenic activity, and the carcinogenic effect of the B-tropic recombinants formed during the preneoplastic period cannot account for the incidence of radiation-induced thymic lymphosarcoma in C57BL or BALB/c mice (Jolicoeur et al, 1978; Declève et al, 1979).

With respect to osteosarcoma, no MuSV has been detected at early stages of the disease. Experiments conceived by Ihle et al (1976b) and Ihle (1977), with the specific purpose of assessing the relationship between viral activation, development of an immune response against virion antigens, and leukemogenesis, are especially relevant to the present problem. In the first place it was found that an exposure to 4×175 rads of x-rays enhanced the rate of appearance of the antibody against MuLV, but did not affect the peak antibody titer. In addition, mice developing high antibody titers had the same probability of becoming leukemic as those which did not show an immune response. This lack of correlation between the development of an immune reaction to the virus and the occurrence of leukemia was further confirmed by the fact that factors which reduced the incidence of thymomas did not preclude antibody production.

The preceding findings support the following conclusions: 1) proviruses are derepressed by irradiation in vivo, 2) virus activation results in the development of an immune response directed against viral proteins, 3) neither viral expression nor antibody production actually correlate with carcinogenesis, and 4) the endogenous viruses and the B recombinants isolated so far during the latency period are unlikely to be the agents actually responsible for radiation carcinogenesis. It must also be emphasized that radiation-induced leukemia occurs in mouse strains that express only xenotropic viruses. (Arnstein et al, 1976; Ihle, 1977; Harvey et al, 1979) and therefore, are prevented from producing any leukemogenic virus by recombination with an ecotropic virus. Likewise, Mayer and Dorsh-Häsler (1982) have demonstrated that infection by endogenous ecotropic or dualtropic MuLV is not a requirement for the development of radioleukemia. Finally, Holmes et al (1981) did not detect any MuLV in CBA mice subjected to a dose of radiation that induced a high frequency of leukemia.

Activation of MuMTV

Unlike MuLV, MuMTV was not detectably expressed in normal mammary glands, or in the liver or spleen of non–tumor-bearing BALB/c mice given 200 rads of x-radiation (Michalides et al, 1979). However, this radiation dose is well below that used to activate MuLV in vitro or in vivo.

EXPRESSION OF RETROVIRUSES IN RADIATION-INDUCED TUMORS

Although the absence of any correlation between viral expression and tumor development is noteworthy, it should not be interpreted as definite proof that MuLV are not involved in radiation carcinogenesis. Further comprehension of the role of viruses requires an accurate characterization of the viruses associated with the different types of tumors and in-depth analysis of the relationships between viral and cellular genomes.

Radiation-Induced Lymphomas

Several studies were carried out on radiation-induced lymphomas between 1976 and 1980 (Table 2). Although various techniques were applied in such studies to detect and characterize viruses, all the results were consistent with the following conclusions: 1) very few tumors produce detectable amounts of ecotropic B-tropic recombinant viruses; 2) N-tropic viruses are less frequently expressed at the stage of overt leukemia than during the preceding preneoplastic period; and 3) xenotropic viruses are regularly detected. It must be noted that only xenotropic viruses were found in lymphomas of C57B, NIH and NZB mice, which do not express ecotropic viruses. Most of the B-tropic viruses so far characterized were recombinants with regard to p30 and p12 (Rassart et al, 1983); besides these *gag* recombinants, some *env* recombinants were described in radiation-induced leukemias by Dorsch-Häsler and Mayer (1983) in RF mice and by Boccara et al (1983) in mice of the BALB/c strain. Special attention was also paid to the possible presence of specific viruses, such as RadLV/VL3 or MCF[S] (Mayer and Duran-Reynals, 1981), which are causative agents of thymic

TABLE 2. Expression of Retroviruses in Radiation-Induced Leukemia

Mouse strain	Type of virus expressed				Reference
	N	B	X	MCF	
C57L	—	—	++	NT[a]	Arnstein et al, 1976
C57BL/6	±	+	++	NT	Ihle et al, 1976a
C57BL/Ka	+	++	++	NT	Lieberman et al, 1976, 1977
C57BL/6	+	+	++	NT	Hass, 1977
ICR/JCL	+	+	NT	NT	Yokoro et al, 1977
NIH	—	—	+	NT	Ihle, 1977
NZB	—	—	+	NT	Harvey et al, 1979
C57BL/Ka	—	++	—	—	Sankar-Mistry and Jolicoeur, 1980
BALB/c	±	++	±	—	Ellis et al, 1980b

[a] NT , not tested

lymphosarcomas. The first can be easily recognized by its unique gp71 (Declève et al, 1978), but attempts to detect it in C57BL/Ka radiation-induced thymomas have been generally unsuccessful. Similarly, no MCF^S has been detected in C57BL or BALB/c thymomas (Table 2), nor was it found in B-cell lymphomas induced by radiation in thymectomized AKR mice (Legrand et al, 1981; Guillemain, unpublished observation); this last result is probably related to the low level of xenotrophic virus expression commonly encountered in thymus-deprived AKR mice (Bedigian et al, 1979).

Finally, it must be recalled that the DNA of MuLV-induced lymphoma cells grown in vitro usually contains a new proviral insert whose localization is specific to the tumor. This characteristic feature has not been detected in C57BL/6 primary radiation-induced thymomas (Janowski et al, 1982), a finding confirmed by Jolicoeur et al (1983), who demonstrated that additional ecotropic recombinant proviruses were inserted at specific sites only in established cell lines or in secondary tumors passaged in vitro.

Radiation-Induced Osteosarcoma

It is well documented that MuLV are expressed in osteosarcomas induced by bone-seeking isotopes (Erfle et al, 1980a). So far, the only evidence that bone tumors release MuSV in addition to MuLV stem from the isolation of FBR-MuSV by Lee et al (1979) and of Os-2 virus by Erfle et al (1979). Both viruses reproduce the original type of osteosarcoma when injected into newborn recipients. This specificity suggests that these MuSV might be the etiologic agents of radiogenic bone sarcomas.

Radiation-Induced Mammary Tumors

Several mouse strains deprived of exogenous milk-born virus are sensitive to the induction of mammary tumor by radiation, and they have been used to assess a possible correlation between MuMTV activation and the incidence of mammary cancer. Molecular hybridization between MuMTV-RNA and viral cDNA, or the synthesis of antibodies directed against viral proteins (p27, gp52) have been used to assess the cellular level of viral expression and the cellular content of viral proteins (Michalides et al, 1979, 1981). In irradiated BALB/c mice, these methods revealed a significant increase of MuMTV expression but did not indicate whether or not this rise had any direct role in mammary carcinogenesis. In addition, it was found that the presence of extra MuMTV proviruses was not required for the development of non-virally induced mammary tumors, as was the case for milk-born mammary tumors.

EXPRESSION OF ONCOGENES IN RADIATION-INDUCED TUMORS

As previously indicated, the genome in normal cells contains genes that exhibit transforming activity when properly activated. More than 20 such genes (protooncogenes) have been identified, either as cellular homologues (c-onc) of the transforming genes of retroviruses (v-onc) or by their biologic properties in transfection assays (Land et al, 1983; Cooper and Lane, 1984; Marshall and

Rigby, 1984). Damage to cellular DNA, such as that induced by radiation, may result in mutations in protooncogenes or in the insertion of retroviral promoters and/or enhancers in aberrant positions in the host genome, thus allowing for the expression of transforming activity. This hypothesis was first tested on radiation-transformed C3HT10½ cells (Kirschmeier et al, 1982) but was not confirmed. Similarily, Boccara et al (1983) did not find any evidence for linkage of viral long terminal repeat-derived (U5) sequences to information of host origin in radiation-induced leukemia. However, the detection of c-onc was reported by Michiels et al (1984), who demonstrated that FBR-MuSV encodes a fos-derived oncogene (the exact relationship between FBR and radiation-induced osteosarcomas remains uncertain), and by Guerrero et al (1984), who detected an activated K-c-*ras* in radioleukemias, whereas chemically induced leukemias expressed N-c-*ras*.

DISCUSSION AND CONCLUSIONS

Data provide evidence that ionizing radiation activates endogenous retroviruses, especially MuLV. Studies in vitro suggest that radiation-induced alterations of cellular DNA are instrumental in releasing proviruses from the control of their repressors (Otten et al, 1976). A similar mechanism also may apply to the initial step of viral induction in vivo. There is a second line of evidence, however, pointing to lack of any correlation between tumor occurrence and expression of endogenous or recombinant viruses; ie, a minority of radiation-induced cancers expresses oncogenic viruses, and those viruses that are most commonly isolated are unlikely to be the causative agents of the tumors (Ihle et al, 1976a; Ellis et al, 1980b; Tress et al, 1982). In addition, new inserts of proviral genome into cellular DNA, which are a characteristic feature of virally induced tumors, are not detected in the cellular DNA of primary radiocancers (Janowski et al, 1982; Michalides et al, 1981). Thus, experimental findings do not validate the simple model originally hypothesized: viral activation, formation of oncogenic recombinant viruses, reinfection, and transformation of cells at early stages of differentiation.

It must be kept in mind that the role originally attributed to retroviruses in radiation carcinogenesis had the purpose of accounting for the discovery of RadLV and explaining the malignant transformation of normal thymus tissue grafted into thymectomized irradiated recipients (Kaplan and Brown, 1954). The discovery of other oncogenic viruses, in addition to RadLV, in radiocancers, has stimulated and justified research along this line. However, it must be stressed that indirect carcinogenic effects are not uncommon in radiobiology, and that most if not all radiation-induced endocrine tumors arise from indirect mechanisms involving primarily target cell stimulation by hormonal imbalance. It has been suggested that a similar mechanism, involving the increased production of thymic "hormones," might apply to radioleukemogenesis. In view of experimental findings indicating that radiation-induced leukemias frequently express *env* protein with xenotropic properties (Fishinger et al, 1981; Tress et al, 1982), it is attractive to postulate that these *env* gene products might provide a blastogenic stimulus to lymphoid cell clones bearing appropriate receptors (McGrath et al, 1978).

It also has been suggested that radiation-induced mutation or genetic transposition of promoter or/and enhancer sequences might result in the activation of protooncogenes (Klein, 1981). There is limited experimental evidence to support this attractive hypothesis so far. It should be kept in mind, however, that radiation may activate the transcription of cellular genes that are not necessarily recognized as oncogenes but may nevertheless play an important role in the multistep process of carcinogenesis.

REFERENCES

Arnstein P, Riggs JL, Oshiro LS, Huebner RJ, Lenette EH (1976) Production of lymphoma and associated xenotropic type C virus in C57L mice by whole-body irradiation. J Natl Cancer Inst 57:1085–1090.

Bedigian MG, Shultz LD, Meier H (1979) Expression of endogenous murine leukemia viruses in AKR/J streaker mice. Nature 279:434–436.

Boccara M, Souyri M, Magarian C, Stavnezer E, Fleissner E (1983) Evidence for a new form of retroviral env transcript in leukemic and normal mouse lymphoid cells. J Virol 48:102–109.

Cooper GM, Lane MA (1984) Cellular transforming genes and oncogenesis. Biochem Biophys Acta 738:9–20

Decleve A, Lieberman M, Boniver J, Kaplan HS (1979) In vivo infectivity of the fibrotropic C-type isolates from' C57BL/Ka mice. Cancer Res 39:4322–4329.

Decleve A, Lieberman M, Ihle JN, Rosenthal PN, Lung ML, Kaplan HS (1978) Physicochemical, biological and serological properties of a leukemogenic virus isolated from cultured RadLV-induced lymphomas of C57BL/Ka mice. Virology 90:23–35.

Decleve A, Niwa O, Gelman E, Kaplan HS (1976) Radiation activation of endogenous leukemia viruses in cell culture: Acute x-ray irradiation. In: Yuhas JW, Tennant RW, Regan JD (eds.), Biology of radiation carcinogenesis. New York: Raven Press, pp 217–225.

Dorsch-Hasler K, Mayer A (1983) Ecotropic MuLV expression in radiation-induced lymphomas of the RF, BALB/c and (BALB/c × RF)F1 mouse strains. Intl J Cancer 32:465–469.

Ellis RW, Hopkins N, Fleissner E (1980a) Biochemical analysis of murine leukemia viruses isolated from radiation-induced leukemias of strain BALB/c. J Virol 33:661–670.

Ellis RW, Stockert E, Fleissner E (1980b) Association of endogenous retroviruses with radiation-induced leukemias of BALB/c mice. J Virol 33:652–660.

Erfle V, Hehlmann R, Schetters H, Meier A, Luz A (1980a) Time course of C-type retrovirus expression in mice submitted to osteosarcomagenic doses of 224-radium. Intl J Cancer 26:107–113.

Erfle V, Hehlmann R, Schetters H, Schmidt J, Luz A (1980b) Time course studies of retrovirus expression in radiation-induced tumors. In: Bachman PA (ed.), Leukaemias, lymphomas and papillomas: Comparative aspects. London: Taylor and Francis, pp 195–204.

Erfle V, Schulte-Overberg S, Marquart KH, Adler ID, Luz A (1979) Establishment and characterization of C-type virus producing cell lines from radiation-induced murine osteosarcomas. J Cancer Res Clin Oncol 94:149–162.

Finkel MP, Reilly CA (1973) Observations suggesting the viral etiology of radiation-induced tumors, particularly osteogenic sarcomas. In: Sanders CL, Brusch RM, Ballon JE, Mahlum DD (eds.), Radionuclide carcinogenesis. US Atomic Energy Commission, Oak Ridge, TN: pp 278–288.

Fishinger PJ, Thiel HJ, Ihle JN, Lee JC, Elder JH (1981) Detection of a recombinant murine leukemia virus-related glycoprotein on virus-negative thymoma cells. Proc Natl Acad Sci USA 78:1920–1924.

Goldfeder A (1972) Electron microscopy study of neoplasms induced by urethan and X-rays in X/Gf mice. Cancer Res 32:2778–2782.

Gross L (1951) "Spontaneous" leukemia developing in C3H mice following inoculation in infancy, with AK leukemic extracts or AK embryos. Proc Soc Exp Biol Med 76:27–32.

Gross L (1958) Attempt to recover a filterable agent from x-ray induced leukemia. Acta Haematol 19:353–361.

Gross L (1970) Oncogenic viruses, 2nd Edition. Oxford: Pergamon Press.

Guerreo I, Calzada P, Mayer A, Pellicer A (1984) A molecular approach to leukemogenesis: Mouse lymphomas contain an activated c-ras oncogene. Proc Natl Acad Sci USA 81:202–205.

Haas M (1977) Transient virus expression during murine leukemia induction by x-irradiation. J Natl Cancer Inst 58:251–257.

Haran-Ghera N (1966) Leukemogenic activity of centrifugates from irradiated mouse thymus and bone marrow. Intl J Cancer 1:81–87.

Haran-Ghera N (1976) Pathways in murine radiation leukemogenesis-coleukemogenesis. In: Yuhas JM, Tennant RW, Regen JD (eds.), Biology of radiation carcinogenesis. New York: Raven Press, pp 245–260.

Haran-Ghera N, Peled A (1967) The mechanism of radiation action in leukaemogenesis. Isolation of a leukaemogenic filtrable agent from tissues of irradiated and normal C57BL mice. Br J Cancer 21:730–738.

Harvey JJ, Tuffrey M, Holmes HC, East J (1979) Absence of ecotropic or recombinant murine leukemia virus in preleukemic and leukaemic x-irradiated NZB mice. Intl J Cancer 24:373–376.

Hilgers J, Bentvelzen P (1978) Interaction between viral and genetic factors in murine mammary cancer. In: Klein G, Weinhouse S (eds.), Advances in Cancer Research Vol. 26. New York: Academic Press, pp 143–195.

Holmes HC, Tuffrey M, Wilson L, Barnes RD (1981) Absence of activated murine leukaemia virus in x-irradiated CBA/H-T6Cr mice. J Gen Virol 53:477–481.

Ihle JN (1977) Serological and biochemical characterization of ecotropic MuLV expression in radiation induced leukemia of mice. In: Duplan JF (ed.), Radiation-induced leukemogenesis and related viruses. Amsterdam: Elsevier/North-Holland Biomedical Press, pp 265–276.

Ihle JN, Joseph DR, Pazmino NH (1976a) Radiation leukemia in C57BL/6 mice. II. Lack of ecotropic virus expression in the majority of lymphomas. J Exp Med 144:1406–1423.

Ihle JN, McEwan R, Bengali K (1976b) Radiation leukemia in C57BL/6 mice. I. Lack of serological evidence for the role of endogenous ecotropic viruses in pathogenesis. J Exp Med 144:1391–1405.

Janowski M, Boniver J, Maisin JR (1982) Common proviral integration sites in C57BL mouse lymphomas induced by radiation leukemia virus and absence of novel virus-related sequences in radiogenic lymphoma DNA. Leukemia Res 6:285–297.

Jolicoeur P, Rassart E, Sankar-Mistry P (1983) Strong selection for cells containing new ecotropic recombinant MuLV provirus after propagation of C57BL/6 radiation-induced thymoma cells in vitro or in vivo. Molec Cell Biol 3:1675–1679.

Jolicoeur P, Rosenberg N, Cotellessa A, Baltimore D (1978) Leukemogenicity of clonal isolates of murine leukemia viruses. J Natl Cancer Inst 60:1473–1476.

Kaplan HS (1978) Review: Etiology of lymphomas and leukemias: Role of C type RNA viruses. Leukemia Res 2:253–271.

Kaplan HS, Brown MB (1954) Development of lymphoid tumors in non irradiated thymic graft in thymectomized irradiated mice. Science 119:439–440.

Kaplan HS, Brown MB (1957) Radiation injury and regeneration in lymphoid tissues. In: Rebuck JW, Bethell FH, Monto RW (eds.), The leukemias: Etiology, pathophysiology and treatment. New York: Academic Press, pp 163–175.

Kaplan HS, Brown MB, Paull J (1953) Influence of bone marrow injection on involution and neoplasia of mouse thymus after systemic irradiation. J Natl Cancer Inst 14:303–316.

Kirschmeier P, Gattoni-Celli S, Dina D, Weinstein IB (1982) Carcinogen and radiation transformed C3H 10T½ cells contain RNAs homologous to the long terminal repeat sequence of murine leukemia virus. Proc Natl Acad Sci USA 79:2773–2777.

Klein G (1981) The role of gene dosage and genetic transpositions in carcinogenesis. Nature 294:313–318.

Land H, Parada LF, Weinberg A (1983) Cellular oncogenes and multistep carcinogenesis. Science 222:771–778.

Latarjet R (1951) Induction, par les rayons X, de la production d'un bactériophage chez B megatherium lysogéne. Ann Inst Pasteur 81:389–393.

Lee CK, Chan EW, Reilly CA, Jr., Pahnke VA, Rockus G, Finkel MP (1979) In vitro properties of FBR murine osteosarcoma virus. Proc Soc Exp Biol Med 162:214–220.

Legrand E, Daculsi R, Bach JP, Duplan JF (1981) Influence of serum thymic factor (FTS) on radiation-induced leukaemogenesis in thymectomized AKR mice. Intl J Cancer 28:59–64.

Lieberman M, Kaplan HS (1959) Leukemogenic activity from radiation-induced lymphoid tumors of mice. Science 130:387–388.

Lieberman M, Kaplan HS, Decleve A (1976) Anomalous viral expression in radiogenic lymphomas of C57BL/Ka mice. In: Yuhas JM, Tennant RW, Regan JD (eds.), Biology of radiation carcinogenesis. New York: Raven Press, pp 237–244.

Lieberman M, Decleve A, Gelmann EP, Kaplan HS (1977) Biological and serological characterization of the C-type RNA viruses isolated from the C57BL/Ka strain of mice. II. Induction and propagation of the isolates. In: Duplan JF (ed.), Radiation-induced leukemogenesis and related viruses. Amsterdam: Elsevier/North Holland Biomedical Press, pp 231–246.

Lwoff A (1953) Lysogeny. Bacteriol Rev 17:269–337.

Lwoff A, Siminovitch L, Kjeldgaard N (1950) Induction de la production de bacteriophages chez une bactérie lysogène. Ann Inst Pasteur 79:815–859.

McGrath MS, Decleve A, Lieberman M, Kaplan HS, Weissman IL (1978) Specificity of cell surface virus receptors on radiation leukemia virus and radiation-induced thymic lymphosarcomas. J Virol 28:819–827.

Marcus SL, Smith SW, Sarkar NH (1981) Quantitation of murine mammary tumor virus-related RNA in mammary tissue of low- and high-mammary-tumor-incidence mouse strains. J Virol 40:87–95.

Marshall CJ, Rigby PW (1984) Viral and cellular genes involved in oncogenesis. Cancer Surv 3:183–214.

Mayer A, Dorsch-Hasler K (1982) Endogenous MuLV infection does not contribute to onset of radiation- or carcinogen-induced murine thymoma. Nature 295:253–255.

Mayer A, Duran-Reynals ML (1981) Xenotropic type-C virus expression in murine thymomas induced by radiation or 3-methylcholantrene. Virology 114:580–584.

Michalides R, Van Deemter L, Nusse R, Hageman P (1979) Induction of mouse mammary tumor virus DNA in mammary tumors of BALB/c mice treated with urethane, x-irradiation, and hormones. J Virol 31:63–72.

Michalides R, Wagenaar E, Groner B, Hynes NE (1981) Mammary tumor virus proviral DNA in normal murine tissue and non-virally induced mammary tumors. J Virol 39:367–376.

Michiels L, Maisin JR, Pedersen FS, Merregaert J (1984) Characterization of the FBR-murine osteosarcoma virus complex: FBR-MuSV encodes a fos-derived oncogene. Intl J Cancer 33:511–517.

Niwa O, Sugahara T (1979) Radiation induction of endogenous type C virus from mouse cells transformed in vitro by murine sarcoma virus. J Natl Cancer Inst 62:329–335.

Otten JA, Quarles JM, Tennant RW (1976) Cell devision requirement for activation of murine leukemia virus in cell culture by irradiation. Virology 70:80–87.

Rassart E, Sankar-Mistry P, Lemay G, Des Roseillers L, Jolicoeur P (1983) New class of leukemogenic ecotropic recombinant murine leukemia virus isolated from radiation-induced thymomas of C57BL/6 mice. J Virol 45:565–575.

Reilly CA, Finkel MP (1971) Evidence of FBJ virus antigen in [90]SR-induced osteosarcomas. Radiat Res 47:252–253.

Rowe WP, Hartley JW, Lander MR, Pugh WE, Teich N (1971) Non-infectious AKR mouse embryos cell lines in which each cell has the capacity to be activated to produce infectious murine leukemia virus. Virology 46:866–876.

Sankar-Mistry P, Jolicoeur P (1980) Frequent isolation of ecotropic murine leukemia virus after x-ray irradiation of C57BL/6 mice and establishment of producer lymphoid cell lines from radiation-induced lymphomas. J Virol 35:270–275.

Stephenson JR (1980) Type C virus structural and transformation-specific proteins. In: Stephenson JR (ed.), Molecular biology of RNA tumor viruses. New York: Academic Press, pp 245–297.

Stockert E, Old LJ (1977) Preleukemic expression of TL antigens in x-irradiated C57BL/6 mice. J Exp Med 146:271–276.

Tennant RW, Rascati RJ, Lavelle GC (1977) Mechanisms in endogenous leukemia virus induction by radiation and chemicals. In: Duplan JF (ed.), Radiation-induced leukemogenesis and related viruses. Amsterdam: Elsevier/North Holland Biomedical Press, pp 179–188.

Timmermans A, Bentvelzen P, Hageman PC, Calafat J (1969) Activation of a mammary tumor virus in 020 strain mice by x-irradiation and urethane. J Gen Virol 4:619–621.

Tress E, Pierotti M, DeLeo AB, O'Donnel PV, Fleissner E (1982) Endogenous murine leukemia virus-encoded proteins in radiation leukemias of BALB/c mice. Virology 117:207–218.

Yokoro K, Nagao K, Ito T, Kawamura Y, Imamura N (1977) A comparative study of radiation, chemical and viral leukemogenesis in mice and rats. In: Duplan JF (ed.), Radiation-induced leukemogenesis and related viruses. Amsterdam: Elsevier/North Holland Biomedical Press, pp 133–148.

EFFECTS OF RADIATION ON THE REPRODUCTIVE CAPACITY AND PROLIFERATION OF CELLS IN RELATION TO CARCINOGENESIS

G.W. BARENDSEN, Ph.D.

The initiation and expression of malignant properties in cells, induced by exposure to ionizing radiation, is a multistep process that depends on a variety of factors. Some of the mechanisms involved in early stages of carcinogenesis can be studied in vitro for various types of cells. Analysis and interpretation of the dose–effect relations for carcinogenesis can benefit from studies on cellular effects, because quantitative assays are available for various end-points, including reproductive death, cell proliferative capacity, and cell transformation.

Some of the processes that constitute the sequence of events of tumor development, and their modification by various agents and conditions, depend not only on responses of single cells, but also on interaction of cells in tissues and on the influence of host factors. The development of tumors may be influenced by immunologic and hormonal factors, as well as by an increase in the rate of cell proliferation caused by tissue damage or cell depletion. It is evident that the influence of these factors will depend on the type of tissue involved. This chapter discusses only some general features of the induction of various types of damage in cultured cells, and their consequences for tumor development.

COMPARISON OF DOSE–RESPONSE RELATIONSHIPS FOR CELL REPRODUCTIVE DEATH, CHROMOSOME ABERRATIONS, MORPHOLOGIC TRANSFORMATION, AND MUTATIONS

General Aspects of Dose–Effect Relations for Cellular Responses to Ionizing Radiation

Ionizing radiation can induce a variety of changes in cells and tissues. Due to the large local energy transfers associated with the discrete events involved in the passage of an ionizing particle through a critical structure or macromole-

From the Radiobiological Institute TNO, Rijswijk, and Laboratory for Radiobiology, Amsterdam, The Netherlands.

cule in a cell, many types of primary physical and chemical changes can be produced. Some of these changes are relatively minor, and most of these are repaired without further consequences. Other changes may result in reproductive death, chromosome aberrations, or cell transformation. The exact nature of the lesions in cells, which are induced as primary biophysical and biochemical changes and which, through a series of steps, lead to observable biological effects, is not yet fully known. It is likely, however, that macromolecular DNA is the major critical target for most of the important cellular effects.

Several types of lesions have been demonstrated in the DNA of irradiated cells, including single-strand breaks, double-strand breaks, base damage, and cross-linking of DNA to DNA or to other molecules. All of these changes might cause observable cellular effects, but the effectiveness per unit dose with which they are induced is likely to depend on the type of DNA lesion and on the region of DNA involved. It is well established that almost all of the single-strand breaks and a large majority of the double-strand breaks of DNA in mammalian cells are repaired. The small minority of lesions that actually lead to damage expressed as reproductive death or chromosomal changes might be more complex and severe at the macromolecular level than simple DNA breaks (Barendsen, 1979). These effective lesions might involve a composite interaction of more than one double-strand DNA break, as suggested on the basis of studies with high linear energy transfer (LET) radiations, which are generally more effective in causing biological effects than are x-rays (Barendsen, 1979).

If primary mechanisms of the induction of damage at the molecular level are similar for different cellular responses, then dose–effect relationships can be expected to exhibit some common characteristics. On the other hand, if primary mechanisms differ, the differences might also be expressed in the dependence of the endpoint on dose, radiation quality, and dose-modifying factors. It is of interest, therefore, to compare the dependence of the effectiveness for induction of different lesions on factors that can be varied in experimental systems; namely, the radiation quality, dose fractionation, dose rate, and cell culture conditions.

The analysis of dose–effect data for different endpoints can be based on two general assumptions concerning biophysical mechanisms:

1. Notwithstanding the presumably complex nature of the induction of cellular damage by ionizing radiation, the local energy transfers involved in the transversal of a single charged particle through a cell are large enough to cause observable biological effects. If a single track can cause sufficient primary damage for the induction of a given type of cellular effect, then the fraction of cells showing a response is expected to increase as a linear function of the dose. This applies to low-LET radiations, but even more to high-LET radiations.

2. In addition to a linear dependence of the frequency of effective lesions on the radiation dose, further damage may be caused by the interaction of sublesions resulting from different particles passing through the same cell. This latter contribution is generally observed to become more important with increasing dose, such that the frequency of many types of cellular effect can be described to a first approximation by

$$F(D) = a_1 D + a_2 D^2 \tag{1}$$

in which a_1 and a_2 are constants with values depending on the effect studied, on the cell type investigated, and on the conditions of exposure to a dose (D) (Barendsen, 1979).

It is of interest to compare the values of a_1, a_2, and their ratio $a_1 : a_2$ for cell lines irradiated with different radiations and assayed for several endpoints. Unfortunately, adequate data are not available in which all endpoints have been assayed for a given cell type irradiated with a wide range of dose, radiation quality, etc. Therefore, a comparison of dose–effect relationships must be based on published data for several types of cells in culture treated with different radiations and assayed with respect to at least two types of effects. In Figure 1 and Table 1, results are presented, derived from dose–effect relationships for the induction of reproductive death, chromosome aberrations, morphologic transformation, and mutations in cultured mammalian cells, as a function of the radiation dose. The data on lethal lesions have been derived from cell survival curves. These curves represent, as a function of the dose, the fraction of cells that have escaped lethal injury. Assuming that these lethal lesions are distributed at random among cells in a population, survival curves can be represented to a first approximation by

$$S(D)/S(O) = \exp - (a_1 D + a_2 D^2) \tag{2}$$

in which a_1 and a_2 have to a first approximation the same meaning as in **(1)** (Barendsen, 1979; Gilbert et al, 1980). A value of $F(D) = 2.3$ corresponds to a fraction surviving cells of $S(D)/S(O) = 0.1$, and a value $F(D) = 4.6$ corresponds to a fraction of surviving cells equal to 0.01.

The data of Figure 1 were selected because of the availability of results for different endpoints in the cell lines assayed after treatment with high-LET radiations, fast neutrons, α-particles, and low-LET radiations, respectively. Data on the comparative effectiveness of high-LET radiations and low-LET radiations are of great importance, because with high-LET radiations evaluation of the linear term of the dose–effect relationship is not complicated by as large a contribution from the quadratic dose term in **(1)** and **(2)** (Barendsen, 1979).

Comparison of the different dose–effect relations for lethal lesions in Figure 1A shows that various types of cells have different sensitivities to low-LET radiation, as well as to high-LET radiation. Values of the various parameters, which can be derived from these curves, are presented in Table 1. Values of a_1 for reproductive death in different types of mammalian cells have been shown to range from about 10^{-1} to 1 Gy^{-1} in the case of photons and between about 1 and 3 Gy^{-1} in the case of the most effective fast neutrons (i.e., those with mean energies in the range of 0.4–1.0 MeV) (Barendsen, 1979). Values of a_2 also vary considerably, with a range of about $10^{-2}–10^{-1}Gy^{-2}$, while a_1/a_2 values vary somewhat less, with a range of 2–10 Gy (Barendsen, 1982).

Relative to the incidence of reproductive death of the cell, the chromosome aberrations most commonly scored in mammalian cells (i.e., dicentrics and centric rings) are induced with a frequency that is lower by a factor ranging

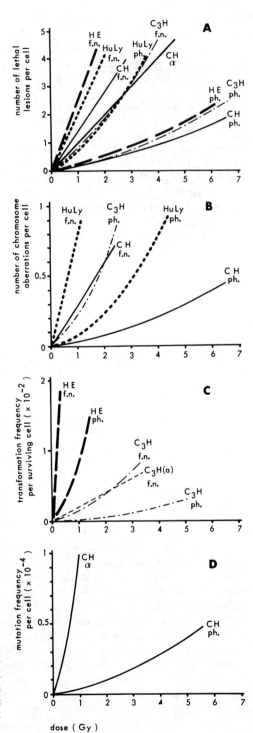

FIGURE 1. Curves showing relationship between the frequency of induction of various types of changes in cultured cells as a function of the radiation dose. (A) Cell lethality, curves derived from survival curves; (B) Chromosome aberrations; (C) cell morphologic transformation; (D) cell mutation, resistance to 6 thioguanine.

Abbreviations: HE, hamster embryo; HuLy, human lymphocytes; CH, Chinese hamster V-79 line; C3H, mouse C3H 10T½ line; fn, fission neutrons, neutrons with mean energies between 0.5 and 1 MeV; ph, photons, x-rays, or gamma rays; α, α-particles of 5–10 MeV energy. (See Table 1 for source notes.)

from 2 to about 10 (Figure 1B and Table 1). It is evident that dicentrics and centric rings constitute only a proportion of all aberration types. Deletions are also potentially lethal, but uncertainty exists about the size of fragments that must be lost to cause lethality. The ratio of dicentrics to deletions varies among different cell types, probably depending on chromosome arm numbers, the location of centromeres, and DNA packing density in the nucleus. Notwithstanding these uncertainties, results of many types of experiments suggest that radiation-induced reproductive death of the cell is due mainly to chromosome structural abnormalities, although not all of these aberrations are readily detectable (Dewey et al, 1971; Nagasawa and Little, 1981; Lloyd and Purrot, 1976).

Data on the morphologic transformation of cells in culture by different types of radiation are available for only two cell types. The curves shown in Figure 1C can be described by the corresponding parameters given in Table 1. The values of a_1 show that this transformation is much less frequently induced than reproductive death or chromosome structural abnormalities (i.e., by a factor of about 50 less for hamster embryo cells and by a factor of about 10^3 less for C3H 10T$\frac{1}{2}$ cells).

The results on mutations, although scarce for high-LET radiations, yield a_1 values, which are a factor 10^4–10^5 smaller than for reproductive death. In the UNSCEAR report (1982), an average value of 4×10^{-5} mutations per lethal event is mentioned, which is similar to the value that can be deduced from the data in Table 1. It can be concluded that specific mutations are induced by a factor of 30–1000 less frequently per unit dose than is cell morphologic transformation.

With respect to the ratio $a_1:a_2$, which represents the dose at which the quadratic term and the linear term contribute equally to the total frequency, no general differences can be deduced between the different types of effect. The values for chromosome aberrations, mutation, and cell transformation are on the average somewhat lower, as compared with $a_1:a_2$ values for reproductive death, but experiments with more cell lines would be required to establish a significant difference.

Implications of Different Yields of Various Cellular Effects for Mechanisms of Induction

Differences among various cellular effects in frequencies per unit dose can be used to derive hypotheses concerning the mechanisms involved. Cell reproductive death and chromosome aberrations presumably can be induced as a result of damage to any one of the chromosomes. Chromosome breaks, leading to lethality of cells and to dicentrics or deletions of chromosomes, may occur at many sites on any chromosome. The probability of breaks may not be uniform along chromosomes, but this is difficult to establish because not all aberrations are observable with the techniques presently available.

Compared with lethal events and chromosome aberrations, specific mutations are less frequently induced by radiation by a factor of 10^4–10^5. This lower frequency can be attributed to the fact that an aberration at a specific site on only one chromosome is presumably required for a given mutagenic event. For

TABLE 1. Parameters of Dose–Effect Relations for Induction of Lethal Lesions, Chromosome Aberrations, Transformation, and Mutations in Mammalian Cells by Different Types of Ionizing Radiation

Frequency $F = a_1D + a_2D$ [a]

Lethal lesions

Cell type	a_1 (Gy^{-1}) ($\times10^{-1}$)	a_2 (Gy^{-2}) ($\times10^{-2}$)	a_1/a_2 (Gy)	Ref.
CH-V79				
photons[c]	1.5	2	7	Cox et al (1977), Zoetelief and Barendsen (1983)
α-particle	10	1	10	Cox et al (1977)
neutrons	14	—	—	Zoetelief and Barendsen (1983)
C3H 10T$\frac{1}{2}$				
photons	1.4	3.6	4	Han and Elkind (1979), Hall et al (1982), Barendsen and Gaiser
neutrons	7	1.1	6	Han and Elkind (1979), Hill et al (1982)

Chromosome aberrations [b]

Cell type	a_1 (Gy^{-1}) ($\times10^{-1}$)	a_2 (Gy^{-2}) ($\times10^{-2}$)	a_1/a_2 (Gy)	Ref.
CH-V79				
photons	0.3	0.6	5	Zoetelief and Barendsen (1983)
neutrons	3	—	—	Zoetelief and Barendsen (1983)
C3H 10T$\frac{1}{2}$				
photons	2	7	3	Nagasawa and Little (1981)

System	Radiation				Reference
human lymphoma	photons	6	15	4	Barendsen (1979)
	neutrons	20	—	—	Barendsen (1979)
human lymphoma	photons	0.4	4	1.0	Lloyd (1976)
	neutrons	8	—	—	Lloyd (1976)
hamster embryo	photons	2	3	7	Hall et al (1982)
	neutrons	25	—	—	Hall et al (1982)
transformation C3H 10T½	photons	0.8	1	0.8	Han and Elkind (1979), Hall et al (1982)
	neutrons	20	—	—	Hill et al (1982)
		8	5	1.6	Han and Elkind (1979)
		6	—	—	Barendsen and Gaiser
mutations[d] Ch-V79	photons	3.5	0.9	4	Cox et al (1977)
	α-particles	60	40	1.5	Cox et al (1977)
hamster embryo	photons	40	40	1.0	Hall et al (1982)
	neutrons	500	—	—	Hall et al (1982)

[a] In case no data on neutrons were available, data on α-particles with LET values of 50 to 100 keV/μm in tissue have been analyzed.

[b] Dicentrics + centric rings for Chinese Hamster cells and Human Lymphocytes, deletions for C3H 10T½ cells.

[c] No distinction is made between X-rays and γ-rays, although differences up to a factor of 2 have been demonstrated for some effects at low doses.

[d] Resistance to 6 thioguanine (g-TG^{R}).

instance, thioguanine resistance in V79 Chinese hamster cells was found at least partly to be associated with structural changes at a specific site on the X chromosome (Cox et al, 1977).

Because cell transformation is more frequently induced by ionizing radiations by a factor of 30–1000 than mutations associated with damage at a specific point on a single chromosome, it may be inferred that many, if not all, chromosomes contain one or more sites with genes that, if damaged, deleted, or transposed to another site, may result in morphologic transformation. This conclusion appears to be in agreement with recent results of molecular biology studies on tumor induction, which indicate that changes occuring at one of 10–20 sites distributed on different chromosomes may be associated with activation of oncogenes and with different types of cancer (Tabin et al, 1982; Heisterkamp et al, 1982; Weinburg, 1982). The very large ratio of $30-10^3$ between the frequency of transformations and of specific mutations, however, suggests that a mechanism of a more general nature than depression or activation of a specific oncogene is involved in the transformation in vitro of cells by radiation, because it is unlikely that as many as 10^3 oncogenes are present in normal cells.

A hypothesis that can account for many features of the sequence of events in carcinogenesis may be based on the assumption that the primary chromosomal changes induced by radiation do not affect transformation genes or oncogenes directly, but that they occur at other sites or in other genes that are present at multiple sites on all chromosomes. The assumption can be made that these primary changes affect functions, which are necessarily performed by all chromosomes. For example, an important function that may be involved is the replication of chromosomes during DNA synthesis. Several genes presumably are present on each chromosome, which are responsible for the stability and order in the replication of DNA. If one of these genes is damaged, deleted, or changed in its expression, then during subsequent cell cycles an instability or fragility of chromosomes could develop which, as a second step, may result in transposition effects on the chromosome involved. In turn, these secondary steps could lead to the derepression or activation of oncogenes. In addition, further mutated clones may be produced at later stages in the development of tumors, due to the induced instability of the replication process. Such a fundamental instability of the DNA replication process induced by a primary change, causing secondary genomic rearrangements in subsequent cell generations, might also be responsible for the development of biological diversity in tumors of unicellular origin, as well as for the evolution and progression of tumors in later stages of their growth and for the development of metastatic characteristics.

This hypothesis of a primary type of chromosomal damage, which increases the probability of activation of oncogenes as a secondary step due to chromosomal fragility during replication, might also provide an interpretation of the observation that the expression of cell transformation can be modified during subsequent generations. The actual transformation process becomes more probable as a result of the initially induced fragility, but tumor development is not a necessary consequence of the primary change (Kennedy et al, 1981; Terasima et al, 1981; Little, 1981; Smith and Sager, 1982; Straus, 1981).

THE RELATIONSHIP BETWEEN TUMOR DEVELOPMENT AND CELL REPRODUCTIVE INTEGRITY

General Aspects of the Influence of Cell Reproductive Death on Tumor Yield

In addition to the differences and similarities between dose–effect relations for induction of cell lethality and transformation, and their implications for mechanisms of tumor induction, the influence of cell survival curves on the probability of tumor development are of interest. If a cell that is transformed by radiation is to develop into a tumor, it obviously must retain the capacity for unlimited proliferation. Thus, the frequency of tumors that actually develop after irradiation as a result of the transformation of normal cells depends on the probability of cell survival. As a consequence, the tumor yield as a function of the dose can be represented by

$$Y = (p_0 + p_1 D + p_2 D^2) \times \exp - (a_1 D + a_2 D^2) \tag{3}$$

in which p_0 is the incidence without radiation, $p_1 D$ and $p_2 D$ are the linear and quadratic terms for the malignant transformation process, and $a_1 D$ and $a_2 D$ are the linear and quadratic terms that determine induction of cell reproductive death. From this formula it can be deduced that the yield of tumors as a function of the dose has a complex shape with the general features illustrated in Figure 2. At low doses of low-LET radiation, where the influence of cell death is small, the yield increases linearly with the dose, whereas at somewhat larger doses the quadratic term may start to contribute significantly. The dose at which the term $p_2 D$ contributes a number of transformations equal to $p_1 D$ is given by $D = p_1/p_2$. The available data, illustrated in Table 1, indicate that for low-LET radiation, values of p_1/p_2 may vary over a range of 0.5–2 Gy. The value of p_1/p_2 depends on the radiation quality, mainly because of the increase in p_1 with LET (Hill et al, 1982; Han and Elkind, 1979).

The influence of cell reproductive death generally becomes significant only at doses in excess of a few grays of low-LET radiation. At a dose that depends on the actual values of a_1 and a_2 for induction of cell reproductive death, the yield of tumors will reach a maximum (Figure 2), and subsequently a decrease of the yield will be observed as cell killing becomes a dominant factor. For high LET radiations, only the parameters p_1 and a_1 are important, and the shape of the yield-versus-dose curve is less complicated (Figure 2). The general shape of the yield-versus-dose curve, first suggested by Gray (1965), has been subsequently analyzed by other investigators (Barendsen, 1978). The yield of tumors, as well as the values of the dose at which the maximum yield is obtained, depends on parameters of the cell survival curves. Some of the characteristics of survival curves will be discussed in more detail.

Characteristics of Mammalian Cell Survival Curves

Differences in Sensitivity to Single Doses of Radiation. Many reports in the literature demonstrate that bone marrow stem cells exhibit a higher sensitivity to x-rays than intestinal crypt stem cells or skin stem cells (Barendsen, 1982). For these different types of stem cells, the survival curves mainly represent the

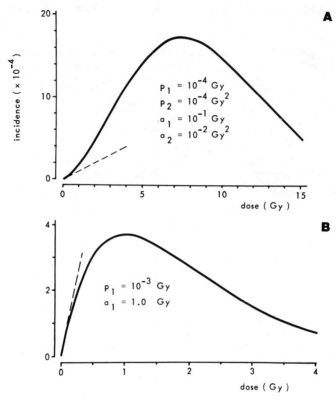

FIGURE 2. Examples of incidence-versus-dose relationships for tumors induced by low-LET radiation and high-LET radiation. Parameters have been chosen to demonstrate the importance of linear and quadratic terms in the induction of transformation and cell lethality. Broken lines represent initial slopes determined by the parameter p_1. (A) low-LET radiation $I = (P_1D + P_2D^2) \cdot \exp - (a_1D + a_2D^2)$ (B) high-LET radiation, $I = P_1D \cdot \exp - a_1D$.

sensitivity of non-cycling cells, and the differences cannot be attributed to different distributions of cells in the replication cycle, the influence of hypoxia, or to other conditions. Furthermore, the three cell types are present in the same animal, contain the same amount of DNA distributed over the same number of chromosomes and with the same genetic information. Consequently, for lack of better insight, the observed differences in survival curves can only be ascribed to differences in intrinsic radiosensivity. Hence, it is evident that, in addition to differences in susceptibility to malignant transformation, differences in the survival curves of normal cells in different tissues may cause large variations in the yield of tumors as a function of dose.

As mentioned earlier, the survival curves, which are commonly presented as fractions of clonogenic cells on a logarithmic scale as a function of the dose on a linear scale, actually show the fractions of cells that have escaped reproductive death as a function of the dose. Many survival curves for low-LET radiations can be described adequately by (2) in the dose region, where the fraction of surviving cells lies between 1 and 0.1. For higher doses, corresponding to surviving fractions of less than 0.1, more complex multihit models provide a better description (Barendsen, 1979). For high-LET radiations, the term $\exp$-$a_1 D$ dominates, and $\exp$-$a_2 D^2$ is of lesser importance. In Figure 3, a few examples of survival curves show considerable differences for cells from different normal tissues. As mentioned earlier, published data show that a_1 values may vary between 10^{-1} and 1 per Gy of low-LET radiation, and between approximately 1 and 3 per Gy of high-LET radiation.

Dose Fractionation. The administration of a given total dose in two or more fractions separated by intervals of a few hours generally decreases the yield of cellular effects per unit dose; e.g. the yield of cell reproductive death or chromosome aberrations. As a consequence, the fraction of surviving cells generally increases with dose fractionation, provided the total dose is kept the same. The decrease in the frequency of lesions or the increase in survival generally is attributed to repair of sublethal or subeffective lesions, which can interact only during a limited time interval after their production to cause lethal or effective lesions. The terms effective and subeffective lesions must be used to replace

FIGURE 3. Examples of survival curves of cells from different normal tissues for different radiations.

Abbreviations: MBM, mouse bone marrow stem cells (Broerse et al, 1977); MS, mouse skin stem cells (Douglas and Fowler, 1976); MJ, mouse jejunal crypt cells (Broerse et al, 1977); RE, rat endothelial cells (Reinhold and Buisman, 1973).

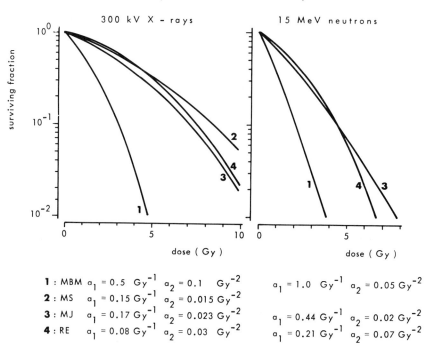

1 : MBM $a_1 = 0.5 \ Gy^{-1}$ $a_2 = 0.1 \ Gy^{-2}$ $a_1 = 1.0 \ Gy^{-1}$ $a_2 = 0.05 \ Gy^{-2}$

2 : MS $a_1 = 0.15 \ Gy^{-1}$ $a_2 = 0.015 \ Gy^{-2}$

3 : MJ $a_1 = 0.17 \ Gy^{-1}$ $a_2 = 0.023 \ Gy^{-2}$ $a_1 = 0.44 \ Gy^{-1}$ $a_2 = 0.02 \ Gy^{-2}$

4 : RE $a_1 = 0.08 \ Gy^{-1}$ $a_2 = 0.03 \ Gy^{-2}$ $a_1 = 0.21 \ Gy^{-1}$ $a_2 = 0.07 \ Gy^{-2}$

the terms lethal and sublethal lesions if other effects than lethality are considered. The repair processes, which decrease the probability of interaction among sublesions, only affect the terms that increase with the square of the dose in **(1)**, **(2)**, and **(3)**. As noted earlier, the linear term represents the frequency of damage induced by individual ionizing particles and is not dependent on the interaction of sublethal or subeffective lesions that are produced by two or more independent particles. It is important to note, however, that the effective lesions produced as a result of the passage of a single ionizing particle, may be due to a composite interaction of subeffective changes produced along the same track (Barendsen 1979). The effect of fractionation on dose-effect relationships occurs with low-LET radiations most markedly, as illustrated in Figure 4. For high-LET radiations, the influence of fractionation is reduced or absent and the induction of lesions is generally proportional to the dose, as shown in Figure 1; the corresponding survival curves are exponential, and the influence of fractionation on survival is also reduced or absent.

Most survival curves for mammalian cells irradiated with single doses of low-LET radiation have a_1/a_2 values ranging from 2 to 10 Gy. A survival curve with $a_1/a_2 = 5$ Gy is presented in Figure 4A. The influence of dose fractionation on the percentage of surviving cells is shown to be smaller at low doses than at high doses. For instance, at a total dose of 8 Gy, division of the dose into two equal fractions is shown to cause an increase in the percentage of cells surviving by a factor of about 3.6 and division of the dose into four equal fractions causes an increase in survival by a factor of about 6.8 relative to the percentage of cells surviving after a single dose. At a total dose of 4 Gy, division of the dose into two equal fractions increases the percentage of cells surviving by a factor of only 1.4. As a consequence of the increasing effect of fractionation with increasing dose, the influence of fractionation on the yield of tumor development depends on the range of doses considered. The example shown in Figure 4 can provide a simple illustration. A single dose of 8 Gy yields a surviving fraction of 0.016. Division of this dose into four equal increments yields a fraction of surviving cells of about 0.106, corresponding to an increase by a factor of about 7. The yield of transformed cells after fractionated irradiation with four doses of 2 Gy is smaller than after a single dose of 8 Gy; but in the example illustrated in Figure 4, the difference is smaller than a factor 7. If $p_1/p_2 = 1$ Gy for transformation, as in the example in Figure 4B, the yield of transformed cells after four doses of 2 Gy would be a factor of about 3 less than after a single dose of 8 Gy. If cell transformation and reproductive death are independent phenomena, and if tumor incidence can be described by **3**, then the total effect of fractionating a dose of 8 Gy into four equal increments would increase the yield of developing tumors by a factor of $7/3 = 2.3$, assuming sufficiently long intervals between exposures to allow complete repair of sublethal and subeffective damage. At lower doses (e.g., at a total dose of 4 Gy fractionated in two doses of 2 Gy), however, the influence of fractionation would be to increase the proportion of surviving cells from 0.24 to 0.33 (i.e., by a factor 1.4), whereas, the number of transformed cells would decrease by a factor 1.7. Thus, the yield of developing tumors according to **(3)** would decrease by a factor $1.4/1.7 = 0.8$. Further fractionation of a total dose of 4 Gy into still smaller fractions would decrease the yield of developing tumors even

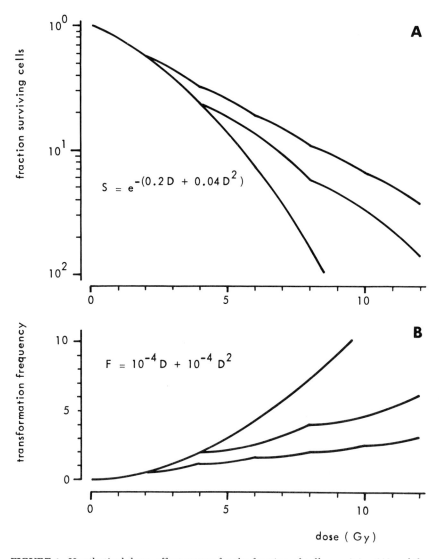

FIGURE 4. Hypthetical dose–effect curves for the fraction of cells surviving (A) and the frequency of cell transformation (B), to illustrate the effects of dose fractionation on both types of effect and their possible influence on tumor induction.

further. Experimental data showing such a variable influence of fractionation with the total dose have been published by Burns and Vanderlaan (1977).

With high-LET radiations, fractionation of a total dose into many fractions would not be expected to change the yield of developing tumors, because no repair of subeffective or sublethal damage occurs between fractions.

This example indicates that unless the actual doses employed and values of the parameters p_1/p_2 and a_1/a_2 in (3) are evaluated quantitatively, the influence of dose fractionation in tumor incidence cannot be predicted. An application of these considerations to published experimental results, described in the next section, may serve as a further illustration (Barendsen, 1978).

Analysis of Data on the Yield of Myeloid Leukemia in Mice

Data on tumor induction for a wide range of single and fractionated doses of high-LET and low-LET radiation, and for tissues in which the survival curves of stem cells are known, are extremely scarce. An important series of results on the induction of myeloid leukemia in mice has been published by Upton et al (1970). For this leukemia, the radiosensitivity with respect to reproductive death of the susceptible normal cell type can be assumed to be equal to the sensitivity of bone marrow stem cells, for which data are available (Barendsen, 1979). In order to analyze whether or not (3) can adequately represent the yield of these leukaemias as a function of dose, dose rate, dose fractionation, and radiation quality, appropriate values of parameters a_1, a_2, p_1, and p_2 have been adopted on the basis of experimental data available from the other sources (Barendsen, 1978). For mouse bone marrow stem cells, values of a_1 and a_2 equal to 4×10^{-1} Gy^{-1} and 8×10^{-2}, respectively, have been derived from experimental data for gamma rays. Assuming an analogy with chromosome aberration induction and morphologic transformation of cells in vitro, values of p_1/p_2 equal to 1 Gy for 200–3000 kV x-rays and 0.5 Gy for ^{60}Co gamma rays have been adopted for the induction of malignant transformation. On the basis of these values, shapes of the dose–response curves were calculated and compared with the experimental results. The only parameter that remained to be selected, to obtain a fit to the experimental data, was p_1 (Barendsen, 1978). It was demonstrated that the application of parameters derived on the basis of other types of experimental evidence provided a good fit to the model for expressing the data on leukemia induction.

In addition to the experimental data on induction of leukemia by a single acute dose of x-rays, and by low-dose rate irradiation with gamma rays, results have been published on the effectiveness of fractionated treatments (Upton et al, 1958). With the same parameters as adopted for interpretating the effectiveness of single doses, calculations were made to predict the effect of fractionated doses, yielding results that are in fair agreement with the observed incidence (Table 2). It is evident that the incidence observed after three fractions of 1.5 Gy is not significantly different from the incidence after a single dose of 4.5 Gy. This result, at first glance surprising, is in good agreement with predictions on the basis of (3), using the same values of parameters as adopted for describing the single-dose data. For the long intervals of 5 days, some repopulation of the surviving bone marrow stem cells to 0.5 of the initial number was assumed on the basis of observations by Lahiri et al (1970).

It can be concluded that the model described by (3), with parameters adopted on the basis of analogy with other radiobiologic data, can adequately describe variations in the effectiveness of radiation for leukemogenesis in mice as a function of dose, dose rate, dose fractionation, and radiation quality (Barendsen, 1978).

TABLE 2. Effect of Fractionation on Leukemia Incidence Induced by X-Rays in RF Mice

Model: $I = (20 D + 20 D^2)$. $(\exp. (-4 \times 10^{-1}D - 8 \times 10^{-2}D^2)$

	Incidence (%)	
	Calculated	Observed
0.75 Gy, single dose	19	8 ± 3
1.5 Gy, single dose	34	32 ± 6
1.5 Gy, two fractions 2 days interval	26	15 ± 5
1.5 Gy, two fractions 6 days interval	26	22 ± 5
4.5 Gy, single dose	16	25 ± 6
4.5 Gy, three fractions 2 days interval	22	20 ± 6
4.5 Gy, three fractions 5 days interval	32	26 ± 7

Calculation:	Induced leukemia (%)	Cell reproductive integrity
Effect of first dose of 0.75 Gy	18.6	0.71
Effect of second dose of 0.75 Gy	$18.6 \times 0.71 + 0.71 \times 18.6 = 26.4$	0.50
Effect of first dose of 1.5 Gy	34.4	0.46
Effect of second dose of 1.5 Gy	$34.4 \times 0.46 + 0.46 \times 34.4 = 31.7$	0.21
Effect of third dose of 1.5 Gy, assuming repopulation to 0.5	$31.7 \times 0.46 + 0.5 \times 34.4 = 31.8$	0.25

INFLUENCE OF TISSUE RESPONSES ON TUMOR DEVELOPMENT

Cell Proliferation in Tissues

In addition to the effectiveness of radiation for induction of malignant transformation of cells and cell reproductive death, tumor development can be influenced by the collective responses of cells in tissues after irradiation. An important response is acceleration of the proliferation of surviving cells after irradiation with relatively high doses. In many tissues, functioning cells have a limited life span, and loss of these cells is compensated for by the proliferation and subsequent differentiation of cells produced by division of surviving stem cells. Under normal conditions an equilibrium is maintained by homeostatic mechanisms. After irradiation, however, proliferation of stem cells is impaired, while loss of functioning cells continues. As a consequence, the surviving stem cells may be induced to start proliferating at an accelerated rate in order to restore tissue integrity and function. Since experimental evidence indicates that cell transformation is a multistep process that may depend on continued proliferation, a tissue response causing accelerated proliferation may promote tumor development.

Not all normal tissues depend to the same extent on cell proliferation for their integrity and function. It is possible to distinguish three types of systems:

1. *Rapid cell renewal systems*, which are characterized by a relatively high rate of cell turnover. These systems depend strongly on cell production, and the differentiated functional cells have a mean life span of a few days to a few weeks. Examples include the epithelium of the gastrointestinal tract and urinary tract, bone marrow, skin, and testis.

2. *Conditional cell renewal systems*, which show relatively little cell proliferation under normal conditions, because of the long life span of their differentiated functional cells. Examples include the liver, kidney, bone, and blood vessel endothelium. After significant damage to the parenchymal cells, loss of dead cells can result in rapid replacement by induction of accelerated proliferation of surviving stem cells. This replacement can occur early or late, depending on the life span and rate of loss of the functional cells.

3. *Static systems*, which consist of cells that are not replaced in the normal adult organism. The best example is the central nervous system. It is of interest to note, however, that the supporting neuroglial cells in the nervous system must be regarded as a conditional cell renewal system.

It is evident that the influence of tissue repopulation on tumor development must depend strongly on the type of tissue concerned. Moreover, different types of cells are commonly present in any given tissue. It is impossible, to therefore, give a specific formula for the dependence of tumor yield on the influence of cell proliferation. It can be assumed that this dependence behaves as a nonstochastic effect and that a threshold dose may exist below which this influence is negligible (Columbano et al, 1981).

An example of a tissue in which the proliferation of surviving cells may be an important determinant of the tumor yield is the skin. In Figure 5, data published by Albert et al (1967, 1972), Burns et al (1968), and Hulse (1967) for skin tumor induction in rats and mice have been replotted on a log–log scale. The resulting curves all show an increase in the slope of the yield-versus-dose curve at rather large doses (Figure 5). The slopes in the steepest parts of the curves correspond to a power function with an exponent in excess of 2. This applies even to the curve for α-particle irradiation. It is likely, therefore, that the increase in slope at higher doses is due to compensatory proliferation of surviving cells in the skin. Experiments by Burns et al with different electron penetrations in rat skin led these investigators to the same conclusion (Burns et al, 1976).

Another example of a tissue in which cell proliferation may greatly enhance tumor development is the skeleton (Marshall and Groer, 1977). The analysis of tumor induction by α-radiation from radium has led Marshall and Groer to the conclusion that two effective events are required for the malignant transformation of an endosteal cell. Because the dependence of stimulated proliferation on the dose and the influence of the proliferation on tumor development are not known, however, quantitative analysis and conclusions about mechanisms must be tentative.

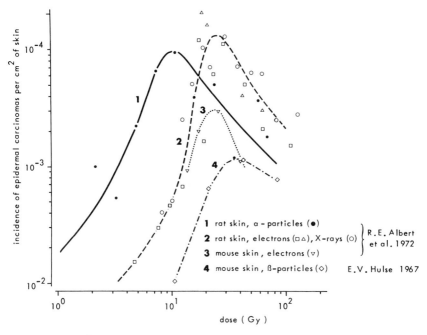

FIGURE 5. Incidence of epidermal carcinomas per centimeter squared of skin in rats and mice irradiated with different radiations. At doses in excess of 20 Gy of low-LET radiation and 2 Gy of high-LET radiation, a steep increase in incidence is observed, which can be attributed to stimulation of proliferation in surviving cells.

Hormonal Modification of Tumor Development

It has been amply demonstrated that the administration of estrogens to rats irradiated with x-rays or neutrons increases the incidence of mammary adenocarcinomas (Shellabarger et al, 1976; Broerse et al, 1978). These results exemplify a situation in which hormones act synergistically with radiation to increase the frequency of tumors.

The administration of hormones alone, as well as of x-rays alone, increases the incidence of mammary tumors in various strains of rats. It is not known, however, whether or not the increase by hormones is due to actual malignant transformation, to the promotion of transformation of cells, or to promotion of the development of tumors. Furthermore, an accurate dose–response curve for a range of hormone concentrations is not known. In experiments with one rat strain having a high natural incidence, the effects of hormonal stimulation on mammary cancer incidence could be adequately described in terms of a forward shift in time of the occurence of tumors. In experiments with another strain of rats, however, which exhibit a low control incidence, this could not be established (Broerse et al, 1978).

The influence of hormonal balance has also been implicated as a factor in the induction of other tumors and in the modifying effects of the dose rate of low-LET and high-LET radiations (Ullrich et al, 1977). Without further information, however, it is not possible to evaluate the mechanisms by which hormones promote or inhibit the incidence of various types of tumors. It is possible that the influence of hormones is merely to cause accelerated proliferation of cells, thereby enhancing malignant transformation, but the action of hormones might also be to increase or inhibit the proliferation of cells that have already been transformed.

Immunologic Influence on Tumor Development

Impairment of immunological defense mechanisms is known to increase the probability of development of certain neoplasms in laboratory animals and in humans (e.g., those treated with immunosuppressive agents for kidney transplantation). It is possible that this effect becomes important only after a large decrease in immunologic competence (e.g., a 50% decrease in the number of immune competent cells). It is noteworthy that irradiation may depress immunological responses significantly at doses in excess of a few grays of x-rays (UNSCEAR, 1982).

General Formula For Tumor Yield

Because the effects of changes in hormonal balance, immunologic resistance, and tissue homeostasis or carcinogenesis are not known precisely, the incidence of tumors as a function of radiation dose can only be approximated by an expression of the following type

$$Y = (p_0 + p_1D + p_2D^2)\cdot\exp - (a_1D + a_2 D^2)\cdot F\cdot_{imm}(D)\cdot F_{horm}(D)\cdot F_{tiss}(D) \qquad (4)$$

Where the last three factors are unknown functions of the dose. It is evident that much more quantitative data are needed to define the dose-incidence relationship in detail.

CELL PROLIFERATION IN TUMORS AND CANCER DEVELOPMENT

General Cell Kinetic Aspects of Tumor Growth

The rate of growth of tumors depends on the excess of cell proliferation over cell loss. A tumor that grows extremely slowly may not become detectable within the life-span of the host; consequently, the observed incidence depends on the growth rate.

The growth rate of primary tumors varies widely among different types of tumors, as well as among tumors of the same histologic characteristics. A first important factor is the growth fraction (i.e., the fraction of tumor cells actually in progress through the intermitotic cycle—P-cells). It is generally observed that tumors, like normal tissues, contain cells in a resting state—Q-cells (Steel, 1977). A fraction of Q-cells may be capable of starting a new cycle of proliferation, and these cells are denoted G_o-cells. In addition, like differentiated functional cells in normal tissues, tumor cells may include those that have lost the capacity to proliferate. Cells in tumors may die and be lost through exfoliation, perish in necrotic areas with inadequate oxygen supply, or lose their capacity to proliferate as a result of spontaneous chromosome aberrations. As a consequence of variations in all these processes, tumors may show widely varying growth rates, even though cell cycle times of the proliferating cells commonly are in the range of 10–50 hr.

For a tumor to become detectable at a minimum volume of about 0.1 cm^3 a mass of about 10^8 cells must accumulate. If this number of cells results as a clonal derivative from the initial transformation of a single cell, the number of cell-doubling times or volume-doubling times is at least 26. For an experimental animal with a life span of 700–1400 days, it is evident that the average growth rate of a tumor must be at least equivalent to a volume-doubling time of 30 days, to detect the tumor within the life span of the animal. For some experimental leukemias and lymphomas in animals, volume-doubling times of 10–30 hr have been observed; whereas for some carcinomas, doubling times of 10–20 days have been measured. In humans, some fast growing embryonal tumors have volume-doubling times ranging between 20 and 40 days; whereas for some adenocarcinomas doubling-times between 40 and 1000 days have been reported. It is evident that the growth rates of radiation-induced tumors during the time interval between irradiation and tumor observation may play an important part in the dose–effect relationship. If tumors induced by low doses tended to grow more slowly, due to either intrinsic properties of the induction process, or to less late damage to surrounding tissues, the dose–response relationship would be modified accordingly. As a consequence, a threshold might be observed. This would apply in particular to experiments in which animals live less than their natural life span or are killed at specific ages (Broerse et al, 1982; Ullrich et al, 1979). Even if animals are observed until the end of their natural life span, the observed incidence may not truly reflect the rate of tumor induction. Consequently, analysis of dose–incidence relationships must be used with great caution in attempts to derive information about the mechanisms of carcinogenesis at the cellular level.

REFERENCES

Albert RE, Burns FJ, Heimback RD (1967) The association between radiation damage of the hair follicles and tumour formation in the rat. Radiat Res 30:590–599.

Albert RE, Burns FJ, Bennett P (1972) Radiation-induced hair-follicle damage and tumor formation in mouse and rat skin. J Natl Cancer Inst 49:1131–1137.

Barendsen GW (1978) Fundamental aspects of cancer induction in relation to the effectiveness of small doses of radiation. In, Late biological effects of ionizing radiation, Vol. II. Vienna: International Atomic Energy Agency.

Barendsen GW (1979) Influence of radiation quality on the effectiveness of small doses for induction of reproductive death and chromsome aberrations in mammalian cells. Intl J Radiat Biol 36:49–63.

Barendsen GW (1982) Dose fractionation, dose rate and iso-effect relationships for normal tissue responses. Int J Radiat Oncol Biol Phys 8:1981–1997.

Barendsen GW, Aten JA, Wilder M, Gaiser JF (1985) Cell transformation in vitro by different radiations. Intl J Radiat Biol 48:291.

Barendsen GW, Gaiser JF (1985), Cell transformation in vitro by fast neutrons of different energies: implications for mechanisms. Radiat Prot Donmetry (in press).

Broerse JJ, Barendsen GW, Gaiser JF, Zoetelief J (1977) The importance of differences in intrinsic cellular sensitivity for the effectiveness of neutron radiotherapie treatments.

In, Radiobiological research and radiotherapy, Vol. II. Vienna: International Atomic Energy Agency.

Broerse JJ, Knaan S, Van Bekkum DW, Hollander CJ, Nooteboom AL, Van Zwieten MJ (1978) Mammary carcinogenesis in rats after x- and neutron irradiation and hormone administration. In, Late biological effects of ionizing radiation, Vol. II. Vienna: International Atomic Energy Agency, pp 13–27.

Burns FJ, Sinclair IP, Albert RE, Vanderlaan M (1976) Tumor induction and hair follicle damage for different electron penetrations in rat skin. Radiat Res 67:474–481.

Burns FJ, Vanderlaan M (1977) Split-dose recovery for radiation-induced tumours in rat skin. Intl J Radiat Biol 32:135–144.

Columbano A, Rajalakshmi S, Sarma DSR (1981) Requirement of cell proliferation for the initiation of liver carcinogenesis as assayed by three different procedures. Cancer Res 41:2097–2083.

Cox R, Thacker J, Goodhead DT, Munson RJ (1977) Mutation and inactivation of mammalian cells by various ionising radiations. Nature 267:425–427.

Dewey WC, Miller HH, Leeper DB (1971) Chromosomal aberrations and mortality of x-irradiated mammalian cells: Emphasis on repair. Proc Natl Acad Sci 68:667–671.

Douglas BG, Fowler JF (1976) The effect of multiple small doses of x-rays on skin reactions in the mouse and a basic interpretation. Radiat Res 66:401–426.

Gilbert CW, Hendry JH, Major D (1980) The approximation in the formulation for survival $S = \exp-(\alpha D + \beta D^2)$. Intl J Radiat Biol 37:469–471.

Gray LH (1965) Radiation biology and cancer. In, Cellular radiation biology. Proc 18th Ann Symp Fund Cancer Res 7–25, M.D. Anderson Inst. Oct 1964 Baltimore: Williams and Wilkins. 1965

Hall EJ, Rossi HH, Zaider M, Miller RC, Bork C (1982) The role of the neutrons in cell transformation research. In Proc Semin Broerse JJ, Gerber GB (eds.), Neutron carcinogenesis.

Han A, Elkind MM (1979) Transformation of mouse C3H/10T½ cells by single and fractionated doses of x-rays and fission spectrum neutrons. Cancer Res 39:123–130.

Heisterkamp N, Groffer J, Stephenson JR, Spurr NK, Goodfellow PN, Solomon E, Carritt B, Bodmer WF (1982) Chromosomal localization of human cellular homologues of two viral oncogenes. Nature 299:747–749.

Hill CK, Buonoguro FM, Myers CP, Han A, Elkind MM (1982) Fission-spectrum neutrons at reduced dose rates enhance neoplastic transformation. Nature 298:67–69.

Hulse EV (1967) Incidence of pathogenesis of skin tumours in mice irradiated with single external doses of low energy beta particles. Cancer XXI:531.

Kennedy AR, Fox M, Murphy G, Little JB (1980) Relationship between x-ray exposure and malignant transformation in C3H 10T½ cells. Proc Natl Acad Sci, USA, 77:7262–7266.

Lahari SK, Keizer HJ, Van Putten LM (1970) The efficiency of the assay for haemopoietic colony forming cells. Cell Tiss Kinet 3:355.

Little JB (1981) Influence of noncarcinogenic secondary factors on radiation carcinogenesis. Radiat Res 87:240–250.

Lloyd DC, Purrott RJ, Dolphin GW, Edwards AA (1976) Chromosome aberrations induced in human lymphocytes by neutron irradiation. Intl J Radiat Biol 29:169–182.

Marshall JH, Groer GG (1977) A theory of the induction of bone cancer by alpha radiation. Radiat Res 71:149–192.

Nagasawa H, Little JB (1981) Induction of chromosome aberrations and sister chromatid exchanges by x-rays in density-inhibited cultures of mouse 10T½ cells. Radiat Res 87:538–551.

Randolph ML, Slater M, Upton AC, Conklin JW (1967) Late effect of fast neutrons and gamma rays in mice as influenced by the dose rate of irradiation: Methodology of irradiation and dosimetry. Radiat Res 32:475–492.

Reinhold HS, Buisman GH (1973) Radiosensitivity of capillary endothelium. Br J Radiol 46:54–57.

Shellabarger CJ, Stone JP, Holtzman S (1976) Synergism between neutron radiation and diethylstilbestrol in the production of mammary adenocarcinomas in the rat. Cancer Res 36:1019–1022.

Smith BL, Sager R (1982) Multistep origin of tumor-forming ability in Chinese hamster embryo fibroblast cells. Cancer Res 42:389–396.

Steel GG (1977) Growth kinetics of tumours. Oxford: Clarendon Press.

Straus DS (1981) Somatic mutation, cellular differentiation, and cancer causation. Natl Cancer Inst 67:233–241.

Tabin CJ, Bradley SM, Bargman CI, Weinberg RA, Papogeorge AG, Scolnick EM, Dhar R, Lowy DR, Chang EH (1982) Mechanism of activation of a human oncogene. Nature 300:143–149.

Terasima T, Yasukawa M, Kimura M (1981) Radiation-induced transformation of 10T½ mouse cells in the plateau phase: Post-irradiation changes and serum dependence. Gann 72:762–768.

Ullrich RL, Jernigan MC, Storer JB (1977) Neutron carcinogenesis: Dose and dose-rate effects in BALB/c mice. Radiat Res 72:487–498.

Ullrich RL, Jernigan MC, Adams LM (1979) Induction of lung tumors in RFM mice after localized exposures to x-rays or neutrons. Radiat Res 80:464–473.

UNSCEAR (1982) Report on ionizing radiation. Sources and biological effects. New York: United Nations, 37th Session, Supplement No. 45 (A/37/45).

Upton AC, Wolff FF, Furth T, Kimball AW (1958) A comparison of the induction of myeloid and lymphoid leukemias in x-radiated RF mice. Cancer Res 18:842–848.

Upton AC, Randolph ML, Conklin JW, Kastenbaum MA, Slater M, Melville GS, Conte FP, Sproul JA (1970) Late effects of fast neutrons and gamma-rays in mice as influenced by the dose rate irradiation: Induction of neoplasia. Radiat Res 41:467–491.

Weinberg RA (1982) Oncogenes of spontaneous and chemically induced tumours. Adv Cancer Res 36:149–163.

Zoetelief J, Barendsen GW (1983) Dose–effect relationships for induction of cell inactivation and chromosome exchanges in three cell lines by photons and neutrons of different energy. Intl J Radiat Biol 43:349–362.

NEOPLASTIC TRANSFORMATION IN VITRO

GERALD L. CHAN, Ph.D AND JOHN B. LITTLE, M.D.

With few exceptions, human cancers have been shown to be clonal in origin (Fialkow, 1976). All of the cells within a tumor are the progenies of a single cell that has undergone the process of neoplastic transformation. In terms of carcinogenic mechanisms, cell transformation or the conversion of a normal cell to one with the malignant phenotype may be regarded as the first step in the total process. Whether or not such a transformed cell can successfully give rise to a tumor depends on subsequent tissue and systemic factors, of which a major influence is likely to be the immune response.

In the study of experimental carcinogenesis with laboratory animals, these tissue and systemic factors are clearly important determinants. Furthermore, with ionizing radiation, exposure of the target cells, themselves, may be accompanied by significant radiation-induced systemic effects. Cell transformation in vitro, thus, offers an experimental approach complementary to animal studies in radiation carcinogenesis. Whereas in vivo studies emphasize the whole process of carcinogenesis, rather than the individual components, in vitro cell transformation focuses exclusively on events at the level of the irradiated target cells.

Cell transformation systems offer a controlled environment in which cellular processes may be examined in the absence of many experimental uncertainties and complicating factors. However, such an environment must be recognized as an artificial one. First, the cell culture medium is only a general approximation of the nutrient milieu in vivo, particularly as concerns hormones or growth factors, for example. Second, two-dimensional growth in a cell culture dish with the plastic substratum does not reproduce the three-dimensional architecture of cells within tissues. Finally, the growth of a single cell type within a culture precludes any interactions among different cell types found in intact tissues.

From the Laboratory of Radiobiology, Harvard School of Public Health, Boston, Massachusetts.

Notwithstanding, there are also many indications that cell transformation in vitro is a valid model system for studying carcinogenesis. These include the following:

1. Most in vitro cell transformation systems conform to the criterion of conversion from non-tumorigenic to tumorigenic cells.
2. A large number of carcinogenic and non-carcinogenic chemicals have been tested in both animals and cell transformation systems; the correlation for carcinogenicity is very high. Similar correlations hold for the effects of many inhibitors and promoters of carcinogenesis that have been tested in vitro and in vivo.
3. Transformation in vitro responds to initiation and promotion in the same way that two-stage carcinogenesis has been demonstrated in many tissues in experimental animals.
4. Mouse cells transformed in vitro by ultraviolet (UV) light exhibit the same antigenic determinants as those found specifically and ubiquitously in UV-induced mouse skin tumors. These same mouse cells, transformed in vitro by any other agent, do not have these antigenic determinants, as is the case of mouse skin tumors induced by agents other than UV light (Fisher, Kripke, and Chan, 1984).
5. Mouse cells transformed in vitro have been shown to have activated oncogenes that can be isolated, transfected into recipient cells and will transform them. The oncogenes of the parental non-transformed cells are inactive. This is analogous to human tumors and normal human cells, which have been studied in the same DNA transfection assay (Shilo and Weinberg, 1981).

DESCRIPTION OF CELL TRANSFORMATION SYSTEMS IN VITRO

The ideal in vitro cell transformation system is one consisting of human epithelial cells, because over 90% of human cancers are of nonmesenchymal origin. For technical as well as historical reasons, however, most studies of radiation-induced transformation in vitro have utilized either hamster embryo fibroblasts or mouse embryo-derived fibroblast cell lines.

The hamster system involves the use of primary fibroblast cultures. These are obtained by culturing cells that grow out from minced embryos. The cells are diploid and have a limited life span in vitro. Transformation is usually measured by a colony assay. Cells are plated in low density, treated with a carcinogen and allowed to grow to macroscopic colonies. The whole experiment usually requires about 10 days. After fixation and staining, the morphology of each colony is examined. Non-transformed colonies display a flat orderly morphology, whereas cells in the transformed colonies are piled up. Such transformants, as routinely scored in this assay system, were found to be non-tumorigenic in syngeneic mice (Barrett and T'so, 1978a). When these morphologic transformants were cloned and serially passaged in culture, however, they exhibited a sequential acquisition of the various phenotypes that were characteristic of malignantly transformed cells, including the acquisition of tumorigenic potential at the end of extensive passaging. Considering the relatively high frequency of morphologic transformation in this system, typically one to two orders of magnitude higher than the frequency of single gene muta-tions after identical carcinogenic treatments (Barrett and T'so, 1978b), it may be concluded that the event of morphologic transformation in the hamster system reflects only initial steps in the total carcinogenic process.

In contrast to the hamster cells, fibroblasts derived from mouse embryos frequently develop into immortal cell lines in culture. Cell lines that are highly sensitive to "contact" or density inhibition of growth can be selected by impos-ing appropriate culture conditions prior to establishment of immortality (To-daro and Green, 1963; Reznikoff et al, 1973a). Although these normal cell lines are immortal and aneuploid in karyotype, they exhibit almost all the morpho-logic and growth characteristics of non-transformed cells, including non-tu-morigenicity in the appropriate animal hosts.

Transformation in these mouse cell lines is detected and measured by a focus assay in contrast to the colony assay used in the hamster system. Cells are plated in low density, exposed to a carcinogen, grown to confluence, and held in that culture condition for about 4 wk, during which time the transformed cells grow up as foci of piled up cells on top of the density-inhibited back-ground monolayer of normal cells (Figure 1). Provided that low-passage cells

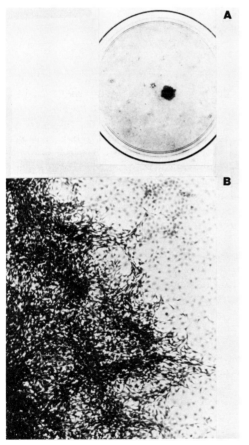

A

B

FIGURE 1. Appearance of trans-formed foci of mouse embryo fibro-blasts line. (A) Petri dish with large transformed focus overlying the normal monolayer of BALT/3T3 cells; (B) View of the edge of a trans-formed focus of C3H × 10T½ cells. Note the normal monolayer in the upper right hand corner, being in-vaded by the transformed cells, which are stellate in appearance and grow in a piled-up, criss-crossed, and swirling pattern.

are used in this protocol, spontaneous transformation is a rare event. Cells isolated from transformed foci in these mouse cell systems have been shown to exhibit a full complement of transformed phenotypes, including ubiquitous tumorigenicity in appropriate hosts (Reznikoff et al, 1973b; Jones et al, 1976; Bertram, 1977; Chan and Little, 1979; Hahn, 1980). The mouse cell lines most commonly used in radiation transformation studies are the C3H 10T$\frac{1}{2}$ clone 8 system (Reznikoff et al, 1973a,b) and the Balb/3T3 A31-1-1 system (Little, 1979). The initiation of transformation in these cell systems also appears to be a high-frequency event (Kennedy et al, 1980a).

It is important to recognize that there are fundamental differences in the biology underlying the hamster and the mouse cell transformation systems. If the hamster system reflects transformation from the normal to a premalignant state, the mouse systems may be regarded as reflecting transformation from a premalignant to a malignant state. The processes underlying transformation in the hamster system should be proximal in the multistep carcinogenic process, whereas the processes underlying transformation in the mouse systems should be distal and consumating. Because transformation by chemicals in both systems correlates highly with animal carcinogenicity, the transformation events in both systems must be regarded as relevent to carcinogenesis.

FACTORS INFLUENCING TRANSFORMATION BY IONIZING RADIATION

Dose–Response Relationships

Borek and Hall (1973) measured the dose-response of x-ray induced transformation in Syrian hamster embryo cells. They found that in the dose range from 1 to 100 rads, single-hit kinetics were observed. Larger doses resulted in a leveling off and then a decline in the frequency of transformation. In the same system, Borek et al (1978) found that the dose–response curve for 430-kev monoenergenic neutrons was also linear in the dose range of 0.1–100 rads. The induction of transformation in these hamster cells by polycyclic hydrocarbons also followed a linear dose–response relationship (Huberman and Sachs, 1966).

The dose–response for radiation-induced transformation in the mouse 10T$\frac{1}{2}$ cells is more complex. When the transformation frequencies are expressed on a per survivor basis, the general shape of the curve in this system is consistently the same (i.e., an ascending portion at lower doses followed by a plateau at higher doses) (Terzaghi and Little, 1976a). When such a dose–response relationship is expressed in terms of the transformation frequency per irradiated cell, the curve becomes one consisting of an ascending portion at lower doses followed by a descending portion at higher doses (Little, 1977; Han et al, 1980). Such an ascending–descending curve resembles the dose–response seen in radiation-induced neoplasms in experimental animals, and has been suggested by Gray (1968) to represent the two competitive processes of transformation induction and cell killing. At lower doses, the induction effect predominates, whereas, at higher doses, cell killing predominates.

Using the 10T$\frac{1}{2}$ system, several groups of investigators have measured transformation frequencies at low doses. Han et al (1980) showed that for ^{60}Co gamma rays delivered at a dose-rate of 100 rads/min, the transformation frequency on a per survivor basis had a slope of unity in the dose range of 0–100 rads. Other measurements made by these investigators showed that in the dose range of 150–400 rads the transformation dose–response curve approximates a slope of 2 on a log–log plot, suggesting a quadratic relationship (Han and Elkind, 1979). This quadratic relationship is also evident in the data of Terzaghi and Little (1976a).

The data of Miller et al (1979) are in agreement with those of Terzaghi and Little (1976a) and Han and Elkind (1979) with respect to the quadratic relationship in the dose range of 100–400 rads; however, their results show that in the dose range of 10–100 rads the dose–response relationship is not simply a linear one. In the extreme low range of 10–30 rads linearity is approximated, whereas, in the range of 30–100 rads the slope of the transformation dose–response curve is extremely small, about 0.2. Thus, the complete dose–response curve is quadriphasic, consisting of a linear phase, an almost horizontal phase, a quadratic phase, and finally a plateau phase (Figures 2 and 3). The data of Terzaghi and Little (1976a) are generally consistent with such a shape of the transformation dose–response curve, but these investigators did not study

FIGURE 2. Dose-response relationship for the induction of neoplastic transformation in mouse 10T$\frac{1}{2}$ cells by single and split doses of x-rays. The solid circles (●) are for single, acute x-ray exposures. The open circles (○) represent similar total doses, split into equal fractions with an interval of 5 hr between them. The spontaneous transformation frequency in these experiments was approximately 10^{-5}.

Reproduced from Miller et al (1979), by permission.

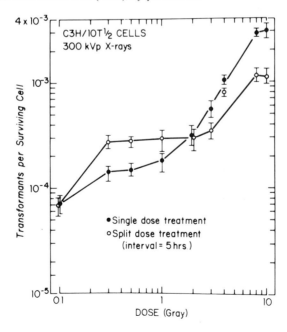

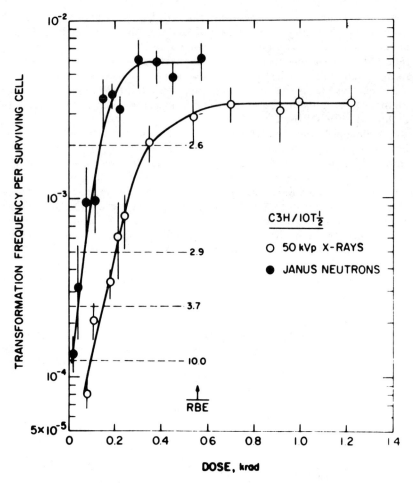

FIGURE 3. Dose–response relationship for the induction of neoplastic transformation in mouse 10T½ cells by 50 kVp x-rays (○) and fission spectrum neutrons (●). Reproduced from Han and Elkind (1979), by permission.

transformation at doses below 50 rads. In addition to corroborating the quadratic and the plateau phases at high doses, they demonstrated a shallow slope of about 0.3 between 50 and 100 rads. Although the results of Little (1979) on x-ray transformation of mouse 3T3 cells suggest a nearly linear increase of transformation frequency with doses of 10–400 rads, on close examination, the data in chart 5 of that paper are consistent with the dose–response characteristics described by Miller et al (1979).

The complexity of the dose–response curve for cell transformation is by no means a unique phenomenon. Single gene mutations in bacteria induced by UV light have been shown to follow multiphasic dose–response relationships. For example, Doudney (1976) showed that mutation in tryptophan prototrophy in *Escherichia coli* followed dose-square kinetics at low doses; at intermediate doses, the response was linear; at higher doses, dose-square kinetics was again observed. As noted by Witkin (1976), the explanation for such complexities in the dose–response curve for bacterial mutation have been a subject of debate and conjecture for several decades, and no fully satisfactory explanation has emerged. The process of cell transformation is likely to be at least as complex as mutagenesis in *E. coli*. It may be prudent, therefore, to refrain from suggesting mechanistic explanations for the observed dose–response relationships at this time.

Dose Fractionation

Miller et al (1979) measured the transformation frequencies of $10T\frac{1}{2}$ cells following fractionation of x-ray doses into two equal halves separated by 5 hr. Their measurements extended from total doses of 10–1000 rads. The survival data indicated that fractionated doses were less cytotoxic than single doses. The transformation data, as shown in Figure 2, indicate that below 150 rads dose fractionation was more effective for inducing transformation by a factor of about 2, whereas above 150 rads dose fractionation was less effective. If one assumes recovery from the transforming effect of the first dose in the 5-hr interval, these results of dose fractionation are a direct consequence of the shape of the dose–response curve observed by these investigators for single dose transformation. Thus, the opposing effects of dose fractionation at large and small doses need not reflect opposing underlying processes.

The assumption that there is recovery from the transforming effect of the first dose in a split dose transformation protocol is supported by the analysis of Han and Elkind (1979), who studied transformation of $10T\frac{1}{2}$ cells by 700 rads of x-rays administered as either a single dose or as two fractions separated by varying time intervals, including 5 hr. Terzaghi and Little (1976b) also measured transformation of $10T\frac{1}{2}$ cells by fractionated x-ray doses down to 150 rads. The results of these two latter groups are in essential agreement with that of Miller et al (1979), as are the results of split dose x-ray transformation experiments in mouse 3T3 cells irradiated with total doses of 10–400 rads (Little, 1979).

Borek and Hall (1974) and Borek (1979) studied transformation in the hamster embryo system by single and fractionated doses of x-ray. Their results are in complete agreement with those from the 3T3 and $10T\frac{1}{2}$ systems. For total doses of less than 150 rads, two doses separated by 5 hr resulted in enhanced transformation, whereas reduced transformation was observed when the total dose exceeded 150 rads. In fact, when the ratios of transformation frequencies for split and single doses were plotted against total dose, the data from the mouse and the hamster systems completely coincided (Hall and Miller, 1981). This coincidence is most remarkable considering 1) transformations in the hamster and the mouse $10T\frac{1}{2}$ cells represent different biological processes and 2) the dose–response curves for single dose transformation in the two systems are different. For the hamster cells, induction of transformation by single x-ray doses below 150 rads follows single-hit kinetics. Recovery from such single-hit events is usually not expected. In spite of the observed coincidence in the data, therefore, the mechanisms responsible for the split dose transformation effects in the hamster and $10T\frac{1}{2}$ systems may differ. Because there is negligible cell killing in the dose range below 150 rads, the effects of dose fractionation observed in the low-dose range may not be applicable to higher doses. Indeed, there are cases in animal studies that bespeak of this same point.

Dose-Rate Effects

In most experimental animal models, protraction of an x-ray dose by decreasing the dose-rate results in a reduction in its carcinogenic potential (Fry, 1981; Ulrich 1980). Transformation of $10T\frac{1}{2}$ cells is no exception. Han et al (1980) studied the transformation of $10T\frac{1}{2}$ cells by x-rays administered at dose rates of 100, 2.5, 0.5, and 0.1 rads/min. In all cases, the dose–response curve followed the same general shape: a rising portion followed by a plateau. As the dose-rate was decreased, the plateau value of transformation frequency per survivor diminished. As for the low-dose region, they examined particularly the dose–response curve for 100 and 0.1 rads/min in the total dose range of 0–150 rads. Their results indicate that for the high-dose rate, the induction of transformation was linear with dose with a slope of 1 on a linear–linear plot. The induction of transformation was also linear with dose for the dose-rate of 0.1 rads/min, but the slope was about 0.5.

These results suggest two discrepancies between the endpoints of cell survival and transformation. First, with respect to the endpoint of cell survival, a single-hit phenomenon usually has not been accompanied by recovery due to dose protraction. With respect to transformation, however, apparently there is recovery even though the induction kinetics at the acute dose-rate are single-hit. Second, where recovery is observed for cell survival, it is usually observed whether the total dose is protracted by lowering the dose rate or by dose fractionation. Indeed, this is the case with $10T\frac{1}{2}$ cells (Han et al, 1980; Miller et al, 1979). At low total doses, however, fractionation appears to result in enhanced transformation. These apparent discrepancies remain to be explained.

High-LET Radiation

Neutrons. Transformation of hamster embryo cells by neutrons was studied by Borek et al (1978) using monoenergetic neutrons of 430 keV. Comparison was made with transformation induced by 250 kVp x-rays. Han and Elkind (1979) studied transformation of mouse $10T\frac{1}{2}$ cells by fission spectrum neutrons with an average energy of 850 keV. Comparison was made with x-rays of 50 kVp. In both systems, neutron-induced transformed cells were examined and found to have properties no different from cells transformed by x-ray. Thus, the final transformed phenotype does not appear to vary with the type of radiation used to transform the cells.

For the same absorbed dose, neutrons were more effective than x-rays in cell transformation. In both hamster and $10T\frac{1}{2}$ systems, the shape of the neutron transformation dose–response curve resembled the respective x-ray transformation curve with the exception of it being shifted to the left (i.e., to smaller doses). Thus, the neutron transformation dose–response curve in the hamster cells is linear from 0.1 to 100 rads. Data for mouse 10T$\frac{1}{2}$ cells are shown in Figure 3. In this system the slope of doses below 200 rads is very closely approximated by a dose-square model. At larger neutron doses, the transformation frequency per surviving cell assumes a plateau value about twofold higher than the plateau value for x-ray transformation. Whether there are linear or zero slope components at extremely low neutron doses, as was observed in x-ray transformation in this system (Miller et al, 1979), cannot be ascertained from the existing data.

In order to assess the relative biological effectiveness (RBE), which is defined to produce the same biological effect, an endpoint which has relevance to animal or human carcinogenesis data should be used. Thus, we have chosen to compare the induced transformation frequencies per irradiated cell for neutrons and x-rays. This quantity, in fact, is the product of transformation frequency per survivor and the survival fraction. Such a plot of the dose–response data from the hamster embryo system indicates RBE values between 5 and 15 for the 430 keV neutrons, depending on the level of effect selected for comparison (Borek et al, 1978). The variations of RBE with dose appear to be bidirectional. At an x-ray dose of about 15 rads, or a fraction of 6×10^{-4} of the irradiated cells transformed, the RBE value reaches a maximum of about 15. For both larger and smaller doses, the RBE values are smaller. Thus, the generalization that RBE values increase with decreasing dose does not appear to hold true for extremely small doses in the hamster embryo system. With the mouse 10T$\frac{1}{2}$ system, the RBE values for transformation by fission spectrum neutrons generally are smaller than those found in the hamster cells at comparable doses. These values are in the range of 2–5. The RBE values in the 10T$\frac{1}{2}$ cells appear to increase with decreasing dose, though the data at very low doses are less extensive. Of course, the relationship of these RBE values to those for the complete process of radiation carcinogenesis in animals or man remains largely unknown.

In contrast to low-LET radiation, neutron irradiation of 10T$\frac{1}{2}$ cells at low-dose rates (0.43 and 0.086 rad/min) resulted in no survival enhancement, compared with high dose rates of 10.3–38 rads/min (Hill et al, 1982). For total doses of less than 120 rads, however, low dose rate irradiation resulted in enhanced transformation. For example, at a total dose of 10 rads, low dose rate irradiation was almost 20 times more effective in causing transformation than high dose rate irradiation. Interestingly, there are now emerging in vivo data supporting the notion that for low total doses, low dose rate irradiation from neutrons is more carcinogenic than high dose rate irradiation (Vogel and Dickson, 1981; Ulrich et al, 1976, 1977; Kennedy and Little, 1978a). Further substantiation of these observations will no doubt result in profound implications for radiation protection.

Alpha Particles. Robertson et al (1983) studied the induction of transformation by [238]Pu alpha particles in Balb/3T3 cells. Such alpha particles of 5.3 MeV energy were found to be more efficient than x-rays in the induction of transformation. When actively dividing 3T3 cells were exposed to alpha particles or x-rays in the dose range of 25–250 rads, a maximum RBE for transformation was found to be 3. This was in the same range as the RBE for cell killing, which was found to have a value of 3.5 at 50% survival. When the transformation fre-

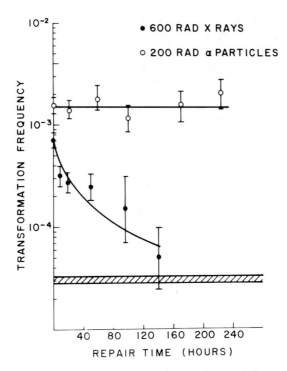

FIGURE 4. Neoplastic transformation induced by 600 rads of x-rays (●) or 200 rads of alpha particles from ^{238}Pu (○) as a function of confluent holding time following irradiation. The cells were irradiated while in density inhibited, confluent growth; they were subsequently maintained in stationary growth for various periods of time after irradiation to allow for the repair of potentially lethal damage. As can be seen, the transformation of x-irradiated cells declined markedly with increasing repair intervals, whereas, there was no change in the transformation frequency among alpha-irradiated cells. This result implies that the RBE for alpha radiation may be very high in noncycling cell populations.

Data from Robertson et al (1983).

quency was expressed on the per irradiated cell basis, the yield of transformants was not significantly higher in alpha-irradiated cultures except at very low doses where cell killing was minimal.

When nonproliferating plateau phase 3T3 cells were exposed to alpha particles, a further property of alpha-induced transformation was discovered (Robertson et al, 1983). Maintenance of x-irradiated 3T3 cells in a nonproliferating state for up to 5 days after exposure resulted in both recovery from potentially lethal damage and a continual decline in the transformation frequency. The same protocol of plateau phase maintenance in alpha-irradiated 3T3 cells resulted in neither survival enhancement nor a decline in transformation. Thus, as the recovery time was prolonged, the ability of alpha particles to transform 3T3 cells relative to x-rays increased markedly due to the decline in transformation in the x-irradiated cultures. This result is shown graphically in Figure

4. As can be seen, for example, the transformation frequencies for 600 rads of x-rays and 200 rads of alpha particles with no plateau holding were approximately equal. With a postirradiation holding time of 5 days, the transformation decline in the x-irradiated cells was in excess of tenfold. In the absence of any concomitant change in the alpha-induced transformation frequency, the RBE value was raised to the proximity of 50. This effect may be compared with a maximum increase in the RBE for cell killing of 2.5–5 with prolonged plateau phase holding.

These results demonstrate that carcinogenic damage induced by alpha particles is inefficiently repaired. Because it seems likely that the target cells for transformation in many organ systems in animals may be nonproliferating stem cells or other quiescent cell populations with the potential for proliferation, the carcinogenic potential of alpha particles may simply be cumulative with dose. Thus, the ultimate carcinogenic effects of alpha particles would be underestimated by measurements made with dividing cells.

Transformation by alpha particles has also been studied by Lloyd et al (1979) using 5.6 MeV alpha particles generated by a Tandem Van de Graaff generator. Their results also confirm that alpha particles are more efficient than x-rays in inducing transformation, though dose–response and recovery data are not available.

Incorporated Radioisotopes

One component of the natural background radiation to which the human population is exposed is internally emitting radionuclides. Because there is little doubt now that DNA is the target macromolecule in carcinogenesis, radionuclides that can be incorporated into DNA are of particular interest. Two of these have been investigated for their potential in inducing neoplastic transformation in vitro.

Tritium (^{3}H) has been most extensively studied in the form of ^{3}H-thymidine. ^{3}H emits a beta particle in each decay with an average energy of 5.7 keV. The track length of this beta particle in water is about 1 micron. When ^{3}H-thymidine is incorporated into the DNA, therefore, most of the energy from the beta particles is deposited within the nucleus. Several studies in vivo have documented the carcinogenicity of ^{3}H-thymidine when injected into mice (Baserga et al, 1966; Armuth and Berenblum, 1979).

^{125}I decays by electron capture, emitting a photon plus on the average 21 very low energy Auger electrons. The transmutation product is ^{125}Te, which is highly charged and causes molecular fragmentation. Thus, the energy deposition from ^{125}I decay is extremely localized, and the LET can be considered to be very high. ^{125}I has been most extensively studied in iododeoxyuridine (IdUrd), which can be incorporated into DNA in place of thymidine. Chan et al (1976) showed that following incorporation into the DNA of V79 Chinese hamster cells, each decay of ^{125}I was 16 times more lethal than a ^{3}H decay. LeMotte and Little (1984) have further shown that in diploid human fibroblasts, incorporated ^{125}IdUrd is six times more efficient in producing double-strand breaks than incorporated ^{3}H-thymidine. Their calculation shows that, on the average, each ^{125}I decay results in one double-strand break.

Transformation studies with incorporated radioisotopes have been carried out by LeMotte et al (1982) with the Balb/3T3 mouse embryo fibroblast system. Two radiolabeled compounds were used, ^{125}IdUrd and ^{3}H-thymidine (labeled in the methyl group). Both are incorporated into the cellular DNA at the same positions. The amount of incorporated label was measured by scintillation counting of a known number of cells for each data point, and the dose expressed as picocuries per cell. The results of these transformation experiments are shown in Figure 5. ^{125}I was approximately 20 times more effective per decay than ^{3}H in transforming 3T3 cells.

Because ^{125}IdUrd was much more cytotoxic than ^{3}H-thymidine, these investigators also examined the transformation data for the two isotopes at equitoxic levels and compared them with the effects of external x-rays. Their data indicate that at equitoxic doses, the effectiveness of transformation was in the order of ^{125}I, ^{3}H, external x-rays. ^{125}I was particularly effective at low doses; in fact, transformation frequencies three times background were induced by ^{125}I doses that yielded no measurable effect on survival. Approximately 300 rads of x-rays were required to induce similar frequencies of transformation, a dose that killed approximately 50% of the cells. This high efficiency of low dose rate, high-LET radiation exposure in the induction of malignant transformation at low total doses is reminiscent of the results of Hill et al (1982) described above with low dose rate, high-LET neutron exposure.

FIGURE 5. Dose–response relationship for the induction of neoplastic transformation in mouse 3T3 cells by ^{125}I and ^{3}H incorporated into cellular DNA as ^{125}IdUrd and ^{3}H-thymidine. The doses are expressed in terms of picocuries per cell based on measurements of incorporated radioactivity at each point.
Reproduced from LeMotte and Little (1982).

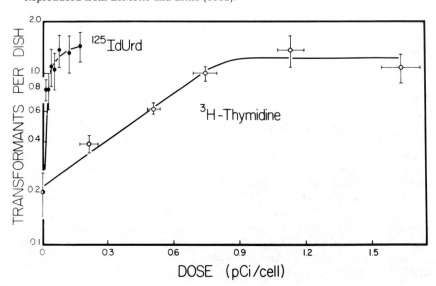

The mechanistic basis for this increased effectiveness of ^{125}I is not clear, although the higher efficiency for inducing DNA double-strand breaks is a reasonable conjecture. Martin and Haseltine (1980) showed that double-strand breaks induced by decay of incorporated [125]IdUrd may not be merely scissions of phosphodiester bonds; rather, up to five bases on both strands in the immediate vicinity of the decay event may be damaged and even eliminated. Such perturbations to the DNA, even if the strands are rejoined, can potentially lead to frameshift mutations. Frameshift mutagens have been suggested to be particularly effective carcinogens.

Influence of Repair Processes

Most of the ultimate biological effects of radiation on living cells are composite results of the initial molecular damage produced by the radiation and its subsequent modulation or repair by cellular processes. Although damage from ionizing radiation can be ubiquitous to all cellular constituents, the lethal effect of radiation has been thought to have its origin in damage to the cellular DNA (Little and Williams, 1977). The same is true of the oncogenic effect of radiation. While there are many lines of indirect evidence in support of an association between DNA damage and oncogenesis (Chan, 1981), recent DNA sequence comparisons between a silent transforming gene in the normal human genome and its activated counterpart in a bladder carcinoma (Reddy et al, 1982) strongly suggests that integrity of the cellular DNA must be restored after damage if oncogenesis is to be averted.

It is known from genetic and biochemical studies of prokaryotes and eukaryotes that multiple enzymatic pathways are available for the repair of DNA damage. It would be ideal if a specific repair process for a specific x-ray–induced DNA adduct could be modulated, and its influence on oncogenesis measured. The case of excision repair of ultraviolet (UV) light-induced pyrimidine dimers in xeroderma pigmentosum patients, or the photoreactivation of the same lesion in the fish, *Poecilia formosa*, provide examples of such an approach (Cleaver and Bootsma, 1975; Hart et al, 1977). As yet, there are no comparable studies of the oncogenic potential of an ionizing radiation-induced DNA adduct. While there are biochemical tools to measure several types of ionizing radiation-induced DNA damage, such as strand breaks and altered bases (Kohn et al, 1976; Hariharan, 1980; Paterson, 1978), it has not yet been possible to specifically modulate the cellular repair processes that deal with these lesions. Consequently, all transformation studies in vitro aimed at assessing the influence of repair have used conditions where cellular recovery from lethality was observed that has been inferred to result from the activity of DNA repair processes. Classical examples of such include dose-fractionation protocols. The molecular repair mechanisms underlying the phenomenologic observations associated with these protocols remain obscure.

Little and Williams (1976) described a very rapid, temperature-dependent, and dose-rate dependent recovery process in x-irradiated plateau phase cells. In subsequent experiments (Little, 1977), mouse $10T\frac{1}{2}$ cells were irradiated at either 37°C or 5°C with 600 rads delivered at a very high dose rate (95 rads/sec). After irradiation, the cells were immediately subcultured from plateau phase and seeded at low density to assay for clonogenic survival or transformation. The cells that were irradiated at 37°C showed both higher survival and a lower transformation frequency than cells irradiated at 5°C; survival was 1.5-fold higher, whereas, transformation was 7-fold lower. Cells irradiated at 5°C and held for 4 hr at 5°C showed no change in transformation, as was also the case for cells irradiated at 37°C and held for 4 hr at 37°C. However, cells irradiated at 5°C and held for 4 hr at 37°C showed a decline in transformation frequency to the level of cells irradiated at 37°C. It would be consistent with these results to hypothesize that at 37°C, but not at 5°C, there is an error-free repair process that is able to ameliorate both the lethal and oncogenic effects of radiation.

Another study by Terzaghi and Little (1975) involves the phenomenon of recovery from potentially lethal damage in plateau phase cells (Little, 1969). X-irradiated 10T½ cells held in the plateau phase before subculturing to reinitiate cell proliferation exhibit a recovery in survival that is complete within about 3 hr. Parallel transformation experiments showed that, concomitant with this recovery there occurred an enhancement in transformation. When the cells were held for more than 3 hr, a decline in the transformation frequency was seen. With long holding times (12–48 hr), the frequency declined below that seen with no plateau phase holding and to nearly background levels—a result similar to that reported previously by Borek and Sachs (1966) with hamster embryo cells and shown graphically for x-irradiated mouse 3T3 cells in Figure 4. These results may be interpreted as suggestive of two qualitatively different types of repair processes—a fast error-prone one operating in short holding times, followed by a slow error-correcting one operating at long holding times.

The molecular nature of these putative DNA repair processes remains unknown. Based on their results, Weichselbaum et al (1978) suggested that recovery from x-ray–induced potentially lethal damage reflects base damage excision repair, because cells from some ataxia telangiectasia patients are deficient in both this kind of recovery and repair activity (Paterson et al, 1976). This suggestion remains conjectural in the light of unresolved conflicting evidence on whether or not base excision repair is important to the highly radiosensitive character of ataxia telangiectasia (Ritter et al, 1977; Painter and Young, 1980; Smith and Paterson, 1980; Painter, 1981).

Radiation Exposure in Utero

Borek et al (1977) devised an in vivo/in vitro combination protocol for studying the oncogenic effects of exposure to x-rays in utero. Pregnant hamsters in the 12th day of gestation were irradiated, and the embryos were explanted immediately following irradiation. The cells derived from these embryos were cultured and serially passaged to assess the effects of exposure to carcinogens in utero. By the 7th–9th passage, transformation was evident, manifested by the appearance of morphologically altered foci. When cloned, cells from such foci exhibited growth properties characteristic of transformed cells. For an equivalent x-ray dose, the frequency of transformation in the case of irradiation in utero was reported to be at least tenfold lower than in the case of irradiation of cultured embryo cells in vitro.

NONCARCINOGENIC MODIFYING FACTORS

It has long been known that carcinogenesis is a process consisting of a number of sequential steps, some of which can be affected by agents or factors that alone are noncarcinogenic. This tenet is classically demonstrated by the two-stage mouse skin carcinogenesis experiments of the initiation-promotion protocol (Berenblum and Shubik, 1947). According to this protocol, a subeffective dose of carcinogen was applied to mouse skin and followed by repeated applications of croton oil, a noncarcinogenic irritant agent. Such a sequential treatment gave rise to many papillomas, whereas no tumors arose if either the carcinogen or the croton oil applications were omitted. Since the initial mouse skin experiments, the two-stage carcinogenesis phenomenon has been demonstrated in a number of other organ systems in experimental animals. The process of initiation and promotion, indeed, may be events general to carcinogenesis. Recent evidence indicates that although initiated cells may remain dormant until they are promoted to form tumors, they can also be inhibited from consumating the carcinogenic process. Several such inhibitors have been identified.

These findings are potentially of considerable importance to the problem of radiation carcinogenesis in the human population. Indeed, most members of the general population are exposed to only low levels of radiation, levels that may be equivalent to the subeffective dose of carcinogen used in the two-stage carcinogenesis experiments. Ultimately, the contribution of low doses including background radiation to the cancer risks of humans may be largely determined by secondary factors that promote radiation-initiated cells to consumate the carcinogenic process. If so, inhibitors of the promotion or expression phase of carcinogenesis offer an avenue for reducing human cancer risks without demanding the sacrifice of the many benefits of radiation to society.

A number of transformation studies in vitro have examined factors involved in the expression phase of radiation carcinogenesis. The following is a summary.

Tumor Promoters

Although many tumor promoters of diverse, unrelated chemical structures have been identified, most transformation studies in vitro have focused on the chemical 12-0-tetradecanoyl-phorbol-13-acetate (TPA). TPA is one of the most active phorbol esters in the classic tumor promoter croton oil. In addition to being a potent tumor promoter, this agent offers many structural analogs with differing degrees of effectiveness for promotion in mouse skin carcinogenesis, including the parent compound phorbol, which is totally inert for mouse skin promotion.

Kennedy et al (1978) showed that TPA can act as a promoter of x-ray transformation of mouse $10T\frac{1}{2}$ cells in vitro if applied repeatedly after x-irradiation. The experimental protocol involved treating $10T\frac{1}{2}$ cells with low doses of x-rays followed by addition of TPA in the weekly or twice weekly medium change during the ensuing 6 wk. The cells were incubated with TPA during the

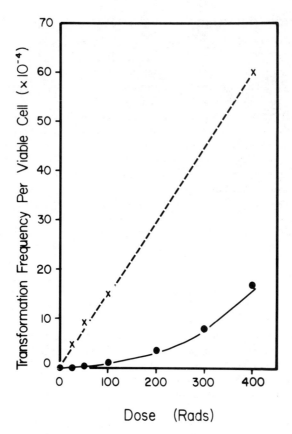

FIGURE 6. Dose-response relationship for the induction of neoplastic transformation in mouse 10T½ cells by x-rays alone (●) or by x-rays followed by treatment with the phorbol ester tumor promoter TPA (X). Incubation with TPA was begun 48 hr after irradiation and continued for the full 6-wk expression period.

Reproduced from Little (1981), by permission.

entire expression phase. TPA by itself was found to be either extremely weak or totally ineffective in transforming 10T½ cells. Kennedy et al (1978) found that the enhancement of transformation by TPA was most marked at low radiation doses. For doses below 100 rads, for example, the transformation frequency was found to be about 20-fold higher in the presence of TPA, whereas at a dose of 400 rads the transformation frequency was enhanced only by a factor of about 3. These results are summarized graphically in Figure 6.

As has been discussed earlier in this chapter, the transformation frequency of 10T½ cells declines when increasing numbers of surviving cells are seeded on each dish. It appears that TPA can partially ameliorate the suppressive effect of high cell density on the expression of transformation (Kennedy et al, 1978). Han and Elkind (1982) have recently confirmed this observation. One possible explanation is that the nontransformed cells exert an inhibitory effect on the growth of the transformed or potentially transformed cells, and that TPA reverses this inhibition. This suggestion is supported by the experiments of Sivak and VanDuuren (1970) who showed in cocultivation experiments that increasing the ratio of normal 3T3 to SV40-transformed 3T3 cells resulted in increasing inhibition of growth of the SV40-transformed cells. In the presence of TPA, however, this growth inhibition was not observed. Yotti et al (1980) also presented evidence that amelioration of cell-to-cell communication by TPA is central to its promotion actions.

Another observation of Kennedy et al (1978) is that the transformed foci arising from TPA promotion of x-ray transformation are predominantly of the type II category. Formation of type III foci was only minimally enhanced by TPA. This observation is interesting in that TPA promotion of mouse skin carcinogenesis produces largely benign papillomas. The parallelism between these in vitro and in vivo observations may eventually be revealing of some aspects of TPA action.

Another parallelism between the in vitro and in vivo action of TPA is that promotion by TPA is effective even when applied long after the initiating event. Kennedy et al (1980b) seeded $10T\frac{1}{2}$ cells at a low density of 300 surviving cells per dish, irradiated them with 400 rads of x-rays and allowed them to undergo 13 divisions to reach confluence. Such confluent cultures were trypsinized, diluted and the cells reseeded at 300 cells per dish. TPA was then added to these subcultured cells, which were allowed to proliferate to confluence and held in confluence for 4 wk as in the standard transformation experiment protocol. The results of these experiments indicate that beginning TPA treatment 13 rounds of cell division after irradiation resulted in transformation enhancement identical to cells exposed to TPA starting immediately after irradiation. Thus, the responsiveness of radiation-initiated cells to TPA promotion appears permanent, self-replicating, and undiluted by as many as 13 rounds of cell division.

Several other features of the promoting action of TPA are also borne out by these subculture experiments. The fact that TPA can be active 13 cell divisions after irradiation precludes the possibility that promotion is due to inhibition of DNA repair, or that TPA alters repair activities so as to convert premutational lesions in the DNA to mutations. This notion is also supported by the observation that exposure of cells to TPA for only 48 hr immediately following irradiation is ineffective for promotion. Furthermore, TPA promotion cannot be due to mere stimulation of cell proliferation by TPA, because cells replated to low cell density but deprived of TPA exposure showed no enhancement of transformation in spite of their being allowed 13 more rounds of cell division.

The expression of transformation in irradiated $10T\frac{1}{2}$ cells consists of a 2-wk active proliferation phase followed by a 4-wk quiescent plateau phase. TPA appears most effective when present during the 2-wk proliferative phase (Kennedy et al, 1980b). When exposure is limited to the quiescent phase, however, its effectiveness is also significant. Recently, Han and Elkind (1982) have shown that $10T\frac{1}{2}$ cells irradiated with neutrons are also subject to promotion by TPA. Thus, the responsiveness to TPA promotion can be initiated not only by low-LET radiation, but also by neutrons.

All of these studies have provided insight into the mode of action of TPA in the promotion of radiation transformation (Little and Kennedy, 1982). However, the understanding of the basic mechanisms of TPA promotion in terms of biochemical and genetic processes is still lacking. In biochemical terms, for example, suggestions have been made recently that TPA promotion acts via free radical processes (Nagasawa and Little, 1981; Emerit and Cerutti, 1981). In genetic terms, it has been suggested that TPA promotion acts by inducing mitotic recombination (Kinsella and Radman, 1978; Nagasawa and Little, 1979). The integration of these observations and hypotheses to provide a unified view of the role of TPA promotion in radiation carcinogenesis remains a much needed task.

Suppression of Transformation

A class of agents called the protease inhibitors have been shown to inhibit mouse skin carcinogenesis (Troll et al, 1970; Hozumi et al, 1972). The effects of these inhibitors of proteolytic enzymes on radiation transformation have been tested in studies in vitro. These studies have centered largely on antipain and leupeptin, two small-molecule protease inhibitors isolated from microbial origins. These compounds are much less cytotoxic than the synthetic protease inhibitors.

Kennedy and Little (1978b) reported that addition of 50 μg/ml of antipain to the culture medium for the entire 6-wk expression period in the 10T$\frac{1}{2}$ cell transformation assay resulted in complete suppression of x-ray—induced transformation, with no effect on cell survival. This was true for transformation induced by 600 rads of x-rays alone, or by 400 rads of x-rays plus continuous TPA treatment. Antipain alone at this concentration was neither cytotoxic nor transforming. Subsequently, Kennedy and Little (1981) reported the commencing exposure to 50 μg/ml of antipain as late as 4 days after irradiation was also effective in the suppression of radiation transformation. Alternatively, exposure to 600 μg/ml of antipain for only 1 day immediately following x-irradiation was partially effective in suppressing transformation. The effects of leupeptin on x-ray transformation were qualitatively similar to antipain, though it appeared slightly less potent and did not inhibit the enhancing effect of TPA as did antipain (Kennedy and Little, 1981). The effect of a large-molecular weight naturally occurring protease inhibitor, soybean trypsin inhibitor (SBTI), differed qualitatively from that of antipain and leupeptin. SBTI was ineffective in suppressing x-ray—induced transformation, but suppressed the enhancement of x-ray transformation induced by TPA. This is not unexpected, as SBTI probably does not enter the cell but acts at the level of the cell membrane, where TPA is also active. Thus, it appears that several proteases are involved in mediating the initiation and expression (promotion) of radiation transformation. The specificities as well as intracellular substrates of these protease inhibitors remain to be determined.

Because proteolytic degradation is involved in many cellular metabolic processes (Holzer and Heinrich, 1980), any protease inhibitor is likely to interfere with a variety of cellular functions. One manifestation of these pleotropic effects of protease inhibitors is the critical importance of the time of exposure to them in relation to radiation exposure. Borek et al (1979) and Geard et al

(1981) reported that exposing 10T$\frac{1}{2}$ cells to antipain for 24 hr prior to and during irradiation, with removal 10 min after irradiation, resulted in a twofold enhancement of radiation transformation. Conversely, if antipain was added 10 min after irradiation for 24 hr, a twofold suppression of transformation was observed. They also reported that the same pattern of enhancement and suppression of transformation occurred in Syrian hamster embryo cells using the same preirradiation and postirradiation antipain treatments.

How protease inhibitors can have such opposing effects on transformation is totally unknown. Hypotheses suggesting explanations for the enhancement of transformation by protease inhibitor pretreatment are particularly lacking. One hypothesis proposed to explain the suppression of transformation by postirradiation protease treatment suggests mechanisms similar to those of UV mutagenesis in E. coli. According to the so-called "SOS hypothesis" (Witkin, 1976), UV mutagenesis in E. coli requires the function of the umuC gene the repressor of which is encoded by the lexA gene. DNA damage by UV-irradiation signals the induction of the recA gene product in ways that are as yet uncertain. One of the functions of the recA protein is to proteolytically cleave the lexA-encoded repressor, which then causes the derepression of (among others) the mutagenic function. Mutations that render the recA protein proteolytically inactive also engender an immutable phenotype. Alternatively, if the proteolytic function of a wild-type recA protein was blocked by the protease inhibitor antipain, mutagenesis was also suppressed (Meyn et al, 1977).

Whether or not transformation in mammalian cells is mediated by similar proteolytic mechanisms of gene depression is unknown, beyond the observation that protease inhibitor treatment postirradiation suppresses transformation. Several lines of evidence, including ones discussed in earlier sections of this chapter, indicate that the phenomenology of transformation of 10T$\frac{1}{2}$ cells in vitro does not conform to expectations for single gene mutations. Thus, there may indeed by fundamental differences between the mechanism of protease inhibitor suppression of transformation in mammalian cells and its suppression of mutagenesis in E. coli.

Vitamins

Analogs of vitamin A, also known as retinoids, have been shown to inhibit oncogenesis, as well as the growth of transformed cells in a number of experimental systems, both in vivo and in vitro (Lotan and Nicholson, 1977; Merriman and Bertram, 1979; Moon et al, 1976). Harisiadis et al, (1978) first showed that in 10T$\frac{1}{2}$ cells the trimethylmethoxyphenyl analog of N-ethylretinemide (TMMP-ERA) inhibited radiation-induced transformation. This particular retinoid was chosen in their study because of earlier reports of its effectiveness as an antitumor agent with little toxicity. In the experiments of Harisiadis et al (1978), a 96-hr exposure of 10T$\frac{1}{2}$ cells to 7.1 μM of the retinoid TMMP-ERA, from 24 hr before to 72 hr after 400 rads of ^{60}Co-radiation, resulted in a greater than threefold suppression of the transformation frequency.

Miller et al (1981) used the same experimental system to show that TMMP-ERA suppressed transformation induced by radiation alone, as well as the enhancement of radiation transformation induced by the tumor promoter TPA.

With a 96-hr exposure to 7.1 μM of TMMP-ERA as just described, TPA was totally ineffective even though it was added immediately after irradiation and for the entire 6-wk duration of the transformation experiment. Thus, it appears that a transient exposure of x-irradiated cells to TMMP-ERA renders the cells permanently refractory to TPA promotion.

Merriman and Bertram (1979) also studied the effects of retinoids on transformation of 10T$\frac{1}{2}$ cells. Their study differed from those just described in two respects: 1) 3-methylcholanthrene, instead of radiation, was used as the carcinogen, and 2) three other retinoids were used instead of TMMP-ERA, namely all-*trans*-retinyl acetate, all-*trans*-retinol, and all-*trans*-retinal. In spite of these differences, it may still be of interest to compare the results of these different studies. Whereas, the results of Miller et al (1981) do not suggest the effect of retinoids to be reversible, the results of Merriman and Bertram (1979) indicate the opposite. They exposed 10T$\frac{1}{2}$ cells to 0.5 μg/ml of all-*trans*-retinyl acetate for 4 wk starting immediately after MCA treatment. The cultures were then maintained for an additional 1–5 wk in retinoid-free medium. The results showed that increasing the duration of this additional period in the absence of retinoid caused a progressive loss of the inhibition of transformation by the earlier exposure to the retinoid. Merriman and Bertram (1979) also showed that exposure of 10T$\frac{1}{2}$ cells to the retinoid from 7 to 14 days after MCA treatment resulted in a 70% inhibition of the MCA-induced transformation, which supports the hypothesis that retinoids act on the expression of transformation rather than on the initiating events.

Another vitamin that has been reported to suppress the expression of transformation in 10T$\frac{1}{2}$ cells is ascorbic acid. However, the effects of this vitamin have been studied only for methylcholanthrene-induced transformation (Benedict et al, 1980; Gol-Winkler et al, 1980) and appear to be reversible. It would be of interest to know whether or not ascorbic acid suppresses radiation-induced transformation, as well.

Hormones, Growth Factors, and Antiinflammatory Agents

There is evidence from animal studies that the hormonal status of the host exerts profound influence on the outcome of a carcinogenic treatment. The observation that the efficiency of transformation varies considerably with the particular lot of fetal calf serum used to supplement the growth medium (Little, 1979) raises the possibility that transformation in vitro is critically dependent on the abundance of certain serum factors, probably hormones or growth factors. However, fractionation of serum components for the identification of a critical factor has proven to be a difficult task.

Based on the observation that tumor growth in rats is suppressed by thyroidectomy, Guernsey et al (1980) examined the effects of the thyroid hormones on x-ray–induced transformation of 10T$\frac{1}{2}$ cells. They employed an ion exchange resin to selectively remove triiodothyronine (T3) and thyroxine (T4) from fetal calf serum. This resin treatment was thought to be specific for these agents, because other low-molecular weight organic anions and cortisol were only minimally depleted, whereas the concentration of T3 and T4 were reduced by

200-fold. The total protein content, as well as the electrophoretic patterns of serum proteins, also remained unchanged by the resin treatment.

Such depletion of T3 and T4 from the serum had no effect on either the growth characteristics of $10T\frac{1}{2}$ cells nor on their survival after x-irradiation. When x-ray transformation experiments were carried out with T3,T4-depleted serum, however, transformation was totally suppressed. Addition of chemically pure T3 to resin-treated serum restored the efficiency of transformation to the same level as was observed with untreated serum. These results suggest that T3 is needed for the expression of radiation transformation in $10T\frac{1}{2}$ cells. Guernsey et al (1980) further showed that in Syrian hamster embryo cells radiation transformation also required T3.

In order to elucidate the mode of action of T3 on transformation, Guernsey et al (1981) examined the time period in which the presence of T3 was obligatory for the support of radiation transformation. By varying the presence or absence of T3 at various time intervals, they found that the time period in which the presence of T3 was obligatory for the support of radiation transformation was the 12 hr prior to irradiation. If cyclohexamide was present together with T3 for this 12-hr period, the support of transformation by T3 was suppressed in a cycloheximide dose dependent manner. These results have led Guernsey et al (1981) to conclude that the initiation of radiation transformation requires cellular proteins the synthesis of which is induced by T3.

While the thyroid hormone T3 has been shown to be required for the expression of radiation transformation, but does not potentiate radiation transformation beyond what is observed in growth medium supplemented with normal serum, the glucocorticoid hormone cortisone has been shown to act synergistically with x-rays. Kennedy and Weichselbaum (1981) showed that continuous exposure of $10T\frac{1}{2}$ cells for 6 wk to $10^{-7}M$ cortisone was sufficient to induce transformation. Combined treatment with x-ray and cortisone led to a higher transformation frequency than the sum of effects from x-ray and cortisone alone. In contrast to cortisone, the glucocorticoid dexamethasone was marginally effective in transforming $10T\frac{1}{2}$ cells and in potentiating transformation by x-rays.

Another hormone-like substance that has been shown to potentiate radiation transformation of $10T\frac{1}{2}$ cells is epidermal growth factor (EGF). Fisher et al (1981) showed that incubation of mouse $10T\frac{1}{2}$ cells with 50 μg/ml of EGF, beginning 48 hr after irradiation with 100 rads of x-rays, and continued for the entire duration of the transformation experiment potentiated radiation-induced transformation by fourfold. On a molar basis, EGF was about ten times more effective than TPA in potentiating radiation transformation. Interestingly, melittin, a potent stimulator of prostaglandin synthesis, appeared to suppress x-ray induced transformation (Little and Kennedy, 1982).

Antiinflammatory agents have been reported to inhibit promotion in vivo. Both steroidal and nonsteroidal agents have been tested for their influence on the expression of x-ray transformation in vitro. Mouse $10T\frac{1}{2}$ cells were incubated with nontoxic or minimally toxic concentrations of these agents for the entire 6-wk postirradiation expression period. The nonsteroidal antiinflammatory agent indomethacin induced transformation by itself, but appeared to suppress x-ray transformation (Little and Kennedy, 1982). Indomethacin also inhibited the TPA enhancement of x-ray transformation. In contradistinction to these results, cortisone, which also induced transformation by itself, enhanced x-ray transformation (Kennedy and Weichselbaum, 1981). The effect of cortisone on the enhancement of x-ray transformation by TPA has not been tested.

Interferon

Brouty-Boye and Little (1977) reported that mouse interferon enhanced radiation transformation of 10T½ cells. A marked increase in the transformation frequency was obtained with continuous interferon treatment after irradiation with 400 rads of x-ray. Preirradiation treatment with interferon for 24 hr produced no statistically significant increase in transformation. Interferon alone was not found to induce transformation in 10T½ cells. Control experiments showed that trypsin or periodate-inactivated mouse interferon, as well as human interferon, were ineffective in enhancing radiation transformation. The mechanism of interferon enhancement of radiation transformation is undetermined. Because transformation of 10T½ cells by carcinogen treatment is not associated with induction of endogenous retroviruses (Rapp et al, 1975), it is possible that the enhancement of radiation transformation by interferon is unrelated to its antiviral activity.

The finding that radiation-transformed 10T½ cells have decreased sensitivity to the growth inhibitory effects of interferon (Brouty-Boye et al, 1979) raises the possibility that interferon facilitates the expression of potentially transformed cells by inhibiting the growth of the nontransformed cells. In this way it might be acting by a similar mechanism as does a reduction in serum concentration in the medium, which has been shown under some conditions to facilitate the expression of radiation transformation presumably by favoring the growth of the potentially transformed cells that have lost their serum dependence (Little, 1977). What is of interest is that the transformation-enhancing activity of interferon is species specific, as is the antiviral activity of interferon, because only mouse—and not human—interferon was effective. The relationship between interferon and transformation by nonviral agents needs to be further elucidated.

Hyperthermia and Radiosensitizers

In recent years, hyperthermia in combination with radiation has evolved as a promising therapeutic modality for cancer. In two separate reports (Harisiadis et al, 1980; Clark et al, 1981), hyperthermia alone was shown not to induce transformation in 10T½ cells. The data on the combination of heat and radiation appear conflicting. Harisiadis et al (1980) reported a twofold suppression of transformation by 2-hr postirradiation hyperthermic treatments ranging from 40°C to 42.2°C. Clark et al (1981) reported that heating the cells for 30 min at 43°C or 15 min at 45°C immediately prior to x-irradiation resulted in a two- to fourfold enhancement of transformation. In a preliminary report, Raaphorst et al (1980) reported that 1 hr at 42°C, either 10 min before or after irradiation, resulted in enhanced transformation. It appears from these data that the duration and temperature of the hyperthermic treatment and the dose of radiation, as well as the temperal relationship between the two are all important variables in determining the effects of heat on radiation-induced transformation. Further experimental classifications are obviously required.

Miller and Hall (1978) reported that exposure of $10T\frac{1}{2}$ cells for 3 or 6 days to the hypoxic cell radiosensitizer misonidazole resulted in significant levels of transformation. When the drug was administered in combination with x-rays, misonidazole potentiated the induction of transformation by the radiation. It is not clear from the data presented whether or not the interaction between the two agents was synergistic or merely additive. Because misonidazole is currently undergoing clinical trials for human use, it is of obvious importance to ascertain the oncogenic potential of this drug.

INTERACTIONS OF RADIATION WITH OTHER CARCINOGENS

Several studies with transformation systems in vitro have addressed the question of interactions between radiation and other carcinogens following sequential exposure. With both the hamster embryo and the mouse $10T\frac{1}{2}$ cells, a common thread that appears in the data is that x-irradiation followed by a chemical carcinogen results in synergistic potentiation of transformation. The degree of synergism increases with time between the treatments and declines after reaching a maximum. In the case of the hamster embryo cells, benzo(a)pyrene treatment following a minimally effective dose of x-rays resulted in a maximum synergism of tenfold when the two treatments were separated by 48 hr; prolonging this time interval to 72 hr resulted in a total decay of any synergistic effects (DiPaolo, Donovan, and Popescu, 1976). In the case of the mouse $10T\frac{1}{2}$ cells, a maximum synergism of a sixfold enhancement in transformation was found when x-irradiation preceded the benzo(a)pyrene treatment by 15 hr (Terzaghi and Little, 1974). These results are shown in Figure 7. When the time interval between treatments was increased from 15 to 25 hr there was a sharp decrease in the synergistic effect. When benzo(a)pyrene treatment was followed by x-irradiation, synergistic potentiation of transformation increased with the time interval between treatments from 0 to 30 hr and declined only slightly with time intervals up to 72 hr. Borek and Ong (1981) found synergistic potentiation of transformation when x-irradiation was followed 24 hr later by exposure to a carcinogenic pyrolysis product of DL-tryptophan. The degree of synergism increased with the x-ray dose.

The mechanisms underlying the synergistic interactions between radiation and chemical carcinogens are undoubtedly complex. Cell cycle related variations in the survival, mutagenic and oncogenic responses of cells to carcinogens are well documented (Watanabe and Horikawa, 1977; Grisham et al, 1980); clearly, additional work is required to define the role of cell cycle effects in the apparent synergistic interactions just described where the time intervals between treatments were short. However, the fact that significant synergistic action was seen in the data of Terzaghi and Little (1974) when the radiation and BP treatments were separated by as long as 72 hr suggests yet another level of interaction; i.e., effects of the second treatment on the process of expression of transformation induced by the first agent.

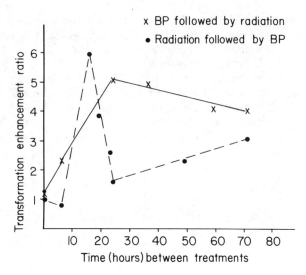

FIGURE 7. Interactions between x-irradiation and benzo(a)pyrene in the induction of neoplastic transformation in mouse 10T½ cells. Cells were treated either with x-rays (200 rads) or BP (2.5 mg/ml) at time 0, followed by the other carcinogen at various intervals of 2–70 hr later. The results are presented as the enhancement observed in the transformation frequency over that expected if the effects of the two carcinogens were simply additive.

Reproduced from Terzaghi and Little (1974), by permission.

CONCLUDING REMARKS

In concluding this review of radiation-induced neoplastic transformation in vitro, it should be emphasized again that cells in culture are but a model system for carcinogenesis in vivo. These experimental systems offer an approach that focuses on the target cells and, thus, the early stages in the carcinogenic process, before recognizable histopathologic changes would be seen in organized tissues. Nevertheless, the elucidation in culture of many phenomena originally associated with carcinogenesis in whole animals, such as the initiation-promotion stages and the dose rate effects for high- and low-LET radiation, lend support to the biological relevance of the systems in vitro. On the other hand, carcinogenesis is a complex multistage process influenced by many factors operating in vivo. Although studies of neoplastic transformation in vitro are particularly useful in examining mechanisms of the early stages of carcinogenesis, care should be taken in extrapolating observations such as dose–response and fractionation effects in cultured cells to the induction of human cancer.

The high frequencies of morphologic transformation observed in vitro, typically one to two orders of magnitude above the frequencies for single gene mutations (Chan and Little, 1978; Landolph and Heidelberger, 1979; Barrett and Elmore, 1982), as well as the evidence in some systems that nearly all of the cells in a culture may be initiated by even moderate doses of carcinogens

(Kennedy and Little, 1980; Kennedy et al, 1980a; Fernandez et al, 1980) remain to be fully explained. The results with recently developed in vivo/in vitro experimental systems suggest that the growth environment in vitro removes certain constraints that operate in the whole animal to halt the progression of an initiated cell into the formation of a full-blown tumor (Terzaghi and Nettesheim, 1979; Terzaghi et al, 1981). In this light, the transformation assays in vitro may be viewed as being optimized for the expression of any carcinogenically initiated cells. Such findings imply that the frequency of initiation in vivo may also be very high. The data of Terzaghi et al (1981), indeed, support this notion.

Another conclusion that emerges from these studies is that factors influencing the expression of the initial carcinogen induced change can greatly alter the ultimate yield of cellular transformation. Indeed, experimental evidence suggests that under some conditions noncarcinogenic secondary factors may be the controlling ones in radiation carcinogenesis (Little, 1981). Such factors include stimuli to and the capacity for cellular proliferation, environmental conditions including the levels of hormones and growth factors, as well as exposure to specific tumor promoters and inhibitors. In the past, these factors were thought to operate largely at the tissue and systemic, rather than the cellular, level. We now know that this is not necessarily the case. Finally, the experimental observations with the various inhibitors of transformation in vitro described in this chapter suggest that the expression phase of the carcinogenic process, rather than the initiation phase, can potentially be a fruitful target for chemoprevention of cancer.

Looking ahead, the development of quantitative transformation systems using cells of human and/or epithelial origins is the logical next step. Such systems will be useful for confirming and extending the results already obtained with rodent fibroblasts. Both in terms of elucidating the mechanisms of radiation carcinogenesis, as well as providing biological bases for the principles of radiation protection, transformation studies in vitro should continue to be a fruitful approach.

REFERENCES

Armuth V, Berenblum I (1979) Tritiated thymidine as a broad spectrum initiator in transplacental two-stage carcinogenesis with phorbol as promoter. Intl J Cancer 24:355–358.

Barrett JC, Elmore E (1982) Comparison of carcinogenesis and mutagenesis of mammalian cells in culture. In: Andrews LS, Lorentzen RJ, and Flamm WG (eds.), Mutagenesis and Carcinogenes. Berlin: Springer Verlag.

Barrett JC, Ts'o POP (1978a) Evidence for the progressive nature of neoplastic transformation in vitro. Proc Natl Acad Sci USA 75:3761–3765.

Barrett JC, Ts'o POP (1978b) Relationship between somatic mutation and neoplastic transformation. Proc Natl Acad Sci USA 75:3297–3301.

Baserga R, Lisco H, Kisieleski WE (1966) Tumor induction in mice by radioactive thymidine. Radiat Res 29:583–596.

Benedict WF, Wheatley WL, Jones PA (1980) Inhibition of chemically induced morphological transformation and reversion of the transformed phenotype by ascorbic acid in C3H/10T½ cells. Cancer Res 40:2796–2801.

Berenblum I, Shubik P (1947) The role of croton oil applications associated with a single painting of a carcinogen in tumour induction of the mouse's skin. Br J Cancer 1:379–391.

Bertram JS (1977) Effects of serum concentration on the expression of carcinogen-induced transformation in the C3H/10T½ Cl 8 cell line. Cancer Res 37:514–523.

Borek C (1979) Neoplastic transformation following split doses of x-rays. Br J Radiol 50:845–846.

Borek C, Hall EJ (1973) Transformation of mammalian cells in vitro by low doses of x-rays. Nature 243:450–453.

Borek C, Hall EJ (1974) Effect of split doses of x-rays on neoplastic transformation of single cells. Nature 252:499–501.

Borek C, Hall EJ, Rossi HH (1978) Malignant transformation in cultured hamster embryo cells produced by x-rays, 430-KeV monoenergetic neutrons, and heavy ions. Cancer Res 38:2997–3005.

Borek C, Miller R, Pain C, Troll W (1979) Condition for exhibiting and enhancing effects of the protease inhibitor antipain on x-ray–induced neoplastic transformation in hamster and mouse cells. Proc Natl Acad Sci USA 76:1800–1803.

Borek C, Ong A (1981) The interaction of ionizing radiation and food pyrolysis products in producing oncogenic transformation in vitro. Cancer Lett 12:61–66.

Borek C, Pain C, Mason H (1977) Neoplastic transformation of hamster embryo cells irradiated in utero and assayed in vitro. Nature 266:452–454.

Borek C, Sachs L (1966) In vitro cell transformation by x-irradiation. Nature 210:276–278.

Brouty-Boye D, Gresser I, Baldwin C (1979) Decreased sensitivity to interferon associated with in vitro transformation of x-ray-transformed C3H/10T½/2 cells. Intl J Cancer 24:261–265.

Brouty-Boye D, Little JB (1977) Enhancement of x-ray induced transformation in C3H/10T½ cells by interferon. Cancer Res 37:2714–2716.

Chan GL (1981) On the nature of oncogenic transformation of cells. Int Rev Cytol 70:101–137.

Chan GL, Little JB (1978) Induction of ouabain resistant mutations in C3H 10T½ mouse cells by ultraviolet light. Proc Natl Acad Sci USA 75:3363–3366.

Chan GL, Little JB (1979) Correlation of in vitro transformation with in vivo tumorigenicity in 10T½ mouse cells exposed to UV light. Br J Cancer 39:590–593.

Chan PC, Lisco E, Lisco H, Adelstein SJ (1976) The radiotoxicity of iodine-125 in mammalian cells. II. A comparative study on cell survival and cytogenetic responses to [125]IUdR, [131]IUdR, and [3]HTdR. Radiat Res 67:332–343.

Clark EP, Hahn GM, Little JB (1981) Hyperthermic modulation of x-ray–induced oncogenic transformation in C3H 10T½ cells. Radiat Res 88:619–622.

Cleaver JE, Bootsma D (1975) Xeroderma pigmentosum: Biochemical and genetic characteristics. Ann Rev Genet 9:19–38.

DiPaolo JA, Donovan PJ, Popescu NC (1976) Kinetics of Syrian hamster cells during x-irradiation enhancement of transformation in vitro by chemical carcinogen. Radiat Res 66:310–325.

Doudney CO (1976) Complexity of the ultraviolet mutation frequency response curve in Escherichia coli B/r: SOS induction, one-lesion and two-lesion mutagenesis. J Bacteriol 128:815–826.

Emerit I, Cerutti PA (1981) Tumor promoter phorbol-12—myristate-13-acetate induces chromosomal damage via indirect action. Nature 293:144–146.

Fernandez A, Mondal S, Heidelberger C (1980) Probabilistic view of the transformation of cultured C3H/10T½ mouse embryo fibroblasts by 3-methylcholanthrene. Proc Natl Acad Sci USA 77:7272–7276.

Fialkow PJ (1976) Clonal origin of human tumors. Biochim Biophys Acta 458:283–321.

Fisher MS, Kripke ML, Chan GL (1984) Antigenic similarity between cells transformed by ultraviolet radiation in vitro and in vivo. Science 223:593–594.

Fisher PB, Mufson RA, Weinstein IB, Little JB (1981) Epidermal growth factor, like tumor promoters, enhances viral and radiation-induced cell transformation. Carcinogenesis 2:183–187.

Fry RJM (1981) Experimental radiation carcinogenesis: What have we learned? Radiat Res 87:224–239.

Geard CR, Rutledge-Freeman M, Miller RC, Borek C (1981) Antipain and radiation effects on oncogenic transformation and sister chromatid exchanges in Syrian hamster embryo and mouse C3H 10T½ cells. Carcinogenesis 2:1229–1233.

Gol-Winkler R, De Clerck Y, Gielen JE (1980) Ascorbic acid effect on methylcholanthrene-induced transformation in C3H 10T½ cells. Toxicology 17:237–239.

Gray LH (1968) Radiation biology and cancer. In: Cellular radiation biology. University of Texas, M.D. Anderson Hospital and Tumor Institute Symposium on Fundamental Cancer Research. Baltimore: Williams and Wilkins Co, pp 7–20.

Girsham JW, Greenberg DS, Kaufman DG, Smith GJ (1980) Cycle-related toxicity and transformation in 10T½ cells treated with N-methyl-N'-nitro-N-nitrosoguanidine. Proc Natl Acad Sci USA 77:4813–4817.

Guernsey DL, Ong A, Borek C (1980) Thyroid hormone modulation of x-ray-induced in vitro neoplastic transformation. Nature 288:591–592.

Guernsey DL, Borek C, Edelman IS (1981) Crucial role of thyroid hormone in x-ray—induced neoplastic transformation in cell culture. Proc Natl Acad Sci USA 78:5708–5711.

Hahn GM (1980) Comparison of the malignant potential of 10T½ cells and transformants with their survival responses to hyperthermia and to amphotericin B. Cancer Res 40:3763–3767.

Hall EJ, Miller RC (1981) The how and why of in vitro oncogenic transformation. Radiat Res 87:208–223.

Han A, Elkind MM (1979) Transformation of mouse C3H/10T½ cells by single and fractionated doses of x-rays and fission-spectrum neutrons. Cancer Res 39:123–130.

Han A, Elkind MM (1982) Enhanced transformation of mouse 10T½ cells by 12-0-tetradecanoyl-phorbol-13-acetate following exposure to x-rays or to fission-spectrum neutrons. Cancer Res 42:477–483.

Han A, Hill CK, Elkind MM (1980) Repair of cell killing and neoplastic transformation at reduced dose rates of ^{60}Co-rays. Cancer Res 40:3328–3332.

Hariharan PV (1980) Determination of thymine ring saturation products of the 5,6-dihydroxydihydrothymine type by the alkali degradation assay. Radiat Res 81:496–498.

Harisiadis L, Miller RC, Hall EJ, Borek C (1978) A vitamin A analogue inhibits radiation-induced oncogenic transformation. Nature 274:486–487.

Harisiadis L, Miller RC, Harisiadis S, Hall EJ (1980) Oncogenic transformation and hyperthermia. Br J Radiol 53:479–482.

Hart RW, Setlow RB, Woodhead AD (1977) Evidence that pyrimidine dimers in DNA can give rise to tumors. Proc Natl Acad Sci USA 74:5574–5578.

Hill CK, Buonaguro FM, Myers CP, Han A, Elkind MM (1982) Fission-spectrum neutrons at reduced dose rates enhance neoplastic transformation. Nature 298:67–69.

Holzer H, Heinrich PC (1980) Control of Proteolysis. Ann Rev Biochem 49:63–91.

Hozumi M, Ogawa M, Sugimura T, Takeuchi T, Umezawa H (1972) Inibition of tumorigenesis in mouse skin by leupeptin, a protease inhibitor from actinomycetes. Cancer Res 32:1725–1728.

Huberman E, Sachs L (1966) Cell susceptibility to transformation and cytotoxicity by the carcinogenic hydrocarbon benzo(a)pyrene. Proc Natl Acad Sci USA 56:1123–1129.

Jones PA, Laug WE, Gardner A, Nye CA, Fink LM, Benedict WF (1976) In vitro correlates of transformation in C3H 10T½ clone 8 mouse cells. Cancer Res 36:2863–2867.

Kennedy AR, Fox M, Murphy G, Little JB (1980a) Relationship between x-ray exposure and malignant transformation in C3H 10T½ cells. Proc Natl Acad Sci USA 77:7262–7266.

Kennedy AR, Little JB (1978a) Radiation carcinogenesis in the respiratory tract. 5 In: Harris CC (ed.), Pathogenesis and therapy of lung cancer, a monograph in the series, "Lung Biology in Health and Disease," edited by C. Lenfant. New York: Marcel Dekker, pp 189–261.

Kennedy AR, Little JB (1978b) Protease inhibitors suppress radiation-induced malignant transformation in vitro. Nature 276:825–826.

Kennedy AR, Little JB (1980) Investigation of the mechanism for enhancement of radiation transformation in vitro by 12-0-tetradecanoylphorbol-13-acetate. Carcinogenesis 1:1039–1047.

Kennedy AR, Little JB (1981) Effects of protease inhibitors on radiation transformation in vitro. Cancer Res 41:2103–2108.

Kennedy AR, Mondal S, Heidelberger C, Little JB (1978) Enhancement of x-ray transformation by 12-0-tetradecanoyl-phorbol-13-acetate in a cloned line of C3H mouse embryo cells. Cancer Res 38:439–443.

Kennedy AR, Murphy G, Little JB (1980b) Effect of time and duration of exposure to 12-0-tetradecanoyl-phorbol-13-acetate on x-ray transformation of C3H 10T$\frac{1}{2}$ cells. Cancer Res 40:1915–1920.

Kennedy AR, Weichselbaum RR (1981) Effects of dexamethasone and cortisone with x-ray irradiation on transformation of C3H 10T$\frac{1}{2}$ cells. Nature 294:97–98.

Kinsella AR, Radman M (1978) Tumor promoter induces sister chromatid exchanges: Relevance to mechanisms of carcinogenesis. Proc Natl Acad Sci USA 75:6149–6153.

Kohn KW, Erickson LC, Ewig RAG, Friedman CA (1976) Fractionation of DNA from mammalian cells by alkaline elution. Biochemistry Washington 15:4629–4637.

Landolph JR, Heidelberger C (1979) Chemical carcinogens produce mutations to ouabain resistance in transformable C3H/10T$\frac{1}{2}$ Cl 8 mouse fibrolabsts. Proc Natl Acad Sci USA 76:930–934.

LeMotte PK, Adelstein SJ, Little JB (1982) Malignant transformation induced by incorporated radionuclides in Balb/3T3 mouse embryo fibroblasts. Proc Natl Acad Sci USA 79:7763–7767.

LeMotte PK, Little JB (1984) DNA damage induced in human diploid cells by decay of incorporated radionuclides. Cancer Res 44:1337–1342.

Little JB (1969) Repair of sub-lethal and potentially lethal radiation damage in plateau phase cultures of human cells. Nature 224:804–806.

Little JB (1977) Radiation carcinogenesis in vitro: Implication for mechanisms. In: Hiatt HH, Watson JD, and Winston JA (eds.), Origins of human cancer. Cold Spring Harbor Conferences on Cell Proliferation, Vol. IV, New York: Cold Spring Harbor Laboratory, pp 923–939.

Little JB (1979) Quantitative studies of radiation transformation with the A31-11 mouse Balb/3T3 cell line. Cancer Res 39:1474–1480.

Little JB (1981) Influence of noncarcinogenic secondary factors on radiation carcinogenesis. Radiat Res 87:240–250.

Little JB, Kennedy AR (1982) Promotion of x-ray transformation in vitro: In: Hecker E, Fusenig NE, Kunz W, Maraks F, and Thielmann HW (eds.), Carcinogenesis, Vol. 7. New York: Raven Press, pp 243–257.

Little JB, Williams JR (1976) Enhancement of survival of irradiated plateau phase cells by Dinitrophenol: Effect of dose-rate and cell strain. Radiat Res 66:90–99.

Little JB, Williams JR (1977) Effects of ionizing radiation on mammalian cells. In: Lee, DHK (ed.), Handbook in physiology, Section 9: Reactions to Environmental Agents. Bethesda: American Physiologic Society, pp 127–156.

Lloyd EL, Gemmell MA, Henning CB, Gemmell DS, Zabransky BJ (1979) Transformation of mammalian cells by alpha particles. Intl J Radiat Biol 36:467–478.

Loton R, Nicholson GL (1977) Inhibitory effects of retinoic acid or retinyl acetate on the growth of untransformed, transformed, and tumor cells in vitro. J Natl Cancer Inst 59:1717–1722.

Martin RF, Haseltine WA (1981) Range of radiochemical damage to DNA with decay of iodine-125. Science 213:896–898.

Merriman RL, Bertram JS (1979) Reversible inhibition by retinoids of 3-methylcholanthrene-induced neoplastic transformation in C3H/10T½ Clone 8 cells. Cancer Res 39:1661–1666.

Meyn MS, Rossman T, Troll W (1977) A protease inhibitor blocks SOS functions in *Escherichia coli:* Antipain prevents repressor inactivation, ultraviolet mutagenesis and filamentous growth. Proc Natl Acad Sci USA 74:1152–1156.

Miller RC, Geard CR, Osmak RS, Rutledge-Freeman M, Ong A, Mason H, Napholz A, Perez N, Harisiadis L, Borek C (1981) Modification of sister chromatid exchanges and radiation-induced transformation in rodent cells by the tumor promoter 12-0-tetradecanoylphorbol-13-acetate and two retinoids. Cancer Res 41:655–659.

Miller RC, Hall EJ (1978) Oncogenic transformation in vitro by the hypoxic cell sensitizer Misonidazole. Br J Cancer 38:411–417.

Miller RC, Hall EJ, Rossi HH (1979) Oncogenic transformation of mammalian cells in vitro with split doses of x-rays. Proc Natl Acad Sci USA 76:5755–5758.

Moon RC, Grubbs CJ, Sporn MB (1976) Inhibition of 7,12-dimethylbenz(a)anthracene-induced mammary carcinogenesis by retinyl acetate. Cancer Res 36:2626–2630.

Nagasawa H, Little JB (1979) Effect of tumor promoters, protease inhibitors and repair processes on x-ray induced sister chromatid exchanges in mouse cells. Proc Natl Acad Sci USA 76:1943–1947.

Nagasawa H, Little JB (1981) Factors influencing the induction of sister chromatid exchanges in mammalian cells by 12-0-tetradecanoyl-phorbol-13-acetate. Carcinogenesis 2:601–607.

Painter RB (1981) Radioresistant DNA Synthesis: An intrinsic feature of ataxia telangiectasia. Mutat Res 84:183–190.

Painter RB, Young BR (1980) Radiosensitivity in ataxia-telangiectasia: A new explanation. Proc Natl Acad Sci USA 77:7315–7317.

Paterson MC (1978) Use of purified lesion-recognizing enzymes to monitor DNA repair in vivo. Adv Radiat Biol 7:1–53.

Paterson MC, Smith BP, Lohman PHM, Anderson AK, Fishman L (1976) Defective excision repair of γ-ray-damaged DNA in human (ataxia telangiectasia) fibroblasts. Nature 260:444–447.

Raaphorst GP, Azzam EI (1980) The comparison of fixation of radiation, heat or radiation plus heat PLD in V79 cells by anisotonic NaCl solutions. Radiation Res 83:427–428.

Rapp UR, Nowinski RC, Reznikoff CA, Heidelberger C (1975) Endogenous oncornaviruses in chemically induced transformation. Virology 65:392–409.

Reddy EP, Reynolds RK, Santos E, Barbacid M (1982) A point mutation is responsible for the acquisition of transforming properties by the T24 human bladder carcinoma oncogene. Nature 300:149–152.

Reznikoff CA, Brankow DW, Heidelberger C (1973a) Establishment and characterization of a cloned line of C3H mouse embryo cells sensitive to postconfluence inhibition of division. Cancer Res 33:3231–3238.

Reznikoff CA, Bertram JS, Brankow DW, Heidelberger C (1973b) Quantitative and qualitative studies of chemical transformation of cloned C3H mouse embryo cells sensitive to postconfluence inhibition of cell division. Cancer Res 33:3239–3249.

Ritter MA, Nove J, Williams J (1979) The oxygen enhancement ratio for radiation lethality in ataxia telangiectasia cells. Intl J Radiat Biol 35:281–285.

Robertson JB, Koehler A, George J, Little JB (1983) Oveogenic transformation of mouse Balb 13T3 cells by Plutonium-238 alpha particles. Radiat Res 96:261–274.

Shilo B-Z, Weinberg RA (1981) Unique transforming gene in carcinogen-transformed mouse cells. Nature 289:607–609.

Sivak A, Van Duuren BL (1970) A cell culture system for the assessment of tumor promoting activity. J Natl Cancer Inst 44:1091–1097.

Smith PJ, Paterson MC (1980) Gamma-ray induced inhibition of DNA synthesis in ataxia telangiectasia fibroblasts is a function of excision repair capacity. Biochem Biophys Res Comm 97:897–905.

Terzaghi M, Little JB (1974) Interactions between radiation and benzo(a)pyrene in an in vitro model for malignant transformation. In: Karbe E and Parks JF (eds.), Experimental lung cancer: Carcinogenesis and bioassays. Heidelberg: Springer-Verlag, pp 497–506.

Terzaghi M, Little JB (1975) Repair of potentially lethal radiation damage in mammalian cells is associated with enhancement of malignant transformation. Nature 253:548–549.

Terzaghi M, Little JB (1976a) X-radiation induced transformation in a C3H mouse embryo-derived cell line. Cancer Res 36:1367–1374.

Terzaghi M, Little JB (1976b) Oncogenic transformation in vitro after split dose x-irradiation. Intl J Radiat Biol 29:583–587.

Terzaghi M, Nettesheim P (1979) Dynamics of neoplastic development in carcinogen-exposed tracheal mucosa. Cancer Res 39:4003–4010.

Terzaghi M, Nettesheim P, Yarita T, Williams ML (1981) Epithelial focus assay for early detection of carcinogen-altered cells in various organs of rats exposed in situ to N-nitrosoheptamethyleneimine. J Natl Cancer Inst 67:1057–1061.

Todaro GJ, Green H (1963) Quantitative studies of the growth of mouse embryo cells in culture and their development into established lines. J Cell Biol 17:299–313.

Troll W, Klassen A, Janoff A (1970) Tumorigenesis in mouse skin: Inhibition by synthetic inhibitors of proteases. Science 169:1211–1213.

Ullrich RL (1980) Carcinogenesis in mice after low doses and dose rates. In: Meyn RE and Withers HR (eds.), Radiation biology in cancer research. New York: Raven Press, pp 309–319.

Ullrich RL, Jernigan MC, Cosgrove GE, Satterfield LC, Bowles ND, Storer JB (1976) The influence of dose and dose rate on the incidence of neoplastic disease in RFM mice after neutron irradiation. Radiat Res 68:115–131.

Ullrich RL, Jernigan MC, Storer JB (1977) Neutron carcinogenesis-dose and dose rate effects in Balb/c mice. Radiat Res 72:487–498.

Vogel HH, Jr, Dickson HW (1981) Mammary neoplasia following acute and protracted irradiation with fission neutrons and ^{60}Cobalt gamma rays. Radiation Res 87:453–454.

Watanabe M, Horikawa M (1977) Analyses of differential sensitivities of synchronized HeLa S3 cells to radiation and chemical carcinogens during the cell cycle. Mutat Res 44:413–426.

Weichselbaum RR, Nove J, Little JB (1978) Deficient recovery from potentially lethal radiation damage in ataxia telangiectasia and xeroderma pigmentosum. Nature 271:261–262.

Witkin EM (1976) Ultraviolet mutagenesis and inducible DNA repair in Escherichia coli. Bacteriolog Rev 40:869–907.

Yotti LP, Chang CC, Trosko JE (1979) Elimination of metabolic cooperation in Chinese hamster cells by tumor promoter. Science 206:1089–1091.

SECTION III
CARCINOGENESIS IN EXPERIMENTAL ANIMALS

EXPERIMENTAL RADIATION LEUKEMOGENESIS IN MICE

KENJIRO YOKORO, Ph.D.

Leukemia is one of the best known neoplasms causally related to radiation exposure, in both humans and laboratory animals. Although experimental studies on radiation-induced leukemogenesis have been pursued in several animal species, studies in mice have been most fruitful in producing many valuable insights into leukemogenesis. This review deals with radiogenic leukemia in mice.

The leukemogenic effect of ionizing radiation in mice was first demonstrated in the early 1930s, in independent studies by Krebs et al (1930), Hueper (1934), and Furth and Furth (1936). These early findings enabled experts to predict the prevalence of leukemia and other neoplasms among the atomic bomb survivors in Hiroshima and Nagasaki, which is now an indisputable fact (Finch, 1984; Schull, 1984; Tokunaga, et al, 1984).

In the meantime, Furth (1978) succeeded in establishing a leukemia-prone mouse strain, Ak (presently known as AKR), and the viral nature of the leukemia in the mice of this strain was later shown by Gross (1951), who isolated a leukemogenic type C RNA virus from the leukemic tissues (passage A virus of Gross). The notion that a virus might be etiologically involved in murine leukemogenesis by ionizing radiation was motivated by this finding. Other epoch-making discoveries in leukemia research are mentioned below and are listed in chronologic order in Table 1.

TYPES OF LEUKEMIA

Thymic Lymphoma (Localized and Generalized)

This type of lymphoma (leukemia), originating in the thymus, is encountered far more frequently than other types of leukemia in most common strains of mice following exposure to ionizing radiation. A detailed histological study by

From the Department of Pathology, Research Institute for Nuclear Medicine and Biology, Hiroshima University, Hiroshima, Japan.

TABLE 1. Epoch-making Discoveries in Leukemia Research

1) Recognition of leukemogenic potency of radiation, chemicals, and hormones
2) Creation of a high-leukemia mouse strain, Ak (AKR), and isolation of a leukemogenic virus from Ak lymphomas
3) Demonstration of the "indirect induction mechanism" in radiation leukemogenesis, and isolation of a leukemogenic virus (Rad LV) from radiation-induced lymphomas of C57BL/Ka mice
4) Isolation of leukemogenic viruses from transplantable, solid mouse tumors
5) Proposal of "oncogene hypothesis"; concept of endogenous RNA viruses and their role in leukemogenesis
6) Role of recombinant virus (MCF virus) in leukemogenesis; mode of its involvement

Siegler et al (1966) revealed the unilateral initiation of the disease. The tumor cells are morphologically lymphoblastic and carry a cell surface antigen (Thy 1), which is one of the specific markers for the T lymphocyte.

Granulocytic (Myeloid) Leukemia

Myeloid leukemia in mice, developing either spontaneously or induced by leukemogenic agents, is much less commonly encountered and has been less extensively studied than lymphoid leukemia. In some cases the leukemic tissue exhibits a yellowish-green color, which is considered to be the counterpart of chloroma or chloroleukemia in humans.

Nonthymic Lymphoma and Reticulum Cell Sarcoma

The influence of radiation in the induction of these types appears to be less conspicuous than in the induction of other types (Upton, 1959; Ullrich and Storer, 1979).

FACTORS INFLUENCING RADIATION-INDUCED LEUKEMOGENESIS

The induction of radiogenic leukemia is modified to a large extent by radiologic, physiologic, and environmental factors. Kaplan et al, using C57BL/Ka mice as a model system, made many contributions to our fundamental knowledge of radiogenic thymic lymphoma (Kaplan, 1967, 1977). On the other hand, studies conducted by Upton et al (1959), Ullrich et al (1976), Hirashima et al (1982), and Mole et al (1983) have furnished much information about the induction of myeloid leukemia.

Radiologic Factors

Dose and Dose Rate. Exposure of 3- to 5-week old C57BL mice to fractionated total-body x-irradiation (four exposures of 150–170 rad each, at 5- to 8-day intervals) is highly efficient for inducing thymic lymphoma, resulting in the development of the disease in approximately 70%–90% of mice, with a mean latent period of approximately 150 days. This procedure also appears to be applicable to mice of most other strains.

In male RF mice, a single total-body x-irradiation of 150, 300, or 450 R, resulted in the induction of myeloid leukemia, as well as thymic lymphoma (Upton, 1959). In similarly irradiated specific pathogen-free RF mice, the incidence of myeloid leukemia was lower and the incidence of thymic lymphoma was higher than in their conventional counterparts (Ullrich and Storer, 1979).

With respect to the influence of dose rate, leukemia induction by low-LET radiation (x-rays or gamma rays) appears to be highly dependent on the dose rate (i.e., a lower dose rate results in a lower incidence), whereas, leukemia induction by high-LET radiation (neutrons) is relatively independent of the dose rate (Upton et al, 1970; Ullrich et al, 1976).

Total-Body versus Partial-Body Irradiation. Total-body irradiation is essential for efficient induction of thymic lymphoma; irradiation of either the upper half or lower half of the body drastically reduces the induction rate. Inhibition of lymphoma development is also achieved by procedures that shield benopietic cells from exposure, such as lead shielding of the exteriorized spleen, the thigh, or the thorax during irradiation (Kaplan, 1949; Lorenz et al, 1953; Kaplan and Brown, 1952a).

Induction of Leukemia by Radioactive Nuclides. Experimental induction of leukemia in mice by radioactive nuclides has been studied to a much lesser extent than induction by external irradiation. Brues et al (1949) were apparently the first to show the leukemogenic effect of radiophosphorus (^{32}P) in mice. Their observation was later reconfirmed by others, and the viral nature of ^{32}P-induced leukemogenesis was suggested by the presence of virus particles in the leukemic tissue and by the cell-free transmissibility of the disease (Holmberg et al, 1964, 1967; Takizawa et al, 1968). Ito et al (1969) observed the induction of nonthymic stem cell leukemia and reticulum cell leukemias, as well as osteogenic sarcomas, following a single intraperitoneal injection of radiostrontium (^{90}Sr, 10 μCi/g body weight).

Physiologic Factors

Age. Fractionated total-body irradiation, initiated at 3–5 wk of age, is most effective for thymic lymphoma induction, and the induction rate decreases rapidly with increasing age at exposure (Kaplan, 1947, 1948). In certain mouse strains, susceptibility to thymic lymphoma development is maximal when irradiation occurs at birth (Upton, 1959; Sasaki and Kasuga, 1981). In contrast, the induction of myeloid leukemia in RF mice is not much influenced by advancing age, up to at least 6 mo.

Sex. Female mice are slightly more susceptible to induction of thymic lymphoma, whereas, myeloid leukemia is more common in male mice. Ovariectomy or orchidectomy has little effect on the induction rate for either type of leukemia (Upton, 1959; Kaplan, 1950). However, administration of estrogens together with irradiation may promote thymic lymphoma, and androgens inhibit its development (Kirschbaum et al, 1949; Kaplan and Brown, 1952b). In RF mice exposed to single doses of gamma rays, there are no significant sex differences in the incidence of all types of leukemia combined (Ullrich and Storer, 1979).

Effect of Thymectomy and Splenectomy. Thymectomy prior to or shortly after irradiation practically eliminates the development of lymphoma, whereas, it has no effect on myeloid leukemia (Kaplan, 1950). On the other hand, splenectomy is highly effective in reducing myeloid leukemia, but has little or no effect on the induction of thymic lymphoma (Upton, 1959).

Immunologic Capability

Irradiation, in addition to any other leukemogenic action, may be expected to create favorable conditions for the development and progression of leukemia through immunosuppressive effects on the host (Haran-Ghera and Peled, 1968). However, the role of immunologic suppression in facilitating the leukemogenic process has not yet been clearly defined. Ito et al (1976) observed a long-standing suppression of both humoral and cellular immune responses in ICR/JCL mice following leukemogenic fractionated x-irradiation, whereas intraperitoneal injection of a leukemogenic dose of ^{90}Sr heightened the humoral immune response. Haran-Ghera (1976) inferred that the transient impairment of immunity following fractionated irradiation did not seem to contribute to the proliferation of preleukemic cells, and Sado (1983) also suggested that the immunosuppressive state is the result of lymphoma development, rather than the cause of the disease.

Recently, it has been reported that leukemogenic irradiation results in severe depression of spontaneous natural killer (NK) cell activity, and that the activity can be restored by bone marrow transplantation from nonirradiated mice (Parkinson et al, 1981). Moreover, the development of radiogenic lymphoma in mice has been significantly inhibited by the injection of a "cloned cell line with NK activity" shortly after irradiation (Warner and Dennert, 1982). The role of NK activity in T-cell lymphomagenesis deserves further exploration.

ROLE OF THE THYMUS AND BONE MARROW

Thymic Lymphomagenesis

The role of the thymus and bone marrow, and their interaction in T-cell lymphomagenesis, have been explored at length by several investigators (Kaplan 1967; Haran-Ghera 1976).

A series of experiments by Kaplan et al (Kaplan et al, 1953a, 1956, 1956, 1956; Carnes et al, 1956) demonstrated that the susceptibility of thymectomized mice to radiation-induced lymphomagenesis is restored by subcutaneous implantation of thymus grafts derived from newborn syngeneic mice. Furthermore, it was shown by them and by Law and Potter (1956) that a certain proportion of the lymphomas that developed at the site of the thymus grafts were actually of "nonirradiated" donor cell origin. Their findings have been reconfirmed recently in a congenic mouse system (Muto et al, 1983).

This "indirect induction mechanism" motivated investigators to speculate that total-body irradiation inactivates an "antileukemic factor" in the body, or activates a latent leukemogenic virus. Similar experiments in rats have appeared to support this idea (Yokoro et al, 1973).

From the preceding findings, it is clear that injury to the bone marrow by total-body irradiation is essential for the efficent induction of radiogenic thymic lymphoma.

Where, then, are the lymphoma cells derived from, and when does their malignant transformation take place? Haran-Ghera (1976, 1977) demonstrated the existence of potentially malignant cells in the bone marrow, but not in the thymus or in the spleen, within 30 days after fractionated irradiation. The results suggest that radiation-induced cell transformation takes place in the bone marrow, rather than in the thymus. On the other hand, a recent report (Boniver et al, 1981) has suggested that the primary site of the neoplastic transformation in irradiated C57BL/Ka mice is the thymus, rather than the bone marrow, in contrast with the findings of Haran-Ghera. At any rate, radiation-transformed cells occur eventually in both the bone marrow and the thymus. The thymic microenvironment, including the epithelial reticular cell network (Hiai et al, 1981; Yanagihara et al, 1981) may be essential for the acquisition of the T-cell phenotype and the initial proliferation of these cells.

Myeloid Leukemogenesis

There are relatively few studies of the mechanisms involved in radiation-induced myeloid leukemia in mice; however, the development of a quantitative assay method for hematopoietic stem cells and a long-term bone marrow cell culture system have permitted analysis of the pathogenesis of myeloid leukemia in connection with stem cell kinetics. Bessho and Hirashima (1982) have reported that overt myeloid leukemia occurred in 24.5% of RFM male mice 4–11 mo after exposure to a single total-body x-irradiation of 300 R, during which the level of colony-forming unit culture stem cells (CFU-C) in the marrow was significantly reduced. The occurrence of the disease ceased as the CFU-C level returned to normal. Potentially neoplastic cells could be detected as early as 18 days after irradiation, and were ultimately observed in 83.3% of mice, as demonstrated by the transplantation assay method. A significant difference in the incidence of overt leukemia and that of potentially neoplastic cells implies the intervention of some unknown host defense mechanism. Bessho and Hirashima have also observed an increased frequency of myeloid leukemia in x-irradiated mice given lipopolysacharide (LPS), which is a potent stimulator for differentiation of CFU-C to granuloid cells through the elevation of serum colony stimulating factor (CSF). A similar promoting effect of turpentine was previously noted by Upton (1959).

SYNERGISM OF RADIATION AND OTHER AGENTS

The synergistic action of radiation with other agents is of practical importance. Furth and Boon (1943) studied the synergism between radiation and methylcholanthrene (MC), and concluded that previous irradiation sensitizes hematopoietic tissue, thereby enhancing the leukemogenic effect of MC. Combined treatment with urethan and radiation is also effective in increasing the frequency of leukemia (Kawamoto et al, 1958). Yokoro et al (1969) have demonstrated synergism between radiation and Gross virus in inducing thymic lymphomas in young adult rats, under conditions in which either agent alone is not leukemogenic.

CYTOGENETIC STUDIES OF RADIATION-INDUCED LEUKEMIA

Various chromosomal aberrations have been observed in leukemic and non-leukemic mice following irradiation (Ford et al, 1958; Nadler, 1963; Joneja and Stich, 1965).

Dofuku et al (1975), using the trypsin–Giemsa banding method, first reported the occurrence of trisomies in several chromosomes, especially of chromosome #15 in spontaneous thymomas of AKR mice. Subsequent studies revealed that the trisomy of chromosome #15 is a nonrandom cytogenetic change commonly associated with mouse T-cell lymphomas induced by leukemogenic agents, such as radiation, chemical carcinogens, and certain viruses (Wiener et al, 1978, 1978; Chan et al, 1979). The significance of trisomy 15 in the pathogenesis of lymphoma may lie in relation to the DNA rearrangements that can result in increased expression of certain normal cellular genes (Klein, 1981).

In the case of myeloid leukemia, Wald et al (1964) found an extra marker chromosome in bone marrow cells of leukemic mice that had been injected with either leukemic cells or cell-free centrifugates originally derived from radiogenic myeloid leukemia in RF mice. They interpreted this, together with other findings (Parsons et al, 1962; Jenkins and Upton, 1963), as evidence that the changes in the chromosome are caused by a virus. Later, Azumi and Sachs (1977) found a consistent partial loss of the chromosome #2 in myeloid leukemic culture clones established from irradiated SJL/J mice. Their findings were soon confirmed and extended in radiation-induced myeloid leukemia in C3H/He and RFM mice (Hayata et al, 1979, 1983).

The consistent occurrence of these type-specific chromosomal changes in leukemic cells strongly suggests that such changes are associated with pathogenesis of the respective leukemias.

CONSIDERATIONS OF THE MECHANISM OF RADIATION LEUKEMOGENESIS

Activation of a Latent Leukemogenic Virus by Radiation?

Although many factors involved in radiation-induced leukemogenesis in mice have been explored, there is as yet no unified concept of the causative mechanism. As pointed out by Kaplan (1967), various findings indicate that the induction of radiogenic thymic lymphoma is difficult to explain simply as a consequence of a mutagenic effect of radiation on the target cells. In the early 1950s many investigators began to focus their attention on the causative implications of leukemia viruses. Interest stemmed initially from the isolation by Gross of a lymphomagenic virus (passage A virus) from spontaneously developing lymphomas of the AKR mouse (Gross, 1951). Gross (1959) was also the first to isolate a lymphomagenic virus (passage X virus) from lymphomas in x-irradiated C3H or C57Br mice. Lieberman and Kaplan (1959) were also successful in isolating a lymphomagenic virus (radiation leukemia virus, Rad LV) from radiogenic lymphomas in C57BL/Ka mice, which led them to conclude that Rad LV is the direct etiologic agent of radiation-induced lymphomas in this mouse strain. Their interpretation was subsequently supported by other investigators (Laterjet, 1962; Jenkins et al, 1963; Ilbery et al, 1964; Hiraki et al, 1964;

Haran-Ghera, 1966; Gross et al, 1968). The demonstration that chemically induced and hormonally induced mouse lymphomas (Toth, 1963; Irino et al,
1963; Ball and McCarter, 1971) were also transmissible by cell-free extracts
gave additional support to the belief that these leukemogenic agents acted
merely as the trigger for the activation of a latent leukemogenic virus already
present in the host. However, the origin, mode of transmission, and site or
mode of residence of the proposed virus remained unknown.

Oncogene Hypothesis and Endogenous RNA Viruses

In 1969, Huebner and Todaro (1969) proposed that the genetic information for
producing C type RNA viruses (murine leukemia virus, MuLV) is preserved in
every vertebrate cell, vertically transmitted from parent to offspring, and that
this viral information (virogene, including oncogene) plays a key role in transforming normal cells into tumor cells. According to this hypothesis, the activation of endogenous viral information is triggered by tumorigenic treatment or
natural aging.

The genetically transmitted endogenous RNA viruses have been subdivided
into three classes, according to their host range (i.e., ecotropic, xenotropic, and
amphotropic). The mink cell focus-inducing (MCF) virus (which is a recombinant virus of ectropic and xenotropic origin with amphotropic host range, is
suspected to be involved in the development of spontaneous lymphomas
(Hartley et al, 1977; Cloyd et al, 1980).

The oncogene hypothesis has had considerable impact on attempts to understand the mechanism of leukemogenesis, and its applicability has been
tested in a variety of experimental systems. Nagao (1977) investigated the appearance of ectropic MuLV infectivity in various tissues of intact, partial-body
shielded, and thymectomized female ICR/JCL mice following fractionated x-
irradiation, to evaluate if there was any correlation between endogenous MuLV
infectivity and the development of lymphomas in each group. The results
indicated that the expression of MuLV may not necessarily be related to the
development of lymphoma.

Decleve et al (1974) studied the appearance of Rad LV-associated antigen-
positive cells in tissues of C57BL/Ka mice following inoculation of Rad LV,
which was thought to be the causative agent of radiogenic lymphomas in
C57BL/Ka mice. They demonstrated that antigen-positive cells emerged only in
the thymus but never in other tissues; the number of positive cells in the
thymus increased gradually during the incubation period and eventually led to
the development of thymic lymphoma. A similar observation was made in W/
Fu rats inoculated at birth with the Gross MuLV (Kawamura, 1976).

In contrast to the above, Rad LV-associated antigen-positive cells were
rarely found in any tissues of C57BL/Ka mice following leukemogenic x-irradiation (Lieberman et al, 1976). Similarly, Ihle et al (1976, 1976) and Mayer and
Dorsch-Häsler (1982) found that expression of endogenous ecotropic MuLV
was not associated with radiation-induced leukemogenesis.

On the other hand, the transient appearance of MuLV group-specific antigen-positive cells in the bone marrow and thymus of mice several weeks after
x-irradiation was interpreted as evidence for viral involvement, even though

there was no viral expression in the established lymphoma cells (Haas, 1977). Jolicoeur et al (1980, 1983) have also reported that a recombinant B-tropic virus with ecotropic host range is regularly released from cell lines derived from radiogenic lymphomas in C57BL/Ka mice, emphasizing the etiologic role of the virus in radiation-induced leukemogenesis. However, our observation that there is no evidence of viral replication in cell lines established from radiation- or chemically-induced lymphomas in NFS/N mice, makes this a somewhat questionable interpretation (Yanagihara et al, 1984). Another report (Lieberman et al, 1971) suggests an inhibitory effect of interferon in radiation- and Rad LV-induced leukemogenesis when the leukemogenic stimuli are submaximal. On the other hand, however, our recent observations that radiation- and chemically-induced mouse leukemogenesis is not affected by intensive treatment with beta-type mouse interferon, whereas leukemia induction with Gross virus is completely inhibited by the same treatment, appears to favor a nonviral mechanism of radiation leukemogenesis (Yokoro et al, unpublished data).

Recently Proposed Hypothesis on Lymphomagenesis

Viral Promoter Insertion Hypothesis. This was first proposed by Hayward et al (1981) in the induction of B-cell lymphomas in chickens by avian leukosis virus, which is devoid of viral oncogenes (v-onc). They inferred that the development of lymphomas was due to the activation of a cellular oncogene (c-onc), through the insertion of a viral promoter sequence adjacent to the c-onc. Repeated virus infection might be required for the insertion of the promoter at an appropriate location, which may account for a long latent period of MuLV-induced leukemogenesis, compared with sarcoma induction by murine sarcoma virus (MuSV), which possesses v-onc. Observations in murine virus-induced lymphomas have also suggested that lymphomagenesis by MuLV can result from insertional mutagenesis of cellular oncogenes (Steffen, 1984).

Receptor-Mediated Leukemogenesis. McGrath and Weissmann (1979; McGrath et al, 1980) have proposed the receptor-mediated leukemogenesis hypothesis in which the continued presentation of MuLV (coding region for viral envelope glycoproteins, that are responsible for determining antigenicity and host range of the virus) determinant to the cell surface receptor acts as a mitogenic stimulus for the replication of MuLV-induced lymphoma cells. Ellis et al (1980) and Tress et al (1982) have observed that leukemogenesis does not show a simple dependence on infectious MuLV expression in radiogenic lymphomas, and that the expression of a recombinant env gene product on the lymphoma cells might play an important role in cell replication. Fischinger et al (1982), analyzing virus-negative radiogenic lymphoma cells of C57BL/Ka origin, emphasized that binding of non–virion-associated permuted gp 70s, which are glycoproteins, and the env gene products of radiation-altered proviral DNA to cell surface receptors might act as the signal for autostimulatory blastogenesis, leading to selective proliferation of receptor-bearing T cells. According to this hypothesis, no complete virus infection or expression of other viral antigens would be required.

Oncogene Activation. In the last few years, the association of oncogene activation and lymphomagenesis has been analysed, using both molecular hybridization and gene transfer techniques. Activation of oncogenes of the *ras* gene family appears rather common in the mouse T-cell lymphoma (Guerrero et al, 1984; Vousden and Marshall, 1984). The T *lym-1* gene also has been isolated from T-cell lymphoma cell lines by molecular cloning (Lane et al, 1984). The molecular approach to lymphomagenesis should be instrumental in elucidating the induction mechanism.

From these hypotheses and observations there is no doubt that investigations of viral oncogenesis have contributed much to exploration of luekemogenic mechanism, in general, and that the distinction between viral leukemogenesis and leukemogenesis by other agents is breaking down.

CLOSING REMARKS

Almost half a century has passed since experimental studies of leukemia—mainly in mice—were introduced as a model system for studying the etiology, pathophysiology, and treatment of human leukemia. At present, a counterpart for almost every form of human leukemia can be induced in rodents by the skillful use of various leukemogens, including ionizing radiation. Furthermore, recent advances in immunology, genetics, tumor virology, and molecular biology have been incorporated into leukemia research, resulting in rapid progress, especially in the investigation of lymphomas and lymphoid leukemias, as reviewed in this chapter. Continued efforts along these lines should enable us to arrive at a unified concept of radiation-induced leukemogenesis in the near future.

REFERENCES

Azumi J, Sachs L (1977) Chromosome mapping of the genes that control differentiation and malignancy in myeloid leukemia cells. Proc Natl Acad Sci USA 74:253–257.

Ball JK, Mc Carter JA (1971) Repeated demonstration of a mouse leukemia virus after treatment with chemical carcinogenes. J Natl Cancer Inst 46:751–762.

Bessho M, Hirashima K (1982) Experimental studies on the mechanism of leukemogenesis following the hemopoietic stem cell kinetics. Acta Haematol Japan 45:1296–1306.

Boniver J, Decle've A, Lieberman M, Honsik C, Travis M, Kaplan HS (1981) Marrow-thymus interactions during radiation leukemogenesis in C57BL/Ka mice. Cancer Res 41:390–392.

Brues AM, Aacher GA, Finkel MP, Lisco H (1949) Comparative carcinogenic effects by x radiation and P^{32}. Cancer Res 9:545.

Carnes WH, Kaplan HS, Brown MB, Hirsch BB (1956) Indirect induction of lymphomas in irradiated mice. III. Role of the thymic graft. Cancer Res 16:429–433.

Chan FPH, Ball JK, Sergovich FR (1979) Trisomy #15 in murine thymomas induced by chemical carcinogens, x-irradiation, and an endogenous murine leukemia virus. J Natl Cancer Inst 62:605–610.

Cloyd MW, Hartley JW, Rowe WP (1980) Lymphomagenicity of recombinant mink cell focus-inducing murine leukemia viruses. J Exp Med 151:542–552.

Decleve A, Sato C, Lieberman M, Kaplan HS (1974) Selective thymic localization of murine leukemia virus-related antigens in C57BL/Ka mice after innoculation with radiation leukemia virus. Proc Natl Acad Sci USA 71:3124–3128.

Dofuku R, Biedler JL, Spengler BA, Old LJ (1975) Trisomy of chromosome 15 in spontaneous leukemias of AKR mice. Proc Natl Acad Sci USA 72:1515–1517.

Ellis RW, Stockert E, Fleissner E (1980) Association of endogenous retroviruses with radiation-induced leukemias of BALB/c mice. J Virol 33:652–660.

Finch SC (1984) Leukemia and lymphoma in atomic bomb survivors. In: Boice JD Jr. and Fraumeni JF Jr. (eds.) Progress in Cancer Research and Therapy. Volume 26 Radiation Carcinogenesis. Epidemiology and Biological Significance. Raven Press, New York, pp. 37–44.

Fischinger PJ, Thiel HJ, Lieberman M, Kaplan HS, Dunlop NM, Robey WG (1982) Presence of a novel recombinant murine leukemia virus-like glycoprotein on the surface of virus-negative C57BL lymphoma cells. Cancer Res 42:4650–4657.

Ford CE, Hamerton JL, Mole RH (1958) Chromosomal changes in primary and transplanted reticular neoplasms of the mouse. J Cell Comp Physiol 1 (suppl):235–269.

Furth J (1978) The creation of the AKR strain, whose DNA contains the genome of a leukemia virus. In: Morse HC, III (ed.), Origins of inbred mice. New York: Academic Press, pp 69–97.

Furth J, Boon MC (1943) Enhancement of leukemogenic action of methylcholanthrene by preirradiation with x-rays. Science 98:133–139.

Furth J, Furth OB (1936) Neoplastic disease produced in mice by general irradiation with x-rays. 1. Incidence and type of neoplasms. Am J Cancer 28:54–65.

Gross L (1951) "Spontaneous" leukemia developing in C3H mice following inoculation, in infancy, with Ak-leukemic extracts, or Ak-embryos. Proc Soc Exp Biol Med 76:27–32.

Gross L (1959) Serial cell-free passage of a radiation-activated mouse leukemia agent. Proc Soc Exp Biol Med 100:102–105.

Gross L, Feldman GG (1968) Electron microscopic studies of radiation-induced leukemia in mice: Virus release following total-body x-ray irradiation. Cancer Res 28:1677–1685.

Guerrero I, Calzada P, Mayer A, Pellicer A (1984) A molecular approach to leukemogenesis: Mouse lymphomas contain an activated c-ras oncogene. Proc Natl Acad Sci USA 81:202–205.

Haas M (1977) Transient virus expression during murine leukemia induction by x-irradiation. J Natl Cancer Inst 58:251–257.

Haran-Ghera N (1966) Leukemogenic activity of centrifugates from irradiated mouse thymus and bone marrow. Int J Cancer 1:81–87.

Haran-Ghera N (1976) Pathways in murine radiation leukemogenesis-coleukemogenesis. In: Yuhas J, Tennant R, and Regen J (eds.), Biology of radiation carcinogenesis. New York: Raven Press, pp 245–260.

Haran-Ghera N (1977) Target cells involved in radiation leukemia virus leukemogenesis. In: Duplan JF (ed.), International symposium on radiation induced leukemogenesis and related viruses. INSERM Symposium No. 4. Amsterdam: Elsevier/North Holland Biomedical Press, pp 79–89.

Haran-Ghera N, Peled A (1968) The mechanism of radiation action in leukemogenesis. IV. Immune impairment as a coleukemogenic factor. Israel J Med Sci 4:1181–1187.

Hartley JW, Wolford NK, Old LJ, Rowe WP (1977) A new class of murine leukemia virus associated with development of spontaneous lymphomas. Proc Natl Acad Sci USA 74:789–792.

Hayata I, Ishihara T, Hirashima K, Sado T, Yamagiwa J (1979) Partial deletion of chromosome #2 in myelocytic leukemias of irradiated C3H/He and RFM mice. J Natl Cancer Inst 63:843–848.

Hayata I, Seki M, Yoshida K, Hirashima K, Sado T, Yamagiwa J, Ishihara T (1983) Chromosomal aberrations observed in 52 mouse myeloid leukemias. Cancer Res 43:367–373.

Hayward WS, Neel BG, Astrin SM (1981) Activation of a cellular onc gene by promoter insertion in ALV-induced lymphoid leukosis. Nature 290:475–480.

Hiai H, Nishi Y, Miyazawa T, Matsudaira Y, Nishizuka Y (1981) Mouse lymphoid leukemias: Symbiotic complexes of neoplastic lymphocytes and their microenvironments. J Natl Cancer Inst 66:713–722.

Hiraki K, Irino S, Sota S, Ikejiri K (1964) Leukemogenic activity of cell-free filtrates of radiation-induced leukemia of RF mice. J Radiat Res 5:1–11.

Holmberg EAD, De Pasqualini CD, Arini E, Pavlovsky A, Rabasa SL (1964) Leukemogenic effect of radioactive phosphorus in adult and fetally exposed BALB mice. Cancer Res 24:1745–1748.

Huebner RJ, Todaro GJ (1969) Oncogenes of RNA tumor viruses as determinants of cancer. Proc Natl Acad Sci USA 64:1087–1094.

Hueper WC (1934) Leukemoid and leukemic condition in white mice with spontaneous mammary carcinoma. Folia Haematol 52:167–178.

Ihle JN, Joseph DR, Pazmino NH (1976) Radiation leukemia in C57BL/6 mice. II. Lack of ecotropic virus expression in the majority of lymphomas. J Exp Med 144:1406–1423.

Ihle JN, Mc Ewan R, Bengali K (1976) Radiation leukemia in C57BL/6 mice. 1. Lack of serological evidence for the role of endogenous ecotropic viruses in pathogenesis. J Exp Med 144:1391–1405.

Ilbery PLT, Winn SM (1964) Indirect transfer of radiogenic lymphoma. Australia J Exp Biol Med Sci 42:133–148.

Irino S, Ota Z, Sezaki T, Suzuki M, Hiraki H (1963) Cell-free transmission of 20-methyl-cholanthrene-induced RF mouse leukemia and electron microscopic demonstration of virus particles in its leukemic tissue. Gann 54:225–237.

Ito T, Nagao K, Kawamura Y, Yokoro K (1976) Studies on the leukemogenic and immuno-logic effects of radiostrontium (^{90}Sr) and x-rays in mice. In: Proceedings of the 14th annual Hanford biology symposium on radiation and the lymphatic system, ERDA Symposium Series 37. Springfield: National Technical Information Service, US Dept. of Commerce, pp 209–217.

Ito T, Yokoro K, Ito A, Nishihara E (1969) A comparative study of the leukemogenic effects of strontium-90 and x-rays in mice. Proc Soc Exp Biol Med 130:345–350.

Jenkins VK, Upton AC (1963) Cell-free transmission of radiogenic myeloid leukemia in the mouse. Cancer Res 23:1748–1755.

Joneja MG, Stich HF (1965) Chromosomes of tumor cells. IV. Cell population changes in thymus, spleen and bone marrow during x-ray-induced leukemogenesis in C57BL/6J mice. J Natl Cancer Inst 35:421–434.

Kaplan HS (1947) Observations on radiation-induced lymphoid tumors of mice. Cancer Res 7:141–147.

Kaplan HS (1948) Comparative susceptibility of the lymphoid tissues of strain C57 Black mice to the induction of lymphoid tumors by irradiation. J Natl Cancer Inst 8:191–197.

Kaplan HS (1949) Preliminary studies on the effectiveness of local irradiation in the induction of lymphoid tumors in mice. J Natl Cancer Inst 10:267–270.

Kaplan HS (1950) Influence of thymectomy, splenectomy and gonadectomy on induction of radiation-induced lymphoid tumors in strain C57 Black mice. J Natl Cancer Inst 11:83–90.

Kaplan HS (1967) On the natural history of the murine leukemias: Presidential address. Cancer Res 27:1325–1340.

Kaplan HS (1977) Interaction between radiation and viruses in the induction of murine thymic lymphomas and lymphatic leukemias. In: Duplan JF (ed.), International sym-posium on radiation-induced leukemogenesis and related viruses. INSERM Sympo-sium No. 4. Amsterdam: Elsevier/North Holland Biomedical Press, pp 1–18.

Kaplan HS, Brown MB (1952a) Protection against radiation-induced lymphoma develop-ment by shielding and partial-body irradiation of mice. Cancer Res 12:441–444.

Kaplan HS, Brown MB (1952b) Testosterone prevention of postirradiation lymphomas in C57 Black mice. Cancer Res 12:445–447.

Kaplan HS, Brown MB, Hirsch BB, Carnes WH (1956) Indirect induction of lymphomas in irradiated mice. II. Factor of irradiation of the host. Cancer Res 16:426–428.

Kaplan HS, Brown MB, Paull J (1953a) Influence of postirradiation thymectomy and of thymic implants on lymphoid tumor incidence in C57BL mice. Cancer Res 13:677–680.

Kaplan HS, Brown MB, Paull J (1953b) Influence of bone marrow injection on involution and neoplasia of mouse thymus after systemic irradiation. J Natl Cancer Inst 14:303–316.

Kaplan HS, Carnes WH, Brown MB, Hirsch BB (1956) Indirect induction of lymphomas in irradiated mice. 1. Tumor incidence and morphology in mice bearing non-irradiated thymic grafts. Cancer Res 16:422–425.

Kaplan HS, Hirsch BB, Brown MB (1956) Indirect induction of lymphomas in irradiated mice. IV. Genetic evidence of the origin of the tumor cells from the thymic grafts. Cancer Res 16:434–436.

Kawamoto S, Ida N, Kirschbaum A, Taylor HG (1958) Urethane and leukemogenesis in mice. Cancer Res 18:725–729.

Kawamura U (1976) Type-C RNA viruses and leukemogenesis: Association of Gross strain of murine leukemia virus infection and leukemogenesis in rats. J Natl Cancer Inst 56:927–930.

Kirschbaum A, Shapiro JR, Mixer HW (1949) Synergistic action of estrogenic hormone and x-rays in inducing thymic lymphosarcoma of mice. Proc Soc Exp Biol Med 72:632–634.

Klein G (1981) The role of gene dosage and genetic transpositions in carcinogenesis. Nature 294:313–318.

Krebs C, Rask-Nielsen HC, Wagner A (1930) The origin of lymphosarcomatosis and its relation to other forms of leucosis in white mice. Acta Radiol 10 (suppl):1–53.

Lane M, Sainten A, Doherty KM, Cooper GM (1984) Isolation and characterization of a stage-specific transforming gene, T lym-1, from T-cell lymphomas. Proc Natl Acad Sci USA 81:2227–2231.

Latarjet R, Duplan JF (1962) Experiment and discussion on leukemogenesis by cell-free extracts of radiation-induced leukemia in mice. Int J Radiat Biol 5:339–344.

Law LW, Potter M (1956) The behavior in transplant of lymphocytic neoplasms arising from parental thymic grafts in irradiated, thymectomized hybrid mice. Proc Natl Acad Sci USA 42:160–167.

Lieberman M, Kaplan HS (1959) Leukemogenic activity of filtrates from radiation-induced lymphoid tumors of mice. Science 130:387–388.

Lieberman M, Kaplan HS, Decleve A (1976) Anomalous viral expression in radiogenic lymphomas of C57BL/Ka mice. In: Yuhas JM, Tennant RW, and Regen JD (eds.), Biology of radiation carcinogenesis. New York: Raven Press, pp 237–244.

Lieberman M, Merigan TC, Kaplan HS (1971) Inhibition of radiogenic lymphoma development in mice by interferon. Proc Soc Exp Biol Med 138:575–578.

Lorenz E, Congdon CC, Uphoff D (1953) Prevention of irradiation induced lymphoid tumors in C57BL mice by spleen protection. J Natl Cancer Inst 14:291–297.

Mayer A, Dorsch-Häsler K (1982) Endogenous MuLV infection does not contribute to onset of radiation- or carcinogen-induced murine thymoma. Nature 295:253–255.

McGrath MS, Pillemer E, Weissman IL (1980) Murine leukemogenesis: Monoclonal antibodies to T-cell determinants arrest T-lymphoma cell proliferation. Nature 285:259–261.

McGrath MS, Weissman IL (1979) AKR leukemogenesis: Identification and biological significance of thymic lymphoma receptors for KAK retroviruses. Cell 17:65–75.

Mole RH, Papworth DG, Corp MJ (1983) The dose-response for x-ray induction of myeloid leukaemia in male CBA/H mice. Br J Cancer 47:285–291.

Muto M, Sado T, Hayata I, Kamisaku H, Nagasawa F, Kubo E (1983) Reconfirmation of indirect induction of radiogenic lymphomas using thymectomized, irradiated B10 mice grafted with neonatal thymuses from Thy 1 congenic donors. Cancer Res 43:3822–3827.

Nadler CF (1963) Chromosomal patterns of irradiated leukemic and nonleukemic C57BL/ 6J mice. J Natl Cancer Inst 30:923–931.

Nagao K (1977) Type-C RNA virus and leukemogenesis: Lack of correlation between expression of endogenous, ecotropic murine leukemia virus and radiation leukemogenesis in mice. Hiroshima J Med Sci 26:177–188.

Parkinson DR, Brightman RP, Waksal SD (1981) Altered natural killer cell biology in C57BL/6 mice after leukemogenic split-dose irradiation. J Immunol 126:1460–1464.

Parsons DF, Upton AC, Bender MA, Jenkins VK, Nelson ES, Johnson RR (1962) Electron microscopic observations on primary and serially passaged radiation-induced myeloid leukemias of the RF mice. Cancer Res 22:728–736.

Rassart E, Sankar-Mistry P, Lemay G, Des Groseillers L, Jolicoeur P (1983) New class of leukemogenic ecotropic recombinant murine leukemia virus isolated from radiation-induced thymomas of C57BL/6 mice. J Virol 45:565–575.

Sado T (1983) Personal communication from National Institute of Radiological Sciences, Chiba, Japan.

Sankar-Mistry P, Jolicoeur P (1980) Frequent isolation of ecotropic murine leukemia virus after x-ray irradiation of C57BL/6 mice and establishment of producer lymphoid cell lines from radiation-induced lymphomas. J Virol 35:270–275.

Sasaki S, Kasuga T (1981) Life-shortening and carcinogenesis in mice irradiated neonatally with x rays. Radiat Res 88:313–325.

Schull WJ (1984) Atomic bomb survivors: Patterns of cancer risk. In: Boice JD Jr. and Fraumeni JF Jr. (eds.) Progress in Cancer Research and Therapy. Volume 26 Radiation Carcinogenesis. Epidemiology and Biological Significance. New York: Raven Press, pp 21–36.

Siegler R, Harrell W, Rich MA (1966) Pathogenesis of radiation-induced thymic lymphoma in mice. J Natl Cancer Inst 37:105–121.

Steffen D (1984) Proviruses are adjacent to c-myc in some murine leukemia virus-induced lymphomas. Proc Natl Acad Sci USA 81:2097–2101.

Takizawa S, Ito A, Kawase A, Yamasaki T, Nishihara H, Yokoro K (1968) Induction of leukemia in mice with radioactive phosphorus (^{32}P) and its modification by thymectomy and splenectomy. J Kyushu Hematol Soc 18:1–7.

Tokunaga M, Land CE, Yamamoto T, Asano M, Tokuoka S, Ezaki H, Nishimori I, Fujikura T (1984) Breast cancer among atomic bomb survivors. In: Boice JD Jr. and Fraumeni JF Jr. (eds.) Progress in Cancer Research and Therapy. Volume 26 Radiation Carcinogenesis. Epidemiology and Biological Significance. New York: Raven Press, pp 45–56.

Toth B (1963) Development of malignant lymphomas by cell-free filtrates prepared from a chemically induced mouse lymphoma. Proc Soc Exp Biol Med 112:873–875.

Tress E, Pierotti M, DeLeo AB, O'Donnell PV, Fleisner E (1982) Endogenous murine leukemia virus-encoded proteins in radiation leukemias of BALB/c mice. Virology 117:207–218.

Ullrich RL, Jernigan MC, Cosgrove GE, Satterfield LC, Bowles ND, Storer JB (1976) The influence of dose and dose rate on the induction of neoplastic disease in RFM mice after neutron irradiation. Radiat Res 68:115–131.

Ullrich RL, Storer JB (1979) Influence of γ irradiation on the development of neoplastic disease in mice. 1. Reticular tissue tumors. Radiat Res 80:303–316.

Upton AC (1959) Studies on the mechanism of leukemogenesis by ionizing radiation. In: Wolstenholm GEW (ed.), Carcinogenesis, mechanism of action. A Ciba Foundation Symposium. Boston: Little Brown, pp 249–268.

Upton AC, Randolph ML, Conklin JW (1970) Late effects of fast neutrons and gamma rays in mice as influenced by the dose rate of irradiation: Induction of neoplasia. Radiat Res 41:467–491.

Vousden KH, Marshall CJ (1984) Three different activated ras genes in mouse tumours; evidence for oncogene activation during progression of a mouse lymphoma. EMBO J 3:913–917.

Wald N, Upton AC, Jenkins VK, Borges WH (1964) Radiation-induced mouse leukemia:

Consistent occurrence of an extra and a marker chromosome. Science 143:810–813.

Warner JF, Dennert G (1982) Effects of a cloned cell line with NK activity on bone marrow transplants, tumour development and metastasis in vivo. Nature 300:31–34.

Wiener F, Ohno S, Spira J, Haran-Ghera N, Klein G (1978) Chromosome changes (Trisomies #15 and 17) associated with tumor progression in leukemia induced by radiation leukemia virus. J Natl Cancer Inst 61:227–237.

Wiener F, Spira J, Ohno S, Haran-Ghera N, Klein G (1978) Chromosome changes (Trisomy 15) in murine T-cell leukemia induced by 7,12-dimethylbenz(a)anthracene (DMBA). Int J Cancer 22:447–453.

Yanagihara K, Kajitani T, Kamiya K, Yokoro K (1981) In vitro studies on the mechanism of leukemogenesis. I. Establishment and characterization of cell lines derived from the thymic epithelial reticulum cell of the mouse. Leukemia Res 5:321–329.

Yanagihara K, Seyama T, Yokoro K (1985) Establishment of virus-negative cell lines derived from radiation- or chemically-induced T-cell lymphomas in NFS/N mice, and generation of oncogenic virus from these cell lines following infection of a non-oncogenic ectropic virus. In: Furmanski P, Hager JC and Rich MA (eds.) Proceedings of the international conference on RNA tumor viruses in human cancer. Boston: Martinus Nijhoff Publishing, pp 372–381.

Yokoro K, Imamura N, Kajihara H, Nakano M, Takizawa S (1973) Association of virus in radiation and chemical leukemogenesis in rats and mice. In: Dutcher RM and Chieco-Bianchi L (eds.), Unifying concepts of leukemia. Basel: Karger, pp 603–616.

Yokoro K, Ito T, Imamura N, Kawase A, Yamasaki T (1969) Synergistic action of radiation and virus in induction of leukemia in rats. Cancer Res 29:1973–1976.

EXPERIMENTAL CARCINOGENESIS IN THE RESPIRATORY TRACT

W. J. BAIR, Ph.D.

Information about respiratory tract carcinogenesis by external irradiation has come mostly from whole-body exposure of animals to x-rays, gamma rays, and neutrons. Because the frequencies of respiratory tract tumors induced in the exposed animals were low, compared with the frequencies of tumors at other sites, little information was obtained regarding the pathogenesis of such tumors. Most of the information about radiation-induced respiratory tract tumors in experimental animals has resulted from studies with radionuclides deposited in the respiratory tract by inhalation or intratracheal instillation. In these experiments, the radionuclides of greatest interest were those having long retention times in the lungs and long radiologic half-lives in relation to the life span of the experimental animals. Thus, even if only one deposition occurred, the lungs and associated tissues were irradiated continuously for long periods. Animal experiments have also been carried out with the short half-lived radon and its decay products, which were identified as the probable cause of the increased incidence of lung cancer in uranium miners and other miners over 30 yr ago. With the exception of the miner experience, animal experiments have yielded the only direct evidence of carcinogenesis in the lung by inhaled radionuclides.

This chapter will identify the respiratory tract tissues irradiated, describe the carcinogenic response, and summarize information about the carcinogenic response in relation to the spatial and temporal distribution of the radiation dose.

To many persons, designation of tumors as malignant or benign is objectionable on the grounds that a clear distinction cannot be drawn between tumors that remain localized, limited in growth potential, noninvasive, and are rarely fatal and those that almost always lead to death through invasion and metasta-

From the Environment, Health, and Safety Research Program, Battelle Pacific Northwest Laboratories, Richland, Washington.

sis. Contributing to this uncertainty is an inconsistency in the classification and terminology of the broad spectrum of tumors occurring in the respiratory tract in experimental animals of many species and strains. To minimize this source of confusion, only tumors clearly considered by the investigators of the original articles as likely or potential causes of death will be considered in this chapter.

TISSUES IRRADIATED

In animals exposed to radiation from external sources, all parts of the respiratory tract are usually assumed to be irradiated relatively uniformly. However, when the radiation sources are radionuclides deposited as particles in the respiratory tract, uniform irradiation is rare, only being approached when the radionuclide emits gamma radiation of sufficient energy to allow penetration throughout the lungs, bronchi, trachea, larynx, and nasopharynx. Usually irradiation by deposited radionuclides is quite nonuniform and becomes even more so as the particles are gradually sequestered in lymphatics and scar tissue. The least uniform irradiation occurs with insoluble radionuclide particles that emit alpha radiation, which will only penetrate for about 50–70 μm in tissue, depending upon the energy of the alpha radiation; the distance of penetration may be extended appreciably if the alpha radiation passes through open spaces (i.e., the lumina of airways). Beta radiation, depending on its energy, may penetrate up to several centimeters from its source and will irradiate respiratory tract structures more uniformly than alpha radiation, but much less uniformly than gamma or x-radiation. Uniformity of dose will also be influenced by the size and number of radioactive particles deposited. Respiratory excursions and any mobilization of radioactive particles that may occur will tend to broaden the distribution of the absorbed energy.

Cells potentially irradiated by radionuclides entering the respiratory tract include all those lining the airways from the nose to sites in the lungs where the radionuclides are deposited, incorporated into cells, or absorbed into the circulating blood and/or lymph. Unless radionuclides are deposited on the walls of the airways, the cells lining the airways are subjected to only brief radiation exposure as the radionuclides pass into the lungs. Further exposure of airways may occur if a radionuclide remains suspended in the air and is exhaled, if it is transported along the surface of the airways from the site of deposition in mucus moved by ciliated lining cells, or if it is moved from the site of deposition by intrapulmonary routes (e.g., lymphatics that are in close proximity to the airways) (Brundelet, 1965). The site of deposition of particles containing radionuclides depends on their size and density, as well as the velocity of the inspired air. Deposition of particles on the surfaces of airways containing ciliated and mucus-secreting cells is usually followed by prompt clearance from the respiratory tract. Deposition in the alveolar region generally decreases the probability of early clearance by the mucociliary escalator and frequently results in phagocytosis of particles by alveolar macrophages and alveolar epithelium, which may lead to long-term retention of a small fraction of highly insoluble particles in bronchiolar, alveolar, and lymphatic structures. A larger portion of the more insoluble particles may be transported to lymph nodes draining the respiratory tract. As solubilization occurs, most of the radionuclide is absorbed into the circulating blood and eventually deposited in other tissues or excreted, but some may be chemically bound in the lungs and retained for long periods.

From the above, it can be concluded that all of the more than 40 different types of cells (Sorokin, 1970) in the respiratory tract may receive radiation from external sources, but that only some of these may be irradiated by internally deposited radionuclides, of which some cell types may be much more heavily irradiated than others. The cell types irradiated by internally deposited radionuclides can be separated into one category that receives transient exposure during passage of particles through the airways or during short-term residence of radionuclides, and a second category of potentially more heavily irradiated cells, such as cells and their progeny that are long-term depots for radionuclides or are adjacent to such depots. Among the types in the first category are ciliated, goblet, basal, brush, small-granule, serous acinar, and mucous acinar cells of the trachea and bronchial epithelium; chondrocytes of the cartilaginous rings lining the larger airways; endothelial cells of blood and lymph vessels; smooth muscle cells; and probably some nerve cells. The more heavily irradiated category would contain epithelial cells of the bronchioloalveolar region, such as nonciliated bronchiolar (Clara) cells, squamous alveolar (type I) pneumocytes, great alveolar (type II) pneumocytes, brush cells, and alveolar macrophages; connective tissue cells, such as fibrocytes, lymphocytes, and macrophages; endothelial cells of blood and lymph vessels, such as arterial, fenestrated, and nonfenestrated capillary, granular and agranular venous, and lymphatic vessel cells; mesothelial cells of visceral pleura; nerve cells such as Schwann and pulmonary glomus cells; and the various cell types of the thoracic lymph nodes.

Of these different cell types, those that appear to be most susceptible to transformation by radiation in experimental animals, and the types of tumors that might result, include basal cells of the epithelium—squamous cell carcinoma; ciliated or goblet mucus-secreting cells—adenocarcinoma; nonciliated secretory bronchiolar cells (Clara cells)—bronchiolar adenocarcinoma or bronchioloalveolar carcinoma; great alveolar cells (type II pneumocytes)—alveolar carcinoma; and endothelial cells of the capillaries and lymphatic vessels—hemangiosarcoma and lymphangiosarcoma, respectively. It should to be noted that the above description is undoubtedly an oversimplification, that not all investigators agree on these concepts, and that research is continuing.

CARCINOGENIC RESPONSE

In animals exposed to radiation from internal or external sources, three kinds of malignant tumors occur most frequently: adenocarcinoma and epidermoid carcinoma, both of epithelial origin, and hemangiosarcoma of endothelial origin. Occasional connective tissue tumors or mesotheliomas are also observed. Adenocarcinoma (bronchioloalveolar carcinoma), the most frequently observed radiation-induced lung cancer, is also the most frequent type occurring spontaneously in most animal species.

In dogs, the most frequent spontaneous lung cancers are peripheral adeno-

carcinoma, with cells resembling those of normal terminal bronchioles or alveolar ducts, and invasive adenocarcinomas, with columnar cells, ciliated or of
glandular origin, which metastasize to bronchial nymph nodes and beyond
(Nielsen, 1970). The reported cumulative incidence of spontaneous primary
lung cancers in a colony of beagle dogs, the breed used in nearly all radionuclide studies, is 4.7% at 16 yr of age (Hahn and Griffith, 1981). Adenocarcinoma
(papillary adenocarcinoma, according to the World Health Organization's classification, and undifferentiated adenocarcinoma, according to Moulton's classification) was observed in five of 77 dogs that died in a population of 225
controls in a life span study; the first such cancer was observed at 11.2 yr of age.
Ten of 11 primary lung tumors in another colony of beagle dogs were classified
as adenocarcinomas (Taylor et al, 1979), and a cumulative incidence of 3% was
calculated for this colony (Hahn and Griffith, 1981).

Because inhaled radionuclides are deposited and retained in regions of the
lungs where cancers originate spontaneously, it is not surprising that the predominant type of radiation-induced tumor is the same type that occurs spontaneously (i.e., peripheral adenocarcinoma). In a completed life span study of 35
dogs that inhaled $^{239}PuO_2$, bronchioloalveolar carcinoma, an adenocarcinoma
originating in the terminal bronchioles and the alveolar regions, occurred in 27
dogs, from about 3–12 yr after a single exposure. In ten of those dogs, 15 other
lung cancers also occurred; these were mostly epidermoid (squamous cell)
carcinoma, but also included mesothelioma in two dogs and hemangiosarcoma
in one (Park et al, 1972). In life span studies of over 1000 dogs that inhaled
plutonium at two laboratories, incomplete results show bronchioloalveolar
carcinoma to be the predominant lung cancer, although other types of epithelial tumors have occurred (Marshall and Guilmette, 1983; Dagle et al, 1985). In
many of the dogs the adenocarcinoma metastasized to lymph nodes, whereas,
some of the epidermoid tumors metastasized to other tissues, such as bone.

Bronchioloalveolar carcinoma, as well as papillary adenocarcinoma and
epidermoid carcinoma, have been observed in beagle dogs that inhaled beta-
gamma emitting radionuclides such as $^{90}SrCl_2$, $^{91}YCl_3$, or insoluble ^{90}Y, ^{91}Y, or
^{144}Ce particles (Marshall and Guilmette, 1983). Hemangiosarcoma and a few
cases of fibrosarcoma were also observed in the lungs of these beagle dogs;
squamous cell carnimoma, adenocarcinoma, and hemangiosarcoma were ob-
served in the nasal cavities of dogs that inhaled $^{91}YCl_3$, $^{144}CeCl_3$, or $^{90}SrCl_2$
(Boecker et al, 1985). Dose-rate may influence the type of lung tumors that
occur. Sarcoma was rare, compared with carcinoma, after inhalation of ^{90}Y
particles and ^{91}Y particles, which had effective half-times in the lungs of 2.5
days and 50 days, respectively and, thus, irradiated the lungs for a relatively
short time at initially high dose-rates of several hundred rads per day. In dogs
that inhaled ^{144}Ce particles, which had an effective half-time of 175 days and
irradiated the lungs for a longer time at a lower dose-rate, the frequencies of
carcinoma and sarcoma were about equal. In dogs that inhaled ^{90}Sr particles,
which had an effective half-time in the lungs of 600 days irradiating the lungs
for a much longer time at a much lower dose-rate, the frequency of sarcoma was
twice that of carcinoma. In this study of nearly 200 dogs, however, it is possible
that total dose could have been a greater influence on tumor type than dose-
rate, because sarcoma tended to occur at the higher doses, although the dose-

rates were relatively low (Hahn et al, 1983). Conflicting results from another study do not help to clarify this point. Low initial dose rates, accomplished by repeated exposures to relatively low concentrations of [144]Ce aerosols, induced bronchioloalveolar carcinoma in two dogs, epidermoid carcinoma in one dog, and hemangiosarcoma in one of 11 dogs that died within about 6 yr after exposure. However, over the same length of time and at comparable total doses high initial dose rates, accomplished by means of a single exposure to [144]Ce particles, induced hemangiosarcomas in eight dogs and carcinoma in seven of 11 dogs that died (Boecker et al, 1980).

Differences in cell turnover times among the target tissues (months to years for pulmonary capillary endothelium, versus 1 wk–2 mo for the epithelial cells of the bronchioles and alveoli) and differences in the spatial as well as temporal distribution of the ionizing events from the two kinds of radiation probably explain why alpha emitters induced predominantly bronchioloalveolar carcinoma, whereas, beta-gamma emitters induced a broader spectrum of tumors, including epidermoid carcinoma and hemangiosarcoma as well as bronchioloalveolar carcinoma (Benjamin et al, 1975). The same explanation may apply to the differences in tumors induced by different beta-gamma emitting radionuclides.

Alpha-emitting radon and radon decay products irradiate the upper and lower respiratory tract (Desrosiers et al, 1978; Cross et al, 1985) even if only a single exposure occurs; however, because of their short range the alpha particles do not penetrate much beyond the basal cells. In 20 dogs that inhaled radon and radon decay products daily for 4.5 yr in total exposures of 9000–~16,000 working level months (WLM)[1], along with uranium ore dust, three had bronchioloalveolar carcinoma, three epidermoid carcinoma, one fibrosarcoma, and two nasal carcinoma, one occurring in a dog that also had epidermoid carcinoma (Cross et al, 1982a). All lung cancers appeared to originate distally, although possibly less so than in dogs that inhaled insoluble radionuclides. Because this was inconsistent with the estimate of radiation dose, 45,000–81,000 rad to the tracheal epithelium and 15–2700 rad to the whole lung, it suggests the pulmonary region of dog lungs is more sensitive to radiation carcinogenesis than the tracheobronchial region. There were too few total cancers in these dogs to draw any conclusions about the spectrum of tumor types except to note that adenocarcinoma (bronchioloalveolar carcinoma) was not the dominant type. Some of the cancers in these dogs appeared to be associated with emphysematous cavities, which were prevalent in the lungs of all of the dogs. A parallel group of 20 dogs was exposed daily to cigarette smoke in addition to radon and uranium ore dust. Only one dog had nasal carcinoma, and one had bronchioloalveolar carcinoma, although the respiratory tracts of the dogs showed lesions similar to those of the nonsmoking dogs that inhaled radon and uranium ore dust. These lesions included vesicular and bullous emphysema, interstitial fibrosis, and pleural fibrosis. The decreased incidence of cancer in the dogs exposed concurrently to cigarette smoke was attributed to

---

[1] The working level (WL), a unit specific for radon and its decay products, is the concentration of short-lived radon decay products in equilibrium with 100 pCi/ℓ of radon. One working level month (WLM) is an exposure equal to breathing 1 WL for 170 hr.

reduction of the radiation dose to the sensitive cells by enhanced particle clearance, increased mucus secretions, and a thickened mucosa induced by cigarette smoke.

In laboratory rats, because spontaneous pulmonary cancers are rare (Kuschner and Laskin, 1970; Pour et al, 1976; Shabad and Pylev, 1970; Hahn and Griffith, 1981; Dagle and Sanders, 1982), ranging from about 0.1% in Wistar strain rats to about 1% in Fischer-344 rats, there is considerable uncertainty about the types that might be considered to occur spontaneously. Experimentally induced lung cancers are epithelial (adenocarcinoma and epidermoid carcinoma), connective tissue (fibrosarcoma, reticulosarcoma, or lymphosarcoma), and endothelial (angiosarcoma or hemangiosarcoma). The adenocarcinoma may have alveolar, bronchiolar, or mucous gland origins, whereas the epidermoid carcinoma may arise from invasive papilloma or metaplastic proliferation of basal cells of the respiratory epithelium.

The principal pulmonary malignancies induced in rats by exposure to alpha-emitting transuranic radionuclides are well-to-poorly differentiated adenocarcinoma, hemangiosarcoma, and epidermoid carcinoma (Dagle and Sanders, 1982). Adenocarcinoma (bronchioloalveolar carcinoma) is usually the dominant type. Of 140 total lung cancers in 982 rats that inhaled either $^{238}PuO_2$, $^{239}PuO_2$, or ^{224}Cm oxide, 72% were adenocarcinoma, 21% were epidermoid carcinoma, 5% were hemangiosarcoma, 1.4% were fibrosarcoma, and 0.7% were mesothelioma. Epidermoid carcinoma is more frequent at high doses than at low doses (Sanders and Mahaffey, 1979; Lafuma et al, 1974; and Morin et al, 1976). Investigators tend to agree that adenocarcinoma originates in the periphery of the lungs (subpleural or peribronchiolar regions). Nonciliated bronchiolar cells (Clara cells) and type II pulmonary epithelial cells appear to be the leading contenders as "cells at risk" for induction of adenocarcinoma by radionuclides in rats (Dagle and Sanders, 1982; Masse, 1980) as well as in hamsters (Kennedy and Little, 1977), and possibly in dogs and baboons (Bair et al, 1980). The cell of origin of epidermoid carcinoma is less certain, although it is sometimes referred to as bronchogenic carcinoma (Lafuma et al, 1974), implying that it "developed directly from focal proliferations of the metaplastic bronchial epithelium" (Shabad and Pylev, 1970).

Of 500 lung tumors in male Sprague-Dawley rats exposed to alpha radiation from radon and radon decay products, 262 were epidermoid carcinoma, 75 adenocarcinoma, 11 anaplastic, 139 bronchioloalveolar, 11 alveolar, and two were angiosarcoma (Chameaud et al, 1982, 1984). Similar frequencies of epidermoid carcinoma and mucus-staining adenocarcinoma (70%) and bronchiolar adenocarcinoma or bronchioloalveolar carcinoma (30%) were observed in 400 rats after inhalation of radon decay products and uranium ore dust (Cross et al, 1985). Of 53 malignant lung cancers, four were epidermoid carcinoma, 25 were adenocarcinoma, ten were adenocarcinoma with squamous differentiation, and 14 were classified bronchioloalveolar carcinoma (described as tumors of Clara cell or type II alveolar cell origin) (Cross et al, 1982b). In experiments with rats, more clearly than in experiments with dogs, the spectrum of tumor types resulting from inhalation of radon and radon decay products seems to reflect a broad distribution of radiation dose throughout the respiratory tract.

Spontaneous pulmonary malignant tumors in hamsters are very rare. Under experimental conditions, adenocarcinoma, epidermoid carcinoma, and anaplastic carcinoma have been reported in Syrian Golden hamsters after intratracheal instillation of many chemicals (Crocker et al, 1970; Smith et al, 1970; Mohr 1970). Mixed epidermoid carcinomas and adenocarcinomas were reported from numerous experiments by Little et al (1975) after intratracheal instillation of alpha-emitting [210]Po with and without hematite. The investigators considered that these tumors probably arose from terminal bronchiolar or alveolar epithelium. These results were confirmed by Anderson et al (1978) and Halliwell et al (1976). Similar cancers were observed in hamsters in which [238]Pu and [239]Pu microspheres were lodged in alveolar capillaries (Anderson et al, 1978). Adenocarcinoma and epidermoid carcinoma were observed in hamsters after single and repeated inhalation exposures to [144]CeO$_2$, a beta-gamma–emitting radionuclide (Lundgren et al, 1982). However, malignant cancers were rarely observed in hamsters that inhaled [238]PuO$_2$ or [239]PuO$_2$ (Sanders, 1977; Hobbs et al, 1976). Clara cells have been identified as the cell of origin in the morphogenesis of adenocarcinoma in hamsters exposed to chemical carcinogens (Reznik-Schuller, 1978); according to Kennedy and Little (1977) this also applies to radiation-induced cancers.

The most common malignant pulmonary tumor in the mouse is the alveologenic carcinoma, which arises from the pulmonary alveolar epithelial cell (Stewart et al, 1970). This tumor has been given various designations: "adenoma, adenoma becoming malignant, carcinoma, alveologenic papillary carcinoma, papillary cystadenoma, adenocarcinoma, bronchiolar cell carcinoma, bronchiolar-alveolar tumor, type A tumor, type B tumor, intermediate type I tumor, or simply the common pulmonary tumor of the mouse." More recent studies indicate that alveolar and papillary tumors arise from different cell types, the papillary tumors arising exclusively from Clara cells (Kauffman, 1981). The frequency of spontaneous pulmonary tumors ranges from 1%–2% to nearly 100% in some strains. Alveologenic carcinoma has been induced experimentally by a number of chemical carcinogens, by alpha radiation from [239]PuO$_2$ (Temple et al, 1959), and by beta-gamma radiation (Gates and Warren, 1960, 1961). This appears to be the type of malignant tumor reported as lung adenoma by Ullrich et al (1979) in mice exposed to x-radiation and neutrons (Ullrich, 1982), and as pulmonary adenoma by Lundgren et al (1980, 1981b) in mice that inhaled insoluble beta-emitting ^{90}Y particles and beta-gamma–emitting [144]CeO$_2$. Spontaneous pulmonary epidermoid carcinoma in mice is rare according to Stewart et al (1970) and is rarely induced experimentally. Among the few cases cited are the epidermoid carcinoma in mice after intratracheal injection of [239]PuO$_2$ (Temple et al, 1959) and also after implantation of gamma-emitting sources (Gates and Warren, 1960, 1961).

Very little is known about spontaneously occurring lung cancers in baboons. Adenocarcinoma (bronchioloalveolar carcinoma) has been observed in baboons after inhalation of [239]PuO$_2$ (Metivier et al, 1972).

DOSE–RESPONSE RELATIONSHIPS

In this section, describing information available on the spatial and temporal distribution of radiation dose and lung cancer response, the radiation dose values are mean values for groups of animals and were calculated on the assumption that the energy was absorbed uniformly throughout the total lung

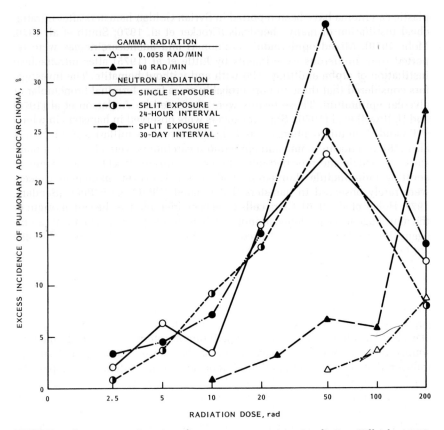

FIGURE 1. Lung cancer in mice after gamma or neutron irradiation (Ullrich, 1982). Published data are adjusted to account for spontaneous tumor incidence. Values are plotted on logarithmic abscissa to spread out the data and are connected by lines to assist the reader.

tissue. Tumor incidence values are simply the percentages of animals in each dose group that died with lung tumors or were killed when death was imminent.

External Irradiation

Studies with germ-free–derived, specific-pathogen–free BALB/c/An NBd female mice resulted in the observation of adenocarcinomas at doses in the range of 10–200 rads of gamma radiation; similar results were obtained with fission neutrons (Ullrich et al, 1979; Ullrich, 1982). The age-adjusted tumor incidence values in Figure 1 are corrected for spontaneous pulmonary adenocarcinomas, the incidence of which was relatively high: 12%–15%. The incidence of pulmonary adenocarcinomas was determined at two dose-rates—40 rad/min and 0.0058 rad/min—in mice exposed to gamma radiation from ^{137}Cs. The lower dose-rate gave a linear response from 50 to 200 rad, whereas, the higher dose-rate showed a greater than linear response beyond 100 rad. The higher dose-rate was more effective at all dose levels tested. The incidence of pulmonary adenocarcinomas was determined after a single exposure to fission neutrons and after split exposures with intervals of 24 hr in one case and 30 days in another. The only suggestion of a dose-rate effect was at 50 rad, the split exposure with the 30-day interval yielded a higher excess incidence of adeno-carcinoma. In all three neutron exposure regimens the excess tumors peaked between 20 and <200 rad. Excess tumors resulting from gamma radiation would have peaked above 200 rad. The author calculated an RBE for neutrons of 18.5 over the linear portions of the dose–response curves, up to about 20 rad.

Irradiation by Inhaled Radionuclides

In experiments with alpha-emitting radionuclides, increased lung cancer has been observed in rats at cumulative mean lung doses less than 10 rad, but with some consistency only above 10 rad. Maximum incidences occurred at mean doses of around 2000. In these experiments many groups of animals, especially hamsters, did not show increases in cancer at mean lung doses of several hundred rad. Attempts to describe the relationship between cancer incidence and cumulative mean lung dose suggested that certain nonlinear functions were more adequate descriptors than linear functions (Bair and Thomas, 1976; Sanders and Mahaffey, 1979; Bair et al, 1980). Combining data from rats and dogs, the risk of lung cancer was given as 25 lung cancer deaths per million animals per rad; a linear model yielded a risk of about 360 lung cancer deaths per million animals per rad. Risk estimates from preliminary analysis of data from an experiment with 128 dogs ranged from 460 to 660 lung cancer deaths per million dogs per rad for inhaled $^{239}PuO_2$ (Fisher et al, 1985).

The data that are available for beta-gamma emitters indicate that as much as 1000 rad or more are required to cause a detectably increased incidence of lung cancer. A task group of the International Commission on Radiological Protec-tion using a nonlinear model estimated the risk of lung cancer in animals after inhalation of beta-gamma emitters as 0.84 lung cancer deaths per million ani-mals per rad (Bair et al, 1980). Values reported by Griffith et al (1985) for inhaled beta-emitters were 5 ± 5 malignant lung tumors per 10^6 per rad for Syrian hamsters, 22 ± 8 for mice, 38 ± 2 for rats, and 21 ± 13 for beagle dogs. Risk estimates reported from a preliminary analysis, using a linear model, of data from a lifetime study of 55 dogs that were exposed once to a ^{144}Ce aerosol, ranged from four to 64 lung cancer deaths per million animals per rad (Boecker et al, 1984). The risk calculated from combined data from 402 dogs 10 yr after exposure to ^{90}Y, ^{91}Y, ^{144}Ce, or ^{90}Sr in fused aluminosilicate particles ranged from five to 55 lung cancer deaths per million per rad (Hahn et al, 1983).

Thus, alpha emitters deposited in the lungs of experimental animals were 10–150 times more effective in causing lung cancer than beta-gamma emitters. This comparison was made using data obtained at relatively high doses, well above those that are likely to apply to human exposures. A few data are avail-able at doses under about 200 rad (Figure 2). The alpha emitters, ^{239}Pu, ^{244}Cm, and ^{253}Es are all about equally effective in causing lung cancer, and all were

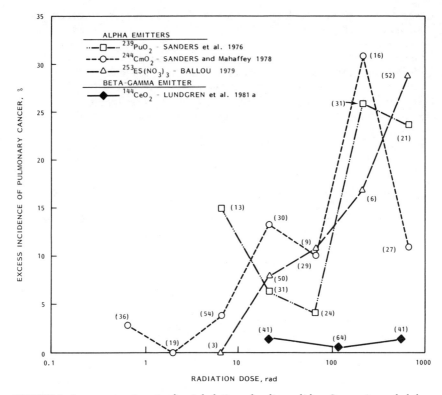

FIGURE 2. Lung cancer in rats after inhalation of radionuclides. Comparison of alpha- and beta-gamma–emitting radionuclides at relatively low radiation doses. Numbers in parentheses represent number of rats in each group. The data are connected by lines to assist the reader. *Alpha emitters:* Data on individual animals provided by investigators were regrouped. One of 447 control rats had a pulmonary adenocarcinoma. *Beta emitters:* Data for equal numbers of male and female Fischer-344 rats were pooled and adjusted for incidence of lung cancer in controls. Two of 142 control male rats had adenocarcinomas; there were none among the 144 females.

much more effective than the beta-gamma emitter, $^{144}CeO_2$, but the difference cannot be assigned a numerical value from these data.

Because the relatively short-half-lived ^{253}Es (20.5 days), which delivered nearly all of its energy at a high rate to lung tissue, was about equally effective as the two long-half-lived alpha emitters, there was no suggestion of a dose-rate effect for alpha emitters. There also was no suggestion of a dose-rate effect in the induction of lung cancer in groups of rats given similar cumulative doses of alpha radiation from $^{239}PuO_2$; however, the temporal distribution of dose was varied by giving two groups a single exposure, another group weekly exposures, and a fourth monthly exposures (Sanders and Mahaffey, 1981). The yield of adenocarcinomas was decreased and that of epidermoid carcinomas was increased by protracting the dose. In experiments with hamsters that inhaled $^{144}CeO_2$ or $^{239}PuO_2$ in single or multiple exposures (Lundgren et al, 1979) the induction of lung tumors appeared to be related to total dose rather than to dose-rate.

In dogs exposed to beta-gamma–emitting insoluble radionuclides (Hahn et al, 1983) dose-rate influenced the type of tumors induced as well as the risk of cancer. The risk of tumor induction was greatest at the highest dose-rate. At comparable total lung doses of about 20,000 rad, the cumulative risk to 10 yr after exposure was 42 lung tumors/10^6/rad for ^{91}Y (50-day effective half-life, 290 rad/day initial dose-rate); 5 lung tumors/10^6/rad for ^{144}Ce (175-day effective half-life, 94 rad/day initial dose-rate); and 12 lung tumors/10^6/rad for ^{90}Sr (600-day effective half-life, 26 rad/day initial dose-rate). In another study, mice given a single inhalation exposure to ^{144}CeO$_2$ were compared with groups given multiple exposures designed to replace the amount of radionuclide reduced in the lungs by biological clearance processes and radioactive decay, thus, maintaining a relatively constant dose rate (Hahn et al, 1980). The frequency of both benign and malignant lung tumors and the time of onset of the tumors were correlated with cumulative radiation dose but not with dose-rate.

While a dose-rate effect for radionuclides deposited and retained largely in the pulmonary region of the lungs is still problematic, this does not appear to be the case for radionuclides with very short radioactive half-lifes, which expend nearly all of their energy at initial sites of deposition in the respiratory tract. Studies of rats exposed daily to radon and radon decay products indicate that the risk of lung cancer is related to the concentration of radon decay products in the air breathed, as well as to the total exposure (Chameaud et al, 1974, 1982). The highest frequency of cancer occurred in rats exposed to radon decay product concentrations of 2500 WL. At comparable total exposures greater than 3000 WLM, the frequency of cancer was greater when the exposure rates were low. At low total exposures the dose-rate effect was less apparent. A trend toward increasing cancer rate with decreasing exposure rate was also observed in other studies (Cross et al, 1985). These same experiments show a reduction of an exposure rate effect at rates less than 50 WLM/wk at a concentration of 250 WL. The lifetime risk of lung cancer calculated from experiments with rats is about 2/10^4/WLM. This would be equivalent to about 1200/10^6/rad, based on 0.17 rad mean lung dose per WLM.

Although the presence of uranium ore dust in air containing radon decay products reduces the fraction of unattached radon daughters in the inhaled air and, thus, reduces the relative amount of energy deposited in upper portions of the respiratory tract, an effect on lung cancer incidence was not observed above 3 mg/m^3 and 300 WLM. Exposure to 1000 WL + 15 mg/m^3 of ore dust resulted in about the same incidence of cancer as exposure to 1000 WL + 3 mg/m^3 of ore dust (Cross et al, 1982b). The presence of ore dust did not eliminate the dose-rate effect. Exposure to 500 WL + 15 mg/m^3 of ore dust resulted in higher frequencies of cancer than 1000 WL + 15 mg/m^3.

Chameaud et al (1976, 1980) also found that inhalation of stable cerium or cigarette smoke increased the induction of lung cancer in rats by exposure to radon decay products. However, the exposure to cigarette smoke only increased the lung cancers induced by radon decay products when the cigarette smoke exposures were begun after completion of the total radon exposures and in this way had a promoting action. As noted before, direct daily inhalation of cigarette smoke decreased the effect of radon decay products in causing lung cancer in beagle dogs exposed daily to 600 WL (> 13,000 WLM lifetime exposure) and uranium ore dust at 13 mg/m^3. The calculated lifetime lung cancer risk was 0.27/10^4/WLM for dogs not exposed to smoke and 0.041/10^4/WLM for dogs exposed to smoke (Cross et al, 1982a, 1985).

It should be noted that, with the exception of a few cancers in the nasopharyngeal region of the respiratory tract, nearly all cancers in experimental animals following exposure to radon decay products occurred in more distal regions than has been observed in human lungs. In both cases, however, the cancers appear to arise where the radiation doses are among the highest, according to dosimetric models (Desrosiers et al, 1978; Harley and Pasternak, 1981).

Although it has been shown that the induction of lung cancer by radon decay products can be increased or decreased by exposure to other materials, the impact of other materials on the effect of radionuclides with long half-lives that remain for long periods in the pulmonary regions of the lungs is more ambiguous. For example, Sanders was unable to show that asbestos increased the carcinogenic response of ^{239}PuO$_2$ in the lungs of rats (Sanders, 1975), whereas, Metivier et al (1979) found that intratracheal injections of benzopyrene after inhalation of ^{239}PuO$_2$ increased the incidence and invasiveness of lung cancer in rats when compared with rats that inhaled only ^{239}PuO$_2$. However, these results may have been influenced by another potential carcinogen, dimethylnitrosamine, given to the rats in their drinking water.

THORACIC LYMPH NODES

Although lung cancer is the subject of this chapter, thoracic lymph nodes may acquire high concentrations of inhaled insoluble radionuclides and accumulate large radiation doses, compared with the average concentrations and doses in the lungs (Bair, 1979). In dogs that inhaled plutonium oxide, primary malignancies were not observed in the thoracic lymph nodes, even though many dogs had primary lung cancers (Dagle et al, 1985). Also, thoracic lymph nodes have not been the sites of primary malignancies in rats that inhaled plutonium (Sanders, 1976). However, primary malignant tumors of tracheobronchial lymph nodes were reported in nine dogs that inhaled insoluble ^{144}Ce particles, and were the cause of death in five of the dogs. The average radiation doses to the lymph nodes were very high: several ten-thousands of rad (Hahn and Boecker, 1980).

CONCLUDING COMMENTS

The results of animal studies suggest that the risk of induction of lung cancer may be highly dependent on delivery of radiation energy to sensitive sites in the respiratory tract in the "right" amount over the "right" time period. The risk of lung cancer did not appear to be greatly influenced by the distribution within the lungs of alpha-emitting radionuclides with relatively long half-lives. However, the potential of alpha-emitting radon decay products, which have short half-lives of a few seconds or minutes and deliver their energy primarily to the sites of initial deposition, to cause lung cancer was subject to influence by a number of factors, including dose-rate and presence of ore dust. Changes in the physiologic state of the respiratory tract caused by exposure to cigarette smoke or other substances that may increase the thickness of the mucous layer also appeared to influence the carcinogenic response.

Results also indicate that the most susceptible sites for cancer induction by irradiation are in the epithelium of the lung parenchyma. Although the question is far from settled, the most frequently mentioned target cell, or cell from which radiation-induced cancers arise, is the nonciliated bronchiolar Clara cell.

What information obtained from studies of radiation-induced lung cancer in experimental animals may be useful in predicting the response of the human lung to radiation exposure? The increased frequency of lung cancer in miners exposed to radon and radon decay products at levels several-fold greater than the average background has been duplicated in experimental animals, providing reassurance of the validity of extrapolating to human beings the results of studies in which experimental animals are exposed not only to radon decay products but also to other sources of radiation, both external and internal. In most cases, it appears that the predominant kinds of lung cancers that are increased by exposure to radiation are those occurring spontaneously in experimental animals. Can it be assumed that in human beings the predominant carcinogenic response following irradiation of the lungs by radionuclides deposited in the lungs or by sources exterior to the body will be an increased incidence of the types of tumors that occur spontaneously and somewhat independent of what cells and tissues receive the highest radiation doses? On the basis of the frequency of occurrence of various types of malignant tumors in human beings (Berg, 1970), the bronchiolar and alveolar tissues (the tissues where radiation-induced cancers originate in animals) appear to be more resistant to cancer induction than the bronchial epithelium, the site of origin of most lung cancers in miners exposed to radon and radon decay products and the most frequent site of human respiratory tumors, whatever the cause. This observation would seem to imply a lesser risk of lung cancer in the human than in experimental animals from insoluble radionuclides deposited in the lung parenchyma. At this time there are no data from humans exposed to radiation that contradict this, nor are there data that preclude applying the results of the extensive studies of radiation-induced lung cancers in experimental animals to the assessment of human risk and the establishment of limits for radiation exposure.

Work performed under U.S. Department of Energy Contract DE-AC06-76RLO 1830.

Completion of this chapter was greatly aided by the generous provision of published papers and advance copies of reports by Drs. R.O. McClellan and B.B. Boecker (Inhalation Toxicology Research Institute); Dr. R.L. Ullrich (Oak Ridge National Laboratory); Drs. J. Lafuma, R. Masse, and H. Metivier (Institut de Protection et Sureté Nucleaire, France); and by my colleagues at Pacific Northwest Laboratory, who also contributed valuable discussions and critical reviews of the manuscript; these include Drs. J.E. Ballou, R.H. Busch, F.T. Cross, G.E. Dagle, J.A. Mahaffey, S. Marks, R.E. Renne, C.L. Sanders, and R.C. Thompson. I am especially indebted to Dr. R.W. Baalman for editorial assistance and to L.N. McKenney for preparation of the manuscript.

REFERENCES

Anderson EC, Holland LM, Prine JR, Smith DM, Thomas RG (1978). Current summary of intravenous microsphere experiments. In: Biomedical and environmental research program of the LASL health division, January-December 1977. Los Alamos, New Mexico: Los Alamos Scientific Laboratory.

Bair WJ (1979). Metabolism and biological effects of alpha-emitting radionuclides. In: Radiation/research. Okada S, Imamura M, Terashima T, and Yamaguchi H (eds.), Tokyo, Japan: Japanese Association for Radiation Research.

Bair WJ, Boecker BB, Cottier H, Morrow PE, Nenof JC, Park JF, Thomas JM, Thomas RG (1980). Annals of the ICRP: Biological effects of inhaled radionuclides. Oxford, England: Pergamon Press.

Bair WJ et al, Boecker BB, Cottier H, Morrow PE, Nenof JC, Park JF, Thomas JM, Thomas RG (1980). Annals of the ICRP: Biological effects of inhaled radionuclides. Oxford, England: Pergamon Press.

Ballou JE, Dagle GE, Giles RA, Smith LG (1979). Late effects of inhaled ^{253}Es $(NO_3)_3$ in rats. Health Phys 37:301–309.

Benjamin SA, Hahn FF, Chiffelle TL, Boecker BB, Hobbs CH, Jones RK, McClellan RO, Snipes MB (1975). Occurrence of hemangiosarcomas in beagles with internally deposited radionuclides. Cancer Res 35:1745–1755.

Berg JW (1970). Epidemiology of the different historical types of lung cancer. In: Nettelsheim P, Hanna MG Jr., and Deatherage JW Jr. (eds.), Morphology of experimental respiratory carcinogenesis. U.S. Atomic Energy Commission Division of Technical Information.

Boecker BB, Muggenburg BA, Hahn FF, Jones RK, McClellan RO (1984). Inhalation toxicology of ^{144}CeCl$_3$ in the beagle dog. In: Kaul A, Neider R, Pensko J, Stieve F-E, and Brunner H (eds.), Proceedings of the 6th International Congress on International Radiation Protection Association. Radiation-Risk-Protection, Compacts Volume I.

Boecker BB, Hahn FF, Cuddihu RG, Snipes MB, McClellen RO (1985). Is the human nasal cavity at risk from inhaled radionuclides? In: Life-span radiation effects studies in animals: What can they tell us? Proceedings of the Twenty-Third Hanford Life Sciences Symposium, Richland, WA (in press).

Boecker BB, Hahn FF, Mauderly JL, McClellan RO (1980). Tumorigenic responses from single or repeated inhalation exposures to relatively insoluble aerosols of ^{144}Ce. In: Radiation protection, a systemic approach to safety. New York: Pergamon Press.

Brundelet PJ (1965). An intra-pulmonary route of dust elimination in rats. In: Inhaled particles and vapors II. Davies CN (ed.), Oxford, England: Pergamon Press.

Chameaud J, Perraud R, Masse R, LaFuma J (1982). Cancers induced by Rn-222 in the rat. In: Clement GE, Nero AB, Steinhausler F, and Wrenn ME (eds.), Proceedings of Specialist Meeting on Assessment of Radon and Daughter Exposure and Related Biological Effects. Salt Lake City: R.D. Press.

Chameaud J, Masse R, LaFuma J (1984). Influence of radon daughter exposure at low doses on occurrence of lung cancer in rats. In: Clemente GF, Eriskat H, O'Riordan MC, and Sinnaeve J (eds.), Radiation protection dosimetry: Indoor exposure to natural radiation and associated risk assessment, Vol. 7. Proceedings of an International Seminar held at Anacapri (Italy), October 3-5, 1983.

Chameaud J, Perraud R, LaFuma J, Masse K, Pradel J (1974). Lesions and lung cancers induced in rats by inhaled radon-222 at various equilibriums with radon daughters. In: Karbe E and Park JF (eds.), Experimental lung cancer: Carcinogenesis and bioassays. New York: Springer-Verlag.

Crocker TT, Chase JE, Wells SA, Nunes LL (1970). Preliminary report on experimental squamous carcinoma of the lung in hamsters and in a primate (galago crassicaudahis). In: Nettelsheim P, Hanna MG, Jr., and Deatherage JW, Jr (eds.), Morphology of experimental respiratory carcinogenesis. U.S. Atomic Energy Commission Division of Technical Information.

Cross FT, Palmer RF, Busch RH, Dagle GE, Filipy RE, Ragan HA (1986). An overview of the PNL radon experiments with reference to epidemiological data. In: Life-span radiation effects studies in animals: What can they tell us? Proceedings of the Twenty-Third Hanford Life Sciences Symposium, Richland, Wa.

Cross FT, Palmer RF, Filipy RE, Dagle GE, Stuart BO (1982a). Carcinogenic effects of radon daughters, uranium ore dust and cigarette smoke in beagle dogs. Health Phys 42: 33–52.

Cross FT, Busch RH, Buschbom RL, Dagle GE, Filipy RE, Loscutoff SM, Mihalko PJ, Palmer RF (1982b). Inhalation hazards to uranium miners. In: Pacific northwest laboratory annual report for 1981 to the DOE office of energy research, Part I, Biomedical Sciences. Richland, Washington: Battelle, Pacific Northwest Laboratories.

Dagle GE, Sanders CL (1982). Radionuclide injury to the lung. In: Hook G (ed.), Pulmonary toxicology. New York: Raven Press.

Dagle GE, Park JF, Weller RE, Ragan HA, Stevens DL (1985). Pathology associated with inhaled plutonium in beagles. In: Life-span radiation effects studies in animals: What can they tell us? Proceedings of the Twenty-Third Hanford Life Sciences Symposium, Richland, Wa (in press).

Desrosiers AE, Kennedy A, Little JB (1978). ^{222}Rn daughter dosimetry in the Syrian golden hamster lung. Health Phys 35:607.

Fisher DR, Cannon WC, Hadley RT, Park JF (1985). Preliminary evaluation of lung doses for dogs exposed to ^{239}PuO$_2$. In: Life-span radiation effects studies in animals: What can they tell us? Proceedings of the Twenty-Third Hanford Life Sciences Symposium, Richland, Wa (in press).

Gates O, Warren S (1961). Histogenesis of lung carcinoma in mice. Arch Pathol 71:103–121.

Gates O, Warren S (1960). The production of bronchial carcinomas in mice. Am J Pathol 36:653–671.

Griffith WC, Lundgnen DL, Hahn FF, Boecker BB, McClellan RO (1985). An interspecies comparison of the biological effects of an inhaled, relatively insoluble beta emitter. In: Life-span radiation effects studies in animals: What can they tell us? Proceedings of the Twenty-Third Hanford Life Sciences Symposium, Richland, Wa (in press).

Hahn FF, Boecker BB (1980). Tumors of the tracheobronchial lymph nodes in beagle dogs after inhalation of a relatively insoluble form of cerium-144. In: Sanders CL, Cross FT, Dagle GE, Mahaffey JA (eds.), Pulmonary toxicology of respirable particles. Springfield, Virginia: Technical Information Center, U.S. Department of Energy.

Hahn FF, Griffith WC (1981). Spontaneous primary lung tumors in the Lovelace ITRI beagle dog colony. In: Bice DE, Snipes MB, and Martinez BS (eds.), Annual report of the inhalation toxicology research institute. Springfield, Virginia: National Technical Information Service.

Hahn FF, Boecker BB, Cuddihy RG, Hobbs CH, McClellan RO, Snipes MB (1983). Influence of radiation dose patterns on lung tumor incidence in dogs that inhaled beta emitters: A preliminary report. Radiat Res 96:505–517.

Hahn FF, Lundgren DL, McClellan RO (1980). Repeated inhalation exposure of mice to ^{144}CeO$_2$. II. Biological effects. Radiat Res 82:123–137.

Halliwell WH, Mewhinney JA, Hobbs CH, Slauson DO (1976). Occurrence and lobar distribution of lung cancer in Syrian hamsters induced by intratracheal administration of ^{210}Po (preliminary report). In: Boecker BB, Jones RK, Barnett NJ (eds.), Annual Report of the Inhalation Toxicology Research Institute Lovelace Biomedical and Environmental Research Institute, Inc. Springfield, Virginia: National Technical Information Service.

Harley NH, Pasternack BS (1981). A model for predicting lung cancer risks induced by environmental levels of radon daughters. Health Phys 40:307.

Hobbs CH, Mewhinney JA, McClellan RO, Mo T (1976). Toxicity of inhaled ^{239}PuO$_2$ in immature, young adult and aged Syrian hamsters. IV. In: Boecker BB, Jones RK,

Barnett NJ (eds.), Annual Report of the Inhalation Toxicology Research Institute Lovelace Biomedical and Environmental Research Institute, Inc. Springfield, Virginia: National Technical Information Service.

Kauffman SL (1981). Histogenesis of the papillary Clara cell ademoma. Am J Path 103:174–180.

Kennedy AR, Little JB (1977). Histochemistry of normal lungs and ^{210}Po induced pulmonary tumors in hamsters. Acta Histochem 58:353–359.

Kuschner M, Laskin S (1970). Pulmonary epithelial tumors and tumor-like proliferation in the rat. In: Nettelsheim P, Hanna MG, Jr., Deatherage JW, Jr. (eds.), Morphology of experimental respiratory carcinogenesis. U.S. Atomic Energy Commission Division of Technical Information.

LaFuma J, Nénot JC, Morin M, Masse R, Mehvier H, Nolibe D, Skupinski W (1974). Respiratory carcinogenesis in rats after inhalation of radioactive aerosols of actinides and lanthanides in various physicochemical forms. In: Karbe E and Park JF (eds.), Experimental lung cancer: Carcinogenesis and bioassays. New York: Springer-Verlag.

Little JB, Kennedy AR, McGandy RB (1975). Lung Cancer induced in hamsters by low doses of alpha radiation from polonium-210. Science 188:737–738.

Lundgren DL, Hahn FF, McClellan RO (1982). Effects of single and repeated inhalation exposure of Syrian hamsters to aerosols of ^{144}CeO$_2$. Radiat Res 90:374–394.

Lundgren DL, Hahn FF, McClellan RO (1980). Influence of age at the time of inhalation exposure to aerosols of ^{144}CeO$_2$ on ^{144}Ce retention, dosimetry and toxicity in mice. Health Phys 38:643–655.

Lundgren DL, Hahn FF, McClellan RO (1981a). Repeated inhalation exposure of rats to aerosols of ^{144}CeO$_2$. V. In: Bice DE, Snipes MB, Martinez BS (eds.), Annual Report of the Inhalation Toxicology Research Institute. Springfield, Virginia: National Technical Information Service.

Lundgren DL, Hahn FF, Rebar AH, McClellan KO (1979). Toxic effects of repeated inhalation exposure of Syrian hamsters to aerosols of ^{144}CeO$_2$ or ^{239}PuO$_2$. In: Biological implications of radionuclides released from nuclear industries. Vienna: International Atomic Energy Agency.

Lundgren DL, Hahn FF, McClellen RO (1981b). Toxicity of ^{90}Y in relatively insoluble fused aluminosilicate particles when inhaled by mice. Radiat Res 88:510–523.

Masse R (1980). Histogenesis of lung tumors induced in rats by inhalation of alpha emitters: An overview. In: Sanders CL, Cross FT, Dagle GE and Mahaffey JA (eds.), Pulmonary Toxicology of Respirable Particles. Technical Information Center, U.S. Department of Energy.

Marshall TC, Guilmette RA eds. (1983). The Annual Report of Inhalation Toxicology Research Institute 1982-1983, Albuquerque, NM: Lovelace Biomedical and Environmental Research Institute LMF-107.

Metivier H, Nolibé D, Masse R, LaFuma J (1972). Cancer provoqués chez le singe babouin (Papio papio) par inhalation de PuO$_2$. CR Acad Sci Sér D 275:3069–3071.

Metivier H, Masse R, L'Hallier I, LaFuma J (1979). Etude de l'action combinée de l'oxyde de plutonium inhalé et de deux cancerogènes chimiques de l'environnement. In: Biological implications of radionuclides released from nuclear industries. Vienna: International Atomic Energy Agency.

Mohr U (1970). Effects of diethylnitrosamine in the respiratory system of Syrian golden hamsters. In: Nettelsheim P, Hanna MG, Jr., Deatherage JW, Jr. (eds.), Morphology of experimental respiratory carcinogenesis. U.S. Atomic Energy Commission Division of Technical Information.

Morin M, Nénot JC, Masse R, Nolibe D, Metivier H, LaFuma J (1976). Induction de cancers chez le rat après inhalation de radióeléments émetteurs alpha. In: Biological and environmental effects of low-level radiation, Vol. II. Vienna: International Atomic Energy Agency.

Nielsen SW (1970). Pulmonary neoplasis in domestic animals. In: Nettelsheim P, Hanna MG, Jr., Deatherage JW, Jr. (eds.), Morphology of experimental respiratory carcinogenesis. U.S. Atomic Energy Commission Division of Technical Information.

Park JF, Bair WJ, Busch RH (1972). Progress in beagle dog studies with transuranium elements at Battelle-Northwest. In: Thompson RC and Bair WJ (eds.), The biological implications of the transuranium elements. Belfast: Universities Press.

Pour P, Stanton MF, Kuschner M, Laskin S, Shabad LM (1976). Tumours of the respiratory tract. In: Turusov VS, Chesterman FC, Della Porta G, Hollander CF, Mohr U, Shabad LM, Sobin LH and Stanton MF (eds.), Pathology of tumours in laboratory animals, Vol. I, Lyon, France: International Agency for Research on Cancer.

Reznik-Schuller H (1978). Ultrastructures of nitrosoheptamethyleneimine-induced tumors in European hamsters. Am J Pathol 93:45–48.

Sanders CL (1975). Dose distribution and neoplasia in the lung following intratracheal instillation of $^{239}PuO_2$ and asbestos. Health Phys 28:383–386.

Sanders CL (1976). Effects of transuranics on pulmonary lymph nodes of rodents. In: Radiation and the Lymphatic System. Oak Ridge, Tennessee: ERDA Technical Information Center.

Sanders CL (1977). Inhalation toxicology of $^{238}PuO_2$ and $^{239}PuO_2$ in Syrian Golden hamsters. Radiat Res 70:334–344.

Sanders CL, Mahaffey JA (1978). Inhalation carcinogenesis of high-fired $^{244}CmO_2$ in rats. Radiat Res 76:384.

Sanders CL, Mahaffey JA (1981). Inhalation carcinogenesis of repeated exposures to high-fired $^{239}PuO_2$ in rats. Health Phys 41:629–644.

Sanders CL, Mahaffey JA (1979). Inhalation toxicology of transuranics in rodents. In: Biological implications of radionuclides released from nuclear industries. Vienna: International Atomic Energy Agency.

Sanders CL, Dagle GE, Cannon WC, Craig DK, Powers GJ, Meier DM (1976). Inhalation carcinogenesis of high-fired $^{239}PuO_2$ in rats. Radiat Res 68:349–360.

Shabad LM, Pylev LN (1970). Morphological lesions in rat lungs induced by polycyclic hydrocarbons. In: Nettelsheim P, Hanna MG, Jr., and Deatherage, JW, Jr. (eds.), Morphology of experimental respiratory carcinogenesis. U.S. Atomic Energy Commission Division of Technical Information.

Smith WE, Miller L, Churg J (1970). An experimental model for study of cocarcinogenesis in the respiratory tract. In: Nettelsheim P, Hanna MG Jr., Deatherage JW, Jr., (eds.), Morphology of experimental respiratory carcinogenesis. U.S. Atomic Energy Commission Division of Technical Information.

Sorokin SP (1970). The cells of the lungs. In: Nettelsheim P, Hanna MG Jr., Deatherage JW Jr., (eds.), Morphology of experimental respiratory carcinogenesis. U.S. Atomic Energy Commission Division of Technical Information.

Stewart HL, Dunn TB, Snell KC (1970). Pathology of tumors and nonneoplastic proliferative lesions of the lungs of mice. In: Nettelsheim P, Hanna MG JR., Deatherage JW Jr., (eds.), Morphology of experimental respiratory carcinogenesis. U.S. Atomic Energy Commission Division of Technical Information.

Stuart BO, Palmer RF, Filipy RE, Gaven J (1978). Inhaled radon daughters and uranium ore dust in rodents. In: Pacific Northwest Laboratory Annual Report for 1977 to the DOE Assistant Secretary for Environment, Part I, Biomedical Sciences. Richland, WA: Battelle, Pacific Northwest Laboratories.

Taylor GN, Shabestar L, Angus W, Lloyd RD, Mays CW (1979). Primary pulmonic tumors in beagles. Am J Vet Res 40:1316–1318.

Temple LA, Willard DH, Marks S, Bair WJ (1959). Induction of lung tumors by radioactive particles. Nature 183:408–409.

Ullrich RL (1982). Lung tumor induction in mice: Neutron RBE at low doses. In: Broerse JJ, Gerber GW (eds.), Proceedings of the European Seminar on Neutron Carcinogenesis. CEC, Luxembourg.

Ullrich RL, Jernigan MC, Adams LM (1979). Induction of lung tumors in RFM mice after localized exposures to x rays or neutrons. Radiat Res 80:464–473.

EXPERIMENTAL CARCINOGENESIS IN THE BREAST

C.J. SHELLABARGER, Ph.D., J.P. STONE, Ph.D.,
AND S. HOLTZMAN Ph.D.

The first reports of mammary carcinogenesis in irradiated animal models were made after observations on mice by Furth and Furth (1936) and Furth and Butterworth (1936). Subsequently, an association between exposure to ionizing radiation and mammary carcinogenesis has been made for guinea pigs, dogs, and rats. The first report of an increased risk for breast cancer in irradiated women was made by MacKenzie in 1965.

GUINEA PIG

All information on mammary carcinogenesis in the irradiated guinea pig comes from a single study (Lorenz et al, 1954). Gamma radiation given 8 hr/day (0.11–8.8 R/day) over the life span produced mammary carcinomas in both sexes. The greatest number of tumors was found in animals exposed to 1.1 R/8-hr day, though tumors appeared earlier with higher daily doses.

DOG

Data from irradiated dogs come from a few ongoing experiments. Andersen and Rosenblatt (1969) gave beagles single or fractionated 250 kVp x-ray exposures of either 100 or 300 R. In an analysis of these data, Chrisp et al (1977) found increased dose-related cumulative incidence rates of deaths due to mammary tumors in the nulliparous dogs but not in the parous dogs. Thomassen et al (1978) gave 1680 beagles either 20 or 100 R of ^{60}Co gamma radiation at various times before or after birth. During the initial 10 yr only two dogs had mammary adenocarcinomas. Fritz et al (1982) studied 267 beagles that received 600 or 1400 R of ^{60}Co gamma irradiation at 5, 10, 17, or 35 R/22-hr day. The frequency of malignant mammary tumors was similar in both the irradiated and control groups, but the tumors occurred at a significantly earlier age in the irradiated dogs.

From the Medical Department, Brookhaven National Laboratory, Upton, New York.

MOUSE

Mammary carcinogenesis in inbred strains of mice is highly dependent on viral, hormonal, genetic, immunologic, dietary, and environmental factors (Nandi and McGrath, 1973). Irradiation of mice may affect mammary carcinogenesis in any of the following ways: 1) directly, by causing neoplastic changes within breast cells; 2) indirectly, by causing functional changes in the endocrine glands; or 3) indirectly, by activating mammary tumor virus (MTV) or other viral agents. In some mouse strains there is good evidence that ionizing radiation usually produces mammary neoplasia by an *abscopal* mechanism. That is, mammary tumors are produced in the breast tissue irrespective of the area irradiated. In fact, Boot et al (1970), using C57BL mice free of both mammary tumor virus (MTV) and nodule-inducing virus (NIV or MTV-L), found that direct x-irradiation (200 rad) of the exteriorized spleen was as effective as whole-body irradiation in inducing mammary tumors in pituitary isograft-bearing animals. However, a direct effect of x-irradiation on mammary carcinogenesis was suggested by an experiment using RIIIfB/Pu (MTV-free) mice to which a dose of 3000–6000 R was confined to two nipple areas (Pullinger, 1954). This direct effect should be investigated further, and techniques similar to those used by Ethier and Ullrich (1982) and Fauklin et al (1982), wherein mammary tissue (intact or dissociated) from an irradiated mouse is transplanted into a cleared fat pad of another mouse for growth, should be useful in obtaining basic information about the scopal effects of radiation on mouse breast tissue.

The induction of mammary tumors in mice by ionizing radiation is highly strain dependent. Strains that have no free MTV or NIV have a low spontaneous incidence of mammary neoplasia and low susceptibility to low-LET radiation (Boot et al, 1970). Every mouse strain studied immunologically by Schlom et al (1978), however, had a strain of MTV present either endogenously or exogenously. Thus, probably *all* mice have MTV present in some form in their mammary tissue, and the role of this virus in radiation carcinogenesis should be established for each strain studied.

The viruses important in mammary carcinoma in mice are RNA retroviruses which, by reverse transcription, can integrate proviral DNA into the host genome (Schlom et al, 1978). At least 11 different MTV strains in 11 different mouse strains have been characterized by their virulence or by the histologic type of tumor induced. A complete description of these strains is beyond the scope of this discussion [see reviews by Bentvelzen (1974) and Schlom et al (1978)].

An all-viral etiology for non–viral-induced mouse mammary carcinogenesis has been postulated, because antigens or virus-specific RNA has been detected in mammary tumors after various carcinogenic treatments (Bentvelzen, 1974). It has been proposed that the transformation of normal mammary tissue into tumor cells by irradiation, chemical carcinogens, or hormones may involve a transforming protein that is encoded by the MTV genome. Thus, induced mammary carcinogenesis in mice free of exogenous MTV would require the expression of endogenous MTV. In support of this postulate, Timmermans et al (1969) found that 200 rad of x-irradiation given to the 02 strain mice (later force-bred and administered urethane in the drinking water) induced mammary tumors (adenocarcinomas?) and gave rise to free MTV and NIV.

Experiments designed to determine the dose-effect or dose-rate effect relationship for whole-body radiation-induced mouse mammary neoplasia have been performed with a variety of strains in which the viral status was not reported. Upton et al (1960), using $(C57LXA/He)F_1$ mice, found that doses of 223–697 rad gamma radiation from an atomic bomb test produced a minimal dose–effect relationship for mammary adenocarcinomas that peaked at 368 rad. In CF-1 female mice exposed to 100, 200, or 400 rad of x-irradiation, Boone (1960) found no increase in mammary tumors over that seen in untreated mice. Boot et al (1970) reported that, in $(C57BLXC3Hf)F_1$ mice treated with either 200 or 400 rad of x-irradiation there was no apparent dose-effect. Vesselinovitch et al (1971), in a similar experiment using $(C57BL/6XC3H)F_1$ mice irradiated with 320 or 480 R, found a mammary tumor incidence of only four of 556 animals for all groups combined.

In an early study of dose-rate effects and relative biological effectiveness (RBE), Ullrich et al (1976) exposed female RFM/Un (a low spontaneous mammary tumor strain) to doses of 0, 24, 47, 94, or 188 rad of neutrons (^{252}Cf) at either 25 rad/min or 1 rad/day. They reported mammary tumor incidences of 2.6, 8.0, 8.4, 9.6, and 3.9, respectively at 25 rad/min and 2.6, 7.3, 7.6, 5.4, and 8.9 at 1 rad/day. In a parallel study using ^{137}Cs gamma irradiation at 0, 10, 25, 50, 100, 150, or 300 rad doses, there was no significant effect of irradiation on mammary neoplasia. They concluded that in this mouse strain the neutron irradiation was more efficient at inducing mammary tumors than gamma irradiation, but no clear dose or dose-rate effects were observed over the dose range used. No RBE could be calculated because of the lack of effect of gamma irradiation. In a later study using BALB/c mice, Ullrich et al (1977) found dose-rate effects for neutron irradiation. They found that for mammary tumorigenesis the low-dose rate (1 rad/day) was less effective than high dose rate (25 rad/day) at low total doses but more effective at high total doses. In the same study using two doses of gamma irradiation, the apparent RBE varied from about 20 at low doses to about 4 at high doses.

Continuing the study of the dose-rate effects of gamma irradiation on BALB/c mice, Ullrich and Storer (1978, 1979) found a dose-rate effect for mammary adenocarcinomas, which indicated some type of sparing effect for low-dose rates of gamma irradiation. Because this sparing effect was also seen for ovarian tumors, this dose-rate effect may only reflect a radiation effect on the ovaries. In a unique study, Ullrich (1983) using BALB/c mice examined very low doses of neutron radiation (0–200 rad) and ^{137}Cs gamma radiation (0–200 rad). He found that for neutron irradiation the mammary tumor incidence curve bends over at 10–20 rad and then plateaus. For gamma irradiation the incidence curve has a steep slope from 0 to 25 rad and then plateaus from 50 to 200 rad. The apparent RBE varied from 4 to 10 in a nonuniform manner, possibly due to radiation-induced ovarian dysfunction. For neutron irradiation at doses of 20 rad or less, the ovarian tumor incidence was lower than the mammary tumor incidence. Conversely, for gamma irradiation from 25 to 200 rad, the ovarian tumor incidence was greater than the mammary tumor incidence. A clear explanation of these results must await additional studies.

Fry et al (1976) irradiated B6CF mice with fission neutrons or gamma radiation. The maximum response with this low-incidence strain was a 3.8% incidence for 80 rad of neutrons and 3.1% for 269 rad of gamma radiation. This indicated an RBE of about 3–4, which is in agreement with the studies by Ullrich et al (1977; 1983) just mentioned, which indicated an RBE of about 4 at slightly lower doses.

The radiation dose and dose-rate dependent neoplastic responses of mouse mammary tissue have not been well characterized. Recent mechanistic studies indicate that radiation-induced mammary carcinogenesis in mice probably is partly the result of a scopal effect but is extremely dependent on viral, hormonal, genetic, and other unknown factors. The destruction of the ovary's capacity to secrete hormones is the most probable cause of decreases in mammary tumor incidence at whole-body irradiation doses over 50 rad. Many more basic data are needed before a clear picture of radiation-induced mouse mammary cancer can emerge.

RAT

Rat mammary neoplasms can be classified as fibroadenomas or adenocarcinomas (Young and Hallowes, 1973). The incidence and proportion of fibroadenomas and adenocarcinomas depends on the strain of rat that is irradiated (Shellabarger, 1972; Broerse et al, 1977; van Zwieten et al, 1977; Gross and Dreyfuss, 1979; van Bekkum et al, 1979; Vogel and Turner, 1982). Adenocarcinomas tend to occur relatively soon after irradiation in female Sprague–Dawley rats (Shellabarger et al, 1957). In nonirradiated female rats, adenocarcinomas tend to appear relatively late in life and with a relatively low frequency. Thus, it is possible to demonstrate that radiation *both* accelerates the appearance of adenocarcinomas (early onset) and causes a higher incidence of adenocarcinomas (extra onset).

There are many reports of a positive association between exposure of female rats to ionizing radiation of several types and the subsequent development of mammary neoplasia. We suggest that all of these reports in rats may be reconciled with a scopal mechanism of radiation-induced mammary carcinogenesis. Evidence for a scopal mechanism has been provided by two types of experiments. First, in partially shielded rats, most mammary neoplasms were found in the irradiated portion of the rat (Bond et al, 1960a; Moskalev, 1973). Secondly, when mammary tissue was removed from a rat and irradiated, and then autografted ectopically, mammary neoplasia was found in these grafts irradiated in vitro (Shellabarger, 1971). The scopal mechanism of radiation-induced mammary neoplasia in the rat is in accord with the proposed mechanism of radiation-induced breast cancer in the human female (MacKenzie, 1965).

Because mammary tissue is subject to hormonal control it would be expected that many—if not all—of the biological modifiers were to act by a common endocrine pathway. For example, male Sprague–Dawley rats, Long–Evans rats, "albino" rats, and WF rats exhibited a smaller mammary carcinogenic response to radiation than female rats of the same strains (Shellabarger et al, 1960; Moskalev, 1973; Gross and Dreyfuss, 1979; Sumi et al, 1980). Three strains of ovariectomized female rats studied in a single experiment exhibited a smaller carcinogenic response to radiation than intact female rats (Broerse et al, 1978), suggesting that a functioning ovary is required for a maximum response of mammary carcinogenesis in the irradiated rats. This conclusion is in accord with the report of Welsch et al (1981), who found fewer mammary adenocarci-nomas in irradiated Sprague–Dawley female rats treated with tamoxifen, an estrogen antagonist, than in rats that were irradiated but not treated with ta-moxifen.

The effect of estrogen administration on the rat mammary carcinogenic re-sponse to radiation depends on the strain of rat studied. In female Sprague–Dawley rats, diethylstilbestrol (DES) alone had no effect on the development of mammary fibroadenomas or mammary adenocarcinomas, but DES *inhibited* both the fibroadenoma and adenocarcinoma responses to x-radiation (Shella-barger et al, 1962a). In contrast, Segaloff and Maxfield (1971) showed that in ACI female rats, DES alone increased the development of mammary adenocar-cinomas and acted in a *synergistic* fashion with x-rays on mammary adenocar-cinoma formation. Subsequently, it was shown that this synergistic interaction in female ACI rats could be extended to DES with neutrons (Shellabarger et al, 1976). When the interaction of DES and radiation was compared in both ACI rats and Sprague–Dawley rats (in a single experiment), it was shown that the interaction between DES and radiation was synergistic in ACI rats and inhibi-tory in Sprague–Dawley rats (Shellabarger et al, 1978). Later, Stone et al (1979) found that circulating prolactin levels were at least 20 times greater in DES-treated ACI rats than in DES-treated Sprague–Dawley rats, thus, implicating prolactin as a significant factor in the synergistic interaction between DES and radiation in ACI rats. Additionally, Stone et al (1980) showed that the synergis-tic interaction between DES and radiation on mammary adenocarcinoma for-mation in female ACI rats was DES dose dependent. From these data it was concluded that DES appeared to act, via prolactin, primarily as a "promoter" stimulating the growth of either spontaneously occurring mammary adenocar-cinoma foci or foci produced by x-irradiation. Holtzman et al (1981) showed that 17-ethinylestradiol (EE2) also interacted in a synergistic fashion with radi-ation on mammary adenocarcinoma formation in female ACI rats. These results with EE2 demonstrate that the synergistic interaction between DES and radia-tion is probably an example of an interaction between an "estrogen" and radia-tion, because the synergistic interaction is not limited to DES.

A third strain of rats, F-344, show a somewhat different response to DES than the ACI or Sprague–Dawley strains. In female F344 rats, DES alone in-duced no mammary adenocarcinomas, but interacted synergistically with radi-ation on mammary adenocarcinoma formation, particularly with regard to inci-dence of rats with mammary adenocarcinomas (Holtzman et al, 1979). Additional data concerned with the interaction of estrogen and radiation on rat mammary carcinogenesis is expected to be forthcoming from a large experi-ment being performed in the Netherlands (Broerse et al, 1978, 1982; van Bek-kum et al, 1979) on three strains of rats that have received estradiol with and without radiation. Their interim reports indicate some estrogen enhancement of radiation-induced mammary neoplasia.

The role of prolactin in radiation-induced mammary carcinogenesis was alluded to in the aforementioned discussion of findings of Stone et al, (1979). However, the role of prolactin in radiation-induced rat mammary carcinogene-sis has a long history. In classical experiments Yokoro and Furth (1961) and Yokoro et al (1961) found that total-body x-rays and mammotrophic (prolactin) hormones administered in the form of isologous functional mammotropic pituitary grafts interacted synergistically with radiation in W/Fu rats for both adenocarcinomas and fibroadenomas. Clifton et al (1976) extended these findings to female Fischer rats, in which they reported that both fibroadenoma and adenocarcinoma formation were increased by pituitary grafts to either gamma- or neutron-irradiated rats. In two important reports Yokoro et al (1977 and 1980) showed that the enhancing (promoting?) effect of pituitary prolactin-secreting tumors on radiation-induced and chemically-induced mammary carcinogenesis in W/Fu rats was still evident when the pituitary tumor grafts were not made until 7–12 mo after administration of x-rays, neutrons, or chemical carcinogens. Following the reasoning of Yokoro et al (1977), we agree that enhancing factors, such as DES and prolactin, can "rescue" long-dormant initiated cells and turn them into tumors. This concept is in accord with the initiation-promotion hypothesis of Berenblum.

Other endocrine factors, in addition to estrogens and prolactin, undoubtedly influence radiation-induced mammary carcinogenesis. For example, Segaloff (1973) showed that progesterone, given after irradiation, inhibited the synergistic interaction of DES and x-rays on mammary carcinogenesis in female ACI rats. Also, Segaloff (1974) noted that the synergism between DES and radiation did not occur if the ACI rats were ovariectomized. Clifton et al (1975) reported that adrenalectomy enhanced mammary carcinogenesis in multiparous Fischer rats grafted with pituitary tumor MtT-F4 after irradiation. Gould and Clifton (1978) found that adrenalectomy and MtT-F4 implantation before irradiation had a similar effect. Jacrot et al (1979) reported that pregnancy plus lactation, after neutron irradiation, enhanced mammary carcinogenesis in Sprague–Dawley rats; however, Shellabarger et al (1962a) reported that pregnancy and lactation had no effect on mammary carcinogenesis in the same strain. At present, the role of the endocrine system in radiation-induced mammary carcinogenesis is far from being understood.

Concerning internal radiation, Durbin et al (1958) found an increased incidence of mammary neoplasia in Sprague–Dawley female rats that received injections of the alpha-emitting radionuclide Astatine[211]. [211]At is a halogen-like element similar to iodine, and it is known that rat mammary tissue has the capacity to concentrate [211]At (Asling et al, 1959).

Astatine[211] in the mammary gland delivers an alpha particle dose that is thought to be sufficient to induce mammary gland neoplasia (Yokoro et al, 1964). Cahill et al (1975a) reported that female Sprague–Dawley rats given equilibrium levels of tritated water (HTO) during pregnancy had an increased incidence of mammary fibroadenomas and adenocarcinomas in the dams. The female offspring had reduced incidences of mammary fibroadenomas (Cahill et al, 1975b). Mahlum and Sikov (1974) found an increased incidence of mammary neoplasia in female Charles River CD rats that were administered [239]Pu intravenously as either weanlings or adults. Studies by Sanders and Mahaffey (1978) indicate that inhaled Curium[244] increased the incidende of mammary tumors in female Wistar rats. Spiess et al (1978) have associated breast cancer in human female patients with the injection of [224]Ra. Adams and Brues (1980) have noted excess breast cancer in women radium dial workers, although these women may have received both external radiation from the bench as well as internal radiation from ingestion.

Concerning x-ray and gamma-ray radiation, some investigators have concluded that the dose–response relationship appears to be linear (Bond et al, 1960b; Shellabarger et al, 1969; Moskalev and Petrovich, 1972; Hellman et al, 1982), although rigorous statistical analyses have not been used to exclude other forms of dose–response relationships. Interpretation of these dose–response relationships is additionally complicated by the fact that experimental conditions differ from experiment to experiment. It is important to determine if the dose–response relationship for low-LET radiation-induced mammary neoplasia in rats is truly linear.

The data on the effect of fractionation and protraction of low-LET radiation and the data on lowering dose-rate of low-LET radiation on radiation-induced mammary carcinogenesis in rats are difficult to interpret, again, because of differences in experimental design. Some investigators have reported that fractionation and protraction or the lowering of dose-rate of low-LET radiation (Shellabarger et al, 1962b; Shellabarger et al, 1966; Shellabarger and Brown, 1972; Moskalev and Petrovich, 1972; Hellman et al, 1982) have little effect on the yield of mammary neoplasia, whereas, others report a smaller yield of mammary neoplasia (Vogel and Dickson, 1981). The lack of effect of spreading the low-LET dose over increasing time found in most studies on radiation-induced mammary neoplasia in rats is consistent with breast cancer data for human female patients (NCRP Report No. 64, 1980), but inconsistent with most studies in other non-mammary tumor systems. Most data for low-LET radiation-induced non-mammary neoplasia in animals and in humans show a reduced carcinogenic effect when the dose is protracted (NCRP Report No. 64, 1980). The data would suggest, therefore, that for low-LET radiation the influence of dose-rate on mammary tumor induction may be less than for tumor induction in most other tissues.

Concerning mammary neoplasia induced in rats by neutrons, all investigators present data consistent with the finding that, unit dose for unit dose, neutron radiation is more effective than low-LET x- or gamma-radiation (Vogel, 1969; Vogel and Zaldivar, 1969; Vogel and Zaldivar, 1972; Shellabarger et al, 1974; Vogel, 1974; Clifton et al, 1975; Clifton et al, 1976; Montour et al, 1977; Yokoro et al, 1977; Vogel, 1978; Broerse et al, 1978; van Bekkum et al, 1979; Shellabarger et al, 1980; Yokoro et al, 1980; Vogel and Dickson, 1981; Shellabarger et al, 1982). In terms of the relevance of the rat RBE studies to the human breast cancer situation, it must be pointed out that none of the rat RBE studies has successfully analyzed the measure of mammary adenocarcinoma formation in non-hormonally treated female rats studied over the life span of the animals. Again, because of differences in experimental conditions, it is difficult to obtain in the rat mammary tumor system a consensus on the RBE value or on whether or not the RBE value increases with decreasing dose. Additional complications come from preliminary reports that neutron irradiation at low-dose rates may be more effective than at high-dose rates (Vogel and Dickson, 1981) and that fractionated neutron doses may be more effective than single neutron doses (Broerse et al, 1982); although other studies report no change in neutron effectiveness on fractionation (Vogel, 1978; Shellabarger et al, 1978). The finding of reasonably large (4–100+) values of the RBE of neutrons for radiation-induced rat mammary neoplasia is in contrast with findings in the Japanese A-bomb survivors (McGregor et al, 1977), in whom the RBE has not seemed to be different from 1; however, uncertainties of the neutron dosimetry for the A-bomb survivors have (at least for now) placed in jeopardy our only source of human data on low-dose neutron-induced breast cancer in the human female. Hence, this situation suggests that it is important to study further low-dose neutron-induced mammary neoplasia in the rat and other appropriate experimental model systems.

FUTURE

Clifton (1978) has summarized the current situation in regard to radiation-induced breast cancer in the human female:

> "Is the lower end of the dose-response curve linear or curvilinear? What is the effect on carcinoma incidence of fractionated low doses? It strikes me that the human studies currently in progress are unlikely to come up with the answers to these two questions with any degree of statistical reliability in the near future. It is almost surely true that absolute dose extrapolation cannot be made from experimental animals to man. However, it seems very likely that the nature of the dose-response curve and probably the effects of dose fractionation will be found to be similar across species lines."

Broakhaven National Laboratory is operated by Associated Universities, Inc., under Contract (DE-AC02-76 CH 00016) to the U.S. Department of Energy. The authors thank Mrs. Doris J. Pion for her secretarial assistance.

REFERENCES

Adams EE, Brues AM (1980) Breast cancer in female radium dial workers first employed before 1930. JO Med 22:583–587.

Andersen AC, Rosenblatt LS (1969) The effect of whole-body x-irradiation on the median lifespan of female dogs (beagles). Radiat Res 39:177–200.

Asling CW, Durbin PW, Johnston ME, Parrott MW (1959) Demonstration of the concentration of Astatine-211 in the mammary tissue of the rat. Endocrinology 64:579–585.

Bentvelzen P (1974) Host-virus interactions in murine mammary carcinogenesis. Biochem Biophys Acta 355:236–259.

Bond VP, Shellabarger CJ, Cronkite EP, Fliedner TM (1960a) Studies on radiation-induced mammary gland neoplasia in the rat. V. Induction by localized irradiation. Radiat Res 13:318–328.

Bond VP, Cronkite EP, Lippincott SW, Shellabarger CJ (1960b) Studies on radiation-induced mammary gland neoplasia in the rat. III. Relation of the neoplastic response to dose of total-body radiation. Radiat Res 12:276–285.

Boone IU (1960) Incidence of tumors in animals exposed to whole-body radiation. In: Watson BB (ed.), The delayed effects of whole-body radiation: A symposium. Baltimore: Johns Hopkins Press, pp 19–37.

Boot LM, Bentvelzen P, Calafat J, Ropcke G, Timmermans A (1970) Interaction of x-ray treatment, a chemical carcinogen, hormones, and viruses in mammary gland carcinogenesis. In: Clark RL, Cumley RW, McCay JE, Copeland MM (eds.), Oncology 1970, Vol. 1. Chicago: Yearbook Medical Publishers, pp 434–440.

Broerse JJ, Knaan S, van Bekkum DD (1977) Incidence of mammary tumors in rats of different strains after fast neutron irradiation. Int J Radiat Biol 31 (abstr):378–379.

Broerse JJ, Knaan S, van Bekkum DW, Hollander CF, Nooteboom AL, van Zwieten MI (1978) Mammary carcinogenesis in rats after x- and neutron irradiation and hormone administration. In: International Symposium of the Late Biological Effects of Ionizing Radiations. Vienna: International Atomic Energy Agency, pp 13–20.

Broerse JJ, van Bekkum DW, Hennen LA, Hollander CF, van Zwieten MJ (1982) Dose-effect relations for mammary carcinogenesis in three rat strains after single and fractionated x- and neutron irradiations. Radiat Res 91:411–412.

Cahill DF, Wright JF, Godbold JH, Ward JM, Laskey JW, Tomkins EA (1975a) Neoplastic and lifespan effects of chronic exposure to tritium. I. Effects on adult rats exposed during pregnancy. J Natl Cancer Inst 55:371–374.

Cahill DF, Wright JF, Godbold JH, Ward JM, Laskey JW, Tompkins EA (1975b) Neoplastic and lifespan effects of chronic exposure to tritium. II. Rats exposed in utero. J Natl Cancer Inst 55:1165–1169.

Chrisp CE, Phemister RD, Andersen AC, Rosenblatt LS, Goldman M (1977) Pathology in a lifespan study of x-irradiated adult female beagles. In: Biomedical Environmental Research ERDA Research and Development Program, UC-48. Springfield, VA: National Technical Information Service, p. 28.

Clifton KH, Sridharan BN, Douple EB (1975) Mammary carcinogenesis enhancing effect of adrenalectomy in irradiated rats with pituitary tumor MtT-F4. J Natl Cancer Inst 55:485–487.

Clifton KH, Douple EB, Sridharan BN (1976) Effects of grafts of single anterior pituitary glands on the incidence and type of mammary neoplasm in neutron- or gamma-irradiated Fischer female rats. Cancer Res 36:3732–3735.

Clifton KH (1978) Reviewers' comments. J Natl Cancer Inst 61:1544.

Durbin PW, Asling CW, Johnston ME, Parrott MW, Jeung N, Williams MH, Hamilton JG (1958) The induction of tumors in the rat by Astatine-211. Radiat Res 9:378–379.

Ethier SP, Ullrich RL (1982) Detection of ductal dysplasia in mammary outgrowth derived from carcinogen-treated virgin female BALB/c mice. Cancer Res 42:1753–1760.

Faulkin L, Mitchell DJ, Cardiff RD, Goldman M (1982) Survival of mouse mammary gland transplants of normal, hyperplastic, and tumor tissues exposed to x-rays. J Natl Cancer Inst 68, 613–618.

Fritz TE, Lombard LS, Doyle DE, Tolle DV, Poole CM, Seed TM (1982) Late pathologic effects of protracted ^{60}Co irradiation of beagles. Radiat Res (abstr) 91:412–413.

Fry RJM, Garcia AG, Allen KH, Sallese A, Tahmisian TN, Devine RL, Lombard LS, Ainsworth EJ (1976) The effect of pituitary isografts on radiation carcinogenesis in the mammary and harderian glands of mice. In: Biological and Environmental Effects of Low Level Radiation, Vol. 1. Vienna: International Atomic Energy Agency, pp 213–227.

Furth J, Butterworth JS (1936) Neoplastic diseases occurring among mice subjected to general irradiation with x-rays. II. Ovarian tumors and associated lesions. Am J Cancer 28:66–95.

Furth J, Furth OB (1936) Neoplastic diseases produced in mice by general irradiation with x-rays. I. Incidence and types of neoplasms. Am J Cancer 28:54–65.

Gould MN, Clifton KH (1978) The survival of rat mammary cells following irradiation in vivo under different endocrinological conditions. Int J Rad Oncol 4:629–632.

Gross L, Dreyfuss Y (1979) Spontaneous tumors in Sprague–Dawley and Long–Evans rats and their F_1 hybrids: Carcinogenic effect of total-body irradiation. Proc Natl Acad Sci 76:5910–5913.

Hellman S, Maloney WC, Meissner WA (1982) Paradoxical effect of radiation on tumor incidence in the rat: Implications for radiation therapy. Cancer Res 42:433–436.

Holtzman S, Stone JP, Shellabarger CJ (1979) Synergism of diethylstilbestrol and radiation in mammary carcinogenesis in F344 rats. J Natl Cancer Inst 63:1071–1074.

Holtzman S, Stone JP, Shellabarger CJ (1981) Synergism of estrogens and x-rays in mammary carcinogenesis in female ACI rats. J Natl Cancer Inst 67:455–459.

Jacrot M, Mouriquand J, Mouriquand C, Saez S (1979) Mammary carcinogenesis in Sprague–Dawley rats following 3 repeated exposures to 14.8 MeV neutrons and steroid receptor content of these tumor types. Cancer Lett 8:147–153.

Lorenz E, Jacobson LO, Heston WE, Shimkin M, Eschenbrener AB, Deringer MK, Doniger J, Schweisthal R (1954) Effects of long-continued total-body gamma irradiation on mice, guinea pigs, and rabbits. III. Effects on lifespan, weight, blood picture, and carcinogenesis and the role of the intensity of radiation. In: Zirkle RE (ed.), Biological Effects of External X- and Gamma-Radiation. Part I. New York: McGraw-Hill, pp 24–148.

McGregor DH, Land CE, Choi K, Tokuoka S, Liu PI, Wakabayashi T, Beebe GW (1977) Breast cancer incidence among atomic bomb survivors, Hiroshima and Nagasaki 1950–1969. J Natl Cancer Inst 59:799–811.

Mackenzie I (1965) Breast cancer following multiple fluroscopies. Br J Cancer 19:1–9.

Mahlum DD, Sikov MR (1974) Distribution and toxicity of monomeric and polymeric ^{239}Pu in immature and adult rats. Radiat Res 60:75–88.

Montour JL, Hard RC, Jr., Flora RE (1977) Mammary neoplasia in the rat following high-energy neutron irradiation. Cancer Res 37:2619–2623.

Moskalev Yu I (1973) Role of the direct action of radiation in the mechanism of development of mammary gland tumors. Byull Eksper noi Biol Med 75:68–70.

Moskalev Yu, Petrovich IK (1972) Effect of small doses of x-radiation on blood composition, lifetime, frequency and rate of development on mammary gland tumors. AEC-tr-7387, Springfield, VA: National Technical Information Service, U.S. Department of Commerce, pp 568–574.

Nandi S, McGrath CM (1973) Mammary neoplasia in mice. Adv Cancer Res 17:353–403.

NCRP Report No. 64 (1980) Influence of dose and its distribution in time on dose-response relationships for low-LET radiations. Washington, DC: National Council on Radiation Protection and Measurements.

Pullinger BD (1954) Carcinoma and atrophy induced by local surface x-irradiation in the mammary gland in RIII$_b$ mice. Br J Cancer 8:445–450.

Sanders CL, Mahaffey JA (1978) Inhalation carcinogenesis of high-fired ^{244}CmO$_2$ in rats. Radiat Res 76:384–401.

Schlom J, Colcher D, Drohan W, Kufe D, Teramots YA (1978) Viruses and mammary carcinoma. In: McGuire WL (ed.), Breast cancer 2. New York: Plenum, pp 23–46.

Segaloff A (1973) Inhibition by progesterone of radiation-estrogen-induced mammary cancer in the rat. Cancer Res 33:1136–1137.

Segaloff A (1974) The role of the ovary in estrogen production of mammary cancer in the rat. Cancer Res 34:2708–2710.

Segaloff A, Maxfield WS (1971) The synergism between radiation and estrogen in the production of mammary cancer in the rat. Cancer Res 31:166–168.

Shellabarger CJ (1971) Induction of mammary neoplasia after in vitro exposure to x-rays. Proc Soc Exp Biol Med 136:1103–1106.

Shellabarger CJ (1972) Mammary neoplastic response of Lewis and Sprague–Dawley female rats to 7,12-dimethylbenz(a)anthracene or x-ray. Cancer Res 32:883–885.

Shellabarger CJ, Aponte GE, Cronkite EP, Bond VP (1962a) Studies on radiation-induced mammary gland neoplasia in the rat. VI. The effect of changes in thyroid function, ovarian function, and pregnancy. Radiat Res 17:492–507.

Shellabarger CJ, Bond VP, Cronkite EP (1962b) Studies on radiation-induced mammary gland neoplasia in the rat. VII. The effects of fractionation and protraction of sublethal total-body irradiation. Radiat Res 17:101–109.

Shellabarger CJ, Bond VP, Aponte GE, Cronkite EP (1966) Results of fractionation and protraction of total-body radiation on rat mammary neoplasia. Cancer Res 26:509–513.

Shellabarger CJ, Bond VP, Cronkite EP, Aponte GE (1969) Relationship of dose to incidence of mammary neoplasia in female rats. In: Radiation induced cancer. Vienna: International Atomic Energy Agency, pp 161–172.

Shallabarger CJ, Brown RD (1972) Rat mammary neoplasia following ⁶⁰Co irradiation at 0.3R or 10R per minute. Radiat Res 51 (abstr):493.

Shellabarger CJ, Brown RD, Rao AR, Shanley JP, Bond VP, Kellerer AM, Rossi HH, Goodman LJ, Mills RE (1974) Rat mammary carcinogenesis following neutron or x-radiation. In: Biological effects of neutron irradiation. Vienna: International Atomic Energy Agency, pp 391–401.

Shellabarger CJ, Chmelevsky D, Kellerer AM (1980) Induction of mammary neoplasms in the Sprague–Dawley rat by 430 keV neutrons and x-rays. J Natl Cancer Inst 64:821–833.

Shellabarger CJ, Chmelevsky D, Kellerer S, Stone JP, Holtzman S (1982) Induction of mammary neoplasms in the ACI rat by 430 keV neutrons, x-rays, and diethylstilbestrol. J Natl Cancer Inst (in press).

Shellabarger CJ, Cronkite EP, Bond VP, Lippincott SW (1957) The occurrence of mammary tumors in the rat after sublethal whole-body irradiation. Radiat Res 6:501–512.

Shellabarger CJ, Lippincott SW, Cronkite EP, Bond VP (1960) Studies on radiation-induced mammary gland neoplasia in the rat. II. The response of castrate and intact male rats to 400R of total-body irradiation. Radiat Res 12:94–102.

Shellabarger CJ, Stone JP, Holtzman S (1976) Synergism between neutron radiation and diethylstilbestrol in the production of mammary adenocarcinomas in the rat. Cancer Res 36:1019–1022.

Shellabarger CJ, Stone JP, Holtzman S (1978) Rat strain differences in mammary tumor induction with estrogen and neutron radiation. J Natl Cancer Inst 61:1505–1508.

Shellabarger CJ, Stone JP, Holtzman S (1978) Mammary neoplasia in female rats after split doses of neutrons. Radiat Res 74 (abstr):548–549.

Spiess H, Gerspach A, Mays CW (1978) Soft tissue effects following ²²⁴Ra injections into humans. Health Phys 35:61–81.

Stone JP, Holtzman S, Shellabarger CJ (1979) Neoplastic responses and correlated plasma prolactin levels in diethylstilbestrol-treated ACI and Sprague–Dawley rats. Cancer Res 39:773–778.

Stone JP, Holtzman S, Shellabarger CJ (1980) Synergistic interactions of various doses of diethylstilbestrol and x-irradiation on mammary neoplasia in female ACI rats. Cancer Res 40:3966–3972.

Sumi C, Yokoro K, Kajitani T, Ito A (1980) Synergism of diethylstilbestrol and other carcinogens in concurrent development of hepatic, mammary, and pituitary tumors in castrated male rats. J Natl Cancer Inst 65:169–175.

Thomassen RW, Angleton GM, Lee AC, Phemister RD, Benjamin SA (1978) Neoplasms in dogs receiving low-level gamma radiation during pre- and postnatal development. In: Late biological effects of ionizing radiation, Vol. II, Radiation. Vienna: International Atomic Energy Agency, pp 181–189.

Timmermans A, Bentvelzen P, Hageman P, Calafat J (1969) Activation of a mammary tumor virus in 020 strain of mice by x-irradiation and urethane. J Gen Virol 4:619–621.

Ullrich RL (1983) Tumor induction in BALB/c female mice after fission neutron or γ irradiation. Radiat Res 93:506–515.

Ullrich RL, Jernigan MC, Cosgrove GE, Satterfield C, Bowles ND, Storer JB (1976) The influence of dose and dose rate on the incidence of neoplastic disease in RFM mice after neutron irradiation. Radiat Res 68:115–131.

Ullrich RL, Jernigan MC, Storer JB (1977) Neutron carcinogenesis. Dose and dose-rate effects in BALB/c mice. Radiat Res 72:487–498.

Ullrich RL, Storer JB (1978) Influence of dose, dose rate and radiation quality on radiation carcinogenesis and life shortening in RFM and BALB/c mice. In: Late biological effects of ionizing radiation, Vol. I. Vienna: International Atomic Energy Agency, pp 95–113.

Ullrich RL, Storer JB (1979) Influence of γ-irradiation on the development of neoplastic disease in mice. III. Dose rate effects. Radiat Res 80:325–342.

Upton AC, Kimball AW, Furth J, Christenberry KW, Benedict WH (1960) Some delayed effects of atom bomb radiation in mice. Cancer Res 20:1–62.

Upton AC, Randolph ML, Conklin JW, Kastenbaum MA, Slater M, Melville GS Jr., Conte FP, Sproul JA Jr. (1970) Late effects of fast neutrons and gamma-rays in mice as influenced by the dose rate of irradiation induction of neoplasia. Radiat Res 41:467–491.

van Bekkum DW, Broerse JJ, van Zwieten MJ, Hollander CF, Blankenstein MA (1979) Radiation induced mammary cancer in the rat. In: Okada S, Imamura M, Terashima T, and Yamaguchi H (eds.), Radiation Research Proceedings of the Sixth International Congress on Radiation Research. Tokyo: Toppan Co.

van Zwieten MJ, Burek JD, Noateboom AL, Hollander CF, Broerse JJ (1977) Morphological aspects of mammary tumors in irradiated and non-irradiated rats of different strains. Int J Radiat Biol 31 (abstr):379–380.

Vesselinovitch SD, Simmons EL, Mikailovich N, Rao KVN, Lombard LS (1971) The effect of age, fraction, and dose on radiation carcinogenesis in various tissues of mice. Cancer Res 31:2133–2142.

Vogel HH Jr. (1969) Mammary gland neoplasms after fission neutron irradiation. Nature 222:1279–1981.

Vogel HH Jr. (1974) Neutron-induced mammary neoplasms. In: Biological effects of neutron irradiation. Vienna: International Atomic Energy Agency, pp 381–389.

Vogel HH Jr. (1978) High LET irradiation of Sprague–Dawley female rats and mammary neoplasm induction. In: Late biological effects of ionizing radiation, Vol. II. Vienna: International Atomic Energy Agency, pp 147–163.

Vogel HH Jr., Dickson HW (1981) Mammary neoplasia following acute and protracted irradiation with fission neutrons and ^{60}Co gamma-rays. Radiat Res 87 (abstr):453–454.

Vogel HH Jr., Turner JE (1982) Genetic component of rat mammary carcinogenesis. Radiat Res 89:264–273.

Vogel HH Jr., Zaldivar R (1969) Experimental mammary neoplasms: A comparison of effectiveness between neutrons, x- and gamma-radiation. In: Symposium on Neutrons in Radiobiology, Conference 691106. Springfield, VA: Clearinghouse for Federal Scientific and Technical Information, National Bureau of Standards.

Vogel HH Jr., Zaldivar R (1972) Neutron-induced mammary neoplasia in the rat. Cancer Res 32:933–939.

Welsch CW, Goodrich-Smith M, Brown CK, Miglorie N, Clifton KH (1981) Effect of an estrogen antagonist (Tamoxifen) on the initiation and progression of gamma-irradiation-induced mammary tumors in female Sprague–Dawley rats. Eur J Cancer Clin Oncol 17:1225–1258.

Yokoro K, Furth J (1961) Relation of mammotropes to mammary tumors. V. Role of mammotropes in radiation carcinogenesis. Proc Soc Exp Biol Med 107:921–924.

Yokoro K, Furth J, Haran-Ghera N (1961) Induction of mammotropic tumors by x-rays in rats and mice. The role of mammotropes in development of mammary tumors. Cancer Res 21:178–186.

Yokoro K, Kunni A, Furth J, Durbin PW (1964) Tumor induction with Astatine-211 in rats: Characterization of pituitary tumors. Cancer Res 24:683–688.

Yokoro K, Nakano M, Ito A, Nago K, Kodama Y, Hamada K (1977) Role of prolactin in rat mammary carcinogenesis: Detection of carcinogenicity of low-dose carcinogens and of persisting dormant cancer cells. J Natl Cancer Inst 58:1777–1783.

Yokoro K, Sumi C, Ito A, Hamada K, Kanda K, Kobayashi T (1980) Mammary carcinogenic effect of low-dose fission radiation in Wistar/Furth rats and its dependency on prolactin. J Natl Cancer Inst 64:1459–1466.

Ycung S, Hallowes RC (1973) Tumors of the mammary gland. In: Turosov VS (ed.), Pathology of tumors in laboratory animals, Vol. I. Lyon, France: International Agency for Research on Cancer, pp 31–74.

THYROID CANCER: REEVALUATION OF AN EXPERIMENTAL MODEL FOR RADIOGENIC ENDOCRINE CARCINOGENESIS

KELLY H. CLIFTON, Ph.D.

Thyroid carcinoma was the first of the solid malignant tumors noted to be increased in the Japanese atomic bomb survivors (Socolow et al, 1963; Hollingsworth et al, 1963). This discovery followed the observations of Duffy and Fitzgerald (1950) and Simpson et al (1955) of an increase in thyroid cancer risk among those exposed as infants to therapeutic x-rays. To these groups were added the radioactive fallout-exposed Marshall Islanders during the 1960s (Conard et al, 1980). On the basis of continuing studies of the atomic bomb survivors (Sampson et al, 1969; Wood et al, 1969; Parker et al, 1973, 1974) and others (DeGroot et al, 1977; Conard et al, 1980; Dumont et al, 1980) it is now clear that:

1. Radiogenic human thyroid cancer latency is shorter among those exposed before puberty than in those exposed after puberty. In those exposed before puberty, however, the tumors usually do not become apparent until sexual maturation;
2. Women are more susceptible than men to both spontaneous and radiogenic thyroid cancer;
3. Radiogenic thyroid cancer is frequently preceded or accompanied by benign nodules, and intensive irradiation increases the frequency of hypothyroidism and simple goiter in those exposed when young;
4. Radiogenic carcinomas are primarily of papillary, follicular, or mixed histopathology.

The advent of atomic energy and the availability of radionuclides for medical and experimental application have stimulated interest in experimental radiation carcinogenesis. The unique capacity of the thyroid gland to concentrate

From the Departments of Human Oncology and Radiology, Wisconsin Clinical Cancer Center, University of Wisconsin Medical School, Madison, Wisconsin.

iodine, and the early application of iodine nuclides to clinical evaluation of throid function made the thyroid an especially attractive and important organ for experimental radiation biology. Short- and long-term studies involving both acute and chronic radiation exposures were initiated in the first post-war decade. This chapter will selectively review the status of experimental studies of radiogenic thyroid cancer as an example of radiation-endocrine neoplasia, reinterpret some older data in the light of recent findings, and assess the implications for humans. The discussion deals with the thyroxine-triiodothyronine–producing follicular cells from which radiogenic thyroid neoplasms arise; tumors of the calcitonin-producing parafollicular C cells have not been shown to increase in frequency following radiation exposure. For reviews of the literature, see Bielschowsky (1955), Doniach (1963), Lindsay and Chaikoff (1963), Christov and Raichev (1972), Malone (1975), and Dumont et al (1980).

THYROID PHYSIOLOGY

The advantages of thyroid neoplasia as an experimental model extend beyond its practical medical importance. Thyroid cell growth, proliferation, and function can be manipulated by hormonal, dietary, or pharmaceutical means. The functional products of the gland are easily quantified. The gland is accessible for surgical procedures. Alternatively, complete or subtotal radiothyroidectomy can be performed with iodide-131. Given syngeneic animals, thyroid pieces or cells are readily transplantable. And finally, the expression of cellular damage in overt neoplasia is heavily dependent on the functional condition of the gland.

The prime functions of the thyroid follicular cells are the synthesis, storage, and release of the thyroid hormones thyroxine (T4) and 3-5-3' triiodothyronine (T3). In addition, small amounts of reverse T3 (rT3; 3-3'-5' triiodothyronine) are secreted and are formed by peripheral deiodination of T4. Synthesis occurs in three phases, including the uptake and concentration of inorganic iodide, the preceding or concurrent synthesis of thyroglobulin (TG), and iodine organification and iodothyronine formation in the TG molecule. The iodinated TG is then stored in the thyroid follicle as colloid.

The concentration of inorganic iodide across the basal thyroid epithelial cell membrane is ATP-dependent and occurs against a gradient of 7:1 in euthyroid animals, and more than 100:1 in animals in which iodide organification is blocked by thiocarbamides, such as propylthiouracil (DeGroot, 1965). The iodide passes to the microvillar follicular apex of the epithelial cell where organification takes place. Inorganic iodide oxidation and organification, and coupling of iodinated tyrosine residues to form iodothyronines within TG molecules occurs in this complex apical region (DeGroot, 1965; Dumont et al, 1980).

The secretion of T4 and T3 involves endocytosis of vacuoles of colloid containing TG at the epithelial cell apices, the hydrolysis of TG with release of T4, T3, monoiodotyrosine (MIT), diiodotyrosine (DIT), and I by enzymes of lysosomes that fuse with the TG vacuoles during their transport through the cells, and the release of T3 and T4 at the basal cell surface. Some MIT, DIT, I and even TG is also released, but most is recycled intracellularly (Deme et al, 1979).

Recent data indicate an active step in the sequence of end-organ cellular T3 uptake, passage through the cytosol and binding to the nuclear receptors (Halpern and Hinkle, 1982). The mitochondria also contain specific receptor sites. As a result of presumed chromatin-receptor T4 or T3 interaction, specific mRNA molecules are synthesized, protein synthesis including NA-K-ATP-ase is increased, and oxygen consumption is stimulated. ATP production is stimulated in the mitochondria (Sterling, 1979). No function has been ascribed to rT3, which is catabolized.

The steps mentioned in thyroid function are subject to feedback regulation through the hypothalamico-hypophyseal system (Figure 1). T4 and T3 levels are monitored via receptors in the hypothalamus and perhaps elsewhere in the central nervous system (Clifton, 1977). If such levels drop below optimum, secretion by the hypothalamus of thyrotropin-stimulating hormone (TRH) results. TRH reaches the anterior pituitary thyrotropin (thyroid stimulating hormone, TSH) secreting cells directly via the hypophyseal portal sinusoids, where it stimulates secretion and synthesis of TSH.

TSH is released into the general circulation whence it reaches the thyroid follicular cells, to stimulate T4 and T3 release and synthesis. As circulating levels of the latter increase, TRH and TSH release are reduced, and the "long loop feedback" circuit is completed (Clifton, 1977).

This long loop feedback is supplemented by two short-loop systems (Figure 1). TSH directly inhibits TRH release, and T3 and T4 directly suppress TSH production by the pituitary thyrotropes. Finally, the system may be further modulated by neural stimulation and by other hormones.

TSH acts on the various stages of thyroid hormone synthesis and release in a time-dependent fashion (Dumont et al, 1980). The initial steps are combination

FIGURE 1. Single long loop (LL) and two short loop (SL) feedback systems in regulation of the hypothalmico-hypophyseal-thyroid system. T4: thyroxine; T3: triiodiothyronine; TRH: thyrotropin releasing hormone; TSH: thyroid stimulating hormone; HHPS: hypothalamico-hypophyseal portal system; GC: general circulation.

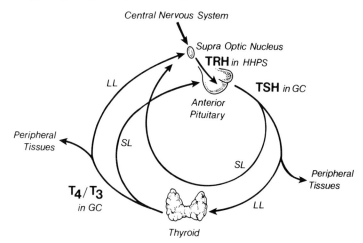

of TSH with specific thyroid cell receptor sites, activation of adenyl cyclase, and formation of 3'-5' cyclic adenosine monophosphate (cAMP) (Rodesch et al, 1969; Knopp et al, 1970; Bowers, 1971; Dumont et al, 1971). Within minutes, colloid droplets are engulfed at the cell apices, and T4 and T3 secretion ensues.

An elevation in iodide uptake and organification occurs a few to several tens of minutes later; mRNA and protein synthesis are required. Finally, TSH stimulates thyroid epithelial cell proliferation, as well as function (Fukuda et al, 1975; Dumont et al, 1980).

Feedback regulation of the thyroid is vulnerable to disruption by natural, therapeutic, or experimental means at virtually every step (Bielschowsky, 1955; Dumont et al, 1980). The goitrogenic effect of iodide deficiency has been recognized since antiquity, and experimental hypothyroidism is readily induced by diets low in iodine. Pharmacologic disruption of iodide concentration by perchlorate, and of iodide oxidation and iodothyronine synthesis by thiocarbamides and other goitrogens are common experimental techniques used to block T4 and T3 synthesis. Partial or total destruction of the thyroid epithelial cells may be induced by administration of radioiodide. A TSH-mimicking molecule, long-acting thyroid-stimulating protein (LATS), results in hyperthyroidism in some humans. Many of these observations have been exploited experimentally in studies of thyroid radiobiology and carcinogenesis.

DOSIMETRY PROBLEMS

For those studying the effects of external photon radiations, the dosimetry problem is important but usually not difficult (Dumont et al, 1980). Doses can be measured directly by implanted microchambers or thermoluminescent dosimeters, and it can usually be assumed that dose distribution to the epithelial cells is uniform. Uniformity of dose distribution can also usually be assumed for exposure to external sources of accelerated particulate radiations, though the physical aspects of dose measurement may be complex (Malone et al, 1974; Malone, 1975; Higgins et al, 1981).

In contrast, dosimetry calculations for radiation from internal thyroid-seeking nuclides is complex and subject to several sources of error (Dumont et al, 1980). Biological variables include: a) the fraction of the internally deposited nuclide concentrated in the thyroid; b) the biological residence time of the nuclide in the gland; c) the uniformity of distribution of the nuclide throughout the gland; and d) glandular and cellular dimensions relative to the mean path length of radiation from the nuclide. In turn, these depend on the physiologic state and, particularly, the dietary iodide intake of the animal.

In much of the literature, ^{131}I uptake has been calculated from a few measurements on small numbers of animals, and the release of the nuclide from the gland has been assumed to be well described by a single exponential function (Lee et al, 1979; Malone, 1975). Lee et al (1979) recently measured the thyroidal uptake and release of ^{131}I at three dose levels in rats sacrificed at intervals during 2 wk after administration. The nuclide clearance was a complex function and the effective nuclide half-lives in the glands were 30%–50% less than those calculated by conventional methods; the estimated total doses calculated according to a refined method (Loevinger and Berman, 1968) were approximately 60% of those in most previous studies (Lee et al, 1979; Dumont et al, 1980). The time of maximum uptake varied with dose; small doses are more effectively incorporated and retained (Malone, 1975).

It is safe to assume that the dose to small animal thyroid glands from ^{131}I and most other thyroid-seeking nuclides is derived from the accelerated electrons released by decay (i.e., the gamma rays are of such energy as to be little absorbed within the small thyroid glands of rats and mice). The loss of beta ray energy from the surface of the gland decreases inversely with gland size; the more the dimensions of gland exceed the mean beta ray path length, the smaller the fraction of beta rays that escape from the gland surface. Corrections for this loss can be made (Loevinger and Berman, 1968; Lee et al, 1979).

A related source of error is due to dose inhomogeneity. Cells in the center of the gland will be irradiated with beta rays from all directions; those near the surface will receive fewer from the surface side. In a mouse, thyroid cells near the surface may receive as little as 50% of the dose to the central cells (Dumont et al, 1980). This error also decreases as gland size increases. These latter two sources of error decrease with nuclides such as ^{125}I, the accelerated electrons of which have such short path lengths as to be absorbed within one cell dimension. However, Greig et al (1970) calculated that, because of the low energy of the electrons emitted during ^{125}I decay, the dose to the basally oriented thyroid epithelial cell nucleus is about 50% that of the dose to the apical cytoplasm.

And finally, none of the overall dose calculation procedures take into account inhomogeneities due to irregular distribution of nuclide within the gland, or even within follicles (Dumont et al, 1980).

In view of the limitations and disagreements within and among the various radionuclide dose estimates, our emphasis in the remainder of this discussion is placed on the effects of exposure to external radiation beams.

PHASES OF EXPERIMENTAL THYROID CARCINOGENESIS

The sequence of events in thyroid carcinogenesis may be divided for discussion into three phases: a) an acute phase including radiogenic damage, intracellular repair and neoplastic initiation; b) the latent phase, from the acute phase until overt tumor formation; and c) the phase of tumor growth.

Acute Phase Carcinogenesis

The first step in radiogenic thyroid cancer induction is generally presumed to be formation of one or more heritable intracellular precancerous changes in one to many of the thyroid epithelial cells; i.e., initiation (Dumont et al, 1980). The nature of initiation is not known; Heidelberger (1981) notes, however, that in the widely studied mouse 10T$\frac{1}{2}$ cell line, mutagenesis may be essential, but is not sufficient for oncogenic transformation in vitro. In turn, it seems to me that the process of transformation in vitro is homologous to but only a portion of the oncogenic process in vivo. In any event, it seems likely that initiation involves direct or indirect effects on the genetic apparatus (Heidelberger, 1981; Knudson, 1981). Perhaps one form of initiation is a genetic or epigenetic change that results in chromosome instability followed by clonal selection of more neoplastic gene imbalances (see Beierwaltes and Al Saadi, 1968).

A problem in thyroid neoplasia is the difficulty in determining if a change is primary to neoplasia or a secondary effect of neoplasia. Furthermore, there is as yet no method for distinguishing initiated cells from their normal neighbors in the thyroid in vivo. A recently designed quantitative thyroid epithelial cell transplantation system, however, has yielded information on the potentialities of normal and irradiated thyroid epithelial cell clonogens (Clifton et al, 1978; Clifton, 1980) and may be applicable to this problem. This method is based on the ability of monodispersed rat thyroid cells to give rise to morphologically and functionally normal thyroid follicles after inoculation into the subcutaneous white fat pads of histocompatible recipients. The cumulative evidence indicates that under appropriate hormonal conditions, follicle(s) can be derived from a single thyroid clonogen (Mulcahy et al, 1980a, 1980b; Clifton, 1980). The proportion of grafted clonogens triggered to follicle formation is dependent on the levels of TSH (Mulcahy et al, 1980b, Watanabe et al, 1983). Furthermore, the majority of untriggered clonogens may survive for at least 1 mo at the site of transplantation in the absence of elevated TSH levels; when such cells are then subjected to increased TSH, they give rise to follicles (Mulcahy et al, 1980b). A similar capacity of thyroid cells to remain dormant in the lungs of mice for up to 1 yr after intravenous injection of monodispersed thyroid cell suspensions was reported by Taptiklis (1968). The clonogenic efficiency of thyroid cells from 1 yr old rats is less than that of young animals (Watanabe et al, 1983).

The capacity of transplanted thyroid cells to form follicles has been used as the endpoint in a dilution assay for thyroid clonogenic cell survival following irradiation with low-LET x-rays in vitro or in vivo (DeMott et al, 1979; Mulcahy et al, 1980c). The resulting survival data were analyzed according to the multi-target, single-hit model (Elkind and Whitmore, 1967). The D_0 value (a measure of inherent radiosensitivity) for thyroid cells exposed to low-LET radiation in vivo or in vitro and assayed by transplantation immediately thereafter was 195–200 rad, near the upper, resistant limit reported for mammalian cells of other types; the n value (a measure of postirradiation intracellular repair of sublethal damage) was 4.

When left in their normal tissue environs for 24 hr after irradiation before removal for cell survival assay, thyroid clonogens were found capable of a high degree of intracellular repair of radiation-induced potentially lethal damage. This type of repair process (in situ repair, ISR) (Gould and Clifton 1979) affects the n value, increasing it to 10–12 in thyroid cells, but not the D_0, which remained 195–200 rad (Figure 2) (Mulcahy et al, 1980c; Gould and Clifton, 1979). In mammary cells, kinetic studies have shown that such repair is complete by 4 hr after exposure (Mahler et al, 1983). It is of interest that mammary epithelial clonogens are significantly more sensitive to low-LET radiation (D_0 = 130 rad) than thyroid clonogens (DeMott et al, 1979), whereas, hepatocytes (D_0 = 250 rad) are more resistant than thyroid clonogens (Jirtle et al, 1981).

On the completion of ISR, the irradiated thyroid epithelial cell population is comprised of three classes: a) a normal cell population, including cells that escaped significant radiation injury, and cells in which any such injury has been completely and correctly repaired; b) "terminally damaged" cells, includ-

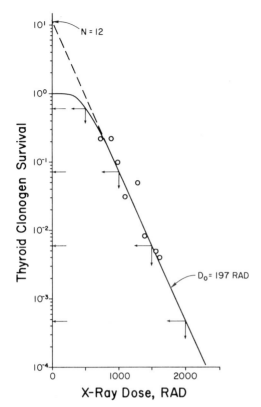

FIGURE 2. Rat thyroid clonogen survival after x-irradiation in vivo followed by in situ repair. Data points from Mulcahy et al (1980c). Arrows indicate survival fractions at 500-rad intervals.

ing those cells that have lost clonogenic capacity but which may persist and function for prolonged periods; and c) reproductively viable but permanently altered cells, including initiated cells.

There is little biochemical evidence of acute impairment of thyroid gland function soon after external radiation doses in the range usually used in carcinogenesis studies; i.e., up to 2000 rad external gamma or x-rays (Dumont et al, 1980). As Doniach (1967, p. 259) has stated:

> The notion that the thyroid gland is resistant to radiation is based on the lack of effect on secretory function. The major damage of radiation is on cell renewal. Since cell renewal is at a very low level in the normal adult thyroid, radiation damage is not immediately manifest functionally.

Thus, animals locally irradiated with carcinogenic doses but otherwise untreated enter the latent phase in a euthyroid condition.

Latent Phase

Given the three cell classes in the thyroid at the end of the acute phase, tumor growth *is not* an inevitability to become manifest after a predetermined period. Rather, whether or not the radiogenic damage is expressed in frank tumor formation, and if so, when, depends on the interaction of internal environmental factors with the cells of the three classes. The importance of the events during latency is underscored by the duration of this phase—10 mo to more than 2 yr in otherwise untreated rats, and proportionately longer in longer-lived species—and the fact that rarely, if ever, is overt cancer observed in 100% of irradiated, otherwise untreated animals.

Under normal circumstances, the thyroid epithelial cell division rate is low, as Doniach (1967) noted, but it is not nil. Tritiated thymidine labeling indices in mature rats generally have been found to 1–3:1000 thyroid cells (Grieg et al, 1969; Sheline, 1969; Christov et al, 1973). Recent studies with grafted thyroid cells have demonstrated that in euthyroid rats, TSH in concert with other factors is adequate at titers that, by definition, are within the normal range to trigger a small portion of the inoculated clonogens to follicle formation (Mulcahy et al, 1980b). The efficiency of such thyroid clonogen triggering is dependent on the age and sex of the host, as are mean TSH levels (Watanabe et al, 1983). The triggering of follicle formation from grafted thyroid clonogens in euthyroid animals likely reflects the homeostatic fluctuations in TSH necessary to support normal gland growth and replacement of cells.

In the early latent phase, cells of all three subpopulations in the irradiated thyroid, thus, will be subjected a few at a time to mitosis-triggering stimuli. Triggered normal cells will respond with normal mitosis. Triggered altered but reproductively viable, including initiated cells, as noted, are not distinguishable from normal; in this discussion, they will be presumed to proliferate in response to triggering stimuli. Triggered terminally damaged cells may pass successfully through one or two mitoses, or survive without division but with persistence of secretory function for several months. Ultimately, however, the proportion of terminally damaged cells will slowly decrease through cell death, and triggering stimuli will again increase to bring about their replacement. Cells of all three classes will again be triggered. Depending on radiation dose and, hence, the fraction of the population comprised of terminally damaged cells, this process of triggering and cell death may continue very slowly, perhaps undetectably, over many months in rats. Or, it may accelerate over time from the slow beginning.

Assuming the thyroid clonogen survival parameters illustrated in Figure 2, no detectable change in gland function or morphology would be expected after 250 rad or less; this is consistent with the report by Doniach (1967) of a threshold between 250 and 500 rad for histologically detectable radiogenic damage. After 1000 rad, however, when only ~7% of clonogens would be expected to retain reproductive capacity (Figure 2), partial glandular atrophy was found to occur with time and was coupled with epithelial cell hypertrophy and interstitial fibrosis, although the animals remained euthyroid (Doniach, 1967). Similar changes were observed after injection of 30 μCi [131]I (Doniach and Logothetopoulos, 1955). Higher doses (> 1500–2000 rad) result in widespread evidence of epithelial cell damage, including mitochondrial swelling, disruption of the endoplasmic reticulum, formation of cytoplasmic vesicles, and nuclear fragmentation (Lindsay and Chaikoff, 1963). Epithelial cell degeneration, follicle disruption, and interstitial and vascular fibrosis develop. These changes are qualitatively similar following exposure to external radiations or internal [131]I (Lindsay and Chaikoff, 1963; Garner, 1963; Doniach, 1977). They occur soon after exposure to very high single doses, or are delayed for weeks to months in smaller animals and years in large species at external doses closer to 2000 rad. If such damage is extensive, hypothyroidism develops as a result of ultimate total or subtotal radiothyroidectomy. It is of importance to note, however, that neoplasia is a less common result in extensively damaged glands than in glands that received radiation doses after which 1%–50% of the epithelial clonogens would be expected to survive.

Goitrogenic drugs, such as aminotriazole, methimazole, and methyl- and propylthiouracil, have been widely used in studies of rat thyroid radiobiology and carcinogenesis, and much has been learned from their use (Dumont et al, 1980). An attempt is made below to reconcile aspects of the interpretation of such data with the recent thyroid clonogen results.

Administration of goitrogenic drugs, alone or in combination with an iodine deficient diet, leads to a period of TSH-stimulated rapid thyroid growth. In unirradiated rats, this hyperplasia proceeds for 8–12 days after a lag of about 2 days, and is followed by a glandular growth plateau. If the thyroid has been exposed to acute irradiation at doses less than 1200–1500 rad before goitro-genic challenge, glandular hypertrophy occurs, but the weight plateau reached is decreased in relation to the dose of radiation. At higher doses, no prolifera-tive growth occurs, although there is some gland enlargement due to non-proliferative cellular hypertrophy (Dumont et al, 1980).

On the one hand, the pattern of growth of the goitrogen-treated rat thyroid has led several investigators to conclude that thyroid cells are inherently lim-ited to one to two serial cell divisions (Doniach and Logothetopoulos, 1955; Grieg et al, 1969; Christov, 1975; Dumont et al, 1980). The degree of inhibition of goitrous growth by radiation, thus, has been taken as a direct measure of cell survival, and has led to D_o estimates of more than 400 rad (Malone, 1975; Dumont et al, 1980). On the other hand, transplantation results, as noted, have shown that a high proportion of normal thyroid epithelial cells are clono-genic, capable of individually giving rise to multicellular functional follicles, and that this clonogenic cell population is considerably more radiosensitive than has been implied by the estimates from goitrogen-treated animals (Clifton, 1980).

This apparent contradiction may be attributable to functional survival of terminally damaged cells, and to the requirement of thyroid cells for factors in addition to elevated TSH for sustained mitotic activity. Sellers and Schonbaum (1962) found that thyroxine in small amounts promotes goitrogenesis in pro-pylthiouracil-treated rats, and a small amount of iodine is necessary for opti-mal mitotic triggering of transplanted clonogens in iodine-depleted rats (Mulcahy et al, 1980b). Finally, the time of appearance of the growth plateau after the initial period of rapid growth during a goitrogenic regimen corre-sponds well with the 2–3 wk required for serum T4 levels to fall below normal after initiation of an iodine deficient diet (Mulcahy et al, 1980b).

In irradiated glands, the population of terminally damaged cells has a radia-tion-induced limit to its proliferative capacity. Despite this limit, terminally damaged cells, which by clonogen assay comprise the majority of the cell population in glands irradiated with 600 rad or more (Figure 2), continue to function and contribute to the non-proliferative cellular hypertrophy seen in the response of irradiated glands to goitrogens.

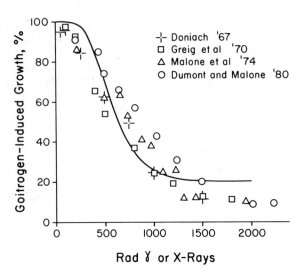

FIGURE 3. Inhibition of goitrogen-induced maximal thyroid growth as a function of radiation dose. Data points are from the literature as indicated. The solid line was calculated from the clonogen survival curve of Figure 2 (see text).

For the purpose of discussion, four sets of data on inhibition by low-LET radiation of goitrogen-induced thyroid growth in rats are plotted in Figure 3. These gave rise to D_o estimates of 450 rad (Grieg et al, 1970), 405 rad (Malone et al, 1974) and 540 rad (Dumont et al, 1980). Doniach (1967) did not estimate the D_o. A linear plot of the formula

$$G = [H + S(1 - H)]\ 100$$

is superimposed. In this model, G is goitrogen-induced thyroid growth expressed as a percentage of the unirradiated maximum; H is the fraction of that growth due to non-proliferative cellular hypertrophy (Dumont et al, 1980), here arbitrarily taken as 0.2; S is the fraction of thyroid clonogens surviving, assuming $D_o = 197$ rad and n=12 (Figure 2); and (1-H) is a constant reflecting the weight increase due to the same number of divisions in the surviving cells at each dose. This model does not take into account cell loss, edema, or proliferation on the part of cells other than surviving epithelial clonogens. It does, however, illustrate that the results of the clonogen transplantation survival assay are reasonably consistent with the inhibition of goitrogen-induced thyroid growth.

From the standpoint of carcinogenesis, the important process during the latent phase is amplification of the radiation-altered initiated cell population under repeated mitosis-triggering stimuli. And during this process, insofar as repeated rounds of DNA synthesis and mitosis play a role in progression of initiated cells, progression as well as amplification occurs. In endocrine-responsive cell populations, progression is frequently associated with quantitative or qualitative changes in hormone responsiveness (Furth, 1961; Clifton and Sriharan, 1975; Furth 1975). However, thyroid tumors often arise in severely hypothyroid animals. Perhaps progression in thyroid neoplasia involves changes in thyroid hormone requirements.

The normal cell population is also amplified during the latent phase; the terminally damaged population is diminished and ultimately completely eliminated.

Any condition that serves to increase triggering stimuli, particularly TSH, will accelerate these shifts in cell populations, shorten the latent period, and increase tumor incidence (Dumont et al, 1980). In fact, chronic iodine deficiency alone was sufficient to induce adenomas and carcinomas in Fischer rats (Beierwaltes and Al-Saadi, 1968) and chronic exposure of mouse thyroid tissue to elevated TSH from grafted secretory thyrotropic pituitary tumors led to TSH-dependent thyroid adenomas (Haran-Ghera et al, 1960) and to an autonomous thyroid carcinoma (Sinha et al, 1965). Goitrogenic drugs are themselves oncogenic (Dumont et al, 1980); however, it is not certain if this effect is mediated exclusively through elevated TSH titers.

Finally, sex-related normal differences in circulating TSH titers probably account for the greater susceptibility of male rats and female humans to thyroid cancer, compared with their respective sexual opposites. Conversely, suppression of TSH levels by thyroid hormone treatment suppresses oncogenesis (Doniach, 1977; Dumont et al, 1980).

In sum, elevated TSH levels accelerate and increase the frequency of radiogenic thyroid tumors; but both adenomas and carcinomas occur in the absence of experimental manipulation other than radiation exposure.

Tumor Growth Phase: Aspects of Dose–Response Relationships

Radiation-induced thyroid tumors first appear as localized hyperplastic nodules. They are often multifocal, suggesting origin from randomly distributed initiated clonogens. Adenomas are more common than carcinomas, occurring 10–16 mo after exposure in rats and increasing in frequency with time thereafter (Doniach, 1963). Carcinomas appear after 18–24 mo in rats and are frequently found within adenomas. Adenomas are predominantly follicular, although papillary types are seen. Carcinomas are predominantly follicular, papillary, of mixed architectures, or are poorly differentiated.

Beierwaltes and Al-Saadi (1968) described dependent, transitional, and autonomous thyroid tumors induced in rats by prolonged iodine deficiency. Growth of the dependent and transitional tumors was stimulated by thyroid hormone deficiency. Dependent tumors were adenocarcinomas or follicular carcinomas; 4% of their cells lacked one chromosome #15, and about 2% bore other marker chromosomes. Transitional tumors were follicular or papillary; 39% of their cells lacked a chromosome #15, and 5% had markers. Autonomous tumors were anaplastic carcinomas, 64% of the cells of which lacked one chromosome #15, and 70% bore marker chromosomes.

Though the relationship between x-ray dose and thyroid oncogenesis in rats is beclouded by the small numbers of animals studied to date, the long latent period, and the differences among experiments in rat strain, age, sex, and postexposure treatment, it is clear that tumor frequency reaches maximum following doses of about 1100 rad (Doniach, 1963; Lindsay and Chaikoff, 1963;

Dumont et al, 1980). Because thyroid clonogen survival is 7×10^{-2} at 1000 rad and 5×10^{-4} at 2000 rad (Figure 2), it is not surprising that tumor induction decreases at higher doses.

Lee et al (1982) have recently reported results of a large-scale study involving a total of 3000 Long–Evans female rats that were irradiated and maintained without further treatment for 2 yr. Acute x-ray doses of 0, 94, 410, and 1060 rad were delivered locally to the thyroid. There was no evidence of thresholds in the resulting carcinoma incidence curve and total tumor incidence curve. In agreement with Malone and Greig (1975), they found that local irradiation of the pituitary gland with or without concurrent exposure of the thyroid had no significant effect on thyroid tumor incidence.

One aim of the study by Lee et al was to compare the neoplastic effect of external x-irradiation with comparable radiation doses from internally administered ^{131}I. They gave 0.48, 1.9, and 5.4 μCi ^{131}I to achieve calculated radiation doses of 80, 330, and 850 rad (Lee et al, 1979, 1982). The range of carcinoma risk per rad was $0.7–2.3 \times 10^{-4}$ for both radiation types, with a somewhat higher risk at lower radiation doses. These findings call into question the previous conclusions that acute external x-radiation exposure is as much as ten times as effective in tumor induction as radiation from internally administered ^{131}I.

A striking aspect of the findings of Lee et al (1982) is the absence of a dose-rate effect between the high rate of x-rays and the low rate from radioiodide. In view of the high intracellular repair capacity of thyroid clonogens (Mulcahy et al, 1980c), it would seem likely that the proportion of terminally damaged cells in the radionuclide irradiated thyroids would be much lower than in the x-irradiated glands. One might then expect a high proportion of initiated cells to survive, unless the initiating events are also subject to repair.

The development of the quantitative thyroid cell transplantation technique for the first time has permitted carcinogenesis in vivo to be studied in terms of surviving clonogens. The results of the first such experiment, aimed at determining the relationship between transplanted surviving thyroid clonogen number and tumor incidence after exposure in vitro to 0 or 500 rad x-rays, are summarized in Figure 4. In this study, the rats were thyroidectomized one day before transplantation and were maintained on a low-iodine regimen from the day of transplantation until death or sacrifice 2.5 yr after grafting. The number of "morphologically intact" cells per inoculation site, corrected for postirradiation survival, varied from 3.7×10^3 to 5.9×10^4. This corresponds to 26–411 surviving thyroid clonogens per graft site, respectively (Mulcahy et al, 1984).

As expected, carcinomas and adenomas occurred in graft sites that received unirradiated cells, as well as in those that received irradiated clonogens. Surprisingly, however, neither carcinomas nor total tumors increased markedly with grafted cell number. The overall increase in risk due to irradiation with 500 rad was about 3.5, compared with unirradiated controls. This compares reasonably well with risk estimates calculated from the in situ thyroid carcinogenesis data of other investigators (Mulcahy et al, 1984).

At the lowest grafted cell number, the risk of carcinoma initiation at 500 rad corresponds to about one initiated clonogen per 1000 clonogens grafted. Gould (1983) has suggested that if all clonogen inocula contained the same proportion

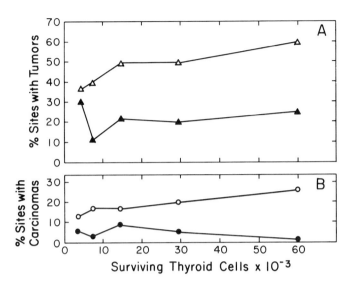

FIGURE 4. (A) Percentage of thyroid clonogen transplant sites with tumors (adenomas or carcinomas). (B) Percentage of thyroid clonogen transplant sites with carcinomas. *Abscissa:* "Surviving thyroid cells" = number of morphologically intact cells inoculated per site corrected for post irradiation survival. *Open symbols:* Thryoid cells were irradiated in vitro with 500 rad x-rays before grafting (clonogen survival approximately 30%). *Closed symbols:* Thryoid cells were unirradiated. All recipient rats were thyroidectomized one day before transplantation and were maintained thereafter on an iodine deficient diet.
Data from Mulcahy et al (1984).

of initiated cells, and if amplification during latency led to the same approximate total cell number, the final numbers of initiated cells would be similar in grafts originating from inocula of different sizes. In any event, the data indicate that initiation is a more frequent event than has generally been considered (Gould, 1983; Mulcahy et al, 1984). Thus, they add further emphasis to the importance of the events that occur during the latent phase, which determine if the initiated cells progress to full neoplasia.

PRESENT AND FUTURE IMPLICATIONS FOR HUMANS

Analysis of the data from atomic bomb survivors and other irradiated groups yielded an overall thyroid cancer risk estimate of 4–5 cases per 10^6 person-yr-rem (CBEIR, 1980). As in experimental animals, the risk of adenomas was greater, about $12–18/10^6$/yr-rem. The cancer risk for women was about three times that for men.

Radiation doses so high as to cause extensive thyroid damage are less apt than lower doses to lead to neoplasia (Dumont et al, 1980). As a consequence, in radiotherapy the greatest risk is likely in those situations where the thyroid is not in the radiation field, but adjacent to it; in the case of individuals who have recieved ^{131}I, the greatest risk is in those in whom the dose was half or less that required for thyroidectomy. Finally, as in experimental animals, human thyroid carcinoma latency is long, occupying a significant fraction of the life span.

The role of radiation as a cause of benign human thyroid disease, and in turn, the possible role of benign disease in human thyroid carcinogenesis deserves further attention. Transient or chronic elevation of TSH or TSH-mimicking substances is a common feature of benign thyroid disease, with the exception of that due to hypopituitarism. Given that irradiated human thyroids contain initiated cells, one would expect most benign human thyroid disease to increase the thyroid cancer risk in irradiated populations.

Hypothyroidism, as well as cancer, has been reported as a late event in the Marshallese fallout victims (Larsen et al, 1978). Hyperthyroidism was more frequent among atomic bomb survivors who received the higher radiation doses, but a causal effect of radiation exposure was not established (Hollingsworth et al, 1963). Simple nontoxic goiter was the most common thyroid disorder generally among the Hiroshima and Nagasaki survivors, and was markedly more common in women than in men (Hollingsworth et al, 1963; Parker et al, 1973). Thus, thyroid diseases other than neoplasia occur among the atomic bomb survivors. Elevated TG titers have been found to be associated with thyroid cancer (Van Herle and Uller, 1975; Lo Gerfo et al, 1977; Black et al, 1981), subacute thyroiditis, and Graves' disease (Izumi and Larsen, 1979; Izumi et al, 1980). A thorough medical study of such a population with modern clinical and laboratory techniques would yield data of great value on the interrelationships among radiation exposure, benign thyroid disease and thyroid neoplasia.

As the experimental studies suggest that thyroid cancer risk increases with the time of exposure to TSH, TSH suppressive therapy would expected to decrease risk. Indeed, in a double-blind study of 396 patients with radiation related nodular thyroids, complete regression of nodules was seen in 29% of those who received thyroid hormone therapy; an additional 38% had partial nodule regression (Tamura et al, 1981).

At the fundamental level, improvements in techniques have made it possible to culture and transplant normal and diseased human epithelial cells. For example, Cathers and Gould (1983) have examined the radiation dose-cell survival response of cultured normal human mammary epithelial cells. Smeds et al (1980) have successfully grafted human toxic thyroid cells in immunodeficient nu/nu mice, and normal human thyroid tissue grew and concentrated radioiodide in a thyroidectomized nu/nu mouse (T. Hiraoka and K.H. Clifton, unpublished). Studies such as these will extend the findings from experimental animal models to humans, and help to establish the limits within which interspecies extrapolations are valid.

CONCLUDING REMARKS

The role of hormones in the etiology of cancer has been known and exploited therapeutically since Beatson's recognition (1896) of an association between breast carcinoma and the ovaries. What the ensuing years have established is that hormones generally act to stimulate neoplastic progression in those cell populations in which they normally play a mitosis-stimulating function. This is clearly the case in radiogenic thyroid carcinoma. Whether or not natural hormones can be considered as initiators in those situations in which tumors arise as a result of prolonged hormone imbalance, as for example thyroid carcinomas following long-term iodine deficiency and consequent chronic TSH stimulation, is perhaps a semantic question. If by initiator it is meant that the agent in question brings about a heritable change by direct physical or chemical interaction, the author thinks not. If however, the term initiator is expanded to include agents that increase the probability of oncogenic error in the genetic apparatus and, once initiation has occurred, cause its amplification by stimulating mitosis, then hormones do qualify. In this sense, hormones might be termed *opportunistic initiators*.

The recently developed thyroid clonogen transplantation technique in rats and the currently developing human cell heterograft and culture systems offer great promise. By their application, the nature of the primary radiation-induced initiating event, and of the events that follow during the long latent period, may be greatly clarified. The understanding so gained will contribute to the diagnosis, therapy, and prevention of thyroid cancer, in particular, and to definition of the processes of radiation and endocrine oncogenesis in general.

Work in the University of Wisconsin laboratories was supported in part by American Cancer Society Grants PDT-86 and RD-179, by National Cancer Institute Grant R01-CA13881, and by Department of Energy Contract DE-AC02-84ER60195.

I am indebted to my friends and colleagues for many fruitful discussions, in particular, Drs. T. Hiraoka and R. Miller (RERF-Hiroshima) and Drs. M.N. Gould, P.A. Mahler, R.T. Mulcahy, and H. Watanabe (University of Wisconsin).

REFERENCES

Beatson GT (1896) On treatment of inoperable cases of carcinoma of the mamma: Suggestions for a new method of treatment, with illustrative cases. Lancet ii:104–107.

Beierwaltes WH, Al-Saadi A (1968) Sequential cytogenetic changes in development of metastatic thyroid acarcinoma. In: Young S and Inman DR (eds.), Thyroid neoplasia. New York: Academic Press.

Bielschowsky F (1955) Neoplasia and internal environment. Br J Cancer 9:80–116.

Black EG, Cassoni A, Gimlette TMD, Harmer CL, Maisey MN, Oates GD, Hoffenberg R (1981) Serum thyroglobulin in thyroid cancer. Lancet ii:443–445.

Bowers CY (1971) Studies on the role of cyclic AMP in the release of anterior pituitary hormones. Ann NY Acad Sci 185:263–290.

Cathers LE, Gould MN (1983) Human mammary cell survival following ionizing radiation. Intl J Radiat Biol 44:1–6.

Christov K (1975) Thyroid cell proliferation in rats and induction of tumors by x-rays. Cancer Res 35:1256–1262.

Christov K, Raichev R (1972) Experimental thyroid carcinogenesis. Current Topics in Pathology. 56:79–114.

Christov K, Bollmann R, Thomas C (1973) Thyroid follicular cell proliferation as a function of age. Beitr Path Bd 148:152–164.

Clifton KH (1977) The physiology of endocrine therapy. In: Becker FF (ed.), Cancer, a comprehensive treatise, Vol. 5. New York: Plenum Press.

Clifton KH (1980) Quantitative studies of the radiobiology of hormone responsive normal cell populations. In: Meyn RE and Withers HR (eds.), Radiation biology in cancer research, 32nd M.D. Anderson Symposium on Fundamental Cancer Research. New York: Raven Press.

Clifton KH, Furth J (1961) Changes in hormone sensitivity of pituitary mammotropes during progression from normal to autonomous. Cancer Res 21:913–920.

Clifton KH, DeMott RK, Mulcahy RT, Gould MN (1978) Thyroid gland formation from inocula of monodispersed cells: Early results on quantification, function, neoplasia and radiation effects. Intl J Radiat Oncol 4:987–990.

Clifton KH, Sridharan BN (1975) In: Becker FF (ed.), Cancer, A comprehensive treatise, Vol. 3. New York: Plenum Press.

Committee on the Biological Effects of Ionizing Radiations (1980) The effects on populations of exposure to low levels of ionizing radiation ("BEIR III") Washington, DC: National Academy Press.

Conard RA, Paglia DE, Larsen PR, Sutow WW, Dobyns BM, Robbins J, Krotosky WA, Field JB, Rall JE, Wolff J (1980) Review of medical findings twenty-six years after accidental exposure to radioactive fallout. BNL 51261 (Biology and Medical TID-4500). Upton, New York: Brookhaven National Laboratory.

DeGroot LJ (1965) Current views of formation of thyroid hormones. N Engl J Med 272:243–250, 297–303, 355–362.

DeGroot LJ, Frohmann LA, Kaplan EL, Refetoff S (1977) Radiation-associated thyroid carcinoma. New York: Grune and Stratton.

DeMott RK, Mulcahy RT, Clifton KH (1979) The survival of thyroid cells following irradiation: A directly generated single-dose-survival curve. Radiat Res 77:395–403.

Doniach I (1950) The effect of radioactive iodine alone and in combination with methylthiouracil and acetylaminofluorene upon tumour production in the rat's thyroid gland. Br J Cancer 4:223–234.

Doniach I (1963) Effects including carcinogenesis of I^{131} and x-rays on the thyroid of experimental animals: A review. Health Phys 9:1357–1362.

Doniach I (1967) Damaging effect of x-irradiation of less than 1000 rads on goitrogenic capacity of rat thyroid gland. In: Young S and Inman DR (eds.), Thyroid neoplasia. New York: Academic Press.

Doniach I (1977) Pathology of irradiation thyroid damage. In: DeGroot LJ, Grohman LA, Kaplan EL, and Refetoff S (eds.), Radiation-associated thyroid carcinoma. New York: Grune and Stratton.

Doniach I, Logothetopoulos JH (1955) Effects of radioactive iodine on the rat thyroids function, regeneration and response to goitrogens. Br J Cancer 9:117–127.

Duffy BJ, Jr., Fitzgerald PJ (1950) Cancer of the thyroid in children: A report of 28 cases. J Clin Endocrinol 10:1296–1308.

Dumont JE, Malone JF, Van Herle AJ (1980) Irradiation and thyroid disease: Dosimetric, clinical and carcinogenic aspects (EUR 6713ER). Luxemborg: Commission of the European Communities.

Dumont JE, Willem C, Sande JV, Neve P (1971) Regulation of the release of thyroid hormones: Role of cyclic AMP. In: Robison GA, Nahas GG, and Triner L (eds.), Cyclic AMP and cell function. Ann New York Acad Sci. 185:291–316.

Elkind MM, Whitmore GF (1967) The radiobiology of cultured mammalian cells. New York: Gordon and Breach.

Fukuda H, Greer MA, Roberts L, Allen CF, Critchlow V, Wilson M (1975) Nyctohemeral and sex-related variations in plasma thyrotropin, thyroxine, and triiodothyronine. Endocrinology 97:1424–1431.

Furth J (1975) Hormones as etiological agents in neoplasia. In: Becker FF (ed.), Cancer, a comprehensive treatise, Vol. 1. New York: Plenum Press.

Garner RJ (1963) Comparative early and late effects of single and prolonged exposure to radioiodine in young and adults of various animal species—A review. Health Phys 9:1333–1339.

Goldberg RC, Chaikoff IL (1951) Development of thyroid neoplasms in the rat following a single injection of radioactive iodine. Proc Soc Exp Biol Med 76:563–566.

Gould MN (1984) Radiation initiation of carcinogenesis *in vivo*: A rare or common cellular event? In: Boice J, Fraumeni JF Jr. (eds.), Radiation carcinogenesis. New York: Raven Press.

Gould MN, Clifton KH (1979) Evidence for a unique *in situ* component of the repair of radiation damage. Radiat Res 77:149–155.

Greig WR et al (1969) Assessment of rat thyroid as a radiobiological model. The effects of x-irradiation on cell proliferation and DNA synthesis *in vivo*. Intl J Radiat Biol 16:211–225.

Greig WR, Smith JFB, Orr JS, Foster CJ (1970) Comparative survivals of rat thyroid cells *in vivo* after ^{131}I, ^{125}I and x-irradiations. Br J Radiol 43:542–548.

Halpern J, Hinkle PM (1982) Evidence for an active step in thyroid hormone transport to nuclei: Drug inhibition of L-^{125}I-triiiodothyronine binding to nuclear receptors in rat pituitary tumor cells. Endocrinology 110:1070–1072.

Haran-Ghera N, Puller P, Furth J (1960) Induction of thyrotropin-dependent thyroid tumors by thyrotropes. Endocrinology 66:694–701.

Heidelberger C (1981) Initiation and promotion, mutagenesis and transformation of C3H/10T1/2 mouse embryo fibroblasts. Gann Monog Cancer Res 27:207–219.

Higgins PD et al (1981) Measurement of OER and RBE for monoenergetic 2.5 and 14.3 MeV neutrons. Intl J Radiat Biol 40:313–319.

Hollingsworth DR, Hamilton HB, Tamagaki H, Beebe GW (1963) Thyroid disease: a study in Hiroshima, Japan. Medicine 42:47–71.

Izumi M, Larsen PR (1979) Correlation of sequential changes in serum thyroglobulin, triiodothyronine and thyroxine in patients with Graves disease and subacute thyroiditis. Metabolism 27:449–460.

Izumi M, Ishimaru T, Takamura K, Usa T, Maeda R, Sato K, Morimoto I (1980) Relationship between human serum thyroglobulin and serum T3, T4, TSH and thyroid size in hyperthyroid and hypothyroid patients. Radiation Effects Research Foundation Technical Report RERF TR 15-80. Hiroshima: Radiation Effects Research Foundation.

Jirtle RL, Michelopoulous G, McLuin JR, Crowley J (1981) Transplantation system for determining the clonogenic survival of parenchymal hepatocytes exposed to ionizing radiation. Cancer Res 41:3512–3518.

Knopp J, Stoloc V, Tong W (1970) Evidence for the induction of iodide transport in bovine thyroid cells treated with thyroid-stimulating hormone or dibutyryl cyclic adenosine 3',5'-monophosphate. J Biol Chem 245:4403–4408.

Knudson AG (1981) Human cancer genes. In: Arrighi FE, Rao PN, and Stubblefield E (eds.), Genes, chromosomes and neoplasia. New York: Raven Press.

Larsen PR et al (1978) Thyroid hypofunction appearing as a delayed manifestation of accidental exposure to radioactive fall-out in a Marshallese population. In: Late biological effects of ionizing radiation, Vol. 1. Vienna: International Atomic Energy Agency.

Lee W, Shleien B, Telles NC, Chiacchierini RP (1979) An accurate method of ^{131}I dosimetry in the rat thyroid. Radiation Res 79:55–62.

Lee W et al (1982) Thyroid tumors following I-131 or localized x-irradiation to the thyroid and the pituitary glands in rats. Radiat Res (in press).

Lindsay S, Chiakoff IL (1963) The effects of irradiation on the thyroid gland with particular reference to the induction of thyroid neoplasms: A review. Cancer Res 24:1099–1107.

Loevinger R, Berman M (1968) A scheme for absorbed dose calculations for biologically distributed radionuclides. J Nucl Med 1 (suppl):8–14.

Lo Gerfo P et al (1977) Serum thyroglobulin and recurrent thyroid cancer. Lancet i:881–882.

Mahler PA, Gould MN, Clifton KH (1983) The kinetics of *in situ* repair in rat mammary cells. Int J Radiat Biol

Malone JF (1975) The radiation biology of the thyroid. Curr Topics Radiat Res Quart 10:263–368.

Malone JF, Greig WR (1975) Effect of pituitary irradiation on the response of rat thyroid to goitrogenic stimulation. Br J Radiol 48:410–411.

Malone JF et al (1974) The response of rat thyroid, a highly differentiated tissue, to single and multiple doses of gamma or fast neutron irradiation. Br J Radiol 47:608–615.

Mulcahy RT, DeMott RK, Clifton KH (1980a) Transplantation of monodispersed rat thyroid cells: Hormonal effects on follicular unit development and morphology. Proc Soc Exp Biol Med 163:100–110.

Mulcahy RT, Rose DP, Mitchen JM, Clifton KH (1980b) Hormonal effects on the quantitative transplantation of monodispersed rat thyroid cells. Endocrinology 106:1769–1775.

Mulcahy RT et al (1980c) The survival of thyroid cells: In vivo irradiation and in situ repair. Radiat Res 84:523–528.

Mulcahy RT et al (1984) Radiogenic initiation of thyroid cancer: A common cellular event. Intl J Radiat Res 45:419–426.

Parker LN, Belsky JL, Mandai T, Blot WJ, Kawate R (1973) Serum thyrotropin level and goiter in relation to childhood exposure to atomic radiation. J Clin Endocrin and Metab 37:797–804.

Parker LN et al (1974) Thyroid carcinoma after exposure to atomic radiation. Ann Intern Med 80:600–604.

Rodesch F, Neve P, Willems C, Dumont JE (1969) Stimulation of thyroid metabolism by thyrotropin; cyclic $3':5'$-AMP, dibutyryl cyclic $3':5'$-AMP and prostaglandin E_1. Eur J Biochem 8:26–32.

Sampson RJ, Key CR, Buncher CR, Iljima S (1969) Thyroid carcinoma in Hiroshima and Nagasaki I. Prevalence of thyroid carcinoma at autopsy. J Am Med Assoc 209:65–70.

Schimmel M, Utiger RD (1977) Thyroidal and peripheral production of thyroid hormones. Ann Intern Med 87:760–768.

Sellers EA, Schonbaum E (1962) Goitrogenic action of thyroxine administered with propylthiouracil. Acta Endocrinolog 40:39–50.

Sheline GE (1969) Thyroid proliferative potential as a function of age. Cell Tiss Kinet 2:123–132.

Simpson CL, Hempelmann LH, Fuller LM (1955) Neoplasia in children treated with x-rays in infancy for thymic enlargement. Radiology 64:840–845.

Sinha D, Pascol R, Furth J (1965) Transplantable thyroid carcinoma induced by thyrotropin. Arch Pathol 79:192–198.

Smeds S, Anderberg B, Boeryd B (1980) Studies of human toxic thyroid tissue in nude mice. Thyroid Res 8:777–780.

Socolow EL, Hashizume A, Nerilishi S, Niitani R (1963) Thyroid carcinoma in man after exposure to ionizing radiation. N Engl J Med 268:406–410.

Sterling K (1979) Thyroid hormone action at the cell level. N Engl J Med 300:117–123 (part I); 173–177 (part 2).

Tamura K, Shimaoka K, Tsukada Y, Razack MS, Sciascia M (1981) Suppressive therapy for radiation-associated nodular thyroid disease: Double-blind study with T3 and dessiccated thyroid. Japanese J Clin Oncol 11:457–462.

Taptiklis N (1968) Dormancy by dissociated thyroid cells in the lungs of mice. Eur J Cancer 4:59–66.

Van Herle AJ, Uller RP (1975) Elevated serum thyroglobulin. A marker of metastases in differentiated thyroid carcinomas. J Clin Invest 56:272–277.

Watanabe H, Gould MN, Mahler PA, Mulcahy RT, Clifton KH (1983) The influence of donor and recipient age and sex on the quantitative transplantation of monodispersed rat thyroid cells. Endocrinolgy 112:172–177.

Wood JW, Tamagaki H, Neriishi S, et al (1969) Thyroid carcinoma in atomic bomb survivors Hiroshima and Nagasaki. Am J Epidemiol 89:4–14.

RADIATION CARCINOGENESIS IN RAT SKIN

FREDRIC J. BURNS Ph.D. AND ROY E. ALBERT M.D.

The skin has been utilized extensively for studying the toxic and carcinogenic effects of environmental and industrial agents (Bock, 1977). In comparison with reactions in internal organs, skin reactions are relatively easy to observe, and skin tumors are detectible at earlier times in their development than tumors in most other organs. The skin contains several cell types, many of which are susceptible to carcinogenesis by exposure to radiation or chemical carcinogens. As a result of exposure to ionizing radiation, rat skin develops several different types of tumors including squamous and basal cell carcinomas, sarcomas, and keratosebaceous tumors. Each type of tumor probably arises from a distinct cell population in the skin. Rat skin develops tumors in response to a number of environmentally important carcinogens other than ionizing radiation, including polycyclic aromatic hydrocarbons and ultraviolet (UV) radiation. Skin is one of the organs in which extensive comparisons of animal results with human epidemiologic data are available (Albert, Burns, and Shore, 1978; Modan, Baidatz, and Mart, 1974). Rat skin, in particular, has proved to be a sensitive and reproducible system for studying the dose-response and time-response characteristics of radiation carcinogenesis and for investigating the mechanisms relating the absorption of the radiation by the cells to the ultimate development of cancer (Albert, Neuman, and Altshuler, 1961).

TIME-RESPONSE FUNCTION OF TUMOR OCCURRENCE

Following exposure of rat skin to single doses of ionizing radiation, epithelial tumors generally begin appearing about 10 wk after irradiation, and new tumors continue to appear at an accelerating rate throughout life. The reproduc-

From the Institute of Environmental Medicine, New York University Medical Center, New York, New York.

ibility of this time pattern is remarkable and by comparing responses at specific times after irradiation, the dose–response relationship can be determined. A time-independent dose–response relationship is possible only if the tumor yield is described by a function where time and dose are separable; i.e., the overall function is a product of two functions one being only a function of time and one being only a function of dose (Whittemore and Keller, 1978). This important idea can be expressed as follows

$$Y(D,t)=f(D)g(t) \tag{1}$$

where the overall yield [Y(D,t)], in tumors per animal for any dose (D), or time after irradiation (t), is a product of function of dose only [f(D)] and function of time only [g(t)].

Figure 1 shows examples of tumor occurrence as a function of time in experiments where rat skin was irradiated with electron radiation penetrating to a depth of about 1.0 mm. The occurrence time of each tumor was the earliest time of visual detection, generally when the tumor was about 1.0 mm diameter. Each tumor was confirmed histologically. Analysis of data alone so far has not been adequate for deriving the analytic forms of f(D) and g(t). Although data provide guidance, the selection of appropriate analytic forms is best derived from basic biological and statistical considerations.

Because of compatibility with the multistage theory of carcinogenesis, the following form has been chosen for g(t) (Armitage and Doll, 1954; Foulds, 1975)

$$g(t)=cx(t-w)^n \tag{2}$$

This form, sometimes referred to as a Weibull function, has often been used to fit a variety of temporal data for events occurring randomly in time. Specifically, the Weibull function has been found to be useful for describing the relation between tumor incidence and time in human populations.

Unfortunately, even the most complete data currently available for rat skin are not adequate for estimating w and n unambiguously. While noninteger values of n are conceivable, consistency with the multistage model requires the use of integers. Restricting n to an integer means that it can only be 1 or 2, because higher values are excluded as inconsistent with the data. The value of w is close to 0 wk and independent of the radiation dose if $n=2$, so we have generally used the latter value in the model.

The data in Figure 1 indicate that new tumors continue to occur at very long times after single doses of radiation. They probably continue to appear for as long as the animals are alive. A carcinogenic alteration in the target cells presumably occurred at the time of or within a few hours after irradiation, yet, a palpable tumor is not seen until many months or even years later. The distribution of appearance times seems not to depend on the distribution of growth rates of the tumors. Tumor growth rates as a function of the time of detection (generally when the tumors are about 1.0 mm in diameter) have indicated no difference between the late and early tumors (Albert et al, 1969; Burns, Vanderlaan, and Albert, 1973). Moreover, the distribution of histologic types of tumors has been approximately the same among early and late occurring tumors.

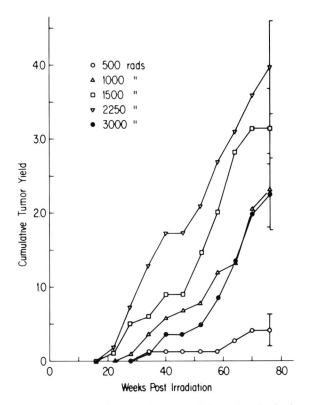

FIGURE 1. Tumor yield in rat skin as a function of time after single doses of electron radiation, as indicated.

DOSE–RESPONSE FUNCTION

Perhaps the most widely used analytic form of the dose–response function, f(D), describing the response of cells to radiation, especially for endpoints such as cell lethality and chromosomal aberration induction, is the quadratic (sometimes called linear-quadratic) function derived from the dual action theory (NAS, 1980; Kellerer and Rossi, 1978). The hypothesis underlying the dual action theory states that the yield of any biological endpoint requiring two radiation-induced events is proportional to the square of the radiation dose in a microscopic region of space that essentially defines the target region within the cell (Kellerer and Rossi, 1978). The form of the expected function is

$$f(D) = AD + BD^2 \tag{3}$$

Equation **3** can be derived from biophysical considerations of the way radiation dose is distributed statistically in small regions of space or from various biological hit theories predicated on the assumption that breaks in the DNA are the primary event in the carcinogenic mechanism (Kellerer and Rossi, 1978; Burns and Vanderlaan, 1977).

Figure 2 shows the tumor yield as a function of dose, i.e. f(D), at 80 wk after irradiation for skin in rats irradiated at 28 days of age with monoenergetic electrons to a depth of 1.0 mm or greater (Vanderlaan, Burns, and Albert, 1976; Burns, Albert, and Heimbach, 1968; Albert, Burns, and Heimbach, 1967a; Burns et al, 1973). The ascending part of the solid curve in Figure 2 is fitted with the function in **3** with A=0. The data in Figure 2 are perhaps the most complete set presently available on the dose–response function of radiation carcinogenesis in a specific organ system.

It is typical of radiation carcinogenesis that the dose–response relationship rises to a peak and then declines at higher doses. The downturn of response at higher doses may reflect the reduced numbers of cells at risk for carcinogenesis, because of the cell-killing effects of radiation. If the alterations relevant to carcinogenesis are transmitted to daughter cells during cell division, then cell lethality that is compensated by regeneration should not affect the cancer incidence. On the other hand if cell lethality is not compensated by regeneration or if regeneration is incomplete, the cancer yield would be reduced because of fewer cells at risk for carcinogenic expression.

Proportionality between the coefficient A and the linear energy transfer (LET) of the radiation is one of the more important expectations of the linear quadratic theory. To examine this question, rat skin was exposed to an argon ion beam at the Lawrence Radiation Laboratory Bevalac Accelerator (Burns and Albert, 1980). The LET of this beam is so high (125 kev/micron) that only a few tracks per nucleus are sufficient to produce a dose of several hundred rads. The results were a striking confirmation of the dual action hypothesis and are shown in Figure 3. In contrast to the data for the electron beam, the dose–response relationship is nearly linear below approximately 900 rads. At higher doses, the yield declined in association with ulceration and loss of tissue. The

FIGURE 2. The yield of tumors as a function of dose at 80 wk after exposure of rat skin to single doses of electron radiation. The error bars were estimated from the square roots of the numbers of tumors.

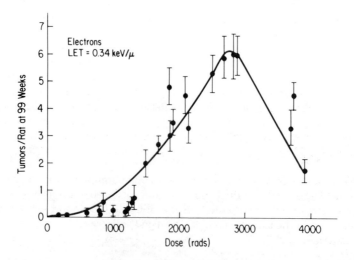

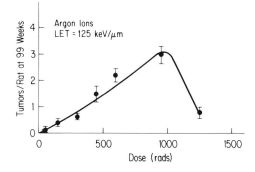

FIGURE 3. The yield of tumors at 80 wk as a function of dose of argon ions. The rats were irradiated at the Bevalac at University of California.

data from Figures 2 and 3 can be combined to provide estimates of the relative biological effectiveness (RBE) as a function of dose. The RBE is about 2.5 near the peak yield dose, and increases as the dose is reduced, reaching about 50 at the lowest dose where data are available (i.e., an argon ion dose of about 75 rads).

RECOVERY AND REPAIR FOR RADIATION CARCINOGENESIS OF SKIN

Generally, mammalian cells are capable of repairing part of the damage related to cell lethality produced by low-LET ionizing radiation. Certainly, if multiple events are involved in carcinogenesis, one might expect carcinogenic alterations to be subject to comparable repair mechanisms. A series of experiments was designed to establish in rat skin whether or not splitting a given dose into two fractions separated in time has a bearing on the carcinogenic effect of a given dose. Carcinogenicity was reduced with increasing time between doses, indicating that the tissue was capable of repairing radiation damage relevant to carcinogenesis (Burns et al, 1975). The repair half-time of the repairing event relevant to carcinogenesis was estimated to be about 3 hr (Burns and Vanderlaan, 1977). These data are shown in Figure 4, which shows a plot of the function P (percentage of damage not repaired). P was determined from the equation

$$P=(f(D,0)-f(D,t)/(f(D,0)-f(D,+))) \qquad (4)$$

where $f(D,0)$ is the cancer yield when two equal doses of magnitude $D/2$ were given with no separation in time (single dose of magnitude D), $f(D,+)$ is the response when two exposures were separated by 24 hr or more, and $f(D,t)$ is the cancer yield when the two exposures were separated by time, t.

Having observed repair for two doses, we asked whether or not a similar degree of repair occurs irrespective of how many individual doses are given. Daily fractions of electrons were given to the same region of skin. A given dose D was split into n equal fractions of magnitude D/n. Because the time between fractions is long in comparison with the repair half-time, the expected yield, y_n, from n fractions equals n times the yield from one fraction $Y(D/n)$ [i.e., $Y_n =nY(D/n)$]. Y_n is measurable, and dividing it by the fraction number and plotting against the dose per fraction (D/n) gives $Y(D/n)$ (i.e., the single dose yield

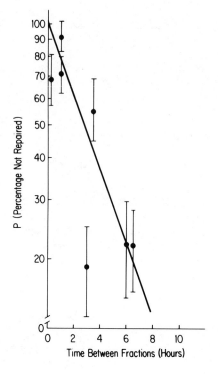

FIGURE 4. The proportion of unrepaired carcinogenic damage as a function of dose at 80 wk after single doses of argon ions in rat skin. See text for an explanation of how these data were derived from the tumor yields.

FIGURE 5. The dose–response relationship for tumor induction in rat skin given multiple daily exposures to electron radiation, as indicated. The data are plotted as tumor yield per fraction as a function of the dose per fraction (see text).

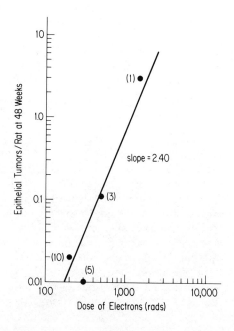

for a dose of D/n). The data are shown in Figure 5. The tumor yield per fraction at 48 wk after irradiation is plotted against the dose of electrons per fraction on a log–log scale. The slope of 2.4 is an estimate of the dose exponent of the second term in **3**.

The question was addressed whether or not the cancer yield is affected when the radiation exposures include times when tumor cells from previous exposures are present and consequently are exposed to additional radiation. In these experiments, the radiation doses were given weekly for the duration of life. The results are shown in Figure 6 for doses of 75 and 150 rads/wk. Also included in Figure 6, for comparison, are results for a single dose. The log–log plot reveals the time exponents to be about 2 for single doses and more than 6 for the lifetime exposures. At 75 rads/wk the exponent was only 2.9, but the data are based on a relatively small number of tumors.

The increased exponent for the multiple doses is much greater than would be expected if the effects of each individual dose were simply additive in each time increment. Simple additivity means that the yield from multiple exposures can be derived by integrating the yields from many small single exposures. Integration of the single-dose function gives an expected exponent of about 3 (i.e., 1 more than about 2). In the multistage theory, the increased value of the exponent could mean either that the number of events increased or that clonal growth expanded the number of early stage cells. Split-dose repair seen for two doses appeared to be operative for as many as 60 exposures, although its effect was partially compensated by the increased time exponent.

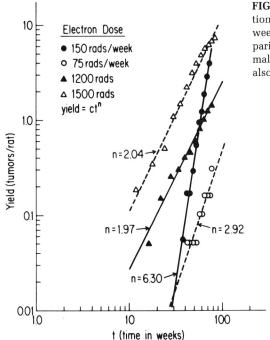

FIGURE 6. Tumor yield as a function of time for rats irradiated weekly for duration of life. For comparison, comparable data for animals exposed to single doses are also shown.

Electron Dose
- ● 150 rads/week
- ○ 75 rads/week
- ▲ 1200 rads
- △ 1500 rads

yield = ct^n

$n = 2.04$

$n = 1.97$

$n = 2.92$

$n = 6.30$

Yield (tumors/rat)

t (time in weeks)

GEOMETRICAL DISTRIBUTION OF DOSE

One surprising result of studies of radiation carcinogenesis in rat skin has been the finding that the yield of tumors is not always proportional to the amount of tissue (number of cells) irradiated (Albert, Burns, Heimbach, 1967a; Albert and Burns, 1976). To study the question of how the geometrical distribution of dose affects the cancer yield, rat skin was irradiated with low energy x-rays in either a sieve pattern or in a uniform pattern. The resulting tumor yields were expressed in units of numbers of tumors per unit area of tissue exposed. Tumor occurrence was markedly delayed when the skin was irradiated through sieves or pores in comparison to uniform exposure. Moreover, when the tissue between the heavily irradiated pores was irradiated with a low dose, the delayed onset was eliminated. We interpreted these results to mean that proximity of unirradiated cells somehow affected the rate of progression of irradiated cells to cancer. Based on geometrical considerations, the protective effect was equivalent to a nonresponse in an annular ring extending for a distance of about 200 u from the edge of the unirradiated region.

Other studies have shown that the yield of tumors is decreased for a given surface dose as the penetration of the radiation is decreased. If the penetration was less than about 180 microns, no tumors at all were observed in groups of about 20 rats (Burns et al, 1975; Albert, Burns, and Heimbach, 1967b). If the radiation penetrated deeper than 180 microns, tumors of all histologic types, including squamous carincomas and adnexal tumors were produced. Overall the yield of tumors was more closely related to the dose at about 300 microns than to the surface dose. Because the bulbs of the resting phase hair follicles are located at a depth of about 300 microns, the results suggested that the entire hair follicle or perhaps only the hair germ near the distal end of the hair follicle needs to be irradiated for carcinogenesis to occur. A test of this hypothesis by selective irradiation at 300 microns with an alpha particle Bragg peak was negative (i.e., no additional tumors were induced over the number expected from the Bragg curve plateau region) (Heimbach, Burns, and Albert, 1969). Unfortunately the width of the Bragg peak may have been too narrow to irradiate a sufficient number of cells to produce a detectible yield of tumors, so the question of whether or not a special target cell population exists at 300 microns remains unresolved.

HAIR FOLLICLE CELL PROLIFERATION AND CARCINOGENESIS

To test if the cell proliferation rate affects the tumor yield, rat skin was exposed in the growing phase of the hair cycle, when the epithelial cell populations in the hair follicles and epidermis are in a relatively rapid state of proliferation (Burns et al, 1976). The yield of tumors in growing phase skin was only slightly higher than in similarly-exposed resting phase skin, in spite of the great differences between the proliferation rates at the time of irradiation. Furthermore, when cell proliferation in the skin was stimulated by plucking the hair repeatedly or by stripping the skin surface with cellophane tape repeatedly, the tumor yield was unaffected. Perhaps not all cells in the hair follicles or the epidermis are at risk for radiation carcinogenesis. If the cells at risk are only a small proportion of the total cells (e.g., the germ cells) the proliferation of the entire organ may not be relevant to the stimulation of carcinogenesis.

The location of the carcinogenically sensitive cells in the anagen phase was determined by varying the penetration of the radiation. The depth found to be most closely correlated with tumor yield was about 0.4 mm; a value not very different from the comparable value found for resting phase skin. In spite of the great difference between the depth of anagen (1.0 mm) and telogen (0.3 mm) follicles, the locations of the critical region did not differ greatly. Perhaps the follicular stem cells (the presumptive target cells) remain at about the same level in the skin throughout the entire hair cycle. Such a possibility is plausible, because during the transition from the large growing follicle to the smaller resting follicle (a transition known as catagen), the entire follicle below the level of the germ cells is resorbed. Presumably, cells with carcinogenic alterations existing below the hair germ level in a growing follicle are resorbed before their carcinogenic potential has a chance to be expressed.

DNA DAMAGE AND REPAIR IN RELATION TO CARCINOGENESIS

There are numerous candidates for the initial lesion in DNA that sets a cell on the path to cancer. Some of the most frequently cited are DNA strand breaks, base damage in the form of adducts, base deletion, DNA–DNA cross links, and others. Breaks in the deoxyribophosphate strand structure are one important way that ionizing radiation damages DNA, and we decided to examine whether or not their induction and repair kinetics were consistent with our knowledge about carcinogenesis in the rat skin (Ormerod, 1976). If such breaks occur in only one strand (single-strand breaks), they are readily repairable, presumably correctly, because of the availability of an unbroken homologous template. However, if breaks occur in both strands (double-strand breaks), the consequence may be a break in the chromosome, which may not be repairable or may repair in a way that causes chromosomal rearrangements (Leenhouts and Chadwick, 1974).

Because two single-strand breaks on opposite strands could produce a double-strand break, it was important to determine if the kinetics of single-strand break repair correlated with repair of carcinogenic damage. It was known that mammalian fibroblasts in tissue culture generally are able to repair radiation-induced single-strand breaks with a half-time of about 20 min, which is much less than the half-time for the repair of the carcinogenic effect. Because the rate of single-strand break repair could be different in vivo, we applied existing techniques to measure the rate of repair of DNA single-strand breaks in the rat epidermis (Burns and Sargent, 1981). Utilizing alkaline unwinding, we obtained data indicating that single-strand breaks were produced in proportion to dose, and that the repair half-time was about 21 min, not very different from values found for a variety of cell lines in vitro. These data are shown in Figures 7 and 8. The discrepancy between half-time for repair and half-time for tumor induction is significant and indicates that single-strand breaks do not fulfill the requirements of the initial lesion in carcinogenesis.

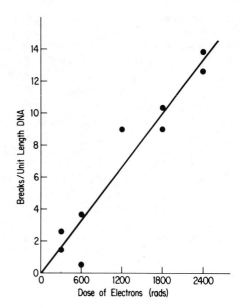

FIGURE 7. The yield of single-strand breaks in rat epidermis as a function of radiation dose for electron radiation. The rats were 28 days old at the time of exposure.

FIGURE 8. The removal of DNA breaks in the epidermis as a function of time after irradiation of rat skin with electrons. The number of breaks was estimated by an alkaline unwinding procedure described in the text.

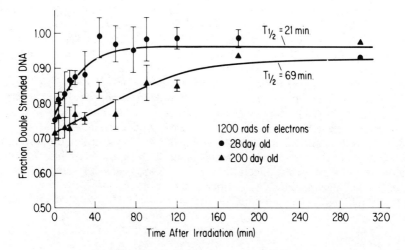

UV CARCINOGENESIS IN COMBINATION WITH IONIZING RADIATION

A large part of the skin cancer burden in humans is associated with exposure to the UV component of sunlight. Furthermore, there is an indication that humans exposed to both UV light and ionizing radiation run a significantly higher risk of developing skin tumors than individuals exposed to either of these agents alone (Shore, Albert, and Pasternack, 1976). In an attempt to determine if rat skin exhibited a similar response synergism, we exposed rats to single doses of ionizing radiation (electrons) followed by multiple weekly doses of germicidal (254 nm) or solar spectrum (greater than 290 nm) UV light. The yield of skin tumors was then determined for at least 18 mo after the final radiation dose.

To obtain an estimate of the UV radiation dose, pyrimidine dimers were measured in the epidermal DNA. Dimers exhibited a linear dependence on exposure dose. The UV alone produced a large number of benign keratoachanthomas but no malignant tumors. The yield of keratoachanthomas was proportional to the dose of UV light and to the number of dimers in the epidermis, for both wavelength regions tested (Strickland, Burns, and Albert, 1979).

The addition of UV to the ionizing radiation yielded more tumors at low doses of ionizing radiation. However, there were fewer tumors at higher doses of ionizing radiation, where the greatest number of tumors is normally expected to occur. The reduction in tumor yield seemed to reflect a sterilizing effect on the development of small tumors, because when the UV exposures were stopped, tumors began to appear at about the same rate as observed in the groups that received ionizing radiation without subsequent UV. It was especially interesting that the UV prevented the onset of all types of tumors, including squamous cell carcinomas and adnexal (hair follicle) tumors. Because more than 80% of the solar spectrum UV dose was absorbed in the epidermis, and because virtually none penetrated as deep as the sebaceous glands, the hair follicle germ cells received little, if any, dose. If the sterilizing effect resulted from a direct action of the UV, one must assume that the presumptive tumor cells were in or just below the surface epidermis at the time of exposure to the UV. This interpretation conflicts with the results indicating that critical targets for radiation carcinogenesis may be located about 300 microns below the skin surface. The enhancement by UV of the induction of malignant tumors at lower doses of ionizing radiation may be comparable with the syngerism observed in human skin.

A MODEL OF RADIATION CARCINOGENESIS

One theory concerning the molecular effects of radiation on living cells is the dual action hypothesis. In this hypothesis, events or hits resulting in molecular changes are postulated as the starting point for several measurable endpoints of biological damage. The radiation may act by altering the cell, to establish the potential for subsequent carcinogenic alterations that do not require further action of the radiation. The conversion of the altered cells to cancer cells can be thought of as a form of progression, a process whereby cells advance in a series of discrete steps to malignancy. We have been attempting to explain radiation carcinogenesis data in terms of a two-event or dual action postulate (Figure 9) (Burns and Vanderlaan, 1977). An interaction is assumed to occur between two primary events, somehow forming an aberrant cell, which progresses in a presumably stepwise manner to acquire malignant properties. The interaction between events is envisioned to proceed quickly when they are in close geometrical and temporal proximity. Furthermore, the events are assumed to be reparable, so that an interaction may be averted if one event is repaired before the second occurs. Unfortunately, the identity of the primary event is unknown, although it is presumably a molecular alteration in a DNA molecule because the neoplastic properties must be propagated to daughter cells. As mentioned, one plausible candidate is a break in the deoxyribophosphate strand structure, which could be the initial event in a cascade that leads to additional mutational and karyotypic changes or mutations.

Certain conclusions about the nature of the initial events can be derived from information now available. We must assume that the hypothetical events are a direct or indirect result of the molecular absorption events (ionizations) produced by the radiation. This assumption infers that the geometrical distribution of the hypothetical lesions in the cells must be directly related to the distribution of the primary ionizations.

Consequently, the distribution of carcinogenic events (hypothetical) must be determined by the physical location of the ionizations, which can be markedly altered by varying the LET of the radiation. As an ionizing particle (e.g., electron) passes through a cell, it leaves a track of ionizations, which are spaced in a manner that depends on the velocity, mass, and charge of the particle. The LET is proportional to the number of ionizations per unit length of track. At extremely low LET values, where many individual tracks are necessary to produce a given dose, most ionizations in a given nucleus are produced

FIGURE 9. A schematic diagram of the model showing the two routes by which radiation may produce molecular damage leading to carcinogenesis. The pathways show the major modes of action of radiation of different LET values. The upper panel indicates interactions between events in different tracks and the lower panel indicates interactions between events in the same track.

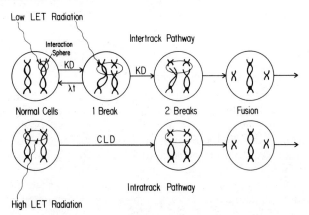

by different particle tracks. For example, high-energy electrons produce only about 3 ions in traversing an epidermal nucleus, and as many as 3000 tracks are required to produce a dose of a few hundred rad. As the LET increases, the number of tracks necessary to produce a given dose declines proportionally, until at very high LET values (e.g., 100 kev/micron or higher) hundreds of rads can be delivered by only one or two tracks per nucleus. In the latter circumstance, the primary ionizations and any events derived from them follow a geometrical alignment along particle tracks. Consequently, at high LET the chance that members of an interacting pair of events are contained within the same track is quite high. Because as the LET increases the chance of events being within an interaction distance of one another increases proportionately, intratrack interactions are proportional to LET as well as dose. Moreover, because events in a given track are produced almost simultaneously, intratrack interactions proceed quickly, without the possibility of significant repair.

At extremely low LET values, many individual tracks are necessary to produce a given dose, and the two members of any interacting pair of events were likely to have been produced by events in different tracks. Since events associated with different tracks are independent, the probability of two occurring within an interaction distance is the product of the individual occurence probabilities. Events are assumed to be proportional to primary ionizations (either single ionizations or clusters) and to dose. Hence, the yield of interactions between events in different tracks must be proportional to dose squared. When two events interact, it is assumed that an irreparable lesion is formed.

Without specifying the nature of the primary events, the considerations just mentioned lead to the following dose-response function when the time of exposure is so short that the repair during the exposure can be neglected

$$Y_1(D) = aLD + bD^2 \qquad (5)$$

and to the following function when the dose rate is much less than the repair rate (i.e., r/D is much less than c) and the repair constant in the equation $L = L_0 e^{-ct}$

$$Y_2(D) = aLD + (bDr)/c \qquad (6)$$

The similarity of **5** and **3,** derived from the dual action theory, is obvious.

Equation **6** is an expression of the expected dose-response function at low dose rates. Equations **5** and **6** imply that the dose–response characteristics of the carcinogenic response to radiation can be specified by three constants: a, b, and c. The three parameters are measurable as follows: b in dose-response studies with low-LET radiation, a in dose response studies with high-LET radiation, and c in fractionation studies with low-LET radiation. Relevant experiments have already been carried out for rat skin, and the results are as follows: $a = 2.5 \times 10^{-5}$ tumor micron/rad/kev/rat, $b = 1.3 \times 10^{-6}$ tumors/rat/rad^2, and $c = 0.24$ hr^{-1}. In **5** the ratio of axL to b is the dose, D_e, where the linear and dose-squared terms make equal contributions to the total response. On the basis of the numerical evaluations above

$$D_e = (axL)/b = 19L \qquad (7)$$

where L is the LET of the radiation in kev/micron. For argon ions, $L = 125$ kev/

micron and D_e is 2875 rad; whereas, for electrons, $L = 0.34$ kev/micron and D_e is 6 rad.

It is recognized that the approach outlined here is overly simplified in that it neglects a number of potentially important factors, such as the cytotoxic effect of the radiation and the likelihood that a variety of biological or hormonal factors may modify the expression of neoplastic and potentially neoplastic cells. Certainly, cytotoxicity cannot be ignored at doses above the peak yield, where further dose increases lead to unregenerated tissue destruction and fewer tumors. Accordingly, the model outlined can only be fitted to data below the peak.

HISTOLOGY AND GROWTH CHARACTERISTICS OF TUMORS

The skin contains a variety of cell types, and the tumors induced by ionizing radiation exhibit a distribution of histologic types that reflect the major types of cells found in the skin. For example, the various types of tumors occur with the following overall relative frequencies: squamous carcinomas, 30%; basal cell carcinomas, 20%; keratosebaceous tumors, 35%; sebaceous tumors, 10%; and sarcomas, 5%. The distribution of tumor types is relatively invariant and does not depend on the type of radiation, the geometrical distribution of the radiation, or the temporal pattern of dose application. A slight excess of squamous cell carcinomas is seen at doses above the peak yield dose.

An important question in environmental carcinogenesis is whether or not and how diverse carcinogens might interact to produce cancer in a given tissue. We examined this question in rats by exposing the skin to single doses of ionizing radiation followed by multiple weekly doses of 7,12-dimethylbenz-(a)anthracene (DMBA). DMBA is a polycyclic aromatic hydrocarbon that requires metabolic activation prior to producing its carcinogenic effect. There was a striking difference in the temporal onset patterns. The tumors induced by DMBA are consistent with a power function having an exponent of about 6, while the same function for radiation has an exponent of about 2. This difference is partly associated with the contrast between multiple exposures and single exposures. The tumor yield when the two carcinogens were given to the same animals was almost exactly the summation of the yields for exposure to each agent individually. Prior irradiation with electrons failed to sensitize the skin to exposure to DMBA.

COMPARISON OF RADIATION SKIN CARCINOGENESIS IN DIFFERENT SPECIES

The usefulness of experimental animals for estimating hazards and risks to humans is clearly dependent on the validity of the implicit assumption that the mechanisms of action are similar if not identical in different species. At the present time it is not possible to specify the mechanism of radiation damage in human tissue, but it is possible to draw inferences of similarities between species by comparisons respective of dose–response and time–response functions.

A comparison of radiation carcinogenesis in rat and mouse skin reveals some striking differences (Albert, Burns, and Bennett, 1972) when the tumor yields are compared under conditions of exposure to radiation that are as identical as possible (i.e., the yield of tumors in the rat is about 40 times greater than that in the mouse for the same number of animals exposed).

The great excess of tumors in the rat can be attributed to two principal factors 1) the greater size of the rat and 2) the presence of hair follicle tumors in the rat that are not present in the mouse. By comparing the results in terms of tumor yield per unit area, the rat excess is reduced to about eight times that of the mouse. Although a variety of epithelial tumors were expressed in the rat, squamous cell carcinoma is the single predominant tumor in the mouse. Because the latter tumor comprises only about 12% of the rat tumors, comparison of squamous cell carcinomas alone between the two species gives nearly identical yields.

The rat is more sensitive to radiation carcinogenesis, because it has more cells at risk for squamous cell carcinoma induction and because its epithelial cells are at risk for a variety of additional tumors that are presumably of hair follicle origin. Neither of these results could have been predicted a priori, and both deserve further study. Such results emphasize the need to understand mechanisms before making extrapolations between species in any quantitative manner.

Supported by the United States Department of Energy Contract AT(11-1)2737 and Center Grants from the National Institute of Environmental Health Sciences (ES 00260) and the National Cancer Institute (CA 13343).

REFERENCES

Albert RE, Burns FJ (1976) Tumor and injury responses of rat skin after sieve pattern x-irradiation. Radiat Res 67:474–481.

Albert RE, Burns FJ, Bennett P (1972) Radiation-induced hair follicle damage and tumor formation in mouse and rat skin. J Natl Cancer Inst 49:1131–1137.

Albert RE, Burns FJ, Heimbach R (1967a) Skin damage and tumor formation from grid and sieve patterns of electron and beta radiation in the rat. Radiat Res 30:525–540.

Albert RE, Burns FJ, Heimbach R (1967b) The effect of penetration depth of electron radiation on skin tumor formation in the rat. Radiat Res 30:515–524.

Albert RE, Burns FJ, Shore R (1978) Comparison of the incidence and time patterns of radiation-induced skin cancer in humans and rats. In: Late biological effects of ionizing radiation: Proceedings of a symposium, Vol. 2. Vienna, 13–17 March. Vienna: International Atomic Energy Agency, pp 499–505.

Albert RE, Newman W, Altshuler B (1961) The dose–response relationships of beta-ray-induced skin tumors in the rat. Radiat Res 15:410–430.

Albert RE, Phillips P, Bennett P, Burns F, Heimbach R (1969) The morphology and growth characteristics of radiation-induced epithelial skin tumors in the rat. Cancer Res 29:658–668.

Armitage P, Doll R (1954) The age of distribution of cancer and a multistage theory of carcinogenesis. Br J Cancer 8:1–12.

Bock FC (1977) Cutaneous carcinogenesis. In: Marzulli FN and Maibach HI (eds.), Advances in modern toxicology, Vol. 4. New York: John Wiley & Sons, pp 473–486.

Burns FJ, Albert RE (1980) Dose–response for rat skin tumors induced by single and split doses of argon ions. In: Biological and medical research with accelerated heavy ions at the bevalac. Berkeley, Ca, University of California.

Burns FJ, Albert RE, Heimbach R (1968) The RBE for skin tumors and hair follicle damage in the rat following irradiation with alpha particles and electrons. Radiat Res 36:225–241.

Burns FJ, Albert RE, Sinclair IP, Bennett P (1973) The effect of fractionation on tumor induction and hair follicle damage in rat skin. Radiat Res 53:235–240.

Burns FJ, Albert RE, Sinclair IP, Vanderlaan M (1975) The Effect of a 24-hour fractionation interval on the induction of rat skin tumors by electron radiation. Radiat Res 62:478–487.

Burns FJ, Albert RE, Vanderlaan M, Strickland P (1975) The dose response curve for tumor induction with single and split doses of 10 Mev protons. Radiat Res 62:598–599.

Burns FJ, Sargent EV (1981) The induction and repair of DNA breaks in rat epidermis irradiated with electrons. Radiat Res 87:137–144.

Burns FJ, Sinclair IP, Albert RE, Vanderlaan M (1976) Tumor induction and hair follicle damage for different electron penetrations in rat skin. Radiat Res 67:474–481.

Burns FJ, Vanderlaan M, Albert RE (1973) Growth rate and induction kinetics of radiation-induced rat skin tumors. Radiat Res 55:531.

Burns FJ, Vanderlaan M (1977) Split-dose recovery for radiation-induced tumors in rat skin. Intl J Radiat Biol 32:135–144.

Foulds L (1975) Neoplastic development-2. New York: Academic Press.

Heimbach R, Burns FJ, Albert RE (1969) An evaluation by alpha particle Bragg peak radiation of the critical depth in the rat skin for tumor induction. Radiat Res 39:332–344.

Kellerer A, Rossi H (1978) A generalized formulation of dual radiation action. Radiat Res 75:471–488.

Leenhouts HP, Chadwick KH (1974) Radiation-induced DNA double strand breaks and chromosome aberration. Theor Appl Genet 44:167–172.

Modan B, Baidatz D, Martz H (1974) Radiation-induced head and neck tumors. Lancet i:277–279.

National Academy of Sciences (1980) The effects on populations of exposure to low levels of ionizing radiation. Washington, DC: Advisory Committee on Biological Effects of Ionizing Radiation (BEIR), National Research Council.

Ormerod MG (1976) Radiation-induced strand breaks in the DNA of mammalian cells. In: Yuhas JM, Tennant RW, and Regan JD (eds.), Biology of radiation carcinogenesis. New York: Raven Press, pp 67–92.

Shore RE, Albert RE, Pasternack BS (1976) Follow-up study of patients treated by x-ray epilation for tinea capitis. Arch Env Health 20:21–28.

Strickland P, Burns FJ, Albert RE (1979) Induction of skin tumors in the rat by single exposure to ultraviolet radiation. Photochem Photobiol 30:683–688.

Vanderlaan M, Burns FJ, Albert RE (1976) A model describing the effects of dose and dose rate on tumor induction by radiation in rat skin. In: Biological and environmental effects of low-level radiation, Vol. I. Vienna: International Atomic Energy Agency, pp 253–263.

Whittemore A, Keller J (1978) Quantitative theories of carcinogenesis. SIAM Rev 20:1–30.

EXPERIMENTAL CARCINOGENESIS IN THE SKELETON

MARVIN GOLDMAN, Ph.D.

The effects of radiation on bone probably constitute the largest body of experimental information on the carcinogenic effects of ionizing radiation on a single tissue. Mammalian radiogenic bone cancers were first seen as a tragic consequence of radium poisoning in workers of the luminous dial industry early in this century. For many years the carcinogenic potential of radium in bone was the cornerstone of radiation protection standards for exposure to internally deposited radionuclides. More recently, both the atomic era with its weapons fallout, including bone-seeking radionuclides, and the concern regarding the long-lived components of the uranium fuel cycle have added political impetus to the scientific questions regarding radiation cancer in bone.

Although we now know that bone is relatively less sensitive to radiation carcinogenesis than some other tissues, its slow mineral turnover rate and its avid uptake and tenacious retention of certain radioactive elements have stimulated a high level of interest in the study of some fundamental comparative radiobiologic questions. As indicated later in this volume, our knowledge of the effects of radiation on the human skeleton is confined mainly to our experience with radium, thorium, and external radiation therapy. The human radium experience is one of the few extensive links between skeletal radiation carcinogenesis in man and that in experimental animals. At least four or five animal species have been used to mimic and "scale" the radium data to the human experience with respect to time, space, and activity.

This chapter discusses factors concerning skeletal radiation carcinogenesis, from the cellular microscopic level to species differences regarding metabolic, anatomic and physiologic differences. The radiation quality, itself, be it from external sources or internally deposited radioactivity, is also important in de-

From the Laboratory for Energy-Related Health Research, University of California, Davis, Davis, California.

termining the quality and quantity of response following irradiation. How radiation is delivered in time and space is significant, as is age at exposure. The relationship between dose and effect can be summarized mathematically by different risk models that attempt to integrate the available data and provide bases for extrapolation. The empirical observations to date still leave unanswered, however, the most basic questions as to exactly which cell it is that initiates a bone cancer and through what subcellular and molecular events the process of neoplasia proceeds.

SKELETAL FACTORS

The anatomy and physiology of the skeleton and its supporting tissues have certain unique features for the study of radiation carcinogenesis. Although there are no known reports of radiation-induced cancer in supporting tissues such as muscles, tendons, and the membranes of joints, radiation from external sources or internally deposited radionuclides has been observed to induce tumors in cartilage, bony tissues, hematopoietic marrow, and the vasculature within the skeleton. The mammalian skeleton contains both cortical bone and cancellous bone; the former constitutes about 80% of the mineral mass of the skeleton, and the remainder is cancellous.

The anatomical and physical characteristics of skeletal growth, maturation, and disease in most mammals are similar to those described for humans in Chapter 20; however, the skeleton in rodents (Loutit et al, 1976) contains a minimum of cancellous, trabecular bone, even in vertebrae, and consists for the most part of tubular, cortical marrow-containing bone which continues to grow throughout life. This difference between species is important, since it is the distribution of potential cells at risk, rather than mineral mass, that is of primary importance in determining radiation cancer risk.

In cancellous bone, cellular and mineral metabolism are about ten times more rapid than in the cortical bone. Trabecular bone may have a greater cell density (and radiation cancer risk) than a comparable volume of cortical bone. In dogs, for example, following uniform skeletal labelling with ^{90}Sr, the trabecular portion of the skeleton has a mineral turnover half-time of about 1.5 yr, whereas, for cortical bone this factor is about 15 yr, and radiation-induced cancers are more frequently associated with trabecular portions of the skeleton than with the cortex (Pool, 1972). Consideration of the pattern of skeletal growth, mineral accretion, and bone remodelling has shown that radiation-induced cancer can appear in all parts of the skeleton, although the tumor probabilities for given radiation exposure are highly influenced by the quality and quantity of cells in the radiation field (Goldman and Bustad, 1972a).

An important consideration in skeletal carcinogenesis is the accurate determination of the specific cells at risk. The most likely cell populations at risk for bone tumor induction are osteoblasts and committed bone progenitor cells. One might also consider pluripotential stem cells of the bone marrow to be at risk for bone cancer, but in chimera studies with mice at least, it has been shown that pluripotent marrow cells do not give rise to radiation-induced bone tumors (Barnes et al, 1970).

Radiation induced bone sarcomas are usually osteogenic sarcomas, although hemangiosarcomas, fibrosarcomas, and, in some instances, chondrosarcomas are also seen. Studies with bone-seeking radionuclides have also shown that the epithelial tissues overlying contaminated bone mineral are at risk for epithelial carcinomas (Nilsson, 1971; Ash and Loutit, 1977; Goldman and Bustad, 1972a). The tumors appear to result from the direct action of ionizing radiation on the cells at risk, and not from some humoral, viral, or other abscopal action. One model suggests that the cancer risk is confined to a layer of endosteal cells within 10 μm of the mineral osteoid (Vaughan, 1973). Although most osteoprogenitor cells are close to the endosteum, it is likely that some mesenchymal cells within adjacent marrow may also contribute to osteosarcoma risk. Studies of ^{90}Sr- and ^{226}Ra-burdened dogs suggest that osteosarcomas which arise within the cortical bone may be associated with microvascular alterations accompanying bone remodelling (Pool et al, 1983).

Although radiation-induced leukemia is discussed elsewhere, it should be noted that bone-seeking radionuclides with radiation emissions sufficiently energetic to deliver a significant dose to the adjacent marrow can induce a spectrum of myeloproliferative disorders, including myeloid leukemia, as has been seen in ^{90}Sr-treated swine, dogs, and rodents (Goldman and Bustad, 1972a). Characteristics of leukemogenesis under these circumstances are the requirement for a continuous high dose rate, a short latent period, and a reasonably short "plateau" of risk, particularly in animals exposed as juveniles (Book et al, 1983). This pattern of radiation has not been effective in inducing myeloid leukemias at low doses and dose rates, or in animals exposed as adults.

Radiation-induced bone tumors in animals have most of the characteristics of the corresponding spontaneous cancers. In mice, for example, ^{90}Sr-induced tumors are accompanied by an expected increased level of alkaline phosphatase prior to roentgenographic confirmation of tumor appearance (Bailey et al, 1976). Histologically, experimentally induced tumors resemble those found naturally in man, ranging from densely ossified osteogenic sarcomas to giant cell-containing osteolytic tumors. Fibrosarcomas and hemangiosarcomas are common to the species tested for radiation carcinogenesis (Finkel et al, 1976). The minimum post-exposure time to tumor appearance (latency period) ranges from 180 days in the mouse to about 600 days in the dog (Goldman et al, 1973).

Radiation-induced osteosarcomas grow rapidly. In rats given ^{144}Ce, the tumor mass doubling time was approximately 17 days (Klein et al, 1977). Radionuclide-induced osteosarcomas in beagle dogs had a doubling time that was independent of dose, of location. of age at appearance, or of radionuclide treatment, and ranged from 5 to 60 days (average 12 days)—similar to that seen in rodents (Thurman et al, 1971).

It appears that radiation-induction of bone cancer requires irradiation of committed progenitor cells, probably preosteoblasts and preosteoclasts, which not only line endosteal and periosteal surfaces but are found in remodelling sites within cortical bone (Pool et al, 1983). Alkaline earth radionuclides (e.g., radium and strontium) will be incorporated within bone mineral, and with time, much of the radiation dose will be absorbed at a greater distance from cells at risk than with radionuclides such as plutonium, which are incorporated into surface osteoid organic matrices (United Nations, 1977).

SPECIES DIFFERENCES

Most information on experimental skeletal carcinogenesis comes from studies with mice, rats, guinea pigs and dogs; limited additional information comes from studies with nonhuman primates and swine (Knowles, 1981). Each species has unique metabolic characteristics. Because many studies attempt to develop qualitative and quantitative information for extrapolating risk to man, it is important to consider factors which bear on the effectiveness of radiation doses and of the radiation responsiveness of the target tissues.

Skeletal metabolism affects the dosimetry of internally deposited radionuclides. Bone-seeking radioactive elements can be described either as volume seekers or as surface seekers (ICRP, 1973). Volume seekers are generally divalent alkaline earth minerals—similar in behavior to calcium—and include barium, radium, and strontium. These cations are incorporated within bone hydroxyapatite and are handled like the mineral itself. These cations resemble calcium in their absorption into the bloodstream from the diet and in their subsequent incorporation into skeletal mineral, but only qualitatively; quantitatively, each is unique (Stara et al, 1971). Other radioactive elements, such as plutonium, americium, and curium, have different metabolic pathways and are generally incorporated into the organic osteoid of bone, increasing the potential for their short-range alpha particle emissions to impinge upon the adjacent cells at risk (Vaughan, 1973; World Health Organization, 1982).

The physical decay characteristics of a radionuclide also constitute a significant dosimetric parameter. The absorbed skeletal dose and its rate of change are integrated products of the biologic processes that govern the retention of the nuclide in the target tissue and the physical processes that determine its rate of decay. Radiologic characteristics of bone-seeking radionuclides are summarized in Tables 1-2 of Chapter 20.

The physical dimensions of skeletal structures are also important dosimetric factors. With energetic bone-seeking radionuclides, for example, the mean size of the marrow cavity influences the magnitude and distribution of the radiation dose to the bone marrow, and it is different for each species. Spiers et al (1972) computed the mineral and marrow dosimetric constants for a range of beta-emitting bone-seeking radionuclides, including the following examples for ^{90}Sr. A uniform deposition of ^{90}Sr in the canine skeleton was estimated to deliver an associated mean beta radiation dose to the marrow 43% as large as that delivered to mineral bone, whereas in humans it was calculated to be 31% as large and in mice only 25% as large, because of the small size of the mouse skeleton relative to the potential path length of ^{90}Sr beta particles. Because of the nonuniform distribution of cells at risk within the skeleton, it is important to consider the specific physical and biologic dosimetric parameters in any calculation of radiation risk. Bone cancer from skeletally-deposited radioactivity is also influenced by the persistence of the radionuclide relative to cells at risk. The retention of volume-seeking radionuclides generally follows species-specific mineral metabolism patterns. For example, retention of radium in humans and dogs follows comparable kinetic patterns, the major deposition variable being the mineral addition rate at the time of intake (Parks and Keane, 1983). Many of the relevant metabolic parameters have been quantified (ICRP, 1973). Assessing the consequences of skeletal irradiation by internal emitters, however, requires a clear understanding of the microscopic, as well as macroscopic metabolic and dosimetric factors related to their deposition (Goldman et al, 1969; Moskalev, 1975).

Most osteosarcomas induced in radium-treated mice contain virus particles, suggesting that the viruses may be a contributory factor in the development of murine osteosarcoma (Lloyd et al, 1975). The influence of viruses in inbred mouse strains (such as the C57Bl, the RFM, and the BALB) may relate to the finding that bone tumors are naturally uncommon in RFM and BALB mice, and that the spontaneous incidence is somewhat higher in C57Bl mice. Interestingly, although RFM mice are well known for their susceptibility to radiation leukemia, they are the least susceptible to bone cancer induction by radiostrontium, as compared with BALB mice, which yield an intermediate response, or C57Bl mice, which show a maximal response at the levels tested (Wright et al, 1972).

The beagle dog has received considerable attention as a model for radionuclide-induced bone cancers. In contrast to the situation in larger breeds, bone cancer is rare in smaller breeds such as the beagle. Hence the quantification and analysis of radiation-induced cancers are simpler in this species (Bustad et al, 1972).

EFFECTS OF EXTERNAL IRRADIATION

Although most of the radiation-induced bone cancer data pertains to bone-seeking radionuclides, the carcinogenic effects of external radiation also have been studied. Woodard (1957) showed that acute x-ray exposure of mice to 900 or 2500 R caused marked skeletal cell killing, with depression of alkaline phosphatase activity and bone mineral uptake of tracer doses of radiostrontium. Post exposure recovery of mineral dynamic parameters followed about a 30-day cyclic pattern after 900 R, and required about 6 mo to return to normal levels after the 2500 R exposure. Finkel (1964) x-irradiated mice locally with 250, 625, or 1000 R and found among the survivors a cancer induction rate of 3 $\times$ 10^{-5} osteosarcomas per Roentgen. The lowest exposure (250 R) corresponded to a skeletal radiation dose of 500 rad (5 Gy) and a cancer risk of about 1.5 $\times$ 10^{-5}/rad.

Although the damaging effects of acute x-irradiation are more severe in the very young, it is not clear that (as postulated for ^{224}Ra carcinogenicity in humans), young experimental animals are markedly more sensitive than adults (Heller, 1948).

In rats, Solheim (1977) found that osteogenic sarcoma induction per rad per cm² of bone was comparable whether from internally deposited bone-seeking radionuclides or from external irradiation. With dose rates up to 2.8 Gy/day, for a 1-yr period, he noted the resulting osteosarcomas to have a 180-day latency. In rabbits given either 1756 R in a single exposure, or fractionated exposures totalling 4650 R, to their hind limbs, the single exposure was twice as effective as the fractionated exposures, even though the total dose from the latter was 2.6 times higher. It was also noted that ^{99m}Tc-pyrophosphate scanning detected the resulting osteosarcomas 2.5 mo earlier than conventional radiography (King et al, 1980; Goldman et al, 1970). Compared with neutrons, photon doses 2.86

times higher were ineffective in inducing osteosarcomas when delivered to the heads of rabbits, but three of five rabbits receiving the lowest neutron dose (1680 rad) developed invasive and metastasizing osteosarcomas within 1 yr (Bradley et al, 1977). The principal cancer risk from external low-LET skeletal irradiation may thus be in the more sensitive marrow elements than in the osteoid elements (Vaughan, 1973).

EFFECTS OF INTERNAL EMITTERS

Skeletal Irradiation by Beta Particles

The skeletal effects of low-LET radiation from beta-emitting radionuclides have been studied in different animal species and with variable doses and dose rates. Several detailed reviews exist (Caldecott and Snyder, 1960; Dougherty et al, 1962; Mays et al, 1969; Stover and Jee, 1972; Goldman and Bustad, 1972; Sanders et al, 1973; Vaughan, 1973; Jee, 1976), along with technical summaries in the reports of the National Academy of Sciences (1980), the United Nations Scientific Committee on the Effects of Atomic Radiation (1977, 1982), the International Atomic Energy Agency (1969, 1976), and the NCRP (1980).

Unlike alpha-emitting radionuclides, the emissions from which penetrate through tissue to distances of only a few cell diameters, energetic beta-emitters in the skeleton deliver a more uniform and penetrating radiation dose to cells in and around the skeleton, thus inducing a spectrum of neoplasia.

In mice, single injections of $^{55}FeCl_3$ induce leukemias, thymic lymphomas, hemangioendotheliomas, reticulum cells sarcomas, and comparable numbers of osteosarcomas. The short-range of the Auger electron radiation from ^{55}Fe, which is restricted mainly to the marrow, implies that the carcinogenic effect on bone may arise within the marrow's bone progenitor cells, rather than from the penetrating but miniscule x-ray dose to the bone cells themselves (Laissue et al, 1977). Phosphorus-32, with a beta energy similar to that of $^{90}Sr/^{90}Y$, but with a much shorter half-life, is a potent inducer of osteogenic sarcomas in rats (Ingelton, 1977). Of the alkaline earths ^{45}Ca and ^{90}Sr, the shorter-lived, less energetic calcium is less potent per unit of radiation exposure in mice (Finkel and Biskis, 1968). Kuzma and Zander (1957) have reported a similar finding for ^{45}Ca and ^{89}Sr in rats.

Radiostrontium carcinogenicity was anticipated over forty years ago (Pecher, 1941). Strontium-90, produced by the fissioning of uranium, has been studied for over 30 yr in mice, rats, rabbits, swine, dogs, and primates. Strontium-90 decays to an energetic short-lived beta emitter, ^{90}Y, with a beta particle range of several millimeters in tissue. It is not surprising, therefore, to find that in addition to inducing osteosarcomas, internally deposited ^{90}Sr causes a spectrum of hematopoietic and epithelial tumors adjacent to bone. Neoplasia of bone and marrow resulting from ^{90}Sr have been reported in CBA mice by Nilsson (1962) and in CF_1 mice by Finkel and Biskis (1968). Strontium-90–induced osteosarcomas have been observed in rabbits injected at different ages (Vaughan, 1973), as well as in ^{90}Sr-fed swine (Howard et al, 1969). In beagle dogs receiving single injections of ^{90}Sr at 1.4 yr of age, bone tumors resulted from average skeletal doses over 5000 rad (Mays and Lloyd, 1972). A lessening

of the effect has been noted when the strontium administration has been protracted by fractionated injections or continual ingestion (NCRP, 1980). In mice
(Wright, 1972) and dogs (Goldman et al, 1969a), chronic irradiation of the
skeleton by ^{90}Sr early in life enhances the risk of leukemogenesis. Comparable
marrow effects have been observed in swine fed ^{90}Sr by Clark et al (1972).

The research on long-lived animals has suggested that myeloproliferative
cancers are likely to appear within short times and mainly with high dose-rates
(i.e., to have a short latency and "plateau" of risk). For osteogenic sarcomas, the
data with beta-emitters best support a non-linear, sigmoid risk model and in
many instances actually fit a "practical threshold" model (Evans, 1974).

A third ^{90}Sr effect in long-lived animals is epithelial carcinomas in tissues
adjacent to ^{90}Sr-labeled mineral (Dungworth et al, 1969; Parks et al, 1984).
Furthermore, when soluble forms of radioactive cerium or strontium are inhaled by dogs, they produce a high yield of hemangiosarcomas, as well as
myelogenous leukemias, osteosarcomas, and fibrosarcomas (Benjamin et al,
1975). Administered by inhalation in the form of nonsoluble, fused clay particles, however, the ^{90}Sr is confined to the lung, and skeletal effects do not result.
In view of the dosimetric characteristics of these radionuclides, abscopal factors do not appear to be involved in the cancers they induce, since the tumors
arise only in tissues receiving measurable doses.

Skeletal Irradiation by Alpha Particles

Studies using short-range alpha particles support the concept that tumor induction by bone-seeking radionuclides is the result of direct cellular irradiation. The early recognition of ^{226}Ra toxicity and the more recent human toxicity
data on short-lived ^{224}Ra confirm the carcinogenic efficiency of bone-seeking
alpha-emitting radionuclides. The high specific ionization of alpha particle
radiation over short path lengths results in high doses to cells. Paradoxically,
alpha particle irradiation is not only highly cytocidal but also highly effective
in tumor induction (Goldman, 1976). The increasing availability of alpha-emitting radioelements (e.g., plutonium) from the proliferation of nuclear weapons
and the development of nuclear energy has stimulated international interest in
understanding and quantifying the toxicity and carcinogenicity of these nuclides. Finkel's (1968) classic experiments at the Argonne National Laboratory
on bone-seeking radionuclides first demonstrated that the alpha-emitting bone-
seekers were ten times more effective as bone carcinogens on an activity basis
than were beta-emitters in mice. Most bone-seeking alpha-emitting radionuclides have energies of about 5 MeV and in unit density tissue deposit about
100 KeV of energy per micron over a path length of 40–50 μm (~4–5 cell
diameters).

The importance of the spatial distribution of the dose is seen by comparing
long-lived ^{226}Ra and short-lived ^{224}Ra with respect to total dose and patterns of
protraction (Müller et al, 1983). A single administration of ^{226}Ra, comparable
with that used by Finkel (1968), was taken as a reference level for osteosarcoma
induction. At a skeletal dose similar to the reference ^{226}Ra dose, achieved by
protracted and fractionated administrations of the short-lived ^{224}Ra isotope, an
increased carcinogenicity per rad was seen with increased protraction, and

also when the unit dosage administered was diminished. The "most efficient" dosimetric pattern had the most sparse distribution of alpha particles on bone surfaces, both in time and in space. With ^{226}Ra, an increasing fraction of the alpha dose is expended in bone mineral, as metabolic processes "bury" the Ra burden and interpose an increasing mass of noncellular mineral between the Ra and the presumed cells at risk. The importance of local dosimetry is also seen in the work of Nilsson and Broome-Karlsson (1976), in which ^{241}Am citrate produced both skeletal and hemopoietic tumors in mice. Furthermore, two lifetime dog studies with ^{226}Ra are now nearing completion. Injections of ^{226}Ra killed marrow cells and induced leukopenia but, unlike ^{90}Sr, did not result in an increased risk for leukemia. However, the ^{226}Ra was equally effective in inducing skeletal osteosarcomas whether administered in fractionated doses or in a single dose. A wide range of doses was used, and the data suggest a greater unit dose efficiency at lower doses than at higher doses where cell killing and "wasted radiation" may be significant (Wrenn et al, 1983; Book et al, 1983).

The 88-yr half-life ^{238}Pu and the 24,000-yr half-life ^{239}Pu were also studied. In rodents (Finkel, 1968) and dogs (Stevens et al, 1976), ^{239}Pu tumor induction increased with increasing dose and showed an associated decrease in latent period with increasing dose. Plutonium has proven to be a most effective carcinogen for bone in all species studied (Jee, 1976).

Variations in deposition pattern, half-life, and animal species for alpha emitters with comparable particle ranges permit evaluation of the relative importance of these parameters. Many of the bone-seeking alpha emitter studies parallel experiments with beta emitters. Spiers (1974) has shown the relative dosimetric importance of radionuclide energy related to bone structure, size, and cell distribution, with respect to alpha- and beta-particles in human and animal bone.

The studies on bone seeking radionuclides have not shown the relative biologic effectiveness (RBE) to be constant over a wide range of doses. In setting radiation protection standards, however, it has been the custom to apply a constant potency or effectiveness factor (RBE) of 10–20 for absorbed alpha radiation doses relative to doses of low-LET beta-irradiation or x-irradiation. Raabe et al (1983) showed that ^{90}Sr (β) and ^{226}Ra (α) were of about equal carcinogenic potency at average skeletal dose rates of 10 rad/day, but the RBE increased with decreasing dose rate to reach a value of 30 at the point where the ^{90}Sr doses had only one-thirtieth the probability of inducing cancers as did the ^{226}Ra. Moskalev et al (1983) also showed that osteosarcomas were induced with equal frequencies in rats by high ^{238}Pu alpha doses and high doses of ^{249}Bk beta irradiation, but that on a dosimetric basis, ^{249}Bk was only 40% as effective as the alpha emitter. Book et al (1983) reported that beagles attained their normal mean life span at skeletal doses less than 284 rad from radium or 2392 rad from ^{90}Sr and that, for both radionuclides, the lower the radiation dose or dose rate, the later the average tumor appearance time, a dose–effect relationship that has been a consistent finding (Goldman et al, 1969). The similarity in pathologic sequelae of ^{226}Ra in dogs and humans (Book, 1980), and the clinical, radiologic, and histologic similarity between the bone lesions in both species (Morgan and Pool, 1982) underscore the utility of the animal model for investigating risks to humans.

EFFECT OF DOSAGE RATE

As mentioned above, skeletal cancers in mice, rats, and dogs have shown a non linear dose–effect relationship following exposure to beta-emitting radionuclides (NCRP, 1980). This was first shown with ^{90}Sr in mice (Finkel et al, 1960). As with carcinogenicity for the lung (NAS, 1976), the carcinogenicity of alpha emitters for the skeleton shows a pattern different from that of beta emitters; i.e., concentrated or "hot-spot" distribution of alpha particle radiation is less effective (e.g., more "energy-wasteful") than are the same number of alpha particles distributed more uniformly in space and time within tissues. For protracted, fractionated ^{224}Ra administrations (Müller et al, 1977), the pattern of alpha flux plays an important role in determining carcinogenic efficiency. Raabe et al (1980), comparing ^{226}Ra effects in humans, dogs, and mice showed that, for each species, ^{226}Ra was more efficient per unit dose at lower dose-rates than at higher dose-rates. This suggests that the carcinogenicity of plutonium would be greater following a pattern of continual administration than following a single administration of the same total dose.

EFFECTS OF AGE AT EXPOSURE

Although age at exposure is important in quantifying radiation risk in other tissues, it does not appear to be the case for the skeleton when dosimetry is taken into account. In humans exposed to ^{224}Ra, bone tumor induction, although elevated, was not markedly different in juveniles or adults. Luz et al (1978) compared alpha-particle-induced osteosarcomas in 1 yr old and 6 mo old mice and found that the age-corrected osteosarcoma incidence was not significantly different. Finkel et al (1972) found no age effect in ^{90}Sr-treated dogs. When the appropriate dose corrections are applied, age does not appear to play a major role in determining subsequent risk. The juvenile growing skeleton, however, incorporates a greater fraction of bone-seeking radionuclides than that of the adult, and, thus, the risk to the young in a contaminated environment would be greater than that to an adult (Della Rosa et al, 1965; UN, 1977).

DOSE–RESPONSE RELATIONSHIPS

The simplest dose–response is a linear relationship (NAS, 1980), but when a sufficient range of dose gradation has been tested, regardless of species, bone cancer risk has not been found to be linear. As Finkel (1968) has shown in the mouse, at high radiation doses where considerable destruction of skeletal tissue occurs, much of the radiation dose is "wasted," with the result that fewer tumors/rad are observed than at lower radiation doses. For both high- and low-LET radiation at exceedingly low doses, an inverse relationship between dose and average tumor latency is seen in mice (Rosenblatt et al, 1971) and dogs (Rosenblatt et al, 1972), which suggests a "practical threshold" (Book et al, 1983) at the dose at which the average latency period equal to the individual's life expectation (Evans, 1974).

The cumulative incidence of osteosarcomas in relation to exposure time and radiation dose can be described by a three-dimensional logistic response surface, which has been shown to be completely nonlinear for both beta emitters and alpha emitters. The log-normal relationship between dose-rate, latency, and bone cancer probability, as reported by Raabe et al (1983), and the linear-quadratic or dose-squared relationship between incidence and total dose (NAS, 1980), both contradict the idea that a single universal empirical relationship can be applied to bone-seeking radionuclides. The data for low-LET emitters best fit a nonlinear response model with a sigmoid or S-shape. The data for alpha emitters can fit either a linear or a curvilinear model. A linear relationship fits the data at higher doses, but as Rowland (1983) and Evans (1974) have shown with ^{226}Ra in humans, the linear response model overestimates the risk at low doses.

SCALING THE SPECIES

To extrapolate the radionuclide carcinogenicity data from animals, for predicting numerical risks to humans, the extrapolation is usually based on the relationship between the cumulative radiation dose and cancer incidence. One model uses a life-table treatment of cumulative tumor incidence data to construct a three-dimensional logistic response surface of dose, time, and effect (Rosenblatt et al, 1976). For ^{226}Ra, where human, canine, and murine data are available, the logistic model was used to estimate maximum cumulative incidence rates for a range of doses in mouse and dog. Based on radioactivity administered, ^{226}Ra was estimated to be 5–10 times more carcinogenic in animals than in humans. When the three species were compared in terms of survival as a function of dose-rate, Raabe et al (1983) showed that tumor latency increased as dose-rate decreased, and that radium was more effective per unit dose at low dose rates than at high dose rates. If life span is accounted for, a lifetime dose of 0.5–1.0 Gy of skeletal irradiation was estimated to be the minimum dose associated with fatal bone cancer induction. Another analysis of these data (Mays et al, 1976) used a linear dose–response model and derived a bone sarcoma risk of 70×10^{-6} in mice, 320×10^{-6} in dogs, and $6–53 \times 10^{-6}/$ rad in humans. Mays et al (1976) also estimated that plutonium was 15 times more carcinogenic per rad than radium.

Rosenblatt et al (1976), using metabolic models for dog, mouse, and humans, and determining maximum cumulative incidence rates for the three nuclides in experimental animals, predicted approximately a 10^3 difference for isoeffectiveness between ^{226}Ra and ^{239}Pu in humans. Their model predicts a maximum cumulative human bone cancer incidence of about 18% in association with the ICRP bone limit of 40 nCi of ^{239}Pu. However, if the plutonium cancers were to show an increase in latent period with decreasing dose, this upper limit of risk might not be achieved until later than the normal life expectation.

The parallel between humans and laboratory animals in the pathogenesis of radium-induced bone lesions was strengthened in the detailed pathology studies of Pool et al (1983) and in the comparison of the temporal progression of osteolytic bone destruction in both species by Morgan et al (1983). Also, Raabe et al (1983), by plotting log-normal tumor appearance time against average skeletal dose rate, estimated a common slope for mice, dogs, and humans.

Mole (1958) compared plutonium and radium following moderate to high doses and found the relationship between the risk and the logarithm of the radiation dose to be similar for both radionuclides (i.e., a nonlinear response model for alpha emitters). He also postulated that the risk of bone tumor production was proportional to the square of the injected dose (Mole, 1963), and for nonskeletal tumors, he suggested that radiation-induced cancer might be caused by two independent cellular events, each of which has a small but constant probability of occurrence. Two comparable events, an initiating event plus a promoting event, have been invoked to explain the shape of the response curve by Casarett (1973). From the low-LET studies, in particular, as well as from certain high-LET studies, it is clear that a simple monotonic proportionality function does not fit the data over the full range of tested doses. Recent analysis of the human ^{226}Ra toxicity data suggests that a dose-squared model fits the data best (NAS, 1980).

PHYSICAL AND BIOLOGICAL FACTORS

Physical as well as biological factors play important roles in understanding cancer risk from skeletal irradiation. The spatial distribution of deposited radionuclides in bone has been shown to follow both a diffuse as well as a hot-spot pattern (Jee, 1976). This local dose distribution has been the subject of speculation and study for carcinogenesis in the lung as well as in bone (NAS, 1976). For alpha particles, the more diffuse their distribution in the tissues at risk both in space and in time, the more efficient and effective they are as carcinogens. Goldman (1976) has suggested that at the cellular level, alpha particle traversals of cell nuclei depositing at least 100 KeV of ionizing radiation were most likely to cause sterilization, if not death, of the cell. Because the likelihood of such energy deposition is minimized with diffuse alpha particle distribution, this relationship may explain differences in osteosarcoma risk as a function of local alpha particle distribution. The spatial deposition of ionizations from 20 to 80 KeV of alpha particle "intrusion" into a cell nucleus, while not lethal to the cell, are likely to cause irreparable nucleic acid damage that might either "initiate" or "promote" a cellular neoplastic change (Goldman, 1976).

Spiers and Vaughan (1976) have taken a dosimetric approach to the estimation of plutonium risks in humans, based on the dosimetric parameters for radium and plutonium in both trabecular and cortical bone. They have estimated plutonium to have a threefold greater potency than radium for equal skeletal radionuclide burdens. This dosimetry-based value is lower than the ratio of Pu to Ra based on animal toxicity ratio, which is 6:9 for equal skeletal burdens (Rosenblatt et al, 1976). The dosimetry of radium and plutonium was also evaluated by Thorne (1977), who estimated an upper effectiveness limit for ^{239}Pu of 15 relative to ^{226}Ra. A most likely Pu/Ra potency ratio is inferred to be 8:10, which is about the same as that derived empirically from animal toxicity studies.

Ever since the early work of Berenblum (1941) on the possible role of chemical agents that either initiate or promote the carcinogenic process, scientists have questioned the extent to which radiation-induced carcinogenesis follows principles posed by Berenblum for chemical carcinogens. Radiation can be a complete carcinogen, in that it can both initiate and promote the steps necessary for the cancer process. For radionuclide-induced osteosarcoma in animals exposed to combinations of short- and long-lived nuclides, Müller et al (1983b) speculated that an apparent synergism resulted if there was an initial high dose rate followed by continuous irradiation at a lower dose rate. They proposed that a high initial dose rate might cause an initiating event and that subsequent long-term low-level irradiation might act as a promoting agent.

In studying osteosarcoma induction from ^{90}Sr in mice, Nilsson and Broome-Karlsson (1976b) found a promoting or synergistic effect with subsequent steroid hormone treatment, including a shortening of the tumor latency period. However, simultaneous administration of the radionuclide with the steroid resulted either in no enhancement or an actual reduction in osteosarcoma incidence. Loutit (1976) suggested that steroid cofactors may also promote the development of nonosteogenic sarcomas (angiosarcomas) in ^{90}Sr-treated mice, speculating that the origin of angiosarcomas might be in radiation-damaged bone marrow stroma adjacent to the sites of radiostrontium deposition, and that bone marrow injury or atrophy, followed by hematopoietic tissue replacement is associated with the appearance of pleomorphic cells suggestive of malignancy. Nilsson (1966) found that ^{90}Sr-induced intramedullary osteosarcoma buds transplanted into syngeneic mice were autonomous and that subsequent bud growth did not depend on the continued presence of ^{90}Sr irradiation.

Goldman et al (1976) compared early radiation effects on bone marrow from different radionuclides, and related the early radiation effects on blood cells to the subsequent risk of osteosarcoma. For ^{90}Sr, [226]Ra, and [239]Pu, they used the reduction in circulating blood neutrophils during the year following injection of the radionuclide as a predictor for the occurrence of osteosarcomas in the same animals 10 yr later.

SYNTHESIS AND SUMMARY

Internal or external irradiation can induce a range of skeletal cancers in experimental animals. An underlying feature of the experiments is that the primary risk resides almost exclusively in the cells that are irradiated, and that is there is no strong support for an abscopal effect in cancer induction (Van Cleave, 1968).

The induction of osteosarcomas in experimental animals is not one of the most sensitive tumorigenic effects of tissue irradiation. High-LET radiations (neutrons and alpha particles) are more effective in inducing such tumors than are low-LET radiations (beta particles and gamma rays).

The experiments with internal emitters show a paradox between the effects of high-LET radiation and those of low-LET radiation with respect to dose-rate and risk. When large numbers of animals are studied over a sufficient range of dose-rates, the risk per unit dose of low-LET radiation is smaller at low dose rates than at high dose rates, which lends support to a dose–effect model variously described as dose-squared, sigmoid, S-shaped, or even as a threshold model (Goldman, 1982). Conversely, with high-LET alpha irradiation, the risk per unit dose is larger at lower doses and dose-rates than at higher doses and dose-rates.

When substantial bone marrow doses are associated with skeletal irradiation from internally deposited radionuclides, the exposed animals may develop angiosarcomas, as well as a spectrum of leukemogenic responses. The induction of myeloid leukemia is more likely to occur in continuously irradiated juvenile bone marrow than in adult bone marrow.

Although the specific cells at risk for osteogenic sarcoma can be presumed to be in or near the endosteal layer of bone, it is quite possible that progenitor cells within the mineral cortex or in marrow also contribute to the risk for bone cancer induction.

As discussed by Casarett (1973), the pathogenesis of radionuclide-induced bone tumors requires consideration of the physical and chemical characteristics of radionuclides, as well as the temporal and spatial relationship of the doses they deliver to particular cells at risk. In view of the dynamic interaction of these physical and biological characteristics, it is not at all surprising that multi-event models seem most consistent with the shapes of the dose-response curves (Moskalev and Streltsova, 1964; United Nations, 1977). The inverse relationship between the latency of osteosarcomas and the radiation dose affords a practical approach for estimating boundary conditions in assessing the potential risks to the human skeleton following low-level ionizing radiation.

REFERENCES

Ash P, Loutit JF (1977) The ultrastructure of skeletal hemangiosarcomas induced in mice by strontium-90. J Pathol 122:209–218.

Bailey JM, Hill WD, Fiscus AG, Reilly CA, Finkel MP (1976) Plasma alkaline phosphatase in mice with experimentally-induced osteosarcomas. Lab Anim Sci 26:66–69.

Barnes DWH, Carr TEF, Evans EP, Loutit JF (1970) ^{90}Sr-induced osteosarcomas in radiation chimeras. Int J Radiat Biol 18:531–537.

Benjamin SA, Hahn FF, Chifelle TL, Boecker BB, Hobbs CH (1975) Occurrence of hemangiosarcomas in beagles with internally deposited radionuclides. Cancer Res 35:1745–1755.

Berenblum I (1941) The mechanism of carcinogenesis. Cancer Res 1:807–814.

Book SA (1980) The canine as a model in radiobiologic research. In: Shifrine M and Wilson FD (eds.), The canine as a biomedical research model: Immunological, hematological, and oncological aspects. Springfield: US Department of Energy.

Book SA, Spangler WL, Parks NJ, Rosenblatt LS, Goldman M (1983) Effects of long-term, low-level exposures from strontium-90 and radium-226 in beagle dogs. In: Broerse JJ, Barendsen YW, Kal HB, and vanderKogel AJ (eds.), Radiation research: Somatic and genetic effects. Amsterdam: Martin Nijhoff.

Bradley EW, Look BC, Casarett GW, Bondelid RO, Maier JG, Rogers CC (1977) Effects of fast neutrons on rabbits—I. Comparison of pathologic effects of fractionated neutron and photon exposures of the head. Intl J Radiat Oncol Biol Phys 2:1133–1139.

Bustad LK, Stitzel KA, Haro EK, Goldman M (1972) The choice of the beagle for radiobiologic studies. In: Stover BJ and Jee WSS (eds.), The radiobiology of plutonium. Salt Lake City: The JW Press.

Caldecott RS, Snyder LA (eds.) (1960) Radioisotopes in the biosphere. Minneapolis: University of Minnesota.

Casarett GW (1973) Pathogenesis of radionuclide-induced tumors. In: Sanders CL, Busch RH, Ballou JE, and Mahlum DD (eds.) Radionuclide Carcinogenesis. (CONF 720505) Springfield: US Department of Commerce.

Clark WJ, Busch RH, Hackett PL, Howard EB, Frazier ME, McClanahan BJ, Ragan HA,

Vogt GS (1972) Strontium-90 effects in swine: a summary to date. In: Goldman M and Bustad LK (eds.), Biomedical implications of radiostrontium exposure. Springfield: US Department of Commerce.

DellaRosa RJ, Goldman M, Andersen AC, Mays CW, Stover BJ (1965) Absorption and retention of ingested strontium and calcium in beagles as a function of age. Nature 205:197–198.

Dougherty TJ, Jee WSS, Mays CW, Stover BJ (eds.) (1962) Some aspects of internal irradiation. Oxford: Pergamon Press.

Dungworth DL, Goldman M, Switzer JW, McKelvie DH (1969) Development of a myelo-proliferative disorder in beagles continuously exposed to ^{90}Sr. Blood 34:610–632.

Evans RD (1974) Radium in man. Health Phys 27:497–510.

Finkel MP, Biskis BO, Bergstrand PJ (1960) Radioisotope toxicity: Significance of chronic administration. In: Caldecott RS and Snyder LA (eds.), Radioisotopes in the bio-sphere. Minneapolis: University of Minnesota.

Finkel MP, Jinkins PB, Biskis BO (1964) Parameters of radiation dosage that influence production of osteogenic sarcomas in mice. In: Control of cell division and the induc-tion of cancer; National Cancer Institute Monograph 14:243–270. Bethesda: US De-partment of Health Education and Welfare.

Finkel MP, Biskis BO (1968) Experimental induction of osteosarcomas. Prog Exp Tumor Res 10:72–111.

Finkel MP, Biskis BO, Greco I, Camden RW (1972) Strontium-90 toxicity in dogs: Status of Argonne study on influence of age and dosage pattern. In: Goldman M and Bustad LK (eds.), Biomedical implications of radiostrontium exposure (CONF710201). Springfield: US Department of Commerce.

Finkel MP, Reilly CA, Biskis BO (1976) Pathogenesis of radiation and virus-induced bone tumors. Recent Results Cancer Res 54:92–103.

Goldman M (1976) An overview of high LET radiation effects in cells. In: Jee WSS (ed.), The health effects of plutonium and radium. Salt Lake City: The JW Press.

Goldman M (1982) Ionizing radiation and its risk. West J Med 137:540–547.

Goldman M, Dungworth DL, Bulgin MS, Rosenblatt LS, Richards WPC, Bustad LK (1969a) Radiation-induced neoplasms in beagles after administrations of ^{90}Sr and ^{226}Ra. In: International Atomic Energy Agency (ed.), Radiation-induced cancer. Vi-enna: International Atomic Energy Agency.

Goldman M, Della Rosa RJ, McKelvie DH (1969b) Metabolic, dosimetric and pathologic consequences in the skeletons of beagles fed ^{90}Sr. In: Mays CW, Jee WSS, Lloyd RD, Stover BJ, Dougherty JH, and Taylor GN (eds.), Delayed effects of bone-seeking radio-nuclides. Salt Lake City: University of Utah Press.

Goldman M, Williams JR, Bulgin MS (1970) Application of ^{18}F to image ^{226}Ra-induced bone lesions. J Nucl Med 11:208–213.

Goldman M, Bustad LK (1972a) Proceedings synthesis. In: Goldman M and Bustad LK (eds.), Biomedical implications of radiostrontium exposure (CONF 710201) Springfield: US Department of Commerce.

Goldman M, Bustad LK (eds.) (1972b) Biomedical implications of radiostrontium expo-sure (CONF 710201). Springfield: US Department of Commerce.

Goldman M, Rosenblatt LS, Hetherington NW, Finkel MP (1973) Scaling of the dose, time and incidence of radium-induced osteosarcomas in mice and dogs to man. In: Sanders CL, Busch RH, Ballou JE, and Mahlum DD (eds.), Radionuclide carcinogenesis (CONF 720505). Springfield: US Department of Commerce.

Goldman M, Wilson FD, Rosenblatt LS, Book SA (1976) Early radiation effects on bone and blood as "predictors" of osteosarcoma: A late effect. In: International Atomic Energy Agency (ed.), Biological and environmental effects of low-level radiation. Vienna: International Atomic Energy Agency.

Heller M (1948) Histopathology of irradiation from external and internal sources. In: Bloom W (ed.), National nuclear energy series div. IV, Vol. 22–1. New York: McGraw-Hill.

Howard EB, Clarke WJ, Karagianes MT, Palmer RF (1969) Strontium-90 induced bone tumors in miniature swine. Radiat Res 39:594–607.

Ingleton PM, Underwood JC, Hunt NH, Atkins D, Giles B, Coulton LA, Martin TJ (1977) Radiation-induced osteogenic sarcoma in the rat as a model of hormone-responsive differentiated cancer. Lab Anim Sci 27:748–756.

International Atomic Energy Agency (1969) Radiation-induced cancer. Vienna: International Atomic Energy Agency.

International Atomic Energy Agency (1976) Biological and environmental effects of low-level radiation. Vienna: International Atomic Energy Agency.

International Commission on Radiological Protection (1973) Alkaline earth metabolism in adult man (ICRP Publ. 20). Oxford: Pergamon Press.

Jee WSS (ed.) (1976) The health effects of plutonium and radium. Salt Lake City: The JW Press.

King MA, Casarett GW, Weber DA, Burgner FA, Omara RE, Wilson GA (1980) A study of irradiated bone. III. Scintigraphic and radiographic detection of radiation-induced osteosarcomas. J Nucl Med 21:426–31.

Klein B, Pals S, Masse R, Lafuma J, Morin M, Binart N, Jasmin JR, Jasmin C (1977) Studies of bone and soft tissue tumors induced in rats with radioactive cerium chloride. Intl J Cancer 20:112–119.

Knowles JF (1981) Radiation-induced bone tumors in the guinea-pig. Intl J Radiat Biol 40:553–555.

Kuzma JF, Zander G (1957) Cancerogenic effects of ^{45}Ca and ^{89}Sr in Sprague Dawley rats. Arch Path 63:198–206.

Laissue JA, Burlington H, Cronkite EP, Reincke U (1977) Induction of osteosarcomas and hematopoietic neoplasms by ^{55}Fe in mice. Cancer Res 37:3545–3550.

Lloyd EL, Loutit JF, MacEvicius F (1975) Viruses in osteosarcomas induced by ^{226}Ra. A study of the induction of bone tumors in mice. Intl J Radiat Biol 28:13–33.

Loutit JF (1976) Vasoformative nonosteogenic (angio)sarcomas of bone-marrow due to strontium-90. Intl J Radiat Biol 30:359–383.

Loutit JF, Corp MJ, Ardran GM (1976) Radiographic features of bone in several strains of laboratory mice and of their tumours induced by bone-seeking radionuclides. J Anat 122:357–375.

Luz A, Müller WA, Gössner W, Hug O (1979) Osteosarcoma induced by short-lived bone-seeking alpha emitters in mice: The role of age. Envir Res 18:115–119.

Marshall JH, Groer PG (1977) A theory of the induction of bone cancer by alpha radiation. Radiat Res 71:149–192.

Mays CW, Lloyd RD (1972) Bone sarcoma risk from ^{90}Sr. In: Goldman M and Bustad LK (eds.), Biomedical implications of radiostrontium exposure (CONF 710201). Springfield: US Department of Commerce.

Mays CW, Jee WSS, Lloyd RD, Stover BJ, Dougherty JH, Taylor GN (eds.) (1969) Delayed effects of bone-seeking radionuclides. Salt Lake City: University of Utah Press.

Mays CW, Spiers H, Taylor GN, Lloyd RD, Jee WSS, McFarland SS, Taysum DH, Brammer TW, Brammer D, Pollard TA (1976) Estimated risk to human bone from ^{239}Pu. In: Jee WSS (ed.), Health effects of plutonium and radium. Salt Lake City: The JW Press.

Mole RH (1958) The dose relationship in radiation carcinogenesis. Br Med Bull 14:184–189.

Mole RH (1963) Carcinogenesis as the result of two independent rare events. In: Harris RJC (ed.), Cellular basis and aetiology of ionizing radiation. London: Academic Press.

Morgan JP, Pool RR (1982) Radium-226-induced bone lesions in beagles. Vet Radiol 23:261–71.

Morgan JP, Pool RR, Kirsh IE (1983) Comparison of radiological changes in humans and beagles with skeletal deposits of radium. Health Phys 44 (suppl 1):353–363.

Moskalev YI, Streltsova VN (1964): The carcinogenic effects of ionizing radiation. A review of current problems. Atomic Energy Rev 2:149–194.

Moskalev YI, Levdik TI, Lyubchanskii ER, Nifatov AP, Erokhin RAS, Buldakov LA, Lemberg VK, Koshurnikova NA, Filippova LG, Ternovskii IA (1975) Metabolism and biological effects in rodents of plutonium and other actinide elements. In: Nygaard OF, Adler HI, and Sinclair WK (eds.), Radiation research: Biomedical, chemical, and physical perspectives. New York: Academic Press.

Müller WA, Luz A (1977) The osteosarcomogenic effectiveness of the short-lived ^{224}Ra compared with that of the long-lived ^{226}Ra in mice. Radiat Res 70:444–448.

Müller WA, Luz A, Schaffer EH, Gossner W (1983a) The role of time-factor and RBE for the induction of osteosarcomas by incorporated short-lived bone-seekers. Health Phys 44 (suppl 1):203–212.

Müller WA, Schaffer EH, Linzner V, Luz A (1983b) Late effects of incorporated radionuclides in mice as occurring with combined application of different radiation qualities and intensivities (α- and β-emitting bone-seekers). In: Broerse JJ, Barendsen GW, Kal HB, and vanderKogel AJ (eds.), Radiation research: Somatic and genetic effects. Amsterdam: Martin Nijhoff Publishers.

National Academy of Sciences (1976) Health effects of alpha-emitting particles in the respiratory tract. Washington: National Academy of Sciences.

National Academy of Sciences (1980) The effects on populations of exposure to low levels of ionizing radiation: 1980. Washington: National Academy Press.

National Council on Radiation Protection and Measurements (1980) Influence of dose and its distribution in time on dose-response relationships for low-LET radiations (NCRP Report 64). Washington: National Council on Radiation Protection and Measurements.

Nilsson A (1962) Strontium-90 induced bone and bone marrow changes. Uppsala: Almquist and Siksells.

Nilsson A (1966) Early development of transplanted 90Sr-induced osteosarcoma buds. Acta Radiol Ther Phys Biol 4:7–16.

Nilsson A (1971) Radiostrontium-induced carcinomas of the external ear. Acta Radiol Ther Phys Biol 10:321–328.

Nilsson A, Broome-Karlsson A (1976a) The pathology of americium-241. Acta Radiol Ther Phys Biol 15:49–70.

Nilsson A, Broome-Karlsson A (1976b) Influence of steroid hormones on the carcinogenicity of ^{90}Sr. Acta Radiol Ther Phys Biol 15:417–426.

Parks NJ, Keane AT (1983) Consideration of age-dependent radium-retention in people on the basis of the beagle model. Health Phys 44 (suppl 1):103–112.

Parks NJ, Book SA, Pool RR (1984) Squamous cell carcinoma in the jaws of beagles exposed to ^{90}Sr throughout life: Beta flux measurements at the mandible and tooth surfaces and a hypothesis for tumorigenesis. Radiat Res 100:139–156.

Pecher C (1941) Biological investigations with radiocalcium and strontium. Proc Soc Exp Biol Med 46:86–94.

Pool RR, Williams JR, Goldman M (1972) Strontium-90 toxicity in adult beagles after continuous ingestion. In: Goldman M and Bustad LK (eds.), Biomedical implications of radiostrontium exposure (CONF 710201). Springfield: US Department of Commerce.

Pool RR, Morgan JP, Parks NJ, Farnham JE, Littman MS (1983) Comparative pathogenesis of radium-induced intracortical bone lesions in humans and beagles. Health Phys 44 (suppl 1):155–177.

Raabe OG, Book SA, Parks NJ (1980) Bone cancer from radium: Canine dose response explains data for mice and humans. Science 208:61–64.

Raabe OG, Book SA, Parks NJ (1983) Lifetime bone cancer dose-response relationships in beagles and people from skeletal burdens of ^{226}Ra and ^{90}Sr. Health Phys 44 (suppl 1):33–48.

Rosenblatt LS, Hetherington NW, Goldman M, Bustad LK (1971) Evaluation of tumor incidence following exposure to internal emitters by application of the logistic dose-response surface. Health Phys 21:869–875.

Rosenblatt LS (1972) Determination of cumulative tumor incidences and their use in quantitative evaluation of radionuclide carcinogenesis. In: Biomedical implications of radiostrontium exposure (CONF 710201). Springfield: US Department of Commerce.

Rosenblatt LS, Goldman M, Book SA, Momeni MH (1976) Extrapolation of radiation-induced tumor incidence from animals to man. In: International Atomic Energy Agency (ed.), Biological and environmental effects of low-level radiation. Vienna: International Atomic Energy Agency.

Rowland RE, Stehney AF, Lucas HF (1983) Dose–response relationships for radium-induced bone sarcomas. Health Phys 44 (suppl 1):15–31.

Sanders CL, Busch RH, Ballou JE, Mahlum DD (eds.) (1973) Radionuclide Carcinogenesis (CONF 720505). Springfield: US Department of Commerce.

Solheim OP (1977) Development of osteosarcoma in rats after irradiation. Acta Radiol Ther Phys Biol 16:433–446.

Spiers FW (1974) Radionuclides and bone—from ^{226}Ra to ^{90}Sr. Br J Radiol 47:833–844.

Spiers FW, Zanelli GD, Darley PJ, Whitwell JR, Goldman M (1972) In: Goldman M and Bustad LK (eds.), Biomedical implications of radiostrontium exposure (CONF 710201). Springfield: US Department of Commerce.

Spiers FW, Vaughan J (1976) Hazards of plutonium with special reference to the skeleton. Nature 259:531–534.

Stara JF, Nelson NS, Della Rosa RJ, Bustad LK (1971) Comparative metabolism of radio-nuclides in mammals: A review. Health Phys 209:113–137.

Stevens W, Atherton DR, Jee WWS, Buster DS, Grube BJ, Bruenger FW, Lindenbaum A (1976) Induction of osteosarcoma by polymeric plutonium (^{239}Pu IV). In: Jee WSS (ed.), The health effects of plutonium and radium. Salt Lake City: The JW Press.

Stover BJ, Jee WSS (eds.) (1972) Radiobiology of plutonium. Salt Lake City: The JW Press.

Thorne MC (1977) Aspects of the dosimetry of alpha-emitting radionuclides in bone with particular reference on ^{226}Ra and ^{239}Pu. Phys Med Biol 22:36–46.

Thurman GB, Mays CW, Taylor GN, Christensen WR, Rehfeld CE, Dougherty TF (1971) Growth dynamics of beagle osteosarcoma. Growth 35:119–125.

United Nations (1977) Sources and Effects of Ionizing Radiation. New York: United Nations.

United Nations (1982) Ionizing radiation: Sources and biological effects. New York: United Nations.

Van Cleave CD (1968) Late somatic effects of ionizing radiation. Washington, DC: US Atomic Energy Commission.

Vaughan JM (1973) The Effects of Irradiation on the Skeleton. Oxford: Clarendon Press.

Woodard HG (1957) Some effects of x-rays on bone. Clinical orthopaedics 9:118–130.

World Health Organization (1982) Nuclear power: Health implications of transuranium elements (WHO European serial no. 11). Copenhagen: World Health Organization.

Wrenn ME, Taylor GN, Stevens W, Mays CW, Jee WSS, Lloyd RD, Atherton DR, Bruenger FW, Kimmel DB, Miller SC, Shabestari L, Smith JM, Stover B (1983) Summary of dosimetry, pathology and dose response for bone sarcomas in beagles injected with ^{226}Ra. In: Broerse JJ, Barendsen GW, Kal HB, and vanderKogel AJ (eds.), Radiation research: Somatic and genetic effects. Amsterdam: Martin Nijhoff Publishers.

Wright JF, Goldman M, Bustad LK (1972) Age strain and dose-rate effects of ^{89}Sr in mice. In: Biomedical implications of radiostrontium exposure (CONF 710201). Springfield: US Department of Commerce.

EXPERIMENTAL CARCINOGENESIS IN THE DIGESTIVE AND GENITOURINARY TRACTS

HIROMITSU WATANABE, M.D., AKIHIRO ITO, M.D., AND FUMIO HIROSE, M.D.

Radiation has been found to induce a variety of gastrointestinal tumors in laboratory animals. The experimental data are summarized briefly in the following.

ESOPHAGUS AND FORESTOMACH

Mice into which ^{60}Co wires had been implanted in the lungs near the esophagus were observed by Gates and Warren (1968) to develop radiation-induced esophageal cancer (1968). The dose-rates at which carcinogenic effects were noted ranged from 220 to 4000 R/day. The cancer incidence rose to a peak after 751–1000 R/day and then decreased with increasing radiation dose. Total carcinogenic doses ranged between 35,000 and 297,000 R. The middle total dose range, 151,000–200,000 R, was most productive for cancer induction. The incidence of esophageal cancer was influenced more by strain than by sex.

Sáxen (1952) described squamous cell carcinoma of the forestomach after x-irradiation of the stomach region in C57BR mice fed 9,10-dimethyl-1,2-benzanthracene. The incidence of such carcinomas was lower in female than in male mice. Upton et al (1960b) noted that squamous cell carcinoma was the most common form of stomach tumor in LAF$_1$ mice, but saw no significant increase in whole-body gamma or neutron irradiated mice. Cosgrove et al (1968) recorded a relatively large increase in squamous cell carcinomas of the forestomach after larger doses of whole-body radiation and reported that neutron irradiation appeared to be more effective in mice of the LAF$_1$ strain, but not in those of the RF strain.

From the Research Institute for Nuclear Medicine and Biology, Hiroshima University, Hiroshima, Japan.

STOMACH

Many investigators have reported that whole-body irradiation induces adeno-carcinomas of the stomach (Nowell et al, 1958; Cosgrove et al, 1968; Castanera et al, 1971). Hence, an observed incidence of gastric adenocarcinoma of less than 5% implies that the radiation dose to the stomach may have been insuffi-cient. Hirose (1969) reported the induction of gastric carcinomas in the glandu-lar stomach of the rat at a relatively high frequency with local x-irradiation of the stomach. The irradiation schedule involved 15-Gy fractions at 1-wk inter-vals, for a total of six exposures, or 20-Gy fractions at 1-wk intervals, for a total of five exposures. Among the exposed animals, gastric adenocarcinomas devel-oped in 20% and precancerous changes in 37%. The incidence of gastric adeno-carcinoma was higher in female than in male mice. In four of eight Donryo rats, adenocarcinomas were induced with 20 Gy of x-rays fractionated in a total of three exposures (Hirose, 1969). Rats appear more susceptible than mice to localized x-irradiation of the gastric region in induction of gastric adenocarci-noma. Whole-body irradiation, bringing about either bone marrow or intestinal death, is not a suitable method by which a dose of radiation sufficient to cause serious damage to the gastric mucosa can be achieved. Thus, Hirose (1969) concluded that localized irradiation of the gastric region would be more appro-priate for induction of cancer in the glandular stomach.

The mechanism of inducing gastric adenocarcinoma by x-irradiation was proposed by Hirose as following:

Low-dose → Atrophy of mucosa → Regeneration

High-dose → Atrophy of mucosa → Ulceration → Delayed atypical
                                                      regeneration

                                  ↘ Atypical hyperplasia → Adenocarcinoma

It has been known that regenerating tissues have a high sensitivity to radia-tion carcinogenesis. Hence, Hirose et al (1976) studied the influence of immune atrophic gastritis on the induction of gastric carcinoma by x-irradiation of ICR mice. Fractionated doses of 20 Gy of x-rays, to total doses of 60 or 80 Gy, were given to the gastric region of ICR female mice that had immune atrophic gastri-tis induced by injection of allogenic stomach antigen. The incidence was in-creased, and the latency of gastric adenocarcinoma was accelerated, in the group of animals that received immunization with allogeneic stomach antigen 2 wk before x-irradiation, compared with animals treated by x-irradiation alone. Irradiation was introduced when there was an increase of regenerating activity in the pyloric gland mucosa caused by immunization (Watanabe et al, 1977).

Watanabe et al (1980) demonstrated that intestinal metaplasia in gastric mucosa was readily induced in rats by fractionated local x-irradiation with 5 Gy daily for six exposures or with 10 Gy x-rays every other day for three exposures. In these experiments, no gastric adenocarcinomas were obtained. Fujii et al (1980) also described the induction of intestinal metaplasia in rats by localized x-irradiation of the stomach combined with oral administration of N-methyl-N'-nitro-N-nitrosoguanidine, and no gastric tumors were induced by this treatment. These data suggest that gastric adenocarcinomas do not necessarily arise from intestinal metaplasia.

Sáxen (1952) attempted to induce gastric adenocarcinoma by x-irradiation of the gastric region with a single dose of 1000 R but was unsuccessful. Moore et al (1953) applied internal radiation to the stomach of mice with beta rays of ^{32}P in a latex balloon. The doses of beta ray were equivalent to about 18,000 R, and most of the animals died of necrosis and perforation of the gastric wall. Thus, it appears that there is an optimum dose range for the induction of cancer in the glandular stomach. Lower doses of radiation may induce intestinal metaplasia, and markedly higher doses of radiation may decrease the incidence of gastric adenocarcinoma. Hirose (1969) considered that an adequate dose for inducing gastric adenocarcinoma by a single exposure to x-rays is approximately 20 Gy.

SMALL INTESTINE

According to the earliest known report (Henshaw et al, 1947), experimental intestinal carcinoma occurred in less than 1% of mice after x-irradiation. Nowell et al (1959) described results in LAF_1 mice that were subjected to whole-body irradiation with sublethal doses of fast neutrons or lethal doses of x-rays followed by implantation of spleen homogenate or performed with one femur shielded. These animals developed small intestinal carcinoma at a rate of about 22%. In the neutron irradiated group, tumors were induced preferentially and were either mucoid or poorly differentiated adenocarcinomas of the small intestine.

Bond et al (1952) found intestinal tumors in the small bowel of the rat, with formation of well differentiated mucus-producing glands, frequently extending into the muscularis after local irradiation with a single dose of 1800–2800 rem of deuterons. The induction of adenocarcinoma of the small bowel in rats was facilitated by parabiosis or p-aminopropiophenone treatment after whole body x-irradiation (Brecher et al, 1953). Osborne et al (1963) have described the induction of intestinal carcinomas by x-irradiation of the exteriorized ileum and jejunum in Holtzman rats, with exposures of 1000–2500 R with or without blood vessel clamping during irradiation. Over 50% of animals that survived exposure above 1400 R because of intestinal vessel clamping developed tumors. In the 1400 R group, the latency of the intestinal tumors ranged from 55 days to 225 days after irradiation. Subsequently, Coop et al (1974) reported that after 2000 R x-ray irradiation of hypoxic, temporarily exteriorized ileum and jejunum, 56% of the rats developed adenocarcimoma somewhere in the irradiated segment. Colloid carcinoma was commonly observed. Metastases and direct invasion of the tumors into the adjacent mesentery, pancreas, and abdominal wall were observed. In a series of interesting reports, Stevens et al (1981) described common antigenic determinants in rat fetal protein and in a perchloric acid-soluble protein isolated from the sera of rats bearing x-ray–induced small bowel adenocarcinoma.

Tsubouchi and Matsuzawa (1973) found visible nodules within 2 mo following irradiation in 100% of the rats in groups that received 1750 or 2000 R abdominal x-rays; 50% after 1500 R; and 3% after 1000 R. The nodules showed adenomatous hyperplasia and vascular fibrosis. Epithelial cells in the glandular tissue invaded the submucosa. Some of them secreted mucin. If the animals had been kept a longer time, some might have developed adenocarcinoma of the mucinous type. Zaldivar (1968) dealt with the sequence of histopathologic events at exposure levels of 600, 1000, and 1400 R, with and without urethan in a total of 1100 albino rats. No carcinomas were induced in this dose range. In addition, Sebes, Zaldivar, and Vogel (1975) described the effects of x-irradiation of an exteriorized segment of the Sprague–Dawley rat ileum with a single dose of 2200 R, with clamping both of the mesenteric artery and vein during exposure. No adenocarcinomas were found in this experiment. Only six of 34 Sprague–Dawley rats survived for 50 days after 2200 R exposure. The discrepancy between Osborne's group and Zaldivar's group might be due to differences in the post irradiation survival period.

Marks and Sullivan (1960) reported the incidence of intestinal tumors among 51 rats that had received x-irradiation of 1500–1900 R to the abdomen or the exteriorized intestine at age 5 mo, and killed between 9 and 30 mo later. The earliest tumor was observed at 9.5 mo. The incidence and latency of mucinous carcinoma (13%) were lower and later, respectively, than those reported by Osborne et al (1963). The number of survivors was smaller than in Osborne's experiment, probably because no clamping of blood vessels was employed. Rostom et al (1978) irradiated 2 cm² of the lower abdomen of C57BL mice with doses of 16–24 Gy. There were some early deaths in the exposed mice, but those which survived 50–240 days developed a high incidence (25%) of invasive adenocarcinoma of the ileum, with mucin-secreting cells. Sensitivity to the induction of small-intestinal cancer by irradiation thus appears dependent on the species and strain of animals in question.

COLON

Radiation has been shown to induce tumors of the colon. Lisco et al (1949) reported that 75% rats fed the beta emitter, ^{91}Yt, developed adenocarcinoma of the colon between 304 and 548 days after the first feeding. In the study of Nowell et al (1956), whole-body irradiation of mice produced a 27% incidence of caecum tumors with mucin-secreting types. Other reports of radiation-induced colon cancers involve external whole-body irradiation of mice, in which the incidence of large-bowel tumors was about 20% (Nowell and Cole, 1959).

In rats protected from acute radiation death by parabiosis before or after whole-body irradiation with 700 or 1000 R of x-rays, adenocarcinoma of the colon developed in about 5% of the cases (Brecher et al, 1953). Denman et al (1978) reported the effects of irradiation of the descending colon, which was irradiated with a collimated x-ray beam. The colon in male Holtzman rats was exposed, starting with 2500 R and increasing by 1000-R increments up through 6500 R. Animals in each irradiated group developed mucoid adenocarcinomas, with the highest incidence (47%) being reached in the 4500 R group, where there was optimal survival of animals (93%). Below 4500 R the survival rate was still good (80%) but the tumor incidence was lower (20%–40%). Above

5500 R, the survival rate was low (33%–40%); even if all the animals which survived were to develop tumors, the overall incidence would still have been less than that of rats exposed to 4500 R. The development of pulmonary metastases in 1 of 12 rats exposed to 3500 R indicated that these induced colon tumors were malignant. The investigators concluded that colon cells are more sensitive to malignant change than skin or kidney cells.

All the neoplasms arising in the large intestine of the mouse have been mucin-secreting (Rostom et al, 1978). In general, intestinal adenocarcinomas induced by irradiation are of the mucoid type; thus, they are different from chemically induced tumors, which tend to be moderatley to well differentiated adenocarcinomas.

RECTUM

Hirose et al (1977) reported the induction of rectal carcinoma in mice by local x-irradiation. The pelvic region of female ICR and CF_1 mice was irradiated with various doses of x-rays at 1-wk intervals, to determine the relationship between the x-ray dose and induction of rectal carcinoma. The incidence of rectal carcinoma in ICR mice was zero after a single dose of 20 Gy x-rays, but 31% after a single dose of 30 Gy, 6% after two doses of 15 Gy, 25% after three doses of 15 Gy, 42% after two doses of 20 Gy, and 95% after three doses of 20 Gy. Similar cancers developed in 70% of CF_1 mice exposed to two doses of 20 Gy. The development of rectal carcinoma, thus, was dose-dependent at the x-ray dose levels used in Hirose's experiment. When the same dose per fraction was employed, the incidence of this cancer increased with the number of fractions given. Comparison of ICR mice with CF_1 mice showed that the incidence of rectal carcinomas differed by strain.

Terada et al (1980) reported on the influence of immunization by rectal antigen on rectal carcinogenesis in male A/HeJ mice. Induction of rectal cancer was accelerated by two doses of 20 Gy of x-ray in the preimmunized mice, and the incidence of rectal cancer in the immunized mice was significantly higher than that in nonimmunized mice. The cell kinetics of the rectal mucosa were also examined after rectal antigen was administered. After immunization, the number of [3]HtdR-labeled cells was found to be increased, with a concomitant spread of the proliferative zone. G_2 and M phases were shorter in the immunized mice than in control mice. With shortening of those phases of the cell cycle, the frequency of DNA synthesis increased and the cell proliferative zone was expanded. Furthermore, the degree of damage of rectal mucosa after x-irradiation of mice given antigen was greater than that of mice without immunization. However, regeneration after damage in immunized mice was also greater than in the controls. The investigator concluded that x-irradiation during the period of active cell proliferation and shortened cell cycle caused by immunization induced the cancerous change more effectively.

Rostom et al (1978) described the influence of misonidazole on the incidence of radiation-induced rectal tumors in C57BL mice. When the radiosensitizer misonidazole was given in a single dose shortly before irradiation, there was a significant increase in the incidence of multiple tumors, largely attributable to tumors arising in the rectum. Black et al (1980) described the late effects of irradiation of the rectum with negative pi measons in Sprague–Dawley rats. Mucoid type adenocarcinomas and poorly differentiated adenocarcinomas were induced, but they were encountered only at the higher dose levels.

LIVER

The studies by Cole and Nowell (1965) have served to emphasize the role of proliferative stimuli in radiation hepatocarcinogenesis. The incidence of hepatomas in LAF_1 mice that had been irradiated with a single, whole-body dose of fission neutrons (165–306 cGy) was markedly greater than that in mice irradiated with x-rays (5 Gy). Carbon tetrachloride (CCl_4) was administered to some groups of mice at various times before and after radiation exposure. This proliferative stimulus further increased hepatoma frequency. The greatest hepatoma incidence (95%) occurred in a group that received neutron irradiation during the first proliferative wave, 1 day after CCl_4 treatment. When CCl_4 was given 1 mo after neutron exposure, the hepatoma incidence was 75%, and the incidence after neutron exposure alone was 7%. In contrast, when x-irradiation was performed 1, 2, or 3 days after CCl_4, the hepatoma incidence was only 10%–23%, whereas, when CCl_4 was given 1 mo after x-irradiation, the incidence of tumors was 43%. Willey et al (1973) found that a single, whole-body 2-Gy dose of ^{137}Cs gamma rays increased the hepatoma incidence by approximately three- to fourfold over the control rates when a pure proliferative stimulus was added. A single, whole-body 2-Gy dose of fission neutron irradiation increased the hepatoma incidence by approximately six- to ninefold over the control rates when combined with partial hepatectomy. Furthermore, both the ^{137}Cs gamma ray and fission neutron hepatocarcinogenesis rates were enhanced, regardless of whether the irradiation was given during liver regeneration or 8–13 wk prior to partial hepatectomy. However, neither ^{137}Cs nor fission neutron irradiation alone (i.e., without partial hepatectomy), significantly increased the incidence of hepatomas. Vesselinovitch et al (1971) reported that exposure of neonatal $B6C3F_1$ mice to 320 cGy of x-rays led to an increased incidence of hepatocellular tumors. Sasaki et al (1981) also reported that hepatocellular tumors developed at a high incidence especially in neonatally x-irradiated $B6WF_1$ mice. Neonatal female mice were more susceptible than 5 wk old mice. Also, hepatocellular tumors developed in excess in the group irradiated at a late intrauterine stage. The incidence of hepatocellular tumors in male mice was higher than in the female mice. The high susceptibility of perinatal mice to x-ray–induced hepatocellular tumorigenesis may be related to the high frequency of mitosis at and/or after x-ray irradiation. The incidence of liver tumors was significantly enhanced in mice irradiated with 200 R within 24 hr after birth, and reached a maximum after 400 R. The incidence at 600 R was lower than that at 400 R.

Witcofski and Pizzarello (1976) compared the carcinogenic potential of a dose of 250 cGy x-rays with similar doses of radiations from ^{113m}In, and ^{198}Au delivered at different dose-rates to rat livers. No significant differences in tumor incidence were observed. N-2-fluorenyldiacetamide (2-FAA) was administered after irradiation to reduce the latent period and increase the number of radiogenic liver tumors. It was concluded that 2-FAA acted as a promoter to enhance radiation tumorigenesis in the liver and to decrease the latent period.

Maisin et al (1978) administered chemical radioprotectors to mice with a single whole-body exposure to ionizing radiation. These chemicals protected against tumorigenesis by 350 R irradiation, but the incidence of liver tumors was not affected after 650 R. Jirtle et al (1981) have used an in vivo transplantation assay to determine the survival of liver cells exposed to sparsely ionizing radiation. Importantly, this model may allow quantitative analysis of carcinogenesis by total-body irradiation.

KIDNEY

Hamilton (1975) summarized the experimental evidence on radiogenic renal tumors in rats and mice. In his review on mice exposed to atomic bomb radiation, dose–response relationships were rarely estimated. Rosen et al (1962) concluded that neutrons were more effective in the induction of renal tumors than x-rays in rats. Carcinomas were recorded, particularly in a group exposed as young adults but never in a group exposed at older ages (Nowell and Cole, 1959). Maldague (1969) concluded that renal neoplasia arose as the result of an interaction of a specific proliferative stimulus with radiation-altered kidney cells.

The tumors just described included both benign and malignant types, and were induced by neutron, gamma, and x-irradiation. They were also induced by both whole- and partial-body irradiation. Strain, sex, and age differences were reported.

Recently, Mahler et al (1982) reported an influence of dietary protein on rat radiation nephropathy. Groups of 14-Gy-irradiated animals fed isocaloric diets of high (50%), normal (20%), or low (4%) protein showed median life spans of 59, 103, and 200 days, respectively. As a result, the investigators concluded that a low protein diet might also be beneficial in delaying or reducing radiation nephropathy in radiotherapy patients. Furthermore, it is conceivable that dietary manipulation might permit a larger therapeutic dose.

PROSTATE

Hirose et al (1976) reported carcinomas of the prostate in male ICR/JCL mice after x-irradiation of the pelvis. The incidence of prostate tumors increased as the interval between x-ray fractions was shortened. The results further suggest that development of prostate carcinomas depends on radiation dose. Hirose et al (1978a, 1978b) performed similar experiments with Wistar rats. Seven-wk-old male mice were irradiated over the pelvic region with a total of 60 Gy (10 × 6) or 40 Gy (10 × 4) x-rays, with several different time intervals between fractions. In the six fraction group, the mean latent period of prostatic adenocarcinomas was short and the frequency of the undifferentiated type of tumor was high. Conversely, in the four-fraction group, the mean latent period of adenocarcinomas was long and the frequency of differentiated adenocarcinomas was as high as that of anaplastic lesions.

Brown and Warren (1978) published an extensive study of 1120 parabiotic NEDH rats in which one partner was total-body irradiated with 1000 R and the other shielded. 1000 R whole-body x-irradiation is weakly carcinogenic for the

rat prostate. The absence of prostatic tumors in the irradiated, intact Sprague–
Dawley rats suggests that they are rather resistant to the tumorigenic action of
x-rays on the prostate gland, compared with Wistar strain rats (Hirose et al,
1979).

Takizawa and Hirose (1978) suggested that replacement treatments with
testosterone, probably in excess of the physiological dose, acted as a promotor
for the development of prostate cancer and precancerous lesions, since Noble
(1977) found that the incidence of prostate adenocarcinoma was increased
from 0.45% to 18.4% in aged Nb strain rats by prolonged treatment with testosterone or testosterone plus estrogen.

TESTIS

Berdjis (1964) found a fourfold increase in interstitial cell tumors in Sprague–
Dawley rats after whole-body exposure to 500 R or 3 × 350 R x-rays. Lindsay et
al (1969) also found that exposing the scrotal area of Long Evans rats to 150 or
500 R of x-rays induced such tumors. They postulated that the probable hormonal imbalance resulting from radiation damage to the testes could have played
a part in the genesis of the interstitial cell tumors. The testes of albino rats
derived from the Alderhey Park (strain 1) were x-irradiated either bilaterally or
unilaterally with doses in the range of 100–1500 R at age 3 mo by Hulse (1977).
All 24 of 239 tumors were of the interstitial cell type. Hulse concluded that
strain differences in susceptibility to radiation-induction of such tumors may
exist.

OVARY

Many papers (Furth and Furth, 1936; Upton et al, 1960a, 1960b; Li and
Gardner, 1947) described the induction of ovarian tumors by radiation. Lick et
al (1949) reported that x-irradiation of a single ovary did not induce ovarian
tumors if the second ovary was not irradiated. Localized irradiation of a single
ovary did not induce ovarian tumors if the second ovary was not irradiated.
Localized irradiation of a single ovary induced ovarian tumor development
only if the second ovary was extirpated. This strongly suggests that the presence of a functioning ovary in the normal position inhibited tumor formation
in the irradiated ovary. Kirschbaum (1956) found that when irradiated ovaries
were grafted into intact as well as castrated male Balb/c mice, ovarian tumorigenesis proceeded. Grafts of functional normal ovary in previously irradiated
Balb/c females inhibited tumorigenesis in the irradiated induced ovaries. It is
likely that estrogenic hormone acts via the pituitary to suppress gonadotropic
stimulation of ovarian tumor development (Clifton, 1959). For example, Kaplan (1950) concluded that the production of granulosa cell ovarian tumors in
x-irradiated mice was related to an indirect effect of hormone stimulation
which follows ovarian atrophy after irradiation.

Yuhas (1974) suggested that dose-rate effects may be a function of two
components; first, age-dependent changes in sensitivity, and second, true repair of potentially carcinogenic injury. Ullrich et al (1976, 1977) observed a
similar two-component process after neutron irradiation. No tumors were in-

duced in ovaries which were grafted subcutaneously after x-ray irradiation of the recipient. These results indicate that hormonal conditions, especially during early stages of tumorigenesis, as well as direct radiation damage to the ovaries, may determine the type of ovarian tumor induced. Prenatal irradiation was found to have a low tumor-inducing effect. The lowest incidence rates were found after x-irradiation during gestational days 17–19, whereas, neonatal irradiation caused an ovary tumor frequency of nearly 66% (Upton et al, 1960a). By contrast, a significant enhancement of ovarian tumorigenesis was observed in mice irradiated at a late intrauterine stage (Sasaki et al, 1978). Similar results were described by Schmahl and Kriegel (1980); they found a remarkable degree of ovarian tumor induction by prenatal x-irradiation during the fetal period, while irradiation in the period of organogenesis was of low efficacy with respect to this disease. Whole-body irradiation with 20 rad at 10 days after birth produced measurable late effects in female mice of the NMRI strain. Ovarian tumors could be induced at virtually any age by x-irradiation, as well as negative pions of peak and plateau regions (Zimmermann et al, 1979). The influence of dose and dose rate on tumorigenicity after neutron irradiation was investigated in female RF/Un mice exposed to various doses of neutrons at dose rates of 5 and 25 rad/min; neutron irradiation at low dose rates was less effective than at high dose rates at all doses tested (Ullrich et al, 1977). Ovarian tumors were induced at near-maximum incidence at 50 rad of whole body irradiation with x-ray or protons (Clapp et al, 1974, 1978). The RBE for ovarian tumor induction appeared to vary in a complex manner depending upon the region of the dose–response curve.

SUMMARY

We have reviewed gastrointestinal and urinary tract tumors in rats and mice induced with localized or whole-body irradiation. In the literature, the dose for the induction of esophageal cancer has been observed to be enormously high (151,000–200,000 R). In the glandular stomach, 20 Gy/fraction for a total of 60–80 Gy has been carcinogenic in our studies. In the stomach, squamous cell carcinoma is more easily induced by radiation than carcinoma of the glandular stomach. For carcinogenesis in the small intestine, 2000 R seems to be the most effective dose, and for carcinogenesis in the colon, 4500 R. In the rectum, a maximal effect has been obtained with 60 Gy. The effective dosage for hepatocarcinogenesis has been observed to be about 400–500 R. In the prostate, 60 Gy was carcinogenic in our studies. The incidence and types of cancer in the gastrointestinal and urinary tracts have been observed to vary markedly among the different organs.

The determining factors for sensitivity to radiation carcinogenesis depend on species, strain, age, and sex. In the induction of tumors by local- or whole-body irradiation, various enhancing factors have been identified. For stomach and rectal cancer, these include immunization; for hepatic tumors, partial hepatectomy; for prostatic tumors, testosterone; and for rectal cancer, radiosensitizers. The effective radiation dose range varies among individual organs.

It is concluded that neutrons are more effective than x-rays for the production of cancers in the various organs, although neutrons are not suitable for localized irradiation.

This work was supported in part by a Grant-in-Aid for Cancer Research for the Ministry of Education, Science and Culture of Japan.

We are greatly indebted to Dr. Kelly H. Clifton (WCCC, University of Wisconsin), for reading the manuscript and to K. Tanaka and M. Shitamiya for their secretarial work.

REFERENCES

Berdjis CC (1964) Testicular tumors in normal and irradiated rats. Oncologia 17:197–220.

Black WC, Gomez LS, Yuhas JM, Kligerman MM (1980) Quantitation of the late effects of x-radiation on the large intestine. Cancer 45:444–451.

Bond VP, Swift MN, Tobias CA, Brecher G (1952) Bowel lesions following single deuteron irradiation. Fed Proc 11:408–409.

Boschetti AE, Maloney WC (1966) Observations on pancreatic islet cell and other radiation-induced tumors in the rat. Lab Invest 15:565–575.

Brecher G, Cronkite EP, Peers JH (1953) Neoplasms in rats protected against lethal doses of irradiation by parabiosis or para aminopropriophenome. J Natl Cancer Inst 14:159–175.

Brown CE, Warren S (1978) Carcinoma of the prostate in irradiated parabiotic rats. Cancer Res 38:159–162.

Casarett GW (1965) Experimental radiation carcinogenesis. Prog Exp Tumor Res 7:49–82.

Castenera TJ, Jones DC, Kimeldorf DJ, Rosen VJ (1971) The effect of age at exposure to sublethal dose of fast neutrons on tumorigenesis in the male rat. Cancer Res 31:1543–1549.

Clapp NK (1978) Ovarian tumor type and their incidence in intact mice following whole body exposure to ionizing radiation. Radiat Res 74:405–414.

Clifton KH (1959) Problems in experimental tumorigenesis of the pituitary gland, gonads, adrenal cortices, and mammary glands: A review. Cancer Res 19:2–22.

Cole LJ, Nowell PC (1965) Radiation carcinogenesis: The sequence of events. Science 150:1782–1786.

Coop KL, Sharp JG, Osborne JW, Zimmerman GR (1974) An animal model for the study of small-bowel tumors. Cancer Res 34:1487–1494.

Cosgrove GE, Walburg HE, Upton AC (1968) Gastrointestinal lesions in aged conventional and germfree mice exposed to radiation as young adults. In: Sullivan ME (ed.), Gastrointestinal radiation injury. Excerpta Medica Foundation Monogr Nucl Med Biol No 1, Amsterdam, 303–312.

Denman DL, Kirchner FR, Osborne JW (1978) Induction of colonic adenocarcinoma in the rat by x-irradiation. Cancer Res 38:1899–1905.

Fujii I, Watanabe H, Terada Y, Naito Y, Naito M, Ito A (1980) Induction of intestinal metaplasia in the glandular stomach of rats by x-irradiation prior to oral administration of N-Methyl-N'-Nitro-N-Nitrosoguanidine. Gann 71:804–810.

Furth J, Furth OB (1936) Neoplastic diseases produced in mice by general irradiation with x-rays; Incidence and types of neoplasms. Am J Cancer 28:54–65.

Gates O, Warren S (1968) Radiation-induced experimental cancer of esophagus. Am J Pathol 53:667–685.

Hamilton JM (1975) Renal carcinogenesis. Adv Cancer Res 22:1–56.

Henshaw PS, Riley EF, Stapleton GE (1947) The biologic effects of pile radiations. Radiology 49:349–360.

Hirose F (1969) Experimental induction of carcinoma in the glandular stomach by localized x-irradiation of gastric region. Gann Monogr 8:75–113.

Hirose F, Fukazawa K, Watanabe H, Terada Y, Fujii I, Ootuska S (1977) Induction of rectal carcinoma in mice by local x-irradiation. Gann 68:669–680.

Hirose F, Takizawa S, Watanabe H, Takeichi N (1976) Development of adenocarcinoma of the prostate in ICR mice locally irradiated with x-ray. Gann 67:407–411.

Hirose F, Takizawa S, Watanabe H, Takeichi N (1979) Prostate tumors in rats induced by repeated local irradiation with 1,000 rad of x-rays. Sixth International Congress of Radiation Research, Abstract 71.

Hirose F, Takizawa S, Watanabe H, Terada Y, Fujii I, Ootsuka S (1978a) Development of experimental prostatic carcinoma caused by radiation. J Hiroshima Med Assoc 31:358–363.

Hirose F, Takizawa S, Watanabe H, Terada Y, Fujii I (1978b) Induction of prostate carcinoma in rats by local x-irradiation. Nagasaki Igaku Z 53:216–222.

Hirose F, Watanabe H, Takeichi N, Naito Y, Inoue S (1976) Effect of experimental immune atrophic gastritis on the induction of gastric carcinoma by x-irradiation in ICR mice. Gann 67:355–364.

Hulse EV (1977) Can radiation induce interstitial-cell (leydig-cell) tumours of the testis? Intl J Radiat Biol 32:185–190.

Jirtle RL, Michalopoulos G, McLain JR, Crowley J (1981) Transplantation system for determining the clonogenic survival of parenchymal hepatocytes exposed to ionized radiation. Cancer Res 41:3512–3518.

Kaplan HS (1950) Influence of ovarian function on incidence of radiation-induced ovarian tumors in mice. J Natl Cancer Inst 11:125–132.

Kirschbaum A, Liebelt AG, Fletcher GH (1956) Influence of testis on induction of ovarian tumors of mice by x-rays. Proc Soc Exp Biol 92:221–224.

Li MH, Gardner WU (1947) Experimental studies on pathogenesis and histogenesis of ovarian tumors in mice. Cancer Res 7:549–566.

Lick L, Kirschbaum A, Mixer H (1949) Mechanism of induction of ovarian tumors by x-rays. Cancer Res 9:532–536.

Lindsay S, Nicholas CW, Sheline GE, Chaikoff IL (1969) Leydig-cell tumors in rat testes subjected to low dose x-irradiation. Radiat Res 40:366–378.

Lisco H, Finkel MP, Brues AM (1947) Carcinogenic properties of radioactive fission products and of plutonium. Radiology 49:361–363.

Mahler PA, Oberley TD, Yatvin MB (1982) Histologic examination of the influence of dietary protein on rat radiation nephropathy. Radiat Res 89:549–558.

Maisin JR, Decleve A, Gerber GV, Mattelin G, Lambiet-Collier M (1978) Chemical protection against the long-term effects of a single whole-body exposure of mice to ionizing radiation. I. Causes of death. Radiat Res 74:415–435.

Maldague P (1969) Comparative study of experimentally induced cancer of the kidney in mice and rats with x-ray. Vienna: IAEA, pp 439–458.

Marks S, Sullivan MF (1960) Tumors of the small intestine in rats after intestine x-irradiation. Nature 188:953.

Moore GE, Smith GA, Brackney EL (1953) The use of intragastric balloons containing P^{32} in an attempt to produce adenocarcinoma of the stomach in the mouse. J Natl Cancer Inst 13:963–977.

Noble RL (1977) The development of prostatic adenocarcinoma in Nb rats following prolonged sex hormone administration. Cancer Res 37:1929–1933.

Nowell PC, Cole LJ, Ellis ME, (1958) Neoplasms of the glandular stomach in mice irradiated with x-rays or fast neutrons. Cancer Res 18:257–261.

Nowell PC, Cole LG (1959) Late effects of fast neutrons versus x-rays in mice: Nephrosclerosis, tumors, longevity. Radiat Res 11:545–556.

Osborne JW, Nicholson DP, Prasad KN (1963) Induction of intestinal carcinoma in the rat by x-irradiation of the small intestine. Radiat Res 18:76–85.

Rosen VJ, Cole LJ (1962) Accelerated induction of kidney neoplasms in mice after x-irradiation (690 r) and unilateral nephrectomy. J Natl Cancer Inst 28:1031–1041.

Rostom AY, Kauffman SL, Steel GG (1978) Influence of misonidazole on the incidence of radiation-induced intestinal tumors in mice. Br J Cancer 38:530–536.

Sasaki S, Kasuga T, Sato F, Kawashima N (1978) Induction of hepatocellular tumor by x-ray irradiation at perinatal state of mice. Gann 69:451–452.

Sasaki S, Kasuga T, (1981) Life-shortening and carcinogenesis in mice irradiated neonatally with x-rays. Radiat Res 88:313–325.

Sáxen EA (1952) Squamous-cell carcinoma of the forestomach in x-irradiated mice fed 9,10-Dimethyl-1,2-benzanthracene, with a note on failure to induce adenocarcinoma. J Natl Cancer Inst 13:491–453.

Schmahl W, Kriegel H, (1980) Ovary tumors in NMRI mice subjected to fractionated x-irradiation during fetal development. J Cancer Res Clin Oncol 98:65–74.

Sebes JI, Zaldivan R, Vogel HH (1975) Histopathologic changes induced in rats by localized x-irradiation of an exteriorized segment of the small intestine. Sthrahlentherapie 150:403–410.

Stevens RH, Cole DA, Cheng HF (1981) Identification of a common oncofactal protein in x-ray and chemically induced rat gastro intestinal tumors. Br J Cancer 43:817–825.

Takizawa S, Hirose F (1978) Role of testosterone in the development of radiation-induced prostate carcinoma in rats. Gann 69:723–726.

Terada Y (1980) Histology and cell kinetics of rectal mucosal of A/HeJ mice administered syngeneic rectal antigen and its effects on radiation-induced rectal cancer. Hiroshima J Med 28:123–164.

Tsubouchi S, Matsuzawa T (1973) Nodular formations in rat small intestine after local abdominal x-irradiation. Cancer Res 33:3155–3158.

Ullrich RL, Jernigan MC, Cosgrove CE, Satterfield LS, Bowles ND, Storer JB (1976) The influence of dose and dose rate on the incidence of neoplastic disease in RF mice after neutron irradiation. Radiat Res 68:115–131.

Ullrich RL, Jernigan MC, Storer JB (1977) Neutron carcinogenesis. Dose and dose-rate effects in BALB/c mice. Radiat Res 72:487–498.

Upton AC, Odell TT, Sniffen EP (1960a) Influence of age at time of irradiation on induction of leukemia and ovarian tumors in RF mice. Proc Soc Exp Biol Med 104:769–771.

Upton AC, Kimball AW, Furth J, Christenberry KW (1960b) Some delayed effects of atom-bomb radiations in mice. Cancer Res 20:1–59.

Vesselinovitch SD, Simmons EL, Mihailovich N, Rao KVN, Lombard LS (1971) The effect of age, fractionation, and dose on radiation carcinogenesis in various tissues of mice. Cancer Res 31:2133–2142.

Watanabe H, Hirose F, Takizawa S, Terada Y (1977) Induction of atrophic gastritis in ICR mice by the administration of an allogenic antigen. Acta Pathol Japan 27:799–808.

Watanabe H, Fujii I, Terada Y (1980) Induction of intestinal metaplasia in rat gastric mucosa by local x-irradiation. Pathol Res Pract 170:104–114.

Willey AL, Vogel HH, Clifton KH (1973) The effect of variations in LET and cell cycle on radiation hepatocarcinogenesis. Radiat Res 54:284–293.

Witcofski RL, Pizzarello DJ (1976) Influence of dose rate on carcinogenesis resulting from x-ray, [133m]In, and [198]Au irradiation. JNM 17:715–718.

Yuhas JM (1974) Recovery from radiation-carcinogenic injury to the mouse ovary. Radiat Res 60:321–332.

Zaldivar R (1968) Sequence of histopathologic events in the rat bowel after localized x-irradiation and urethan. Strahlentherapie 135:241–249.

Zimmermann A, Michel CH, Stoller CH (1979) Long-term effects of negative pions in female mice exposed to whole-body irradiation. Radiat Envir Biophys 16:295–298.

SECTION IV
CARCINOGENIC EFFECTS
IN HUMANS

LEUKEMIA, LYMPHOMA, AND MULTIPLE MYELOMA

ROBERT W. MILLER, M.D. AND GILBERT W. BEEBE, Ph.D.

Leukemia can be induced by ionizing irradiation of the whole body or part of it, from sources that are external or internal (i.e., radioisotopes). Some studies suggest that susceptibility is greatest during the last weeks of fetal life. A brief history follows.

Individual case reports of leukemia among early radiation workers provided the first suggestion that such exposures could induce this neoplasm in humans. An animal counterpart was then found in mice. Simple epidemiologic studies demonstrated an excess mortality from leukemia among radiologists compared with other physicians. From these retrospective studies, it was evident that an excess of leukemia should be sought in the prospective study of Japanese atomic bomb survivors, and the excess was found in 1952 (reviewed by Miller, 1969). Radiogenic leukemia is clinically indistinguishable from "naturally occurring" leukemia. Radiation is implicated by significantly greater frequencies in exposed groups and by their dependency on the radiation dose.

Information on British men given radiotherapy for ankylosing spondylitis (Court Brown and Doll, 1957, 1965; Smith and Doll, 1982) parallels the findings from the study of the atomic bomb survivors, but almost no information is available from this source on women (who develop the disease much less often than men) or children. In occidental people, about 30% of adult leukemia is chronic lymphocytic leukemia (CLL), but no excess of CLL was found in either the British study or the atomic bomb survivors. A main conclusion from these observations is that leukemia other than CLL is induced by whole-body or by partial-body radiation. Other studies of partial-body exposure to external radiation support this generalization (reviewed by UNSCEAR, 1977; National Academy of Science, BIER, 1980).

Stewart et al reported in 1958 that leukemia and all other forms of child-

From the Clinical Epidemiology Branch, National Cancer Institute, National Institutes of Health, Bethesda, Maryland.

hood cancer are increased after diagnostic exposures in utero, as found on p. 380 (Chapter 24: Cancer in Children). Similar results were obtained by MacMahon in 1962 but, since then, considerable doubt has been expressed about the causal nature of the association (for example, see MacMahon, 1981). A notable observation was the failure to confirm the relationship among Japanese exposed in utero to the atomic bomb, among whom no increase in leukemia or other cancers in childhood was found (Jablon and Kato, 1970; Ishimaru et al, 1981).

Two radioisotopes are known to induce leukemia in humans. Thorotrast (thorium dioxide), once used as a contrast medium in radiology, localizes in bone and liver particularly. Constant bombardment of tissue by alpha particles from thorium produces heavy exposures locally (Mole, 1978). Phosphorus-32 used with or without external radiotherapy for polycythemia vera induces leukemia (Modan and Lilienfeld, 1965), but in much higher frequency than was seen in the atomic bomb survivors (Miller, 1967). This greater frequency may be due to the therapy-induced extension of the life span of these patients, so an intrinsic leukemic phase of their illness now has time to become apparent, or the original disease may predispose to leukemia and, in effect, lower the threshold for inducing it by radiation.

DOSE–RESPONSE AND RISK ESTIMATES

The studies of atomic bomb survivors have yielded the largest number of cases for analysis, and all such cases have been carefully reviewed by hematologists and pathologists according to criteria agreed on by panels of experts from the United States and Japan. The other large series with well-documented details about the type of leukemia concerns British men given radiotherapy for ankylosing spondylitis (Court Brown and Doll, 1957). These two series provide the basis for dose–response and risk estimates.

By the mid-1950s, the data on leukemia among the A-bomb survivors and the British patients treated for ankylosing spondylitis, coupled with the results of drosophila experiments on the genetic effects of ionizing radiation, caused authorities increasingly to argue that protection policy, at least, should be based on the linear, nonthreshold hypothesis, which became a cardinal tenet of radiation protection policy (Lewis, 1957; Court Brown and Doll, 1957; NCRP, 1971). It remains so today, although extensive experimental work suggests that the most appropriate dose–response function for the carcinogenic effects of sparsely ionizing (low LET) radiation is a quadratic function of the type indicated below* (National Council on Radiation Protection and Measurements, 1980; NAS, 1980). The reason is largely that the human experience has failed to provide proof that this function, or any other, is superior to the linear, and the linear is generally more conservative (predicts more leukemia at low-dose levels) than the quadratic. At the very high doses, however, experimental studies have consistently shown that the rising curve of cancer incidence with increasing dose tends to flatten out and bend over, perhaps as a reflection of cell-

---

* $y = a_0 + a_1D^2$, where y = total risk, a_0 is the risk without the influence of radiation, a_1 and a_2 are fitted constants, and D = dose.

killing. In consequence, a more complete expression may have an exponential term that brings down the curve in the high-dose region (Upton, 1977):

$$y = (a_0 + a_1 D + a_2 D^2) \exp(-b_1 D - b_2 D^2),$$

where b_1 and b_2 are additional fitted constants. Cell killing by high doses may well be the explanation for the low incidence of radiogenic leukemia following radiation therapy for cervical cancer (Hutchison, 1968; Boice et al, 1984) and for the low risk coefficient obtained for the ankylosing spondylitis patients (Darby et al, 1985), whose spinal marrow dose was on the order of 500–800 rad.

In 1957, Court Brown and Doll first reported on 13,352 patients with ankylosing spondylitis treated by x-ray, and presented linear dose–response data for the 52 patients who developed leukemia in this series. In 1982, Smith and Doll limited their analysis of this series to patients who received only a single course of radiotherapy, and linearity no longer seems so obvious. In fact, the dose–response plot is without coherent form, a fact that Mole and Major (1983) attribute to protraction of dose. Meanwhile, data on leukemia among the atomic bomb survivors (1950–1978) have been intensively studied by Jablon and Kato (1970), Rossi and Kellerer (1974), Kerr and Jones (1976), Ichimaru et al (1978, 1979, 1981), Rossi and Mays (1978). The dose–response relationships in the two cities may be dissimilar, but a definitive statement must await the results of new analyses based on dose estimates that are currently being revised. The data for the large Hiroshima series have seemed reasonably linear, but those for the smaller Nagasaki series have suggested nonlinearity, with respect to the dose assigned in 1965 (T-65).

In Nagasaki, exposure was almost entirely to gamma (low-LET) radiation, whereas, in Hiroshima it was thought until recently that 20%–25% of the radiation was from densely ionizing (high-LET) neutrons. On the basis of T-65 dosimetry, and on the assumption that the dose–response function for neutrons is linear, U.S. experts on the Committee on the Biological Effects of Ionizing Radiation (BEIR III) (National Academy of Sciences, 1980) could not discriminate among linear (L), linear quadratic (LQ), and "pure" quadratic (Q) dose–response forms for low LET radiation in goodness-of-fit tests. At 5 rad to the active bone marrow the BEIR risk-estimates are, respectively, 11, 5.2, and 0.35 excess deaths from leukemia per million persons per year for these three dose–response models. (LQ is a quadratic form with a nonzero linear coefficient, and Q is a quadratic form with the linear coefficient equal to zero.) The Nagasaki data alone are too sparse to support strong inferences as to the shape of the dose–response curve for low-LET radiation.

Both relative and absolute risk estimates are used in radiation biology. Relative risk estimates are especially favored when the excess risk seems tied to the underlying natural incidence, as may be the case for a particular tumor in a cohort that has passed through the latent period and is moving through the older ages. But relative risk estimates derived from one tumor will generally not be applicable for another, or even for the same tumor in another ethnic group in which the natural incidence is different. For this reason chronic lymphocytic leukemia (CLL) should be removed in applying relative risk estimates from Japanese atomic bomb survivors to persons in the United States. As previously noted, CLL is rare in Japan, but not in the United States, a marked ethnic difference. CLL should be removed in any case for another reason: It has not been induced by radiation in susceptible (occidental) people.

For forms of leukemia other than CLL, from 1950 to 1974 atomic bomb survivors exposed to 400+ rad (kerma) experienced a relative risk of 23 (Beebe et al, 1978). This means that the frequency was 23 times the normal incidence for this high-dose group. During the peak period of expression, 1950–1954, the relative risk was 54. The average *absolute* risk estimates were 1.92 and 4.06 excess leukemia deaths per million persons per year per rad for 1950–1974 and 1950–1954, respectively. Risk estimates are very sensitive to the time-period chosen for the computation, because the excess is not constant over time. Recent calculations by Fujita et al (1983) suggest that absolute risk coefficients for leukemia based on the revised dosimetry will be higher, but not by as much as a factor of two.

The British study of patients with ankylosing spondylitis gives absolute risks of 0.9 and 0.6 excess cases per million persons per year per rad for the leukemogenic effect of a single course of treatment, depending on whether the mean marrow dose was taken to be 214 (National Academy of Sciences, 1980) or 321 rads (Smith and Doll, 1982). The United Nations Scientific Committee on the Effects of Atomic Radiation (UNSCEAR) and the International Commission on Radiation Protection (ICRP) give estimates in terms of the average risk over a lifetime. Thus, the 1977 UNSCEAR report gives an estimate of 15 to 25 excess cases of leukemia per million per rad for low LET radiation at relatively low dose-rates.

Low-dose risk estimates are especially controversial because:

1. At low doses risks are so small that they can be estimated only by interpolation between 0 and the relatively high dose levels at which reliable risk estimates can be made, but there is no agreement as to the best mathematical form to employ for the interpolation.
2. The presumed risk of leukemia (and other cancers) at this level will have great influence on radiation protection policy.
3. Small studies have been reported in which the apparent risk of leukemia is much higher than estimates made by BEIR (National Academy of Sciences, 1980) and UNSCEAR (1977).

In a follow-up study of 3224 former military personnel exposed at the Nevada weapons test site, Caldwell et al (1983) found 10 cases of leukemia compared with 4 expected according to U.S. national rates ($p < 0.01$). The average badge reading for the entire cohort was about 0.5 rem (and the marrow dose perhaps 0.3 rem). At these doses, far less than one radiogenic case would be expected according to the UNSCEAR and BEIR estimates. This experience suggests that background radiation alone should produce even more leukemia than we now experience (from all causes), that the dose estimates are wide of the mark, or that the dose–rate effect on the risk of leukemia is far greater than animal experiments suggest (NAS, 1980). Another peculiarity in the study of the military personnel is that the excess does not have the wave-like temporal distribution characteristic of radiogenic leukemia: only one case occurred within 11 yr after exposure. In a preliminary report on their study of about

50,000 veterans exposed at the Nevada Test Site or in the Pacific tests, Robinette and Jablon (1983) independently confirmed the finding of Caldwell et al for the Smoky shot, but for no other test; nor did they observe excess leukemia for all tests combined.

In a study of leukemia among children resident in Utah, Lyon et al (1979) reported a relative risk of 2.4 for those in counties of "high fallout" from atmospheric weapons tests at the Nevada Test Site compared with those in "low fallout" counties. Environmental monitoring data assembled by Schleien (1981) averaged less than 2 R for this area, and the presumptive bone marrow dose, thus, was well below 1 rem, which is unlikely to induce a measurable increase in the frequency of childhood leukemia. Based on soil sampling throughout Utah, Beck and Krey (1983) found that the average bone marrow dose from external radiation in the high fallout counties was actually lower than in the low fallout counties, 280 versus 420 mrad. These doses are equivalent to about 4 and 6 yr of exposure to natural background radiation in the respective areas. They considered dose to bone marrow from ingested or inhaled radionuclides to be neglibible. If, as the results of Lyon et al had suggested originally, 0.5 rad sufficed to double the natural incidence of leukemia, most of the childhood leukemia could be attributed to background radiation unless, again, continuous radiation exposure is much less leukemogenic than the fractionated exposure of the Utah residents (NCRP, 1980).

Land et al (1984) sought to confirm the findings of Lyon et al by using childhood cancer mortality data from the National Center for Health Statistics. The distribution of deaths from leukemia in time and space (counties) did not support the findings reported by Lyon et al and led to the conclusion that the purported association reflected an anomalously low leukemia rate in southern Utah during 1944–1949, which was used as the baseline rate in the Lyon study.

In another study of the effects of fallout from the nuclear weapons tests in Nevada, Johnson (1984) reported an excess incidence of leukemia, as well as other forms of cancer, among Mormons of all ages resident in southwestern Utah. In 1958–1966 and 1972–1980, only seven cases of leukemia were expected compared with 31 observed among 4125 persons in the area. Because an excess of this magnitude would require an exposure of 100 rad or more according to currently accepted risk estimates, either the Johnson data are subject to a substantial response bias or the generally accepted risk coefficients greatly underestimate the risk of leukemia.

The experience of nuclear workers at the Hanford plant in Richland, Washington, has been analyzed in different ways by several groups (Mancuso et al, 1977; Gilbert and Marks, 1979; and Hutchison et al, 1979), but in no instance has excess leukemia been demonstrated. In still another study, based on a telephone survey of next of kin, Najarian and Colton (1978) reported an excess of leukemia deaths among former employees of the Portsmouth Naval Shipyard where atomic submarines are overhauled and radiation workers have received an average dose of about 1.5 rem to bone marrow. Later investigators based on film-badge measurements of exposure revealed no excess mortality from leukemia and showed that the telephone survey was seriously biased (Rinsky et al, 1981). The next of kin of workers who died of cancer were more likely to be interviewed than others, and the decedent was more likely to be identified as a former nuclear worker if he had died of cancer than from some other cause.

QUALITY OF RADIATION

Experimental studies have shown that the pattern of dissipation of radiation in tissues greatly influences the amount of damage per unit of absorbed dose. Thus, particulate forms of radiation, such as electrons and alpha particles, which have high rates of energy deposition (high LET), are generally more damaging than low-LET radiation (x- and gamma rays), which is sparsely ionizing. The effects of 250 kVp x-rays are the usual standard for making estimates of the relative biologic effectiveness (RBE) of each form of radiation. Only fragmentary information is available with regard to the significance of LET in human leukemogenesis. Until 1981, the exposures in Hiroshima and Nagasaki were thought to differ markedly with respect to the neutron component. On this premise, the difference between the cities in the frequency of leukemia was attributed to the dissimilar quality of the radiation. For leukemia of all types combined, Rossi and Mays (1978) derived a variable RBE estimate for neutrons in relation to gamma rays, ranging from about 60 at 1 rad of neutrons to 8 at 23 rads; the BEIR III (NAS, 1980) estimated average over the entire range of doses was about 11. The current reevaluation (Loewe and Mendelsohn, 1981; Kerr, 1981) of the neutron component of the Hiroshima bomb indicates that the neutron dose in Hiroshima was much lower than previously estimated and, thus, the difference between the cities in leukemia incidence is not at present a useful measure of the RBE of neutrons in inducing this form of cancer. The A-bomb dosimetry had seemed a possible source of information on the RBE of neutrons with respect to leukemia, but the revision now underway makes this doubtful. Nevertheless, attempts have been made to anticipate the RBE values that might result from that revision (Dobson and Straume, 1982; Hendry and Chen, 1983).

Quality of radiation has also been associated with type of leukemia (Ishimaru et al, 1971; Mole, 1975) through the fact that the CGL/AL ratio and the neutron/gamma ratio under T-65 dosimetry are both so much higher in Hiroshima than in Nagasaki. With the revision of the dosimetry the concept that CGL is primarily neutron-induced will have to be reassessed.

It is probably the alpha radiation from Thorotrast that produces the excess leukemia that UNSCEAR estimated to be 50–55 per million per rad per lifetime, in contrast to 15-25 for low-LET radiation (United Nations, 1977). A rather lower estimate is provided by Mays et al in their recent review (Mays et al, in press). The dosimetry, however, is too uncertain for close comparison with risk estimates for low-LET radiation.

DOSE RATE

Experimental studies indicate that for low-LET radiation at a given dose the carcinogenic effect will be less at low than at high dose rates (NCRP, 1980). From its survey of the literature, NCRP (1980) has recommended a dose-rate reduction factor of 2–10 as a divisor of low-dose risk estimates based on observations at high doses and at high dose rates. The 1977 UNSCEAR report used a dose-rate reduction factor of about 2 or 3. The reason for reducing the estimated effects at low dose rates is that the opportunity for healing is greater than when the dose is administered quickly. Most observations on human radiogenic leukemia come from high dose-rate exposures.

An earlier generation of U.S. radiologists, whose exposures may be regarded as having generally been at low dose rate, developed an excess of leukemia, 1930–1954, in the range of 0.4–1.0 extra death per million person-years per rad (National Academy of Sciences, 1972). This result suggests that any dose-rate reduction factor for leukemia in humans would be small, closer to 2 than to 10. Some of the excess leukemia cases among radiologists, however, may have resulted from acute exposures that on occasion were exceptionally large.

SENSITIVITY OF TISSUE

The organs of the body apparently vary in their sensitivity to the carcinogenic effects of ionizing radiation in a fashion that does not reflect the differentials in their natural incidence. Estimates of organ sensitivity are just beginning to be made and differences are under study. If the radiogenic excess is considered in relation to the natural incidence of the tumor, then bone marrow appears to be the most sensitive tissue in the body. But if the comparison is in terms of absolute risk-estimates, the risk-coefficients for both breast and thyroid tissue exceed that for bone marrow by about $2:1$. If comparison is based on the different cell types of leukemia in terms of the number of cells of a given type in the body, a different picture will emerge. Myelocytes are highly susceptible, but lymphocytes are not, despite their ample number in the body. In addition, one must be aware of the influence of frequent cell division, and of variations in immunity or hormonal status, among other variables.

TIME PATTERNS

Radiogenic leukemia has a wave-like temporal pattern: it begins to appear 2–4 yr after exposure to external radiation (about 8 yr after Thorotrast injection), rises to a peak 5–7 yr after radiation, and subsides thereafter. The excess of leukemia occurred for about 20 yr in the ankylosing spondylitis series and in the Thorotrast series, but among the survivors of the Hiroshima bomb a slight excess was still seen 30–33 yr after exposure (Kato and Schull, 1982). Acute granulocytic leukemia continued to appear there long after the chronic form of the disease ceased to be excessive. Excess solid tumors, in contrast to leukemia, generally do not begin to appear until 10 or more years after irradiation and their frequency does not follow a wave-like pattern except for bone cancer following exposure to radium-224. The temporal distribution of radiogenic solid tumors seems to follow natural incidence once the latent period has passed (Boice et al, in press).

HOST FACTORS

The frequency of radiogenic leukemia differs markedly by age at exposure. Among A-bomb survivors under 10 yr of age in 1945, the excess was large in terms of absolute and relative risk estimates. Among those who were 50 yr of age or older in 1945, the absolute risk estimate was as high as that for survivors under age 10 at that time, but the relative risk was lower (Figure 1). Few of the ankylosing spondylitis patients were under age 20 at the time of treatment, but otherwise a similar increasing risk with age at exposure was noted (Smith and Doll, 1982).

Age at exposure also influences the temporal pattern of radiogenic leukemia and the patterns are different for acute leukemia versus chronic granulocytic leukemia (Ichimaru et al, 1978). For the youngest members of the population the excess peaks early for both acute and chronic forms of leukemia, and ceases early, at about 15 yr after exposure. For the older cohorts, the peaks for acute leukemia occur later with increasing age at exposure and subsidence of excess risk is slower. Older cohorts have early peaks for CGL but again subsidence of excess risk is slower.

Of special biologic interest is the question whether, as the findings of Stewart et al suggest, the human fetus is especially susceptible in the 6 wk before birth to the leukemogenic (and carcinogenic) influence of ionizing radiation (Stewart and Kneale, 1971). Although the statistical reliability of the reported excess risk is beyond question, the etiologic significance of the radiation exposure remains controversial (MacMahon, 1981; Monson and MacMahon, 1984). If, in fact, radiation is responsible for the elevated risk, then fetal bone marrow is more sensitive by an order of magnitude than that of young children. Among the reasons why radiation may not be responsible are the following

1. The failure to find evidence of such a large effect among the in utero sample of A-bomb survivors (Jablon and Kato, 1970)

FIGURE 1. Measures of leukemogenic effect by age ATB, 1950–1974, average for both cities. Beebe, 1978.

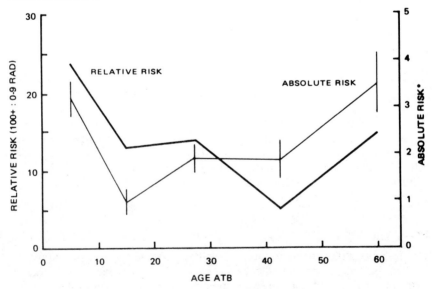

*Excess deaths per million PYR (with 90% confidence intervals)

2. The constancy of the relative risk estimates among all childhood tumor types despite their dissimilar epidemiologic characteristics (Miller, 1969)
3. The failure to reproduce the effect in experimental animals (Sasaki and Kasuga, in press; Brent, 1979)
4. The likelihood of pelvimetry, about 1:10 in MacMahon's series (1962), is so much greater than that of fatal childhood cancer, less than 1:1000, that even a small bias in the selection of women for pelvimetry could have a profound effect on the expectation of childhood cancer (Beebe, 1982)

Favoring the radiogenic hypothesis, on the other hand, is Mole's analysis (1974) of Stewart's data on twins versus singletons for whom radiography was performed. He found that childhood leukemia and solid tumors had similar risks for singletons and twins, indicating that selection of a small percent for x-ray examination could not account for the association with childhood cancers of various sorts.

The risk of radiogenic leukemia among A-bomb survivors is roughly 50% higher in males than in females when risk is measured on an absolute basis, but nearly equal in terms of relative risk (NAS, 1980). Susceptibility according to age and sex parallels that for leukemia in the general population that has not been irradiated. Of special note, acute lymphocytic leukemia was rarely induced by exposure to the atomic bomb after 20 years of age (Ichimaru et al, 1978), and was not induced among British patients given radiotherapy for ankylosing spondylitis, very few of whom were under age 20 when treated.

LYMPHOMA

An early report of excess lymphoma among A-bomb survivors (Anderson and Ishida, 1964) has not been confirmed by later experience. Study of the death certificates of the survivors for 1950–1978 has indicated no real excess of lymphoma, even among the most heavily exposed (Kato and Schull, 1982). CLL, which is clearly not excessive in A-bomb survivors or in British patients given radiotherapy for ankylosing spondylitis, is etiologically and clinically a lymphoma, and different from other forms of leukemia.

Groups at high risk of lymphoma are immunologically deficient, either for genetic reasons (ataxia telangiectasia [AT], X-linked lymphoproliferative syndrome, or Wiskott–Aldrich syndrome, or combined immunodeficiency disorders), or because of therapy, as in immunosuppression for renal transplantation. These groups generally have a normal risk of leukemia, a notable exception being AT in which ALL occurs excessively but with a much lower risk than lymphoma (reviewed by Miller, 1977).

Groups that are genetically at high risk of leukemia (e.g., those with Down's syndrome or Fanconi's anemia) are not usually at high risk of lymphoma. The pathogenesis of lymphoma is apparently different from that of nonlymphocytic leukemia, as indicated by the dissimilar epidemiologic characteristics of the two groups of neoplasms.

Ionizing radiation is strongly clastogenic (breaks chromosomes), but its effects on immunologic defenses are not the sort that predispose to lymphoma. The unequal susceptibility of various tissues to the carcinogenic effects of ionizing radiation illustrates the need to consider influences other than radiation in epidemiologic studies of persons exposed to this physical agent.

MULTIPLE MYELOMA

To evaluate multiple myeloma as a long-delayed effect of exposure to ionizing radiation, Cuzick (1981) reviewed data from all cohorts of radiation-exposed persons whose mortality from cancer is under study by others. He found an excess of myeloma in most of the cohorts and, when the data were pooled, with the exclusion of two cohorts of women who received large doses for uterine cancer (3 observed, 10.71 expected), 50 cases of myeloma were observed compared with 22.21 expected ($p = 2 \times 10^{-7}$). Table 1 shows that these data compared with leukemia occurrence in the same cohort. One would expect that the precursor cells for leukemia and myeloma would lie side by side within the bone marrow and, thus, be equally exposed to radiation. Leukemia, because it has a short latent period, should arise in a cohort first.

Among British patients treated with radiation for ankylosing spondylitis, after an excess of leukemia occurred, an excess of only 1.13 cases of multiple myeloma developed (Smith and Doll, 1982, and personal communication to Cuzick) (Table 1). Among U.S. radiologists, the early excess of leukemia was followed by 11 cases of multiple myeloma versus 7.91 expected, a difference that may well have arisen by chance. Myeloma developed in four Windscale workers (Dolphin, 1976). For three the exposures were known: 3.3, 4, and 59 rems. Among Hanford workers no excess of leukemia has occurred but three workers have developed myeloma after exposures of 20–35 rem, far below doses received by many A-bomb survivors and by the British spondylitics. Radium-dial painters had only a questionable excess of leukemia (Table 1) but, since 1959, six of them are said to have developed multiple myeloma. (According to Stebbings [1983], the published value of 0.86 expected cases of multiple myeloma was an error and the correct value is 2.3.) These three studies fail to show leukemia as a carcinogenic forerunner of excess myeloma and, strangely, the excess myelomas were more numerous than in much more heavily exposed populations. The data from patients given Thorotrast show the expected sequence.

An excess of multiple myeloma was observed in women given radiotherapy for benign gynecologic disorders (mean marrow dose, 40–126 rads) (Wagoner, unpublished), and in another group treated for metropathic hemorrhagica (mean marrow dose, 70–190 rads) (Smith and Doll, 1976). In each of these series there was a small excess of leukemia.

According to Cuzick (1981), the best evidence that radiation induces myeloma is from studies of the atomic-bomb survivors ($p \sim .03$). In the most heavily exposed group, which received 100 rad (Kerma) or more, he cites five cases of multiple myeloma observed versus 1.6 expected. In the next highest exposure category, 50–99 rad, only two cases were observed (Ichimaru et al, 1979). There has been a flurry of recent reports on multiple myeloma from the Radiation Effects Research Foundation (Ichimaru et al, 1979; Ishimaru and Finch, 1979; Ichimaru et al, 1982; Kato and Schull, 1982; Wakabayashi et al,

TABLE 1. Luekemia and Multiple Myeloma Occurrence Compared, in the Radiation-Exposed Cohorts Reviewed by Cuzick (1981)

Cohort	Leukemia		Multiple myeloma[a]		References
	Observed	Expected	Observed	Expected	
Atomic bomb survivors exposure ≥ 100 rads (Kerma)	58	8.24	5	1.59	Ichimaru et al, 1979
Spondylitis:					
British	52[b]	5.48	3	1.87	Court Borwn and Doll, 1965
German	2	0.84	0	0.25	Spiess et al, 1978
Fluorosocpy of chest	2	1.20	0	0.39	Boice, 1979
U.S. radiologists	12	4.02	11	7.91	Lewis, 1963
British radiologists	4	0.65	0	1.04	Smith and Doll, 1981
Windscale workers			4	1.00	Dolphin, 1976
Hanford workers	1	0.70	3	1.10	Gilbert and Marks, 1979
Radium-dial painters	3[c]	1.41	6	0.86	Polednak et al, 1978
Thorotrast					
Denmark	11	<4.70	4	0.77	Faber, 1978
Germany	17	1.0[d]	2	0.93	van Kaick et al, 1978
Portugal	12	0.00[d]	1	0.16	da Silva Horta et al, 1978
Metropathia hemorrhagica	7	2.69	5	2.09	Smith and Doll, 1976
Benign gynecologic, Connecticut	12	9.50	5	1.98	Wagoner, unpublished (cited by Smith and Doll, 1976)
Uranium millers and miners	8	8.00	1	0.27	Wagoner et al, 1964
Total	201	<48.40	50	22.21	

[a] Myeloma data from Cuzick (1981); his myeloma references not always identical with leukemia references used here.
[b] In addition, 15 men died of aplastic anemia (aleukemic leukemia?) versus 0.52 expected.
[c] Additional cases may have been misdiagnosed as aplastic anemia before close surveillance began.
[d] Number observed in the comparison group.

1983), and others are in preparation. In some reports a relationship with dose seems fairly well established, but not so in others; none is entirely negative. The total series of some 30-odd cases is handled differently by different authors, and the most complete analysis, buttressed by a diagnostic evaluation of case material, appears in the two reports of Ichimaru et al (1979, 1982). Although the total series of confirmed cases is small, 29 including controls, with only five observed versus 1.8 expected cases having marrow doses of 50 rad or more, a statistical test of trend with dose returns a reported p-value of less than 0.01.

If the exposure to radiation actually caused the small excess, then several differences between leukemia and multiple myeloma are of interest: 1) the minimal latent period for multiple myeloma is very much longer, perhaps 15 yr in comparison with 2–4 yr for leukemia; 2) excess multiple myeloma has a very different age distribution, being concentrated in the age cohort 20–59 in 1945; and 3) estimated risk coefficients for multiple myeloma are much smaller, perhaps one-fourth or less.

Until recently, as Cuzick noted, the diagnosis of myeloma was much more likely to be made in a cohort under close surveillance than among members of the population in general. Hence, one may be seeing a recent increase in the frequency of myeloma due to improved diagnosis, or perhaps for reasons other than radiation exposure as observed, for example, in the United States (McKay et al, 1982). One might postulate that chronic exposure to internal emitters produces myeloma but not leukemia, as in radium-dial painters, but this possibility seems unlikely. In any event, it appears that impressive statistical differences have been achieved only by merging heterogeneous data.

OVERVIEW

What have we learned about these three types of cancer from the epidemiology of radiation effects? We now know that the granulocytic leukemias are induced by whole- or partial-body radiation at any age. Acute lymphocytic leukemia may be induced by such exposures under 20 yr of age. Susceptibility to radiation-induced leukemia is greatest early in life, late in life, and possibly after exposures in the last 6 wk of gestation. Radiation does not induce chronic lymphocytic leukemia or lymphoma. Data from studies of the Japanese A-bomb survivors indicate that multiple myeloma may occur after a long latent period. If so, the number of excess cases is small. In other radiation-exposed groups, the occurrence of multiple myeloma exhibits an inconsistent pattern that suggests problems with the elusive diagnosis of this disease (i.e., fuller ascertainment among the closely followed exposed cases than in the comparison groups). Radiation exposures, thus, have a much greater or earlier oncogenic effect on certain blood cells than on others. The carcinogenic process, therefore, must be different for the various cells within the hematopoietic system.

REFERENCES

Anderson RE, Ishida K (1964) Malignant lymphoma in survivors of the atomic bomb in Hiroshima. Ann Int Med 61:853–862.

Beck HL, Krey PW (1983) Radiation exposures in Utah from Nevada nuclear tests. Science 220:18–24.

Beebe GW (1982) Ionizing radiation and health. Am Sci 70:35–44.

Beebe GW, Kato H, Land CE (1978) Studies of the mortality of A-bomb survivors: Mortality and radiation dose. 1950–74. Radiat Res 75:138–201.

Boice JD (1979) Multiple chest fluoroscopies and the risk of breast cancer. In: Advances in medical oncology, research and education, Vol. 1. Oxford: Pergamon Press, pp 147–56.

Boice JD, Jr., Beebe GW, Land CE (in press) Absolute and relative time-response models in radiation risk estimation. In: Proceedings of the 20th Meeting, National Council on Radiation. Washington, DC: Protection and Measurements.

Boice JD Jr., Day NE, Andersen A, et al (1984) Cancer risk following radiotherapy of cervical cancer. In: Boice JD, Jr. and Fraumeni JF Jr. (eds.), Radiation carcinogenesis: Epidemiology and biological significance. New York: Raven Press.

Brent RL (1979) Effects of ionizing radiation on growth and development. Cont Epidem Biostat 1:147–183.

Caldwell GG, Kelley DB, Zack M, Falk H, Heath CW (1983) Mortality and cancer frequency among military nuclear test (Smoky) participants, 1957 through 1979. J Am Med, Assoc 250:620–624.

Court Brown WM, Doll R (1957) Leukemia and aplastic anemia in patients irradiated for ankylosing spondylitis. Med Res Council Spec Rep Series no. 295, HMSO, London.

Court Brown WM, Doll R (1965) Mortality from cancer and other causes after radiotherapy for ankylosing spondylitis. Br Med J 2:1327–1332.

Cuzick J (1981) Radiation-induced myelomatosis. N Engl J Med 304:204–210.

Darby SC, Nakashima E, Kato H (1985) A parallel analysis of cancer mortality among atomic bomb survivors and patients with ankylosing spondylitis given x-ray therapy. J Natl Cancer Inst 75:1–21.

da Silva Horta J, da Silva Horta ME, da Motta LC, Tavares MH (1978) Malignancies in portuguese thorotrast patients. Health Phys 35:137–151.

Dobson RL, Straume T (1982) Cancer risks and RBE's from Hiroshima and Nagasaki. In: Broerse JJ and Gerber GB (eds.), Neutron carcinogenesis. Luxembourg: Commission of the European Communities.

Dolphin GW (1976) A comparison of the observed and the expected cancers of the haematopoietic and lymphatic systems among workers at Windscale. London: Her Majesty's Stationery Office.

Faber M (1978) Malignancies in Danish thorotrast patients. Health Phys 35:153–158.

Finch SC, Hoshino T, Itoga T, Ichimaru M, Ingram RH, Jr. (1969) Chronic lymphocytic leukemia in Hiroshima and Nagasaki, Japan. Blood 33:79–86.

Fujita S, Awa AA, Pierce DA, Kato H, Shimizu Y (1983) Re-evaluation of biological effects of atomic-bomb radiation by changes in estimated dose 1983. In: Biological effects of low-level radiation, Proceedings of a Symposium, Venice, 11–15 April 1983. Jointly Organized by IAEA and WHO. Vienna: International Atomic Energy Agency.

Gilbert ES, Marks S (1979) An analysis of the mortality of workers in a nuclear facility. Radiat Res 79:122–148.

Henry JH, Chen FD (1983) Estimates of risk of induced leukemia after neutron or photon radiotherapy 1983. In: Biological effects of low-level radiation, Proceedings of a Symposium, Venice, 11–15 April 1983. Jointly Organized by IAEA and WHO. Vienna: International Atomic Energy Agency.

Hutchison GB (1968) Leukemia in patients with cancer of the cervix uteri treated with radiation. A report covering the first 5 years of an international study. J Natl Cancer Inst 40:951–982.

Hutchinson GW, MacMahon B, Jablon S, Land CE (1979) Review of report by Mancuso, Stewart, and Kneale of radiation exposure of Hanford workers. Health Phys 37:207–220.

Ichimaru M, Ishimaru T, Belsky JL (1978) Incidence of leukemia in atomic bomb survivors belonging to a fixed cohort in Hiroshima and Nagasaki, 1950–1971: Radiation dose, years after exposure, age at exposure, and type of leukemia. J Radiat Res (Japan) 19:262–282.

Ichimaru M, Ishimaru T, Mikami M, Matsunaga M (1979) Multiple myeloma among atomic bomb survivors, Hiroshima and Nagasaki, 1950–1976. Technical Report 9-79. Hiroshima: Radiation Effects Research Foundation.

Ichimaru M, Ishimaru T, Mikami M, Yamada Y, Ohkita T (1981) Incidence of leukemia in a fixed cohort of atomic bomb survivors and controls, Hiroshima and Nagasaki, October 1950–December 1978. Technical Report 13-81. Hiroshima: Radiation Effects Research Foundation.

Ichimaru M, Ishimaru T, Mikami M, Matsunaga M (1982) Multiple myeloma among atomic bomb survivors in Hiroshima and Nagasaki, 1950–76: Relationship to radiation dose absorbed by marrow. J Natl Cancer Inst 69:323–328.

Ishimaru T, Hoshino T, Ichimaru M, Okada H, Tomiyasu T, Tsuchimoto T, Yamamoto T (1971) Leukemia in atomic bomb survivors, Hiroshima and Nagasaki, 1 October 1950–30 September 1966. Radiat Res 45:216–233.

Ishimaru T, Finch SC (1979) More on radiation exposure and multiple myeloma. N Engl J Med 301:439–440.

Ishimaru T, Otake M, Ichimaru M (1979) Dose–response relationship of neutrons and gamma rays to leukemia incidence among atomic bomb survivors in Hiroshima and Nagasaki by type of leukemia, 1950–1971. Radiat Res 77:377–394.

Ishimaru T, Ichimaru M, Mikami M (1981) Leukemia incidence among individuals exposed in utero, children of atomic bomb survivors, and their controls: Hiroshima and Nagasaki, 1945–79. Technical Report 11–81. Hiroshima, Japan: Radiation Effects Research Foundation.

Jablon S, Kato H (1970) Childhood cancer in relation to prenatal exposure to atomic-bomb radiation. Lancet ii:1000–1003.

Johnson CJ (1984) Cancer incidence in an area of radioactive fallout downward from the Nevada Test Site. J Am Med Assoc 251:230–236.

Kato H, Schull WJ (1982) Studies of the mortality of A-bomb survivors. 7. Mortality, 1950-1978: Part 1. Cancer mortality. Radiat Res 90:395–432.

Kerr GD (1981) Findings of a recent ORNL review of dosimetry for the Japanese atomic-bomb survivor. Oak Ridge National Laboratory, Oak Ridge, TN ORNL/TM-8078.

Kerr GD, Jones TD (1976) A reanalysis of leukemia data on atomic-bomb survivors based on estimates of absorbed dose to bone marrow. Health Phys 31:568.

Land CE, McKay FW, Machado SG (1984) Childhood leukemia and fallout from the Nevada nuclear tests. Science 223:139–144.

Lewis EB (1957) Leukemia and ionizing radiation. Science 125:965–972.

Lewis EB (1963) Leukemia, multiple myeloma, and aplastic anemia in American radiologists. Science 142:1492–1494.

Loewe WE, Mendelsohn E (1981) Revised dose estimates at Hiroshima and Nagasaki. Health Phys 41:663–666.

Lyon JL, Klauber MR, Gardner JW, Udall KS (1979) Childhood leukemias associated with fallout from nuclear testing. N Engl J Med 300:397–402.

MacMahon B (1962) Prenatal x-ray exposure and childhood cancer. J Natl Cancer Inst 28:1173–1191.

MacMahon B (1981) Childhood cancer and prenatal irradiation. In: Burchenal JH and Oettgen HF (eds.), Cancer Achievements, challenges, and prospects for the 1980s, Vol 1. New York: Grune & Stratton, pp 223–228.

Mancuso TF, Stewart A, Kneale G (1977) Radiation exposure of Hanford workers dying from cancer and other causes. Health Phys 33:369–385.

Mays CW, Rowland RE, Stehney AF (1985) Cancer risk from the lifetime intake of Ra and U isotopes. Health Phys 48:635–647.

McKay FW, Hanson MR, Miller RW (1982) U.S. Cancer Mortality 1950–1977. Natl Cancer Inst 59 monogr: 475.

Miller RW (1967) Persons with exceptionally high risk of leukemia. Cancer Res 27:2420–2423.

Miller RW (1969) Delayed radiation effects in atomic-bomb survivors. Science 166:569–574.

Miller RW (1977) Cancer and congenital malformations: Another view. In: Mulvihill JJ, Miller RW, Fraumeni JF Jr. (eds.), Genetics of Human Cancer. New York: Raven Press, pp 77–79.

Modan B, Lilienfeld AM (1965) Polycythemia vera and leukemia—The role of radiation treatment. A study of 1222 patients. Medicine 44:305–344.

Mole RH (1974) Antenatal irradiation and childhood cancer: Causation or coincidence? Br J Cancer 30:199–208.

Mole RH (1975) Ionizing radiation as a carcinogen: Practical questions and academic pursuits. Br J Radiol 48:157–169.

Mole RH (1978) The radiobiological significance of the studies with 224-Ra and thorotrast. Health Phys 35:167–174.

Mole RH, Major IR (1983) Myeloid leukemia frequency after protracted exposure to ionizing radiation: Experimental confirmation of the flat dose–response found in ankylosing spondylitis after a single treatment course with x-rays. Leuk Res 7:295–300.

Monson RR, MacMahon B (1984) Pre-natal x-ray exposure and cancer in children. In: Boice JD Jr. and Fraumeni JF Jr. (eds.), Radiation carcinogenesis: Epidemiology and biological significance. New York: Raven Press.

Najarian T, Colton T (1978) Mortality from leukaemia and cancer in shipyard nuclear workers. Lancet i:1018–1020.

National Academy of Sciences Advisory Committee on the Biological Effects of Ionizing Radiation (1972) The effects on populations of exposure to low levels of ionizing radiation. Washington, DC: National Academy of Sciences–National Research Council.

National Academy of Sciences Advisory Committee on the Biological Effects of Ionizing Radiation (1980) The effects on populations of exposure to low levels of ionizing radiation: 1980. Washington, DC: National Academy of Sciences–National Research Council.

National Council on Radiation Protection and Measurements (1971) Basic radiation production criteria, Report no. 39. Washington, DC.

National Council on Radiation Protection and Measurements (1980) Influence of dose and its distribution in time on dose–response relationship for low-LET radiation, Report no. 64. Washington, DC.

Polednak AP, Stehney AF, Rowland RE (1978) Mortality among women first employed before 1930 in the U.S. radium dial painting industry. A group ascertained from employment lists. Am J Epidemiol 107:179–195.

Rinsky RA, Zumwalde RD, Waxweiler RJ, Murray WE Jr, Bierman PJ, Landirgan PJ, Terpilak M, Cox C (1981) Cancer mortality at a naval nuclear shipyard. Lancet i:231–235.

Robinette CD, Jablon S (1983) Studies of participants at tests of nuclear weapons—1. The plumbbob series. In: Broerse JJ, et al (eds.), Radiation research, Proceedings of the Seventh International Congress of Radiation Research, Sessions C, C8-13.

Rossi HH, Kellerer AM (1974) The validity of risk estimates of leukemia incidence based on Japanese data. Radiat Res 58:131–140.

Rossi HH, Mays CW (1978) Leukemia risk from neutrons. Health Phys 34:353–360.

Sasaki S, Kasuga T (in press) Life-shortening and carcinogenesis in mice irradiated at the perinatal period with γ rays. In: Thompson RR and Mahaffey JA (eds.), Proceedings, Twenty-Second Hanford Life Sciences Symposium, 1983, Richland, Washington. Life-span radiation effects studies in animals: What can they tell us? Richland, WA: Battelle Pacific Northwest Laboratories.

Schleien B (1981) External radiation exposure to the offsite population from nuclear tests at the Nevada test site between 1951 and 1970. Health Phys 41:243–254.

Smith PG, Doll R (1976) Late effects of x irradiation in patients treated for metropathia haemorrhagica. Br J Radiol 49:224–232.

Smith PG, Doll R (1982) Mortality among patients with ankylosing spondylitis after a single treatment course with x-rays. Br Med J 284:449–460.

Spiess H, Gerspach A, Mays CW (1958) Soft-tissue effects following [224]Ra injections into humans. Health Phys 35:61–81.

Stebbings JH (1983) Personal communication.

Stewart A, Kneale GW (1971) Prenatal radiation exposure and childhood cancer. Lancet i:42–43.

Stewart A, Webb J, Hewitt D (1958) A survey of childhood malignancies. Br Med J 1:1495–1508.

United Nations Scientific Committee on the Effects of Atomic Radiation: Sources and Effects of Ionizing Radiation, Report to the General Assembly (1977) Publ E77IX1. New York: United Nations.

Upton AC (1977) Radiobiological effects of low doses: Implications for radiological protection. Radiat Res 71:51–74.

van Kaick G, Lorenz D, Muth H, Kaul A (1978) Malignancies in German Thorotrast patients and estimated tissue dose. Health Phys 35:127–136.

Wagoner JK Unpublished data.

Wagoner JK, Archer VE, Carroll VE, Holaday DA, Lawrence PA (1964) Cancer mortality patterns among U.S. uranium miners and millers, 1950 through 1962. J Natl Cancer Inst 32:787–801.

Wakabayashi T, Kato H, Ikeda T, Schull WJ (1983) Studies of the mortality of A-bomb survivors, Report 7. Part III. Incidence of cancer in 1959–1978, based on the Tumor Registry, Nagasaki. Radiat Res 93:112–146.

CARCINOGENIC EFFECTS OF RADIATION ON THE HUMAN RESPIRATORY TRACT

WOLFGANG JACOBI

The respiratory tract is the entrance organ for all inhaled toxic aerosols, gases, and vapors produced by manmade and natural sources in our environment. The combined inhalation exposure resulting from specific occupational sources, from releases into atmospheric air, from indoor sources at home, and from inhalation of tobacco smoke determines the final biological response of the respiratory tract.

The human lung is a sensitive tissue with respect to carcinogenesis. This conclusion is based not only on occupational findings; it is clearly demonstrated by the strong increase of the age-adjusted lung cancer frequency among populations during the last decades. Although this increase can be correlated to a large extent with smoking, there is strong evidence for an additional influence of air pollution due to industrialization and urbanization.

It is also well known that lung cancer can be induced by ionizing radiation. Indeed lung cancer in Rn-exposed underground miners is one of the oldest known occupational, fatal diseases; its occurrence among miners in the Schneeberg–Jachymov region can be followed back for more than 400 yr. But its real cause, the inhalation of the short-lived radioactive decay products (^{218}Po – ^{214}Po) of ^{222}Rn was identified only about 30 yr ago. This radon problem is still the main radiation hazard in mining, particularly uranium mining. Most of our experience on radiation-induced lung cancer described in this chapter results from epidemiologic studies among Rn-exposed miners, which were carried out or started during the last 10–20 yr.

The inhalation of radon daughters is also the most important component of the natural radiation exposure of populations. It results mainly from the enrichment of radon in indoor air. In a not negligible fraction of our houses Rn-levels have been measured that are comparable with those in uranium mines.

From the Gesellschaft für Strahlen- and Umweltforschung, Institute for Radiation Protection, Munich–Neuherberg, Federal Republic of Germany.

Thus, we are confronted not only with a radon problem in mines but also in houses. At the end of the chapter an estimate of the possible lung cancer risk associated with this indoor exposure to radon daughters is given.

EPIDEMIOLOGIC FINDINGS

For assessment of the carcinogenic effects of ionizing radiation on the human respiratory tract, two groups of epidemiologic studies can be quoted, as follows

1. Studies referring to external irradiation of the lung with photons (x- and gamma rays)
2. Studies on Rn-exposed miners who have received a high alpha dose to the bronchial epithelium from inhaled, short-lived $Rn(^{222}Rn)$-daughters.

So far, no excess lung cancer frequency in humans from inhaled, long-lived radioactive materials has been reported; this is also valid for plutonium workers.

Lung Cancer from External Irradiation

An excess lung cancer frequency has been observed among atomic bomb survivors in Hiroshima and Nagasaki and among some groups of X-ray treated patients. These studies are reviewed in the reports of UNSCEAR (1977) and of the U.S. National Academy of Sciences (NAS, 1980). With respect to the studies among x-ray treated patients, only the study of ankylosing spondylitis patients in the U.K. enables an estimate of the magnitude of the radiation-induced lung cancer risk. It must be emphasized that these studies refer to a single irradiation at high-dose rate; no human data for lung cancer from chronic external irradiation at low dose rate are available.

Atomic Bomb Survivors. The published data from this epidemiologic study population now cover a follow up from 1950 until the end of 1978, starting with a time lag of 5 yr after exposure (Kato et al, 1982). The basic data and the estimated lung cancer risk coefficients from this study are listed in Table 1. They refer to those survivors who were exposed to a T65-Kerma in free air exceeding 0.1 and 1 Gy, respectively. Due to ongoing revision of the dosimetric data for the survivors in Hiroshima and Nagasaki, no final dose values can be evaluated at this time. The values of the mean gamma dose to the lung given in Table 1 were estimated from the revised Kerma-values reported by Loewe et al (1981) taking into account a lung dose/kerma ratio of 0.8:1.0, which follows from Monte Carlo calculations. This tentative estimate yields a mean lung dose of about 0.8 and 2 Gy, respectively, for the two groups considered in Table 1.

Ankylosing Spondylitis Patients. Court Brown and Doll have investigated the cancer mortality among ankylosing spondylitis patients in the U.K. who had been treated with x-rays during the period from 1935 to 1954. Recently, Smith and Doll (1982) have reexamined and updated these data to 1970, regarding those 14,111 patients (11,776 male, 2,335 female) who had received only a single course of treatment. The data refer to a mean follow up period of 16.2 yr (until 1970), starting with a time lag of 9 yr after exposure. In Table 1 (right column) the results of this updated study are compared with those for the A-bomb survivors.

TABLE 1. Epidemiologic data and risk coefficients for lung cancer from external photon irradiation*

Quantity or unit		A-bomb survivors H + N (1950–78)[a] T 65-Kerma (old) >0.1 Gy	>1 Gy	Ankylosing spondylitis patients (mean follow-up, 16 yr)
Mean dose { Total lung Gy { Bronchi		0.8	2.0	1.5 2.5
Time lag after exposure (yr)		5.0	5	9
Number of persons		25202	6035	14111
Number of PYR × 10^3		612	148	58
Number of lung cancer deaths {	observed	178	63	88
	expected	149	37	59
	excess	29	26	29
Relative risk (observed/expected)		1.2	1.7	1.5
Mean excess LC-rate per unit dose, cases/10^4 PYR/Gy		0.6 ⎵ 0.7 (0.4; 1.0)	0.9	2.0[b] (1.0; 3)
Relative risk increment per unit dose, percent per Gy		25.0 ⎵ 30.0 (10; 50)	35	20[b] (10; 30)

* 90% confidence limits in brackets.
  [a] Lung dose estimates and risk coefficients refer to revised kerma values, taking into regard a mean lung dose/kerma-ratio of 0.8.
  [b] Risk coefficients refer to mean bronchial dose.

Previous dose estimates for these patients involved large uncertainties. Recently, Drexler et al (1985) have carried out Monte Carlo calculations for the specific irradiation conditions which were applied in the x-ray treatment of the ankylosing spondylitis patients (multiple field irradiation with 200 kV x-rays at 50 cm focus–skin distance). For a mean skin dose at the entrance field of 10–15 Gy, as typical in the treatment of these patients, the calculations yield the following mean dose values: spinal bone marrow, 6–9 Gy; total red bone marrow, 3–5 Gy; total lung, 1–2 Gy; directly irradiated bronchial region, 2,5–4 Gy. It should be emphasized that parts of the bronchial tree were not located in the direct beam; thus, the mean bronchial dose will be somewhat lower, about 2–3 Gy; a mean value of 2.5 Gy is used in this report (Table 1).

Epidemiological Studies Among Rn-Exposed Miners

An excess lung cancer frequency has been observed among several groups of underground uranium, fluorspar, and metal ore miners that were exposed in the past to relatively high levels of ^{222}Rn and its short-lived daughters (^{218}Po–^{214}Po) in the air of the mines. Up to the present time about 25,000 Rn-exposed miners have been included in these epidemiologic studies; about 22,000 of them were uranium miners. The results of these studies have been reviewed in several reports (UNSCEAR, 1977; NAS, 1980; NCRP, 1984; SENES, 1984). Of main relevance are the data from the three large study groups of uranium miners in Colorado, USA (Lundin et al, 1972; Waxweiler et al, 1981; Whittemore et al, 1983), in the CSSR (Sevč et al, 1976; Kunz et al, 1979) and in Ontario, Canada (Muller et al, 1983, 1985, which are summarized in Table 2. These studies enable an estimate of the exposure–risk relationship. The Rn daughter exposure of the miners is defined by the time integral over the potential alpha energy concentration of the short-lived daughter mixture, integrated over the total underground residence time of these workers since their start of mining. This exposure is usually expressed in units of working level-months (WLM); 1 WLM = 3.5×10^{-3} J h/m^3, which corresponds to an equivalent equilibrium (activity) exposure of ^{222}Rn of 6.3×10^5 Bq h/m^3.

In general, the risk analysis for these miners suffers from the following deficiencies of all such studies:

1. The uncertainty of the individual radon daughter exposures
2. The limited follow-up time
3. The possible synergistic or promoting influence of other factors (smoking, nonradioactive air pollutants in mines)
4. The selection of an appropriate control group

The expected lung cancer frequency among the miners is usually evaluated from the observed age-adjusted lung cancer rate among males in the general

TABLE 2. Basic data from epidemiologic studies of uranium miners

Quantity	Colorado, USA 1950–77[a]	Bohemia, CSSR 1948–75[b]	Ontario, Canada 1955–81[c]
Initial number of miners	3,366	2,433	≈13,400
Average follow-up period per miner (yr)	19	26	15
Surviving fraction at end follow-up (%)	72		≈80
Median age at start of uranium mining (yr)	30	35–40	≈25
Average working period in uranium mines, (yr)	9	10	≈2
Number of persons · PYR	62,556	≈60,000	202,795
Mean cumulated exposure (WLM)	820	310	60 ± 25
Fraction of chronic cigarette smokers (%)	≈70	≈70	50–60
Number of lung cancer cases during follow-up { observed	194	≈250	82
expected	40	≈60	57
excess	154	≈190	25
Relative risk (observed/expected cases)	4.8	≈4.2	1.45

[a] White miners only.
[b] Study group A only; the total group involved 4,364 miners.
[c] Only uranium miners without prior gold mining.

population of the considered region, without correction for smoking and other influences.

Histologic Findings

Histological examination of the lung cancers among high-dose atomic bomb survivors indicates an excess of anaplastic small-cell carcinomas, epidermoid carcinomas, and adenocarcinomas (Cihak et al, 1974). Due to the small numbers of excess cases, these studies enable no quantitative estimate of relative frequency of lung cancer as function of dose.

Among Rn-exposed uranium miners, earlier investigations led to the conclusion that the observed increase of bronchogenic carcinoma can be attributed mainly to an excess of anaplastic small-cell ("oat cell") cancers. More recent studies have revealed a significant increase also of epidermoid cancers and of adenocarcinomas, indicating a longer mean latency for the latter types (Horaček et al, 1977; Saccomano et al, 1981). Thus, the frequency of epidermoid cancers, as opposed to small-cell cancers, increases strongly with age. Adenocarcinomas occur predominantly among heavy smokers who started mining at early ages.

In conclusion, the inhalation of radon daughters, as well as external irradiation, leads to an increase of most types of lung cancers. The appearance of these cancers seems to be also strongly related with smoking.

Exposure-Risk Relationship

Low-LET Radiation. Due to statistical uncertainties, the data on lung cancer among atomic bomb survivors allow no definition of the shape of the dose–risk relationship. Kato et al (1982) have carried out a regression analysis of these data, assuming a linear relationship. Based on the revised, preliminary kerma estimates and a minimum latency period of 5 yr, the resulting values and (with their 90% confidence limits in brackets) of the mean excess lung cancer rates and of the relative incremental risk per unit lung dose are given at the bottom of Table 1.

With these assumptions, the data from the atomic bomb survivors yield a mean excess lung cancer rate of about 0.7 (0.4–1.0) 10^{-4} PYR^{-1} per Gy mean lung dose, averaged over the total lung. From the data for the spondylitis patients, a mean excess overall risk of about 3 10^{-4} PYR^{-1} per Gy mean lung dose should be expected; however, if it is assumed that the excess cases are mainly bronchial cancers, one can estimate an absolute risk coefficient of about 2 (1–3) 10^{-4} PYR^{-1} per Gy bronchial dose. The difference in absolute risk coefficients between both groups is probably due partly to their different age and sex distributions.

This is also suggested by the finding that the relative risk increment per unit dose is nearly the same for both groups (Table 1) and is approximately as follows

30% (10–50) per Gy mean lung dose, or
20% (10–30) per Gy mean bronchial dose

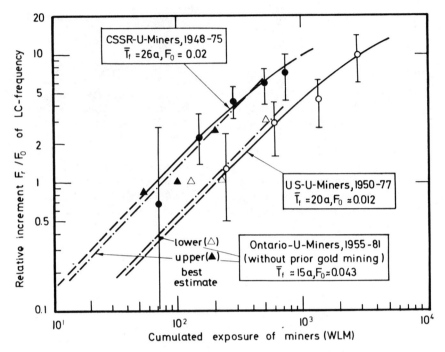

FIGURE 1. Relative increment of lung cancer frequency among uranium miners as a function of their cumulative exposure to Rn daughters (with 95% confidence limits).

As mentioned, these risk coefficients refer to low-LET radiation (gamma and x-rays) at a high dose rate. If one assumes a linear quadratic dose–risk model, which might be more realistic for these exposure conditions, the linear risk term would be lower than the risk/dose ratios given above.

Alpha Radiation (Data from Miners). The data from the three large study groups of Rn-exposed uranium miners (Table 2) enable a direct correlation between cumulative ^{222}Rn daughter exposure and excess lung cancer frequency. Figure 1 shows the observed relative increment of the lung cancer risk among these three groups of uranium miners, averaged over all age groups, as function of their cumulative Rn daughter exposure. Given the indicated 95% confidence limits and the uncertainty of the exposure data, the exposure–risk relationships for these groups are in rather good agreement. The values for the Ontario miners lie between the regression lines for the Colorado and the Czech miners. A statistically significant excess risk results at exposure levels above about 100 WLM, corresponding to a mean bronchial alpha dose of about 0.6 Gy.

These data have been tested for their fit to different exposure–response functions. A linear response was found to yield the best fit in the exposure region below about 1000 WLM. This conclusion is confirmed by the results of experiments with animals exposed to Rn daughters (Chmelesky et al, 1982; Chameaud et al, 1985). The resulting range of the best estimates for the mean excess lung cancer rate and the mean relative risk increment per unit of expo-

Table 3: Mean absolute and relative risk coefficients for lung cancer derived from studies of Rn exposed uranium miners*

Study group (follow-up)	Risk/Exposure ratio	
	Excess risk rate (cases/10^6 PYR/WLM)	Relat. increment of LC-frequency (%/WLM)
Colorado, USA (1950–77)	3–8	0.5–1.0
CSSR, group A (1948–75)	10–20	1.0–2.0
Ontario, Canada (1958–81)[a]	4–10	0.5–1.3

* Averaged over all age groups at start of mining, taking into account a minimum latency of 5–10 yr.
[a] Miners with prior gold mining experience excluded.

sure are summarized in Table 3. They take into account a minimum latency period of 5–10 yr between the start of exposure and the appearance of an excess lung cancer incidence.

The results of other studies of smaller groups of Rn-exposed, nonuranium miners fall into the same range, of about $(2-20)$ 10^{-6} PYR^{-1}/WLM, as do the results from the studies of uranium miners (NAS, 1980; Myers et al, 1981; NCRP, 1984). The only exception seems to be a small group of 150 lead and zinc miners in Sweden, for which an excess rate of 3.0×10^{-6} PYR^{-1}/WLM has been estimated (Axelson et al, 1978); however, the confidence range for this estimate is large.

A comprehensive risk study of various mining groups in Canada (Muller et al, 1983, 1984) indicates that, except in Rn-exposed uranium miners and a small group of gold miners, the observed lung cancer frequency was comparable with the age adjusted frequency in the general male population of the region; the reason for the enhanced risk in the gold miners is still unclear. This finding confirms the conclusion that the enhanced lung cancer frequency in the uranium miners is mainly attributable to their radiation exposure, and that the influence of nonradioactive dusts and vapors in the mines seems to be small. In addition to short-lived radon daughters, these miners were also exposed to enhanced levels of gamma radiation, and they also inhaled long-lived radioactive dusts (uranium ore dust, ^{210}Pb and ^{210}Po). The risk coefficients given in Table 3 include these contributions; however, the estimates indicate that under normal conditions only about 10% of the observed excess of bronchial cancer might be attributable to these other radiation sources.

With this correction, the results from studies of uranium miners listed in Table 3 yield the following average absolute and relative lung cancer risk coefficients, for a minimum latency of 5–10 yr

10 (3–20) excess cases/10^{-6} PYR/WLM, or
1% (0.5–1.5) per WLM

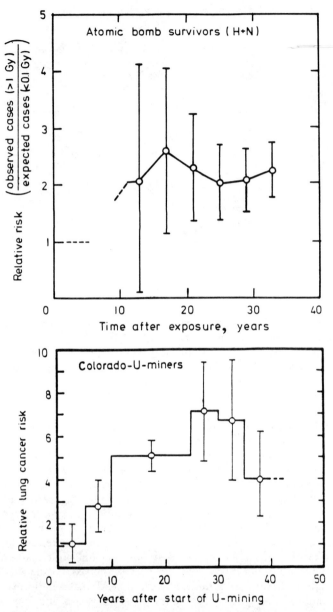

FIGURE 2. Relative lung cancer risk in atomic bomb survivors (upper graph) and Colorado uranium miners (lower graph), as function of the time after exposure or start of uranium mining, respectively (with 95% confidence limits).

The range of uncertainty of this best estimate is given in brackets. It should be recognized that the absolute excess of lung cancer depends on age at the time of exposure and on the length of the follow-up period, although the relative risk seems to be rather constant (Figure 2).

Influence of Smoking

Among the white Colorado miners, a sigificantly higher excess of radiation-induced lung cancer was observed among smokers than among nonsmokers. This finding can be interpreted as a promoting influence of smoking, leading to a shortening of latency for radiation-induced lung cancer (UNSCEAR, 1982). An internal correlation analysis has yielded, as a best fit, a relative risk function

$$R \sim (1 + 0.3 \ 10^{-2}E) \ (1 + 0.5 \ 10^{-3}C)$$
$$\sim 1 + 0.3 \ 10^{-2}E + 0.5 \ 10^{-3}C + 1.5 \ 10^{-6}EC \tag{1}$$

for these miners (Whittemore et al, 1983), showing both an additive and a multiplicative influence of Rn daughter exposure E (in WLM) and cigarette consumption C (in packs). From this relationship, it would follow that at the same level of exposure the relative radiation-induced lung cancer risk should be equal for nonsomokers and smokers, but that the absolute excess risk increases with smoking. For the uranium miners in the CSSR and in Canada a similar analysis is not possible, because no smoking histories are available as yet for those miners who died from lung cancer.

The findings in some smaller groups of non-uranium miners in Sweden are somewhat controversial. In Rn-exposed lead and zinc miners, Axelson et al (1978) found a somewhat lower risk for smokers than for nonsmokers. Another study of a group of Swedish iron miners has yielded only a relatively small reduction of latency among smokers (Radford et al, 1984). A further study of iron miners in Sweden, however, suggested a promoting influence of smoking on underground miners (Damber et al, 1982).

In general, it must be stated that in all these studies the number of lung cancer cases in nonsmokers is too small to enable a clear, quantitative conclusion about the promoting influence of smoking on the rate of radiation-induced lung cancer. To quantify this influence it may be more reasonable to consider the smoking-related promotion of age-specific lung cancer rates, as indicated by comparative studies between nonsmokers and smokers in the general population.

Latency Period and Age Distribution

As already mentioned, the excess lung cancer rate following irradiation depends on age at exposure and the length of followup. Therefore, estimates of the final lifetime risk formulated on the basis of excess risk projection models require additional, simplifying assumptions. A better understanding of the latency distribution and age dependency of radiogenic lung cancer can be obtained by considering the time variation of the relative risk (observed/expected cases). In this context, one should have in mind· that the normal age-specific lung cancer rate $\lambda(t)$ among nonsmokers and chronic smokers increases strongly with age t; i.e., it can be approximated by a Weibul function as follows

$\lambda(t) = k\, t^n$ with $n = 5 - 7$.

In Figure 2 the relative lung cancer risk in atomic bomb survivors and in Colorado uranium miners is plotted as function of time after exposure or after start of uranium mining, respectively, as can be inferred from the data published by Kato et al (1982) and Waxweiler et al (1981). Both studies indicate clearly that after a minimum latency of 5–10 yr the relative risk reaches a rather constant value and that up to 30–40 yr after exposure no significant reduction of the relative risk is observed.

From this general finding, the conclusion can be drawn that the latency period distribution, or the appearance rate of radiation-induced lung cancer as function of time after irradiation, is similar to the age-adjusted distribution of the baseline lung cancer rate in a comparable, nonexposed control population. Or, in other words, irradiation of the lung leads after a transition period to an excess lung cancer rate in subsequent life, the relative age distribution of which is similar to that of the baseline age specific lung cancer rate. On the basis of this finding, a relative risk projection model can be set up that enables an improved estimate of the integral risk as function of exposure or lung dose, respectively, age, and length of followup. It has been shown that such a model fits quite well the results of the epidemiologic studies among Rn-exposed uranium miners (Jacobi et al, 1984).

Furthermore, this finding supports the suggestion that ionizing radiation acts mainly as an initiator, leading to the formation of potentially malignant cells in the critical target tissues of the lung. The manifestation or appearance rate of lung cancer, however, seems to be determined mainly by other factors; namely, susceptibility as function of age and the influence of promoting agents like tobacco smoke.

RISK PROJECTION MODELS

Due to limitations in follow-up time, the epidemiologic studies on radiation-induced lung cancer enable no direct assessment of individual lifetime risks. Different risk projection models can be used for the prediction of this integral risk.

Absolute Risk Projection Model

If a proportional exposure–risk relationship is assumed, the radiation-induced lifetime risk R_r from a single exposure $E(t_e)$ at age t_e is given by the equation

$$R_r(E, t_e) = \int_{t_e+\tau(t_e)}^{\infty} a(t_e,t')E(t_e)p(t_e,t')\, dt' \qquad (2)$$

where the risk is integrated over the remaining lifetime, taking into account a minimum latency $\tau(t_e)$ and the survival probability $p(t_e,t')$ between age t_e at exposure and the considered age t'. The absolute risk coefficient $a(t_e,t')$ gives the excess rate per person multiplied times years at risk (PYR).

The epidemiologic studies, however, enable only an estimate of an age- and time-averaged mean value a of this risk coefficient (Tables 1 and 3) for a restricted followup-period. Normally the absolute risk projection models extrapolate this rate until the end of the lifetime, taking into account the reduction by competing risks. With respect to latency, a time lag τ of 5–10 yr is assumed in these models for exposures occurring after age 40; for exposures at younger ages, the excess rate commences at age 40. If a mean, age averaged excess rate $a = 10(3-20)10^{-6} \ PYR^{-1}/WLM$ (probable uncertainty range in brackets) is assumed, as follows from the uranium miners data (see **2**), and if their age distribution at the start of mining is taken into account, this ARP model yields for these miners a mean lifetime risk of lung cancer of about $2.5(1-5)10^{-4}/WLM$ exposure to Rn daughters, averaged over nonsmokers and smokers. This result is in good agreement with a previous estimate of UNSCEAR (1977).

A somewhat modified version of this ARP model has been proposed in the recently published NCRP-report no. 79 (1984), in which it is assumed that the initial excess lung cancer rate decreases exponentially, with a half-life of 20 yr, due to repair, cell death, or unspecified mechanisms. With this modification, the model predicts an average lifetime risk of only $1(0.4-2)10^{-4}/WLM$ for the exposure conditions of these uranium miners. However, no radiobiologic data are available thus far to justify the assumed removal half-life of 20 yr for potentially malignant cells in the lung. Also, the observed time-dependency of the relative risk of lung cancer in these miners gives no real basis for such an assumption (Figure 2).

Relative Risk Projection Model

The previously considered absolute risk projection model (ARP-model) assumes no correlation between the radiation-induced excess and the highly age dependent baseline rate of lung cancer; however, the epidemiologic findings strongly support such a correlation (Figure 2). Therefore, a relative risk concept seems to be more appropriate for predicting the risk of lung cancer initiated by ionizing radiation (Jacobi, 1984b; Jacobi et al, 1985; Land et al, 1984; Muller et al, 1985, NIH 1985).

In general, the age-specific rate of lung cancer $\lambda_0(t)$ in a nonexposed population can be described by the following relationship

$$\lambda_0(t) = k_0\psi(t) \tag{3}$$

where $\psi(t)$ defines the relative age distribution of the baseline rate. A radiation exposure E can be expected to lead, after a minimum latency τ of 5–10 yr, to an increment during the subsequent lifetime of

$$\lambda_r = f(E) \ \psi_r(t) \tag{4}$$

The observed time invariance of the relative risk leads to the conclusion that the relative age distributions of ψ_r and ψ are similar: $\psi_r(t) \sim \psi(t)$.

Given the assumption of a proportional exposure–risk relationship, $f(E) = a \ E(t-\tau)$, where $E(t-\tau)$ is the cumulated radiation exposure until age $(t-\tau)$, the total age-specific lung cancer rate is equivalent to:

$$\lambda(t) = \lambda_o(t) + \lambda_r(t) = k\psi(t) + aE(t\text{-}\tau)\psi(t)$$
$$= \lambda_o(t)\left[1 + \frac{a}{k}\,E(t - \tau)\right] = \lambda_o(t)[1 + rE(t - \tau)] \tag{5}$$

The relative risk coefficient $r = a/k$ in this equation defines the relative incre-ment of the normal rate per unit of exposure or dose, respectively. Best esti-mates of this value, derived from epidemiologic data, are given in Tables 1 and 3.

The model described by **5** can be denoted as a modified proportional hazard model (MPH model). It implies that the initiating probability of ionizing radia-tion superimposes additively on the initiating potential from other influences, whereas the relative age distribution for the manifestation of lung cancer is determined by other factors, mainly age and the influence of promoting agents, such as tobacco smoke.

The promoting influence of smoking on the normal age-specific lung cancer rate can be expressed by the relationship

$$\lambda_o(t) = \lambda_{o,ns}(t)\,[1 + S(t)] \tag{6}$$

where $\lambda_{o,ns}$ is the rate for nonsmokers and S is the promoting factor due to smoking. If the promoting influence of smoking on radiation-induced bron-chial cancer is assumed to be the same as that for bronchial cancer initiated by other influences, the following total rate is expected

$$\lambda(t) = \lambda_{o,ns}[1 + S(t)][1 + rE(t\text{-}\tau)] \tag{7}$$

The structure of this relationship corresponds to the risk function (see **1**), which was derived by Whittemore et al (1983) from a regression analysis for the Colorado U-miners

By integration over age, taking into account the probability of survival, the individual lifetime risk R_r, or the corresponding integral lung cancer frequency F_r, of radiation-induced lung cancer can be evaluated in the same way as with the ARP model (see **2**). Risk estimates for Rn exposed miners formulated on the basis of the MPH model for chronic exposure conditions yield a lifetime lung cancer risk in the range of $(1\text{-}2)\ 10^{-4}/\text{WLM}$ for nonsmokers and of $(4\text{-}6)\ 10^{-4}/\text{WLM}$ for chronic, heavy smokers (Jacobi et al, 1985). This model also enables an estimate of the lung cancer frequency in populations attributable to indoor exposure to Rn daughters. Some results of this risk analysis are outlined in the following.

LUNG CANCER RISK EXPECTED FROM INDOOR EXPOSURE TO Rn DAUGHTERS

Exposure Levels and Dose to Lung Tissues

The indoor level of ^{222}Rn can vary strongly from house to house; measured levels cover a range from about 2–2000 Bq/m^3. In most houses with greatly enhanced levels, the main source is the Rn entry from soil and not the Rn exhalation from building materials. In some areas with high Rn content in water supplies and natural gas, the Rn entry from these sources also can become important. Recent surveys in various countries indicate a population-averaged, mean indoor level of 20–50 Bq/m^3 for areas with normal background activity (UNSCEAR, 1982). Given a mean equilibrium factor of 0.4–0.5, this corresponds to a mean indoor level of short-lived ^{222}Rn daughters of about 8–25 Bq/m^3 (EEC$_{Rn}$). If a mean indoor residence probability of 0.8, or about 7000 hr/yr, is assumed, then levels correspond to a mean annual indoor exposure of (5–20) 10^{4}Bq h/m^3(Rn-eq.) $\approx$ 0/08–0.3 WLM from Rn daughters.

For the mean bronchial alpha dose, averaged over the basal cell layer in the bronchial tree, a dose conversion coefficient of 4 mGy/WLM has been proposed as reference value for indoor exposure to Rn daughters (NEA, 1983). Given a quality factor of 20 for alpha radiation, a mean per caput value of about 6–25 mSv/yr for the bronchial dose equivalent from indoor exposure to Rn daughters can be estimated. This is about a factor 5–20 higher than the mean natural radiation exposure of other tissues outside the respiratory tract. The mean dose to the pulmonary region from inhaled radon daughters is about a factor 1/5–1/10 lower than the mean bronchial dose.

The available measurements indicate that in about 1% of private dwellings in normal areas the Rn daughter level might exceed 100 Bq/m^3(EEC$_{Rn}$). On the assumption of a mean residence probability of about 0.65 indoors at home, an annual exposure of more than 5×10^5 Bq h/m^3(Rn-eq.) $\approx$ 0.8 WLM, and an annual bronchial dose equivalent of more than 60 mSv, can be estimated to occur under these exposure conditions. These exposure values are comparable with the mean annual occupational exposures of miners in well ventilated underground uranium mines.

Lung Cancer Risk Estimates

So far, no epidemiologic studies of population groups exposed to enhanced Rn levels in houses are available that enable a direct quantitative estimate of the attributable lung cancer risk. Some pilot studies, particularly in Sweden, have been started. Their preliminary results do not exclude a correlation between indoor exposure to Rn daughters and the frequency of lung cancer; but due to the small number of lung cancer cases and other uncertainties, the correlation is not statistically significant.

At the present time, the findings among the three larger groups of Rn-exposed uranium miners (Tables 2 and 3) can be regarded as the most suitable and reliable basis for estimating the lung cancer risk in populations attributable to indoor exposure to Rn daughters. To transfer the risk coefficients for these miners to indoor exposure conditions, appropriate correction factors have to be applied. In view of the different aerosol conditions in mines as compared with houses, the influence of differences in breathing rates, and the risk contributions from other sources, the average risk coefficients for adult numbers of the public are probably about a factor 0.6–0.9 lower than the mean values for miners given in **2.**

Risk evaluations formulated on the basis of ARP models for chronic exposure to Rn daughters in the environment at a constant annual rate of 1 WLM/yr yield, as a best estimate, an attributable lifetime risk of bronchial cancer of about (0.5–1.5) 10^{-2}, or 0.5%–1.5%, for mixed populations, averaged over nonsmokers and smokers (Jacobi, 1984a; NCRP, 1984). Thus at a population averaged, mean exposure rate of 0.2 WLM/yr an attributable risk of about 0.1%–0.3% should be expected. The currently observed lung cancer rates in populations with high life expectancy (70–80 yr) correspond to a mean lifetime lung cancer risk in the range of 1–6%. From this comparison, it would follow that about 3%–10% of the total observed lung cancers in these populations might be associated with the natural exposure to radon daughters. It should be emphasized that the risk data from Rn exposed miners refer to male subjects with a relatively high fraction of smokers (Table 2). The applied ERP models involve no correction for the possible promoting influence of smoking. Thus the estimated absolute risk values given above appear to be more appropriate for male than female subjects; the real values for women are probably lower.

As mentioned, the described MPH model, which is based on a relative risk concept, probably enables a more reliable risk projection from miner's data to the exposure conditions of populations. Preliminary risk estimates using this model were recently published (Jacobi, 1984b). This model leads to the conclusion that at the same exposure conditions the relative, radiation-induced increment R_r/R_0 of the normal lifetime risk R_0, or the corresponding increment F_r/F_0 of the normal lung cancer frequency F_0, is nearly equal in both sexes, as well as in nonsmokers and smokers. The same is valid with respect to the relative attributable fraction, $R_r/R = R_r/R_0 + R_r$ or $F_r/F = F_r/F_0 + F_r$, of the total observed lifetime risk R or frequency F, which include the contribution from inhaled Rn daughters.

In Figure 3, this relative fraction is plotted as function of the Rn daughter level in indoor air (lower abscissa) or the corresponding annual exposure rate (upper scale), as results from the MPH model for chronic exposure at these levels, assuming a mean residence probability $p_{res} = 0.65$ (65%) indoors at home. The shadowed area indicates the range of variation, taking into account a probable uncertainty of ± 50% for the relative risk coefficient. From this figure, it follows that at a mean indoor level of 10–20 Bq/m³(EEC_{Rn}), which seems to be typical for the average population in most countries, 2%–12% (mean value, 6%) of the total lung cancer incidence might be attributable to indoor exposure to Rn daughters at home. Including exposure to Rn daughters in outdoor air and in indoor air elsewhere than at home (i.e., at the work place), increase the total fraction to about 4%–15% (mean value, 8%).

For a reference population with a total lung cancer frequency of

$F_{males} = 60$ LC-cases/10^5 persons per year
$F_{females} = 15$ LC-cases/10^5 persons per year

exposed chronically at a mean indoor level of 10–20 Bq/m³ (EEC_{Rn}), the model predicts an absolute lung cancer frequency attributable to inhaled Rn daughters of

$F_{r,males} \approx 5$ (2–9) LC-cases/10^5 persons per year
$F_{r,females} \approx 1.2$ (0.5–2) LC-cases/10^5 persons per year

$F_{r,total} \approx 3$(1.2–5) LC-cases/10^5 persons per year

This total value averaged over both sexes is in good agreement with the expected range derived from the ARP model. The corresponding loss of life expectancy due to this lung cancer risk from inhaled Rn daughters amounts to about 12 (6–20) days, which is about two orders of magnitude lower than the loss of life expectancy from smoking-related diseases. The values given above refer to a mixed population of nonsmokers and smokers. If allowance is made for a promoting influence of smoking, the absolute lung cancer risk from inhaled radon daughters is lower for nonsmokers than for smokers. For nonsmokers, the MPH model yields an attributable lung cancer risk, which is about 30% of the mean risk values given for the male and female populations, respectively.

Of chief concern is the possible lung cancer hazard for those population groups that are living in houses with greatly enhanced Rn levels. As mentioned, the available indoor measurements indicate that on the average roughly about 1% of the population is living in houses where the current level exceeds 100 Bq/m³(EEC$_{Rn}$), which would lead to an annual exposure above 0.8 WLM. From Figure 3 it follows that in a population group that has received a chronic exposure of 1 WLM/yr, about 15%–40% of the total lung cancers might be initiated by inhaled Rn daughters. This calculated range agrees with the preliminary result of an epidemiological pilot study in Sweden on a population group which is currently exposed to such enhanced indoor levels (Edling et al, 1984); however, the systematic and statistical uncertainties of this small pilot study are quite large.

FIGURE 3. Expected relative fraction (percentage) of the total lung cancer incidence attributable to indoor exposure to Rn daughters, as a function of the mean level of Rn daughters in indoor air at home; estimated with the MPH model for chronic exposure conditions.

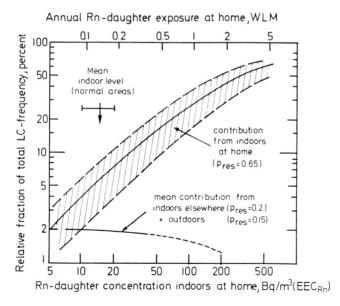

Finally, it must be pointed out that the derived risk estimates refer to a chronic exposure of individuals or populations to Rn daughters at a constant annual rate. Real exposure conditions can differ widely, taking into account individual mobility and living habits, as well as systematic, long-term changes of indoor air quality. There is strong evidence that the average ventilation rates of our houses have decreased during the past decades, due to closed central heating systems and improved air tightness; a mean reduction by a factor of about two has been suggested (Harley, 1984). Due to the reciprocal relationship between the ventilation rate and indoor Rn levels, the currently observed Rn levels are probably higher than in earlier times. This leads to the conclusion that the actual lung cancer frequency from inhaled Rn daughters in the population is probably lower than the risk value estimated from the model for chronic exposure at the current Rn levels.

FINAL REMARKS

The epidemiologic findings indicate that the bronchial epithelium is a rather sensitive tissue of the human body with respect to carcinogenic effects of ionizing radiation. The activity and dose distribution of inhaled radionuclides in the human respiratory tract depends strongly on the radioactive half-lives of the nuclides. With increasing half-life, the ratio of the bronchial dose to the pulmonary dose decreases. This may be one of the reasons for the relatively low carcinogenic efficiency of inhaled long-lived alpha emitters compared with short-lived Rn daughters, on the lung.

Indoor exposure to radon daughters delivers to the general population by far the largest contribution to its present radiation exposure, and radiogenic cancer risk, from natural and artificial radiation sources. Living in houses is essential for human civilization, but the optimization principle of radiation protection should be observed in the construction and ventilation of houses and in personal living habits, since exposure to Rn can be strongly influenced in this way. Principles for limiting exposure of the public to natural sources of radiation were recently outlined by the ICRP (1984). Sufficient ventilation of houses is also necessary, of course, to reduce the health risks from chemotoxic air pollutants which may be released from indoor sources.

REFERENCES

Axelson O, Sundell L (1978) Mining, lung cancer and smoking. Scand J Work Environ Health 4:46–52.

Chameaud J, Masse R, Morin M, Lafuma J (1985) Lung cancer induction by radon daughters in rats; present state of the data on low-dose exposures. p. 350–353 in Proc Int Conf on Radiation Safety in Mining, Toronto/Canada, Oct 1984, Canadian Nuclear Association, Toronto/Canada.

Chmelevsky D, Kellerer AM, Lafuma J, Chameaud J (1982) Maximum likelihood estimation of the prevalence of nonlethal neoplasms—An application to radon daughter inhalation studies. Radiat Res 91:589–614.

Cihak RW, Ishimaru T, Skeer A, et al (1974) Autopsy findings and relation to radiation. Cancer 33:1580–1588.

Damber L, Larsson LG (1982) Combined effects of mining and smoking in the causation of lung carcinoma. Acta Radiolog Oncol 21:305–313.

Drexler G, Williams G (1985) Körperdosen in der strahlentherapie, ein betrag zur quantifizierung des strahlenrisikos. In Hypothesen im strahlenschutz; Strahlenschutz in forschung und praxis Bd. XXV, G. New York: Thieme Verlag, pp 208–220.

Edling C, Wingren G, Axelson O (1984) Radon daughter exposure in dwellings and lung cancer p. 25–34 in Proc Intl Conf Indoor Air Quality, Stockholm, Aug 1984. Swedish Council for Building Research, Stockholm/Sweden

Harley JH (1984) Indoor living, long life and radiation risk. Radiat Protection Dosimetry 7:19–22.

Horaček J, Plaček V, Sevč J (1977) Histological types of bronchogenic cancer in relation to different conditions of radiation exposure. Cancer 40:832–835.

ICRP (1984) Principles for limiting exposure of the public to natural sources of radiation. ICRP publ 39, Pergamon Press.

Jacobi W, Paretzke H and Schindel F (1985) Lung cancer risk assessment for radon-exposed miners on the basis of a proportional hazard model. Proc Int Conf on Occupational Radiation Safety in Mining (H. Stocker, editor); Toronto, Canada: Canadian Nuclear Association, pp 17–24.

Jacobi W (1984a) Possible lung cancer risk from indoor exposure to radon daughters. Radiat Protection Dosimetry 7:353–366.

Jacobi W (1984) Expected lung cancer risk from radon daughter exposure in dwellings. Proc Int Conf on Indoor Air Quality. Stockholm, Sweden: Swedish Council for building research, pp 31–42.

Kato H, Schull WJ (1982) Studies of the mortality of A-bomb survivors. 7. Mortality 1950–78: Part I. Cancer mortality. Radiat Res 90:395–432.

Kunz E, Sevč J, Plaček V, Horaček J (1979) Lung cancer in man in relation to different time distribution of radiation exposure. Health Phys 36:699–706.

Land CE, Tokunaga M (1984) Induction period. In: Boice JD and Fraumeni JF (eds.), Radiation carcinogenesis: Epidemiology and biological significance. New York: Raven Press, pp 421–436.

Loewe WE, Mendelsohn E (1981) Revised dose estimates at Hiroshima and Nagasaki, Health Phys 41:663–666.

Lundin RE, Wagoner JK, Archer VE (1971) Radon daughter exposure and respiratory cancer; quantitative and temporal aspects. Natl Inst Occup Safety and Health, Natl Inst Environ Health Sciences. Joint Monograph no. 1, Washington DC: USDHEW.

Muller J, Wheeler WC, Gentleman JF, Suranyi G, Kusiak RA (1983) Study of mortality of Ontario miners 1955–77, Part I. Report Ontario Ministry of Labour, Ontario Worker's Compensation Board. Toronto: Atomic Energy Control Board of Canada.

Muller J, Wheeler WC, Gentleman JF, Suranyi G, Kusiak RA (1985) Proc Int Conf on Occupational Radiation Safety in Mining (H. Stocker, editor), Toronto, Canada: Canadian Nuclear Association, pp 335–343.

Myers DK, Stewart CG, Johnson JR (1981) Review of epidemiological studies on hazards of radon daughters. In: Proc Intl Conf Radiat Hazards in Mining. New York: Society of Mining Engineers, pp 513–524.

National Institute of Health (1985) Report of the ad hoc working group to develop radioepidemiological tables. Washington DC: Nat Inst of Health Publication No. 85-2748, Jan 1985.

NAS (1980) The effects on populations of exposure to low levels of ionizing radiation. BEIR III-Report. Washington, DC: Natl Acad Sciences, Natl Res Council.

NCRP (1984) Evaluation of occupational and environmental exposures to radon and radon daughters in the United States. Bethesda MD: NCRP Report no. 78.

NEA (1983) Dosimetry aspects of exposure to radon and thoron daughter products. Paris: Report of the OECD Nuclear Energy Agency.

Radford EP, St Clair Renard KG (1984) Lung cancer in Swedish iron miners exposed to low doses of radon daughters. N Engl J Med 310:1485–1495.

Saccomano T, Archer VE, Auerbach O, Kushner M, Egger E, Wood S, Mich R (1981) Age factor in histological type of lung cancer among uranium miners; a preliminary report. In: Proc Intl Conf Radiat Hazards in Mining. New York: Society of Mining Engineers, pp 675–679.

SENES (1984) Assessment of the scientific basis for existing federal limitations on radiation exposure to underground uranium miners. Report for the American Mining Congress, SENES Consultants Ltd., Toronto, Canada, Oct 1984.

Sevč J, Kunz E, Plaček V (1976) Lung cancer in uranium miners and long-term exposure to radon daughter products. Health Phys 30:433–437.

Smith PG, Doll R (1982) Mortality among patients with ankylosing spondylitis after a single treatment course with x-rays. Br Med J 284:449–460.

UNSCEAR (1977) Sources and effects of ionizing radiation. New York: United Nations Sales Publication no. E.77.IX.1.

UNSCEAR (1982) Ionizing radiation: Sources and biological effects. New York: United Nations Sales Publication no. E.82.IX.8.

Waxweiler RJ, Roscoe RJ, Archer VE, Thun MJ, Wagoner JK, Lundin FE (1981) Mortality follow-up through 1977 of the white underground miners cohort examined by the US Public Health Service. In: Proc Intl Conf Radiat Hazards in Mining. New York: Society of Mining Engineers, pp 823–830.

Whittemore AS, McMillan A (1983) Lung cancer mortality among US uranium miners: A reappraisal. J Natl Cancer Inst 71:489–499.

CARCINOGENIC EFFECTS
OF RADIATION ON
THE HUMAN BREAST

ROY E. SHORE, Ph.D., D.P.H.

An association between ionizing radiation and breast cancer was first reported by MacKenzie in 1965. The next major report documenting this association came from the Japanese A-bomb study in 1968 (Wanebo et al) followed soon after by a report of women irradiated for acute postpartum mastitis (Mettler et al, 1969). Although there is now a general consensus that the female breast is one of the most radiosensitive organs, there are not a large number of follow-up studies that document this. Because there is so little that is distinctive in the histopathology of radiation-induced breast cancers (Dvoretsky et al, 1980; Tokuoka et al, 1984), the association has to be documented primarily on a statistical basis. Because the case-fatality rate of breast cancer is only about 40%–45%, mortality studies are generally less satisfactory than incidence studies. The major follow-up studies will be briefly described.

SUMMARY OF MAJOR STUDIES

Follow-up has now been completed for the period 1950–1980 (36 yr since irradiation) for the survivors of the Japanese atomic bombs (Tokunaga at al, 1984, 1979; McGregor et al, 1977). The life span sample (LSS) included 63,300 women among whom breast cancer diagnoses have been ascertained from autopsy records, tumor registries, and the clinical and pathologic records of hospitals in Hiroshima and Nagasaki, plus death certificates from anywhere in Japan. A total of 564 breast cancer cases have been identified among women in the LSS sample, of whom 306 received a dose of at least 1 rad. This study has many strengths, including the wide range of ages at irradiation, the wide range of doses, with large numbers at lower doses, and the fact that women were not selected because of illness as is true of medical irradiation series. On the other

From the Institute of Environmental Medicine, New York University Medical Center, New York, New York.

hand, there are uncertainties in the dosimetry for individuals and in the out-migration patterns; anomalies may also have been introduced by the concomitant irradiation of the ovaries.

In Massachusetts, about 1050 women who received multiple fluorosopic examinations in the course of pneumotherapy for tuberculosis, have been followed for up to 45 yr, as have a group of over 700 women with tuberculosis who had no fluoroscopic exams (Boice and Monson, 1977). The irradiated women ranged in age from 15 to about 50. The women were fluoroscopically examined about 100 times on the average, with a typical breast dose of about 1.5 rad per examination (Boice et al, 1978). The cumulative breast doses ranged from <30 to >600 rad, with a mean of about 150 rad. Follow-up times ranged up to 45 yr, with a mean of 27 yr. Forty-one breast cancers were observed in the irradiated group versus 23.3 expected, for a RR of 1.8. There was no excess in the control group.

Another multiple fluoroscopy study has recently been reported (Howe, 1984) based on records from tuberculosis sanatoria in most of Canada. This study builds upon the earlier, smaller studies (MacKenzie, 1965; Myrden and Hiltz, 1969; Myrden and Quinlan, 1974) of women in Nova Scotia sanatoria. The larger study is based on about 11,300 tubercular women who received multiple fluoroscopic examinations during pneumotherapy and 12,000 tubercular women without fluoroscopy. The breast doses ranged from a few rad to >1000 rad. The women were treated during the 1930s and 1940s, and breast cancer mortality experience was ascertained for 1950–1977 from the computerized Canadian National Death Index. About 170 breast cancer deaths were found in the irradiated group, which was a 60% excess compared with either the control group or population rates.

A particular strength of the two fluoroscopy studies is the fact that the radiation exposures were given in many small fractions, the better to simulate the occupational and diagnostic radiation exposures that people commonly encounter. Perhaps the major limitation of the studies is the uncertainty of individual dose estimates, in spite of major dosimetric evaluations by the respective investigators (Boice et al, 1978; Sherman et al, 1978).

In Rochester, New York, x-ray therapy was used for a number of years in treating acute postpartum mastitis (i.e., infectious breast disease during childbirth and lactation). About 600 irradiated women have been followed for up to 37 yr (Mettler et al, 1969; Shore et al, 1977). Also followed have been a group with acute postpartum mastitis who received no x-ray treatment, and sisters of both the mastitis groups, making a total of about 1300 control women. The breast doses ranged from 50 to >1000 rad, with a mean of about 250 rad. Fifty-seven breast cancer cases have been found in the irradiated group versus 61 in the larger control group, which gives a relative risk of about 2 (Shore and Hildreth, unpublished data, 1984). Among the 69% of the irradiated women who received radiation to only one breast, the elevated risk was confined to the irradiated breast. Among the strengths of this study are the well characterized dosimetry and the inclusion of a control group with the same disease as the irradiated group had. The main limitations lie in the lack of low-dose data, and the fact that the women were postpartum and lactating at the time of irradiation, where the state of the breast differs from the typical nonlactating breast in degree of proliferative activity and hormone stimulation.

In Stockholm, Sweden about 1020 women have been followed who received x-ray therapy during the period 1927–57 for various benign breast conditions (fibroadenomatosis in 77%) (Baral et al, 1977). About 86% were treated in only one breast. The breast doses ranged from a few rad up to about 4000 rad, with a median dose on the order of 700 rad. The patients ranged in age from 10 to 70+ yr at the time of treatment. The subjects were followed for up to 42 yr after irradiation, with an average follow-up of 32 yr. A total of 115 breast cancers were found in irradiated breasts when 28.7 were expected, based on general population rates. This gives a relative risk of 4. By way of comparison, 20 breast cancers were found in the unirradiated breasts when 19.9 were expected. While this study has strengths—principally the adequate dosimetry, the large number of observed tumors, and the wide range of ages at treatment—it also has limitations, notably the lack of a control group of women with similar types of breast disease.

Baverstock et al (1981) followed up about 1100 women with occupational exposure to radium, principally as dial painters. Among the 865 under age 30 at onset of exposure, with an average breast dose estimated as 40 rad, a significant excess of breast cancer was seen (14 observed, 6.8 expected). Stebbings et al (1984) also reported a dose–response relationship for breast cancer among the U.S. radium dial painters. Other smaller and, therefore, less informative studies have been undertaken as well, mostly centering around multiply fluoroscoped women (Cook et al, 1974; Grundy and Uzman, 1973; Delarue et al, 1975; Kitabatake et al, 1975).

TEMPORAL COURSE OF RISK

A rather simplified scheme of the temporal aspects of radiation carcinogenesis is to consider a minimum latent period (between irradiation and the time when the elevated cancer risk begins to appear), an extended plateau period (during which cancer risk is elevated), and perhaps a subsequent period with no excess risk.

The length of the minimum latent period is fairly well defined. Three of the four main studies have reported a minimum latent period of 10–15 yr (Boice and Monson, 1977; Shore et al, 1977; Howe, 1984) before an appreciable cancer excess has been seen. The largest study reported a marginally significant excess between 5 and 9 yr, but a larger excess 10 yr or more postirradiation (Land et al, 1980). Thus, a 10-yr minimal latent period seems to be a reasonable approximation.

A minimum latent period of 10 yr applies only to women who were about 20–25 yr of age or older at irradiation. For those at younger ages the minimum latent period becomes correspondingly longer. For instance, those in the Japanese atomic bomb study who were irradiated at ages 0–9 and those irradiated in infancy for thymic enlargement did not begin to show an excess of breast cancer until 30–35 yr later (Tokunaga et al, 1982; Hildreth et al, 1983). These data support the principle that radiogenic breast cancers will occur almost exclusively at ages at which there is an appreciable natural breast cancer incidence (i.e., beginning at about ages 30–35). Why this should be so is currently unknown, but is an intriguing finding with implications for the biology of cancer.

The question of the length of the period during which radiation-induced breast cancers are expressed (the "plateau period") is currently unresolved. All the studies to date have found an excess risk out to the longest follow-up times. The shortest of these had maximum follow-up times of about 35 yr (Tokunaga et al, 1984; Shore et al, 1977), whereas, the longest were up to 45 yr postirradiation (Howe, 1984; Boice and Monson, 1977). There is no evidence to date that the plateau period for radiogenic breast cancer takes the form of a "wave," with a peak and then a waning phase after a certain number of years (Boice and Monson, 1977). Another question pertaining to temporal patterns is whether or not "tumor acceleration" occurs in response to human irradiation (i.e., whether or not there is an earlier age/time distribution for radiation-induced breast cancers than for spontaneous breast cancers). A related question is whether or not tumor acceleration is dose-dependent. In examining these questions it is important to correct for age at irradiation (AAI) and the varying lengths of follow-up of study subjects, and to distinguish statistically between the radiogenic and the spontaneous components of breast cancer incidence among irradiated subjects, so that temporal variations will not be masked. Although the analyses presented to date have not met all these criteria it seems safe, nevertheless, to say that no important differences have been found between the age distributions of radiogenic and spontaneous breast cancers once AAI has been controlled (Baral et al, 1977; Shore et al, 1977; Land et al, 1980). Nor has any clear relationship between latency interval and dose been seen. Thus, there is no support for radiation as a "tumor accelerator" of breast cancers. Neither was there any indication of a trend toward latencies at lower doses, so a "practical threshold" (Evans, 1966), whereby the latency distribution becomes longer at lower and lower doses until it exceeds the life span, was not supported. In summary, the best current working hypothesis is that radiation produces no appreciable change in the latency distribution of breast cancers; its primary effect is to increment or multiply the natural incidence, at least for ages at risk of 35 yr or more.

DOSIMETRIC DATA AND DOSE–RESPONSE CURVES

Historically, risk calculations have been performed using various surrogates for breast dose (e.g., kerma, entrance dose, 2-cm depth dose, etc). It is now generally thought that the most appropriate calculation is an estimate of the average dose to the epithelial glandular tissue of the breast for each individual.

Epidemiologists' capability of providing precise estimates of individual doses is somewhat limited. Problems in trying to reconstruct doses range from the inaccuracies in determining shielding material thicknesses and configurations in the Japanese atomic bomb study, to questions of the length of exposure and patient orientation (e.g., was the patient rotated?) in the multiple fluoroscopic studies, to individual variations in breast size and in amount and configuration of glandular tissue in all of the studies. Thus, on an individual basis there may be modest to substantial imprecision in the estimated breast dose. What is sometimes not appreciated is that unless there is systematic bias in the dose measurements, the average group doses (whether for a total irradiated group or for subgroups defined by dose ranges) will be substantially accurate even though individual doses may be randomly over- or underestimated. Thus, for epidemiologic purposes, a certain amount of imprecision in dose estimation for individuals will have relatively little effect on the results.

The human dose–response data for breast cancer have been reviewed and analyzed more thoroughly than those of any other type of malignancy, except perhaps for leukemia. All five of the major studies just described have had a reasonably wide range of doses, so that the dose-response curves could be examined. An indepth, parallel examination of three of these studies has been reported (Boice et al, 1979; Land et al, 1980). In general, the functional forms that investigators have tried to fit include some or all of the terms for: linear-quadratic (dose-squared) and high-dose "cell sterilization" effects. It is important in the dose–response analyses to control for AAI, because radiation risk depends on AAI (detailed later in this chapter). In all the analyses performed to date however, it has been assumed that the *shape* of the dose-response curve does not vary by AAI.

Parallel analyses of breast cancer data from the Japanese atomic bomb study (Tokunaga et al, 1979), the Massachusetts multiple fluoroscopy study (Boice and Monson, 1977) and the Rochester postpartum mastitis study (Shore et al, 1977) were performed. The simple linear model fitted all three series adequately. The quadratic term of the linear-quadratic model went to zero for two of the series and was not significant ($p > 0.3$) in the third. The pure quadratic model fit the data sets more poorly than did the linear model; in the case of the largest data set, the Japanese data, the lack of fit for the pure quadratic model was significant. One series (Rochester postpartum mastitis) had a "cell sterilization" term at high doses, but the others did not. Although the dose–response curve in the Swedish series (Baral et al, 1977) has not been as formally evaluated as have the above series, it also appears to be compatible with a linear model. In summary, the evidence from these analyses suggests that a simple linear model is sufficient although a linear-quadratic model cannot be ruled out. A pure quadratic model does not provide a good fit to these data. However, a preliminary report of the large Canadian multiple fluoroscopy series (Howe, 1984) appeared at variance with the above conclusions by seeming to show clear quadratic curvature, so a definite conclusion cannot be reached at this time.

DOSE FRACTIONATION AND DOSE RATE

Radiobiologic theory and a considerable body of experimental data indicate that there is a diminished carcinogenic effect of sparsely ionizing radiation when it is administered at a low dose rate or in a number of small dose fractions, presumably due to the capacity of cells to repair single lesion damage (NCRP, 1980). Although human studies of breast cancer have more variation in degree of dose fractionation than radiation studies of most other cancer sites, most of the variation occurs between studies, rather than within studies. Two studies have had a modest degree of intrastudy variation in dose fractionation (Shore et al, 1977; Baral et al, 1977), but the typical breast dose per fraction was 100 rad or more; at those doses one would probably not expect much if any sparing effect due to dose fractionation.

Inferences about effects based on interstudy comparisons are somewhat tenuous, because many factors beside the one of interest may vary between studies (e.g., medical status of the respective populations at the time of irradiation, or ethnic composition of the populations). Hence, any conclusions must be tempered by these uncertainties. A comparison can be made between the risk estimates from the studies with acute doses and those with substantial dose fractionation or low dose rates. With the largely unfractionated postpartum mastitis, Swedish radiotherapy and Japanese atomic bomb studies, the risk estimates were 8.3, 6.8, and 3.6/MPYR, respectively (Boice et al, 1979). In the multiple fluoroscopy studies (with highly fractionated doses of 0.2–20 rad/ fraction) in Massachusetts, Nova Scotia, and the remainder of Canada, the risk estimates were 6.2, 8.4, and 2–4/MPYR, respectively (Boice et al, 1979; Howe, 1984).

The studies of radium paint luminizers are the only studies with a low dose rate (Baverstock et al, 1981; Stebbings et al, 1984). Although the breast doses are rather uncertain, using their estimated average dose the risk in Baverstock's study is about 8/MPYR, which would not indicate any diminished effect compared with acute exposures. Stebbings et al (1984) found a risk of a similar magnitude, but questioned whether or not the putative risk might be due to methodologic artifacts, instead. Overall, it does not appear that there is an appreciable sparing effect associated with dose fractionation or protraction.

RADIATION QUALITY

Land et al (1980) performed an extensive analysis of the relative biological effectiveness (RBE) of neutron versus gamma irradiation in the Hiroshima and Nagasaki data. The general findings were that an RBE close to one fit the data best and that RBE values greater than about five were statistically incompatible with the data.

Based on the recent reconsiderations of the Hiroshima and Nagasaki dosimetries, it is now believed that the T65 assigned neutron doses erred appreciably on the high side. It is unclear if the neutron component in Hiroshima will still be large enough to examine meaningfully, once the new values are agreed upon. At any rate, conclusions about the RBE of neutrons for breast carcinogenesis should be held in abeyance until the data can be reanalyzed with the new dosimetry. There are no other known sources of epidemiologic information on the RBE of high-LET radiations with respect to breast cancer.

AGE AT IRRADIATION

The effects of AAI are complex in an endocrine system-dependent organ. As such, it is useful to group ages by endocrine status: ages 0–9 (prepubertal), ages 10–19 (perimenarcheal), ages 20–39 (mature ovulatory function), ages 40–54 (perimenopausal), and ages 55+ (postmenopausal). Several studies indicate that irradiation during the perimenarcheal period confers a greater risk of breast cancer than irradiation at later ages. The absolute risk coefficients in the Japanese atomic bomb study and the Massachusetts and Canadian fluoroscopy studies (Boice et al, 1979; Howe, 1984) were generally about twice as large for AAI of 10–19 as for AAI of 20–39 yr. The Swedish study also reported a higher risk at ages 10–19 than at subsequent ages (Baral et al, 1977).

Of the principal studies, only the Japanese atomic bomb study has substantial data for AAI of 0–9. Until recently, no excess had been seen among this group. In the latest report (Tokunaga et al, 1984), however, a significant radiogenic excess has been found, with a magnitude similar to that found in the 10–19 AAI group. The excess was not found before, because of the long latent period associated with young AAI as discussed previously. Excess breast cancer risk among those irradiated at young ages has also been corroborated by the Rochester thymus irradiation study (Hildreth et al, 1983). Among these subjects, who were irradiated during the first year of life, nine breast cancers were observed, whereas 1.9 were expected (p<0.01) based on the sibling control group.

AAI of 40 and beyond are of particular interest because of recent concerns over the risk/benefit ratio of mammographic screening for breast cancer (Bailar, 1976, 1977; Chiacchierini and Lundin, 1979). The most recent Japanese data indicate there is no clear risk at AAI of either 40–49 or 50+ yr (Tokunaga et al, 1984). However, there are two potential complications in interpreting the Japanese perimenopausal and postmenopausal AAI data. First, concomitant irradiation of the ovaries near the time of menopause may have protected against breast cancer development. This interpretation is supported by other studies in which decreased breast cancer was found to be associated with ovarian radiation (Smith and Doll, 1976). Moreover, the ovaries appear to be more sensitive to radiation-induced castration around the age of 40 than at younger ages (Sawada, 1959), and induction of early menopause protects against breast cancer. Secondly, the incidence of breast cancer decreases after menopause among the Japanese, unlike Western countries in which it continues to increase postmenopausally. This suggests there is something fundamentally different between postmenopausal breast cancer in Japan and in the West: perhaps a relative absence of certain hormonal tumor promoters, among the former. Thus, it is not clear that the Japanese data from postmenopausal AAI is directly applicable to predicting risk in Western women.

Fortunately, some data are now available for older AAI in Western series. The Massachusetts fluoroscopy data (Boice and Monson, 1977; Boice et al, 1979) suggest there is little if any radiogenic risk for AAI of 40–49, although the numbers were very small. On the other hand, the Rochester postpartum mastitis data (Shore et al, 1977) suggested that risk was not diminished at AAI of 40–45 but again, the numbers were very small. It should also be noted that in the latter study the breasts were lactating at the time of irradiation; this physiologic state is very different in terms of cell proliferation and hormone stimulation from the normal quiescent, involuting breast at ages 40–49.

The Swedish series (Baral et al, 1977) seems to indicate that radiogenic risk decreases beyond approximately ages 30–35 at irradiation, but a small risk is still present even at postmenopausal ages. The finding of an apparent effect at older ages should be treated with caution, however, since part or all of the observed "effect" may be due to the underlying breast disease at treatment (for which there was no same-disease control group) and not due to radiation.

The Canadian fluoroscopy study (Howe, 1984) showed a clear diminution in risk for irradiation occurring beyond 30 yr of age. In particular, there was no excess risk for AAI of 40–49 or 50+ when the group receiving 100+ rad was compared with population rates; however, the numbers were very small (observed/expected values for AAI 40+ were 1/1.6). In summary, virtually all the studies agree that irradiation at ages 40 and over confers less risk than irradiation in the age range of, say, 20–34. However, they disagree as to whether or not there is at least some risk at the older ages. For radiation protection purposes it should probably be assumed there is some, but diminished, risk at AAI of 40–49 and 50+.

RISK MODELS AND AGE AT RISK

Although one could conceive of a variety of statistical models for the relationship among age at risk, time since irradiation, and breast cancer risk, the two that have been principally considered are the absolute (additive) risk model and the relative (multiplicative) risk model. Both allow for variations in risk depending on dose and on AAI, and both can be tailored to allow for some minimum latency-induction period. The absolute risk model assumes that the excess risk subsequent to irradiation is approximately constant and therefore unrelated to the natural incidence of cancer at successive ages, whereas, the relative risk model assumes that radiogenic risk is proportional to the natural incidence at given ages.

The distinction between absolute and relative risk is important when it comes to projecting our current time-limited data to estimate "lifetime risk," for the following reason. In Western populations breast cancer incidence increases sharply with age. Data are currently available for only limitied lengths of follow-up (mostly <40 yr postirradiation). In projecting to longer lengths of follow-up—and simultaneously to older ages at risk—the relative risk model multiplies the increasingly higher natural incidence rates, whereas, the absolute risk model only adds the same arithmetic increment at older ages. As a result, the relative risk model predicts a lifetime risk several times as high as the absolute risk model.

A recent tabulation was given to compare the absolute and relative risk estimates across ages at risk (but within AAI) for three studies (Land et al, 1980). The coefficients of variation of the age at risk estimates for the AAI-specific absolute risk and relative risk estimates indicate that the relative risk model provides a better fit to the data (i.e., is closer to a constant value across age at risk) than does the absolute risk model. Nevertheless, it is important to recognize that the absolute and relative risk models are simple and convenient approximations that do not incorporate knowledge about the biological mechanism(s) of radiation-induced breast cancer, and which are based on incomplete knowledge as to the temporal distribution of cancers following irradiation. As an example of how they might err, consider a (not unreasonable) hypothetical case in which the true underlying temporal pattern is an extended wave of cancers, like a somewhat flattened normal distribution in which the rate of excess cancers builds up for some years, peaks, and then diminishes. If one has observations only for the first half of this temporal distribution, the observations would seem to favor a relative risk model (because the excess is increasing in parallel with the underlying natural incidence). Of course, the projected relative risk model would grossly exaggerate the risk that would occur on the waning side of the temporal curve. This illustrates the point that a model can be no substitute for lifetime observation of populations at risk.

ENVIRONMENTAL AND HOST MODIFYING FACTORS

Three studies have thus far reported data on factors that may modify the magnitude of radiation induction of breast cancer. This area is no doubt an important one, both for identifying highly susceptible subgroups and for finding preventive measures to lower risk.

Shore et al (1980) reported on two environmental exposures that might alter radiogenic risk. For neither oral contraceptive nor menopausal estrogen exposure, occurring subsequent to irradiation, was there any evidence of a synergism with radiation. Knowing that women of higher socioeconomic status are at higher risk for spontaneous breast cancer, Kato and Schull (1982) studied whether or not there was a synergism between socioeconomic status and radiation exposure in the Japanese atomic bomb study, but found none. These are the only data available on environmental exposures or their surrogates.

Several host-susceptibility factors have been examined. First of all, the Japanese atomic bomb study has found no excess of breast cancer among the male population, indicating that risk is confined to the female breast. AAI is an important moderator of risk (discussed previously).

Age at first childbirth has been documented as an important risk factor for breast cancer, viz, early parity protects against breast cancer (Kelsey, 1979). Thus, something biologically important apparently happens at the time of the first childbirth. Boice and Stone (1978) found in the Massachusetts fluoroscopy data that irradiation at the time of the first pregnancy and childbirth conferred (unsignificantly) more risk (17/MPYR) than irradiation either before or after that time (~1/MPYR). Similarly, Shore et al (1980) examined the Rochester postpartum mastitis data for irradiation at the first childbirth versus irradiation at later childbirths. They found a greater risk (p = 0.05) associated with irradiation at the first childbirth (7/MPYR) than at subsequent childbirths (2/MPYR) with AAI controlled. Thus, both studies indicate that first childbirth is a time of heightened sensitivity to breast irradiation.

Women who are nulliparous or who had their first child at age 30+ are known to be at high risk for breast cancer (Kelsey, 1979), and the question can be asked whether or not these factors also predispose toward radiogenic breast cancer. Boice and Stone (1978) found risk coefficients of about 9 and 2/MPYR for nulliparous and parous women, respectively. It is noteworthy that for those who are nulliparous at irradiation but who subsequently had a child the risk was lower than for those who remained nulliparous (Boice and Hoover, 1981). Shore et at al (1980) compared women with first parity at ages 30+ versus <30 and found risk coefficients of 10 and 4/MPYR, respectively. Thus, the data are consistent with the hypothesis that late/no childbirth is a condition with heightened susceptibility to the effects of breast irradiation. However, larger studies are needed to confirm this interpretation, because the differences were not significant in either study. Several other factors examined but which showed no differences in radiogenic risk included age at menopause, history of ovarian dysfunction, and family history of breast cancer.

IMPLICATIONS FOR RADIOBIOLOGY AND FOR THE EPIDEMIOLOGY OF BREAST CANCER

The variations in radiogenic breast cancer by age, parity, etc. make the point, perhaps better than is made by any other human data, that the relatively simple radiobiologic models based on biophysical and molecular considerations are inadequate in and of themselves to predict cancer risk. Fry (1981) and others have eloquently made the point that tumor promoters, hormone levels, and other modifying factors need to be considered, as well. In the case of breast cancer, it is evident that a radiation insult around the time of menarche or the first childbirth confers greater risk than one at other times. The reasons for this are unknown, although degree of cellular proliferation or degree of breast stimulation by some hormone acting as a cocarcinogen or promoter could be entertained as hypotheses. Similarly, the apparent decline in radiogenic risk past the AAI of 30–35 is currently unexplained.

At this point it is not known if the effects of AAI are only to change the slope of the dose–response curve or if, for example, they also may alter the shape of the dose–response curve or alter the dose-rate and dose fractionation effects. Experimental data indicate that in certain systems with tumor promotion, the promoters change both the height and the shape of the dose–response curve (Little, 1981; Fry, 1981). Human radiation-induced breast cancer might be a good candidate system in which to see such promoter effects, because certain endogenous hormones are thought to serve as tumor promoters. It is to be hoped that it will be possible to analyze human data for such factors within the next few years.

The findings on variations in radiogenic risk according to AAI are also of importance in understanding the biology and epidemiology of breast cancer. They confirm the importance of events related to menarche and age at first childbirth as determinants of breast cancer risk. Interestingly, they do not particularly support the concept that factors having to do with menopause are of importance for breast cancer risk. However, the negative evidence concerning radiation induction of cancer at menopause cannot be construed as ruling out hormonal influences or other factors at that age.

One of the most intriguing findings is that breast irradiation in the first decade of life causes female breast cancer. One might have hypothesized that irradiation to the prepubertal breast—when there is little cellular proliferation and little estrogen stimulation—would lead to little carcinogenic effect. In fact, after a substantial latency period, the opposite was found. The risk appears to be high, comparable with that from irradiation at ages 10–19 (Tokunaga et al, 1982). Thus, it is clear that breast tissue is particularly susceptible to carcinogenic effects before adulthood.

The high sensitivity to radiation at young ages indicates the importance of early environmental exposures for breast cancer risk. This high sensitivity and the accompanying long latency period suggest that radiation affects some early stage of the malignant tranformation process. The diminished breast cancer response for older AAI may reflect a diminution with advancing age in some endogenous factor(s) that translate the early stage lesion into an intermediate stage lesion, or may reflect a diminution in cellular proliferative activity, such that the cells are less sensitive to an initiating event.

Finding that the breast is especially sensitive to radiation at or before the time of the first childbirth augments the oft documented but unexplained epidemiologic finding that young age at first childbirth is somehow protective against breast cancer. Drife (1979, 1981) has recently reported that breast cells from nulliparous women differ in histology and in hormone responsiveness from those of age-matched primiparous women. It would be of interest to compare radiation effects upon breast cells from nulliparous and parous women.

Because the irradiated women who sustained high doses are at considerably heightened risk of breast cancer, they represent prime populations for the study of cofactors in breast cancer and for intervention studies to attempt to diminish risk. While intervention studies might complicate the analyses of the radiation effects, the trade-offs are that they could provide new information on coacting factors and could potentially benefit these women at high risk.

REFERENCES

Bailar JC (1976) Mammography: A contrary view. Ann Intern Med 84:77–84.

Bailar JC (1977) Screening for early breast cancer: Pros and cons. Cancer 39:2783–2795.

Baral E, Larsson L, Mattsson B (1977) Breast cancer following irradiation of the breast. Cancer 40:2905–2910.

Baverstock KF, Papworth D, Vennart J (1981) Risks of radiation at low dose rates. Lancet i 430–433.

Boice JD (1978) Multiple chest fluoroscopies and the risk of breast cancer. Paper presented at the XIIth Intl Cancer Congr, Oct 5–11, Buenos Aires, Argentina.

Boice JD, Hoover R (1981). Radiogenic breast cancer: Age effects and implications for models of human carcinogenesis. In: Burchenal JH and Oettgen H (eds.), Cancer: Achievements, challenges, and prospects for the 1980s. New York: Grune and Stratton, pp 209–221.

Boice JD, Land C, Shore R, Norman J, Tokunga M (1979) Risk of breast cancer following low-dose radiation exposure. Radiology 131:589–597.

Boice JD, Monson R (1977) Breast cancer in women after repeated fluoroscopic examinations of the chest. J Natl Cancer Inst 59:823–832.

Boice JD, Stone B Interaction between radiation and other breast cancer risk factors. In: Late biological effects of ionizing radiation. Vienna: International Atomic Energy Agency, pp 231–247.

Boice JD, Rosenstein M, Trout ED (1978) Estimation of breast doses and breast cancer risk associated with repeated fluoroscopic chest examinations of women with tuberculosis. Radiat Res 73:373–390.

Chiacchierini RP, Lundin F (1979) Risk-benefit analyses for reduced dose mammography. In: Logan W and Muntz E (eds.), Reduced dose mammography. New York: Masson, p. 61.

Cook DC, Dent O, Hewitt D (1974) Breast cancer following multiple chest fluoroscopy: the Ontario experience. Canadian Med Assoc J 111:406–410.

Delarue NC, Gale G, Ronald A (1975) Multiple fluoroscopy of the chest: Carcinogenicity for the female breast and implications for breast cancer screening programs. Canadian Med Assoc J 112:1405–1410.

Drife JO (1979) Evolution, menstruation and breast cancer. In: Bulbrook R and Taylor D (eds.), Commentaries on research in breast disease. New York: Liss, pp 1–23.

Drife JO (1981) Breast cancer, pregnancy, and the pill. Br Med J 283:778–779.

Dvoretsky PM, Woodard E, Bonfiglio T, Hempelmann L, Morse I (1980) The pathology of breast cancer in women irradiated for acute postpartum mastitis. Cancer 46:2257–2262.

Evans RD (1966) The effect of skeletally deposited alpha-ray emitters in man. Br J Radiol 39:881–895.

Fry RJ (1981) Experimental radiation carcinogenesis: What have we learned? Radiat Res 87:224–239.

Grundy GW, Uzman B (1973) Breast cancer associated with repeated fluoroscopy. J Natl Cancer Inst 51:1339–1340.

Hildreth N, Shore R, Hempelmann L (1983) Risk of breast cancer among women receiving radiation treatment in infancy for thymic enlargement. Lancet ii:273.

Howe GR (1984) The epidemiology of radiogenic breast cancer. In: Boice J and Fraumeni J (eds.), Radiation carcinogenesis: Epidemiology and biologic signficance. (1977) New York: Raven Press, pp 119–29.

ICRP (1977) Recommendations of the international commission on radiological protection. ICRP Publ 26. Oxford: Pergamon.

Kato H, Schull W (1982) Studies of the mortality of A-bomb survivors. 7. Mortality, 1950–1978: Part I. Cancer mortality. Radiat Res 90:395–432.

Kelsey JL (1979) A review of the epidemology of human breast cancer. Epidemiol Rev 1:74–109.

Kitabatake T, Kurokawa S, Yamasaki M, Sato T, Kurokawa H (1975) A prospective survey on the incidence of chest malignancies after repeated fluoroscopy during artificial pneumothorax therapy for pulmonary tuberculosis. Nippon Igaku Hoshasen Gakkai Zasshi 35:895–899.

Land CE (1980) Low-dose radiation—A cause of breast cancer? Cancer 46:868–873.

Land CE, Boice J, Shore R, Norman J, Tokunaga (1980) Breast cancer risk low-dose exposures to ionizing radiation: Results of parallel analysis of three exposed populations of women. J Natl Cancer Inst 65:353–376.

Land CE, McGregor D (1979) Breast cancer incidence among atomic bomb survivors: Implications for radiobiologic risk at low doses. J Natl Cancer Inst 62:17–21.

Little JB (1981) Influence of noncarcinogenic secondary factors on radiation carcinogenesis. Radiat Res 87:240–250.

MacKenzie I (1965) Breast cancer following multiple fluoroscopies. Br J Cancer 19:1–8.

McGregor DH, Land C, Choi K, Tokuoka S, Liu P, Wakabayashi T, Beebe G (1977) Breast cancer incidence among atomic bomb survivors, Hiroshima and Nagasaki, 1950–69. J Natl Cancer Inst 59:799–811.

Mettler FA, Hempelmann L, Dutton A, Pifer J, Toyooka E, Ames W (1969) Breast neoplasms in women treated with x-rays for acute postpartum mastitis. A pilot study. J Natl Cancer Inst 43:803–811.

Myrden JA, Hiltz J (1969) Breast cancer following multiple fluoroscopies during artificial pneumothorax treatment of pulmonary tuberculosis. Canadian Med Assoc J 100:1032–1034.

Myrden JA, Quinlan J (1974) Breast carcinoma following multiple fluoroscopies with pneumothorax treatment of pulmonary tuberculosis. Ann R Coll Phys Surg Canada 7:45.

NCRP (1980) Influence of dose and its distribution in time on dose-response relationships for low-LET radiations. Washington, DC: National Council on Radiation Protection and Measurements (NCRP Report no. 64).

Pochin EE (1969) Long term hazards of radioiodine treatment of thyroid carcinoma. UICC Monogr Series 12:293–304.

Sawada H (1959) Sexual function in female atomic bomb survivors 1949–57: Hiroshima. Atomic Bomb Casualty Commission. Technical Report TR 34–59.

Sherman GJ, Howe G, Miller A, Rosenstein M (1978) Organ dose per unit exposure resulting from fluoroscopy for artificial pneumothorax. Health Phys 35:259–269.

Shore RE, Hempelmann L, Kowaluk E, Mansur P, Pasternack B, Albert R, Haughie G (1977) Breast neoplasms in women treated with x-rays for acute postpartum mastitis. J Natl Cancer Inst 59:813–822.

Shore RE, Woodard E, Hempelmann L, Pasternack B (1980) Synergism between radiation and other risk factors for breast cancer. Prev Med 9:815–822.

Smith PG, Doll R (1976) Late effects of x-irradiation in patients treated for metropathia haemorrhagica. Br J Radiol 49:224–232.

Stebbings JH, Lucas H, Stehney A (1984) Mortality from cancers of major sites in female radium dial workers. Am J Indust Med 5:435–459.

Tokunaga M, Norman J, Asano M, Tokuoka S, Ezaki H, Nishimori I, Tsuji Y (1979) Malignant breast tumors among atomic bomb survivors, Hiroshima and Nagasaki 1950–74. J Natl Cancer Inst 62:1347–1359.

Tokunaga M, Land C, Yamamoto T, Asano M, Tokuoka S, Ezaki H, Nishimori I (1982) Breast cancer in Japanese A-bomb survivors. Lancet ii:924.

Tokunaga M, Land C, Yamamoto T, Asano M, Tokuoka S, Ezaki H, Nishimori I (1984) Breast cancer among atomic bomb survivors. In: Boice J and Fraumeni J (eds), Radiation carcinogenesis: New York: Raven Press, pp 45–56.

Tokuoka S, Asano M, Yamamoto T, Tokunaga M, Sakamoto G, Hartmann W, Hutter R, Land C, Henson D (1984) Histologic review of breast cancer cases in survivors of atomic bombs in Hiroshima and Nagasaki, Japan. Cancer 54:849–854.

Wanebo CK, Johnson K, Sato K, Thorslund T (1968) Breast cancer after exposure to the atomic bombings of Hiroshima and Nagasaki. N Engl J Med 279:667–671.

Woodard ED, Hempelmann L, Janus J, Logan W, Dean P (1982) Screening for breast cancer in a high-risk series. J Surg Oncol 19:31–35.

CARCINOGENIC EFFECTS
OF RADIATION ON THE HUMAN
THYROID GLAND

ROY E. SHORE, Ph.D., DR. P.H., LOUIS H. HEMPELMANN, M.D., AND ELIZABETH D. WOODARD, M.D., M.P.H.

Ionizing radiation exposure was first associated with the induction of human thyroid cancer in 1950 (Duffy and Fitzgerald). Since then radiation has been established beyond doubt as a cause of human thyroid neoplasms. Although thyroid neoplasms in animals can also be induced by iodine deficiency, chemical carcinogens, and goitrogens, as well as by exposure to ionizing radiation, the latter is the only known cause of thyroid cancer in humans (Hempelmann and Furth, 1978). Retrospective case studies in human populations first pointed out the association of prior irradiation and thyroid cancer. Although such studies have been enormously valuable in documenting the natural history of the disease and the best methods of management, they provide little information on quantitative aspects of carcinogenesis. Because recent, large scale, long-term prospective studies of thyroid cancer do provide quantitative information about risks, dose-response, and host factors, they will be featured in this chapter.

PROSPECTIVE STUDIES OF THYROID NEOPLASMS SUBSEQUENT TO X-RAY THERAPY

Rochester Thymus Irradiation Study

This study of about 2800 children treated with x-rays for alleged thymic enlargement and their 5000+ nonirradiated control siblings was first reported on in 1955 (Simpson et al). These subjects were almost all less than 1 yr of age at the time of treatment (between 1926 and 1957) and were evenly divided by sex. Thyroid doses were estimated from the factors in the radiation therapy records

From the Department of Environmental Medicine, New York University Medical Center, New York, New York, the Department of Radiology, University of Rochester School of Medicine and Dentistry, Rochester, New York, and the Department of Preventive, Family and Rehabilitation Medicine, University of Rochester School of Medicine and Dentistry.

and ranged from 5 rad to more than 1000 rad with 60% receiving <50 rad (Hempelmann et al, 1967, 1975). Therapy was given in one to eleven treatments, separated by 1–20+ days, with an individual treatment delivering from 5 to >300 rad to the thyroid gland. Thus, there was a modest amount of dose fractionation.

The subjects have been followed for up to 45 yr, with an average follow-up of about 30 yr (Shore et al, 1985). Thirty cases of thyroid carcinoma and 59 benign thyroid neoplasms were diagnosed in the irradiated population, compared with one malignant and eight benign neoplams in almost twice the number of nonirradiated sibling controls. The relative risk in the irradiated series was 45 (90% CI= 32, 61) for thyroid cancer and 15 (90% CI= 8, 28) for benign thyroid neoplasms. The thyroid–cancer induction intervals ranged from 6 to 39 yr.

The strengths of this study are the wide range of doses, the high follow-up rate, and the long length of follow-up. On the other hand, there were uncertainties in the thyroid dose for a subgroup of irradiated subjects who were treated with an intermediate size port; there was a potential surveillance bias due to publicity given to the issue of head and neck irradiation by the press; and there is a question of compromised T-cell mediated immunocompetence in the irradiated group (Reddy et al, 1976).

Cincinnati Study

This is an update of a study of persons given x-ray treatments in childhood for benign diseases, first reported in 1960 (Saenger et al, 1960; Maxon et al, 1980). The 2230 subjects on the original roster had been treated with x-rays for a variety of benign diseases of the head and neck at a mean age of 3.6 yr. About 960 other matched patients with the same diseases—but without x-ray treatment—served as controls. The rate of successful follow-up of the irradiated subjects was low (57%). Sixteen malignant and 15 benign tumors of the thyroid gland were found in the irradiated group, compared with one malignant and two benign thyroid neoplasms found in the controls. Based on a subsample of 312 with recorded radiation treatment factors, the mean thyroid dose for the total group was estimated to be 290 rad per course of treatment, with up to three courses administered. The weakness of this study lies primarily in the poor follow-up rate and the absence of thyroid dose estimates for most irradiated subjects.

Studies of Children Treated with X-rays for Scalp Ringworm

There have been two studies of persons given x-ray treatments to the scalp for tinea capitis infections. The first study of persons in New York City was published in 1968 (Albert and Omran) and the second in Israel appeared in 1974 (Modan et al). In both studies, careful dosimetric measurements were carried out on phantoms to obtain organ-specific doses, particularly for the thyroid gland for the x-ray technique used. In both studies the estimated thyroid doses were of the same order of magnitude (<10 rad), but here the similarity of the two studies ends. The Israeli study was highly positive for thyroid cancer induction, whereas, the New York study was negative.

The Israeli population consisted of 10,842 persons treated with x-rays for tinea capitis between 1948 and 1960 and a like number of carefully matched controls. A second control series was composed of 5400 untreated siblings of the index series, for a total of 16,242 controls. In the irradiated series 29 thyroid cancers have been found versus eight among controls (Ron and Modan, 1980, 1984). The relative risk (RR) of thyroid cancer in the irradiated group was 5.4 (90% CI= 2.7, 10.8) compared with the combined controls. The latent period between treatment and cancer was 4–28 yr (where 31 yr was the maximum length of follow-up for any subject). This is an excellent prospective study with a large population, well controlled except that there was no control group with tinea infection.

The second study, in New York City, involved a smaller population of tinea capitis patients (Albert and Omran, 1968; Shore et al, 1976; Shore, 1982). The irradiated population consisted of about 2200 patients treated for tinea capitis between 1940 and 1959. The controls consisted of about 1400 persons who were treated for tinea capitis by topical medications only. The two groups had almost the same age and follow-up periods (mean, 26 yr) and both were predominantly male. The results show an increased incidence of certain tumors of the head and neck (see Chapter 21), but no cases of thyroid cancer were found in either group. All of the eight cases of thyroid adenoma occurred in the x-irradiated series.

Studies Involving Screening of Neck Irradiated Young Adults

There have been a number of programs throughout the U.S. involving recall of patients treated in radiation therapy departments for various benign diseases (DeGroot et al, 1977), but the greatest interest has been centered in the Chicago area where it is believed that more than 70,000 patients were treated in the 1940s and 1950s (DeGroot and Paloyan, 1973). Despite the fact that the irradiated populations were well defined in x-ray therapy records of the local hospitals, the follow-up rate has usually been poor, and often dependent on mass media publicity with little effort to trace the patients. Although valuable in detecting cases of unsuspected thyroid cancer, the data obtained in these studies usually cannot be used to determine risk estimates or other quantitative factors in carcinogenesis. Only one will be summarized here, the Michael Reese (Chicago) program, because it is the largest and most complete.

A roster of 5266 patients given x-ray treatments (between 1939 and 1962) to the head and neck region, usually to the tonsillar area, was developed using the Michael Reese Hospital's x-ray therapy records (Schneider et al, 1978, 1980). An effort was made to trace these patients in 1974 but only 49% were contacted and only 28% were examined. The work-up included radioimaging of the thyroid gland using Technetium-99m and a gamma camera equipped with a pinhole collimator. This program was unusual in that, when thyroid abnormalities were diagnosed by scintiscan, surgery was performed even in the absence of palpable thyroid nodules. The radiation factors were documented, and the mean thyroid dose was estimated to be about 780 rad of 200 kVp x-rays with a range of about 200–1500 rad (Colman et al, 1976; Schneider et al, 1978).

Of the 2189 subjects who responded, 209 had thyroid surgery before the recall program began in 1974. Of these, 66 patients had malignant thyroid disease, 112 had benign neoplastic disease, and in 31 cases the diagnosis was unknown. An additional 115 carcinomas (including occult cancers <1.5 cm in diameter) and 202 benign neoplasms were discovered by palpation and scintigraphic screening. Combining these data, a total of 181 cases of thyroid cancer occurred in the 2578 subjects seen or contacted (a 7% prevalence), and an additional 314 (12%) had benign neoplastic lesions.

The major strength of the study was the large number of thyroid cancers available for analysis, but the radiation-thyroid publicity, the low follow-up rate, and the absence of a control population with comparable screening make the study potentially subject to biases due to sample selection and nonequivalent surveillance.

PROSPECTIVE STUDIES AFTER EXPOSURE TO [131]I

Cooperative Thyrotoxicosis Therapy Study

In this study, the records of about 30,600 hyperthyroid patients were collected from 25 thyroid clinics (Dobyns et al, 1974). About 19,200 patients had been treated with ^{131}I and 11,400 with surgery or antithyroid drugs between 1946 and 1964. The median age at treatment was 47 yr, with only 2% <20 yr of age. A total of 19 cases of thyroid cancer (0.1%) and 44 adenomas (0.2%) were found in the patients treated with ^{131}I, whereas, eight cases of cancer (0.07%) and 26 adenomas (0.2%) were diagnosed in the patients treated by surgery or drugs. Five of the 19 cases of cancer in the group treated with ^{131}I were anaplastic or spindle cell in type; all had occurred with 5 yr of treatment. The rate of thyroid cancer following ^{131}I therapy was not significantly higher than that after other forms of treatment. Hoffman et al (1984) recently reported on a longer follow-up of about 1000 of these patients.

The interpretation of these data is problematic. First, it is not known how the preexisting thyroid disease may have modified the effect of the radiation. Second, the average follow-up time since treatment with ^{131}I was 8 yr, barely longer than the minimum latent period for thyroid cancer induction. Third, 1280 patients in the surgical category were also treated later with ^{131}I, but were counted as controls (including one case with thyroid cancer).

Swedish Patients Given Therapeutic [131]I

At the Radiumhemmet in Sweden, over 4500 patients were given one to three courses of ^{131}I, with doses estimated at 6000–10,000 rad per course (Holm et al, 1980a; Holm, 1984). Most of the patients were hyperthyroid, and the remainder were euthyroid patients who suffered from heart disease. The patients were 84% female with an average age of treatment of 56 yr. The incidence of thyroid cancer in these patients was determined by searching the records of the Swedish Cancer Registry. A total of four thyroid cancers were observed, where 3.8 were expected (based on general population rates). Thus, the negative results of this study agree with that of the Cooperative Thyrotoxicosis Study. The study is limited by the high thyroid doses and by not having comparison cases as controls; this is especially important because the subjects were treated for a thyroid abnormality.

Ignoring for the moment the methodologic limitations of these therapeutic studies, the high doses of radiation by ^{131}I apparently had little, if any, carcinogenic effect on the diseased thryoid tissue. This supports the generally held impression that the high doses of radiation (many thousands of rads) involved in ^{131}I therapy damage the cells so severely (as evidenced by the prevalence of myxedema in the treated patients) that the capacity for proliferation is lost (i.e., the thyroid cells have been sterilized).

Swedish Study of Patients with Diagnostic Doses of [131]I

A total of 16,575 patients (79% female; mean age, 44 yr) were given diagnostic doses of [131]I (Holm et al, 1980b, 1983). The mean amount of activity used for the test was 60 μCi with 16% of the patients receiving more than one dose. The average radiation dose to the thyroid gland was about 60 rad (Holm et al, 1980c). The patients were followed for 11–29 yr, with a mean of 19 yr. Eleven cases of thyroid cancer were diagnosed in the patient population 5 yr or more after ^{131}I exposure, whereas, 12.2 were expected based on general population rates. Among the approximately 1000 patients who were under age 20 at irradiation (with a mean thyroid dose of 160 rad), no thyroid cancers were observed. Thus, there was no indication of an increase in thyroid cancer incidence among patients given diagnostic doses of [131]I. This is notable in that, based on the thyroid dose and on the PY (person–yr) after a 5-yr minimal latency period, and assuming a risk of $3/10^6$ PY-rad, an excess of about 49 cases of cancer would have been expected. The weakness of the study is that the patients were receiving diagnostic workups for suspected thyroid abnormalities, but no control group of persons with similar abnormalities was available for comparison. A similar study by the Center for Devices and Radiological Health of about 3000 children who received diagnostic[131]I is nearing completion, but the data have not yet been published (Chiachierrini, 1985 personal communication).

STUDIES OF EXPOSURE TO NUCLEAR EXPLOSIONS OR FALLOUT

Residents of Hiroshima and Nagasaki

Less information has historically been available for thyroid cancer than for many other organs from the study of the Japanese atomic bomb survivors. This has occurred because the low case-fatality rate for thyroid cancer makes the extensive mortality data of limited value for the thyroid. However, data have now been reported based on the tumor registries in Nagasaki and Hiroshima (Wakabayashi et al, 1983; Prentice et al, 1982), as well as on those obtained in the biennial examination program (Parker et al, 1974). Wakabayashi et al (1983) have studied the cancers reported in the Nagasaki tumor registry among A-bomb survivors for the years 1959–1978. Of the 71 thyroid cancers observed, 43 were clinically evident and 28 were occult (found at autopsy). For the clinically evident tumors there was a highly significant increasing trend with dose (p < 0.001), but not for the occult tumors; thus, the trend could not be explained away as a bias in the distribution of autopsied individuals. They also reported there was no differential migration away from Nagasaki with respect to dose, which could account for these results.

Prentice et al (1982) studied thyroid cancers among A-bomb survivors in both the Hiroshima (1959–1970) and Nagasaki (1959–1978) tumor registries. The registries documented 62 nonoccult cancers in Hiroshima and 50 in Nagasaki. Their analyses particularly focused on the shape of the dose–response curve for gamma irradiation, and the relative effects of gamma and neutron irradiation. The T65 dose estimates were used with recent minor dosimetric modifications and with dose attenuation to the thyroid gland factored in. It is of interest that the linear risk coefficients for Nagasaki and Hiroshima were very similar—0.36% and 0.43% increases in relative risk per rad, respectively. Another potentially important finding concerned the effects of thyroid screening. Among participants in the Adult Health Study, who had biennial thyroid screening, the diagnosed thyroid cancer incidence was about two times as high as among other subjects (after adjusting for dose and other factors). This provides an estimate of the size of potential biases introduced in studies in which the irradiated group has been screened while the controls have not.

Marshall Islanders Exposed to Radioactive Fallout from Thermonuclear Test in 1954

The Marshallese exposed to radioactive fallout from a thermonuclear test in 1954 are among the most intensely studied of any group subjected to thyroid irradiation (Conard, 1977; Conard et al, 1980). The exposures occurred on three atolls (Rongelap, Ailingnae, and Utirik) that lay in the path of the cloud of radioactive fission products generated by the test explosion. To serve as controls for these irradiated persons, 600 Marshallese were selected on atolls outside the radioactive fallout pattern. The radioisotopes responsible for the irradiation of the thyroid included the short-lived radioisotopes of iodine (^{132}I, ^{133}I, and ^{135}I), as well as the longer-lived ^{131}I. The short-lived isotopes were thought to have delivered about three times as much radiation to the thyroid gland of the Marshallese as did ^{131}I, and at a much higher dose-rate. Gamma irradiation also added to the total dose, so that ^{131}I contributed only about 10%–15% of the total thyroid dose (Adams et. al., 1984). The thyroid doses of these subjects were also difficult to estimate because of the very limited information available retrospectively.

The irradiated subjects were carefully followed first by periodic visits of American medical personnel and in the last decade or so by a resident medical team. The first radiation effect noted was growth retardation in young children; 8 yr after exposure, this was recognized as the result of hypothyroidism. Throughout the intervening years, numerous cases of thyroid nodularity have developed in the irradiated subjects. Children were particularly sensitive to the induction of thyroid nodularity, as is illustrated by the fact that 17 of 22 exposed children on Rongelop, under the age of 10 yr, have developed nodular thyroid glands. Three subjects were in utero at the time of exposure, of whom two have developed thyroid nodules. Women were more susceptible than men to the carcinogenic action of radiation. All seven cases of thyroid cancer in the irradiated population, and two of the five cases in the unirradiated population, occurred in women.

Even though a great amount of effort has been expended on this study, there are major limitations in using it to define quantitative aspects of thyroid cancer induction. The limitations include: the small numbers of people and cancers, uncertainty as to thyroid dose, inclusion of occult thyroid cancers in the tally, unequal intensity of follow-up of the irradiated and control subjects, and the prophylactic thyroid-suppression treatment program begun in 1965.

Children Exposed to Radioactive Fallout from the Nevada Atomic Bomb Tests

In Utah, Nevada, and Arizona a group of 5179 children, 11–18 yr of age, were examined annually from 1965 to 1971 for evidence of thyroid disease (Rallison et al, 1974, 1975). Of these, 1378 lived downwind from the Nevada test site and were believed to be exposed to radioactive iodine. The remaining 3453 children lived in other locations where they were likely to have been exposed to much lower levels of radioactive fallout. The thyroid exposure of the first group was primarily due to ^{131}I in milk from cows that grazed on contaminated forage. (By the time the milk was drunk, the short-lived isotopes of iodine would have largely decayed.) Estimates of the average thyroid doses have ranged from 30 to 300+ rad; the BEIR III (NAS, 1980) report used 120 rad as a best (but by no means certain) estimate.

Twelve thyroid nodules (unaccompanied by goiter or other pathology) were found in the exposed subjects (8.7 of 1000 persons), and 16 nodules were detected in the controls (4.6 of 1000 persons). Benign neoplasms were surgically removed in six exposed subjects and in two controls. Only two thyroid cancers were found, but these were both in the control group (Rallison et al, 1975). This study had certain methodologic limitations, such as major uncertainties as to thyroid dose, a small sample size, and an interval between exposure and examination (10–17 yr), all of which was less than optimal.

DOSE–RESPONSE CURVES AND LOW-DOSE DATA

Shape of the Dose–Response Curve

In spite of the many studies of thyroid neoplasms subsequent to irradiation, only four provide intrastudy dose–response information. Maxon et al (1980) reported their results by number of courses of treatment, where each course on the average delivered about 290 rad to the thyroid. The numbers of thyroid-cancers per persons for one, two, and three courses of treatment, respectively, were 9 of 1157 (0.8%), 3 of 99 (3.0%), and 4 of 10 (40%). They suggested that the curve had quadratic curvature, but presented no statistical evaluation of the dose–response results.

Colman et al (1976) indicated that the Michael Reese thyroid cancer data were compatible with a linear dose–response curve with a slope of about $4/10^6$ PY-rad, where the doses were in the range of about 200–1500 rad (although only a small percentage had doses less than 600 rad). The numbers and rates at each dose point were not given, so it is unclear if other types of curves may have fitted as well or better than the linear curve.

In the most recent analyses of the Rochester thymus irradiation study (Shore et al, 1985) the dose–response curve for thyroid cancers had a strong linear component, but the quadratic component was not significant (p>0.4). The linear dose–response curve gave a risk coefficient of 3.5 ± 0.8/10^6 PY-rad.

The Nagasaki tumor registry data showed a strong dose–response relationship for nonoccult thyroid cancers (Wakabayashi et al, 1983). The linear model provided a good fit to the data and yielded an estimate of 2.2 ± 0.7/10^6 PY-rad. The pure quadratic model could be ruled out, although a linear-quadratic model could not be; however, in the latter model only the linear term was significant.

Prentice et al (1982) analyzed the thyroid cancer data for the LSS (life–span study) in both Nagasaki and Hiroshima, controlling for potential differences related to sex, city, age, and thyroid screening in the biennial health examination program. Their full regression model included terms for gamma, gamma-squared, and neutron dose. In testing for Nagasaki and Hiroshima separately and for both cities together, they found that neutron dose failed to contribute (all p-values >0.3). This will be further discussed under RBE. The linear gamma term was highly significant (p = 0.0001 for both cities), whereas, the gamma-squared term was marginally significant in the negative direction (i.e., a supralinear curve). Inspection of the tabled data indicate that the negative curvature probably came about because of low rates at high doses, compatible with "cell inactivation" when the doses and dose-rates are high. The simple linear model yielded a risk coefficient of a 0.38% increase in the relative risk per rad.

In summary, three of the four studies with dose–response data agree that a linear curve provides a reasonable fit to the data. The remaining study (Maxon et al, 1980) was based on relatively few thyroid cancers, the analysis was by number of courses of treatment (with a wide range of doses at each data point) not dose per se, and the thyroid doses were nearly all high. Thus, its evidence against a linear curve is not compelling. Because of the sparsity of the data in these epidemiologic studies, one cannot choose decisively between a linear and a linear-quadratic curve. However, it seems safe to say that, at least in the high dose-rates in these studies, a pure quadratic curve is very unlikely.

Thyroid Cancer in Low-Dose Studies

Ron and Modan (1980, 1984) reported a clear excess of thyroid cancers among children irradiated for ringworm of the scalp, for whom the estimated average thyroid dose was 9 rad per course of treatment. About 9% of the subjects were known to be treated twice, so the average total dose was about 10 rad. From their data we calculated a risk estimate of 7.7/10^6 PY-rad (95% CI= 3.0, 17.2).

Some investigators have questioned the dosimetry in this series, based on concerns over head size, accurate placement of the ports, squirming of the child, and/or shield slippage during treatment. There have been four dosimetric studies of the scalp-ringworm irradiation procedure (Werner et al, 1968; Lee and Youmans, 1970; Harley et al, 1976; Modan et al, 1977), which shed a certain amount of light on these questions. Lee and Youmans (1970) found that the smaller head size of a 3 yr old child increased the thyroid dose by a factor of about 40% relative to the average 6 yr old child, whereas, it was decreased by a third for a 12 yr old child. Thus, one can estimate thyroid doses of about 13, 9, and 6 rad for children of ages 3, 6, and 12, respectively. Modan et al (1977) found a 50% variation in thyroid doses associated with variations in head and shielding positions. Harley et al (1976) found a 50% increase in dose when the lead-rubber apron was removed from the neck. Taking all these factors into account, one can estimate the probable upper limit of thyroid dose, i.e., a 3 yr old who wiggled so as to receive maximum dose and to displace the lead apron, might have a thyroid dose of about (factors: average dose X head size X right/wrong head position X shielding slipped/in place); 9 X 1.4 X 1.3 X 1.5 = 25 rad. On the other hand, a 12 yr old with ideal beam positioning and no wiggling might have a dose of about: 9 X 0.7 X 0.8 X 1 = 5 rad.

Another question has concerned possible biases in case-finding. Were irradiated subjects sensitized to the possibility of thyroid cancer risk, so that they more often had screening or early detection of the disease? Modan (1979) has indicated that, while this might be true to a degree in recent years, the excess thyroid cancer risk was found before that was the case. In fact, the magnitude of the excess risk was comparable in the earlier report (Modan et al, 1974) and the more recent reports (Ron and Modan, 1980, 1984), so biased case-finding seems to be an unlikely explanation of the excess.

The second potential bias lies in the fact that documentation was poor for possible radiation treatments of scalp ringworm prior to immigration to Israel (Ron and Modan, 1980). Thus, the total thyroid dose to an unknown fraction of subjects could actually have been two or more times as great as the putative dose, which would lead to a spuriously high risk estimate. The magnitude of this possible bias cannot be assessed without further information.

It is a seeming paradox that, while one low-dose study found the highest risk estimate of any study, the other low-dose study found no excess risk of thyroid cancer. Shore et al (1976, 1982) found no thyroid cancers in their series of about 2200 children who were irradiated for ringworm of the scalp, although they did find eight thyroid adenomas (versus 0 among controls). One factor in not finding an effect in this study was the preponderance of males (87%) in the irradiated group; in several studies females have shown two to four times as much radiation-induction of thyroid cancer as males, as noted below. In addition, the irradiated population in the New York study was only 20% as large as in the Israeli study. The question is whether or not the findings of the two studies are compatible with each other. Based on the sex-specific absolute risk estimates from the Rochester thymus irradiation study (plus the expected spontaneous incidence), a total of about 1.2 thyroid cancers would have been expected in the New York study. This is statistically compatible ($p > 0.6$) with the zero observed. The sex-specific absolute risk estimates from the Israeli study yield a total expectation of 1.9 thyroid cancers, which is also statistically compatible ($p > 0.3$) with the zero observed.

While most of the attention concerning low-dose carcinogenic effects on the thyroid has concentrated on the scalp ringworm irradiation studies, two other studies contribute substantial data, as well. The Nagasaki data (Wakabayashi et al, 1983) show six nonoccult thyroid cancers in 66,648 PY in the 0-dose group, and 9 of 117,301 in the 1–9 rad (kerma) group. Based on their reported observed and expected values (controlled for age, sex, and year of diagnosis), the relative risk was 0.81 (i.e., no excess risk was seen). However, a failure to detect an effect given the low thyroid dose (mean of approximately 2.3 rad) and the small number of cancers involved is not too surprising. An analysis shows their result is statistically compatible with absolute risk values even as great as $30/10^6$ PY-rad. A similar examination of the low-dose Hiroshima data could not be undertaken, because Prentice et al (1982) did not report a table with the appropriate dose groupings.

The other study that contributes low-dose information is the Rochester thymus irradiation series. If one examines those with thyroid doses of 1–10 rad, there is only one thyroid cancer. Although this is a numerical excess over the rate in the control group, it is not significant. One has to include doses up to 30 rad (mean dose, 10.5 rad) to achieve significance. The thyroid cancers and PY are then 4 of 25,687 versus 1 of 118,113 among controls. These data give an absolute risk estimate of $14/10^6$ PY-rad, with a lower 95% confidence limit of $1.7/10^6$ PY-rad.

To summarize, of the four sets of low-dose data (average doses of about 10 rad or less), two indicated positive effects and two did not. Thus, the magnitude of low-dose effects is uncertain but, to be prudent, a linear extrapolation from higher doses should probably be assumed.

RADIATION QUALITY AND RBE EFFECTS

Until recently it was thought that variation in radiation quality (i.e., high LET versus low LET) could be studied in the Japanese A-bomb survivors by comparing the Hiroshima data, where there was thought to be a substantial neutron (high-LET) component, with the Nagasaki data, where the exposures were almost exclusively to low-LET gamma rays. The dosimetries are now being reassessed, however, and it appears probable that the neutron component in Hiroshima is substantially less than was formerly assumed. It seems likely, therefore, it will be a tenuous procedure at best to estimate the relative biological effectiveness (RBE) of neutron versus gamma exposures from the Japanese data. Using statistical regression procedures it is difficult or impossible to reliably determine the magnitude and shape of the separate gamma and neutron components when the two are highly correlated, as they were in Hiroshima (i.e., for two predictor variables, if the regression coefficient for one is positive, the other is very likely to be negative when they are highly correlated). Thus, for instance, Prentice et al (1982) were unable to demonstrate simultaneous gamma and neutron effects with their statistical model. To our knowledge, there are no other available data that will allow one to examine radiation quality factors in relation to thyroid cancer, so information on RBE values is not likely to be forthcoming.

DOSE RATE AND DOSE FRACTIONATION EFFECTS

Several experimental studies have reported that ^{131}I, which delivers its radiation dose over the course of 3–4 wk (7-day effective half-life), is several times less effective as a thyroid carcinogen than high dose-rate exposures (Walinder,

1972; Doniach, 1963). However, a recent experimental study reported an equal effectiveness of ^{131}I and x-rays in thyroid cancer induction (Lee et al, 1982).

The results of the human studies of [131] therapy have sometimes been used as evidence for a reduced effect at low dose rates. Unfortunately, these studies do not lend themselves to unambiguous interpretation. The U.S. Cooperative Thyrotoxicosis Study (Dobyns et al, 1974) had too short an average follow-up time to observe much tumor expression. Both that study and the Swedish ^{131}I therapy study (Holm et al, 1980a) had problems in that the doses were in the "cell inactivation" range, and the subjects were largely being treated for thyroid abnormalities that might have altered the thyroid tumor response in unknown ways. However, the Swedish study of diagnostic [131]I (Holm et al, 1980b) obviated the first two criticisms—the thyroid dose was only about 60 rad and the mean follow-up time was 19 yr—and no excess of thyroid cancers was found. Similarly, the Utah study of children who had been exposed to ^{131}I from atomic bomb fallout (with doses on the order of 100 rad) was negative for thyroid cancer (Rallison et al, 1975).

Thus, the data suggest that the thyroid cancer induction by low dose-rate ^{131}I irradiation is substantially lower than for high dose-rate irradiation. However, it should be noted that in most of these studies the irradiation was in adulthood and was given to already abnormal thyroids. One cannot exclude those factors as possible explanations of the apparent diminished response. There is also a "fly in the ointment": in the Marshall Islanders study of ^{131}I exposure a substantial thyroid response was observed. However, the Marshallese had a substantial exposure to gamma radiation and short-lived iodine isotopes, as well, such that 85%–90% of the dose was at high dose rates (Adams et al, 1984). Thus, that study is largely irrelevant to the issue of whether or not exposures at low dose rates have a lower effectiveness than those at high dose rates.

The only study in which dose fractionation effects have been analyzed is the Rochester thymus irradiation study. In the most recent analyses no fractionation effects were seen, but both the number of dose fractions and the number of thyroid cancers at lower doses were too few to have a very powerful test of fractionation effects (Shore et al, 1985).

TEMPORAL PATTERN OF RADIATION EFFECTS

Several studies indicate that thyroid cancer expression following irradiation begins between 5 and 10 yr postirradiation (Shore et al, 1980; Schneider et al, 1978; Ron and Modan, 1980), but the full force of tumor expression is not seen until 10 yr or more postirradiation.

There has been some disagreement in the literature as to the subsequent pattern of tumor expression. Armenian and Lilienfeld (1974) hypothesized that there was a lognormal distribution over time (i.e., a "wave" of excess tumors), which then tapered off to little or no excess by 30–35 yr postirradiation. Earlier reports of the Japanese A-bomb data (Beebe et al, 1977) suggested that this might indeed be the case. But the latest report (Wakabayashi et al, 1983) indicates that the risk continues unabated out to the maximum follow-up time of 33 yr.

The Michael Reese study (Schneider et al, 1978) also indicates an excess risk out to its maximum follow-up time of 33 yr, although the effect appears to be diminishing from its peak at about 20–25 yr postirradiation. Similarly the Rochester thymus irradiation study gives risk estimates for the periods 5–14, 15–24, 25–34, and 35–44 yr postirradiation of 2.0, 4.2, 2.9, and 2.4/10^6 PY-rad, respectively. Thus, excess risk has continued out to at least 40 yr postirradiation, but may be diminishing somewhat as time goes on. In summary, all the recent data agree that radiation induction of thyroid cancer continues for a long period of time, probably more than 40 yr, and a life-long risk appears to be a prudent and reasonable assumption.

Two other aspects of the temporal pattern bear mentioning. Schneider et al (1978) reported an inverse relationship between age at irradiation and tumor latency (i.e., the latency was longer for those irradiated at younger ages). However, other studies have not confirmed this finding. A second question is whether or not there is an inverse relationship between dose and tumor latency (i.e., does irradiation lead to earlier tumor development as well as an increase in rates?). Schneider et al (1978) did not find a significant relationship between dose and tumor latency, nor did the Rochester thymus irradiation study (Shore et al, 1985). Thus, such a relationship, if it exists, must be too small to be detected within the limits of the statistical power of these two studies.

HOST SUSCEPTIBILITY FACTORS AND SYNERGISM

A synergism of radiation with chemicals that stimulate thyroid tissue proliferation has been clearly shown in experimental studies (Christov, 1975; Doniach, 1974) with respect to thyroid tumor induction. Conversely, thyroid suppression diminishes the radiogenic risk (Doniach, 1974). There are no definitive data on proliferation effects in humans, although the apparent reduction in thyroid nodularity consequent to thyroid suppression therapy among the Marshall Islanders (Conard et al, 1980) is a consonant finding. Nothing is currently known from human studies about any other environmental agents that may be synergistic or antagonistic to radiation to the thyroid. The principal host susceptibility factors that have been studied are sex, age at irradiation (AAI), and Jewish ethnicity.

A number of studies have documented sex differences. For example, the Nagasaki A-bomb study (Wakabayashi et al, 1983) reported an excess risk of 2.9/10^6 PY-rad for females and 1.0 for males (values after converting kerma to thyroid dose) for a ratio of 2.9. Similarly, Prentice et al (1982) reported a ratio of about 3 for Hiroshima and Nagasaki combined. In the Rochester thymus series the female and male risk estimates were 5.3 and 2.1/10^6 PY-rad respectively, for a ratio of 2.5. In the Israeli scalp-ringworm series the respective risk estimates were about 18 and 4.7/10^6 PY-rad, for a ratio of 3.9. It is clear that radiation induction of thyroid cancer is greater in females than males. The natural incidence of thyroid cancer is also greater in females than males. This suggests that the effect of radiation may be to multiply the spontaneous risk by a constant (dose dependent) factor or, in other words, the relative risk model may be more appropriate than the absolute (additive) risk model for thyroid cancer.

The effects of AAI are less well documented, because most of the thyroid radiation studies have had a very limited range of AAI. The Marshall Islanders study has sometimes been cited as providing evidence for the increased sensitivity of childhood thyroids to radiation. The rate of thyroid nodules among the highest-dose children was extremely high, but the rate of thyroid cancers was actually comparable in children (<19 yr AAI; 4 of 127 = 3.1%) and in adults (19+ AAI; 3 of 123 = 2.4%), even though the thyroid doses were several times higher among children (Conard et al, 1980). (It should be noted that this comparison may be biased by the selective thyroid suppression therapy.)

Ron and Modan (1984) examined AAI in their scalp-ringworm irradiation study. Their data suggest greater thyroid cancer induction among those irradiated at ages 0–5 than for ages 6–15. However, the thyroid dose was also somewhat greater at younger ages (by approximately a factor of 1.4–2.0 according to Lee and Youmans [1970]), which may account for the difference.

The Japanese A-bomb data, where the AAI covers the lifespan, did show a clear age effect. The excess risk in Nagasaki was about $3.4/10^6$ PY-rad at AAI of 0–19, but only about 0.3 at ages 20+ (Wakabayashi et al, 1983). The analyses of Prentice et al (1982) for both cities corroborated the age effect; the RR per unit dose was clearly higher for AAI <30 than for 30+.

A final host susceptibility factor that has been examined is Jewish ethnicity. Hempelmann et al (1975) first noted that the Jewish subjects in their study apparently had more radiation-induced thyroid cancer than nonJewish subjects. A subsequent formal analysis (Shore et al, 1980) confirmed the interpretation, and the more recent (unpublished) data also support the finding. Although only 9% of the irradiated subjects were Jewish (but, because they tended to get high doses, they contributed 22% of the Py-rad), 47% of the thyroid cancers were in Jewish subjects. It is possible that part of all of this putative Jewish effect may have resulted from more careful thyroid surveillance among Jewish subjects, so it is not necessarily to be taken at face value. Because no other investigators have yet reported data broken down by Jewish ethnicity to corroborate or disconfirm the finding, it should be regarded as tentative at this time.

RISK ESTIMATION

Table 1 gives an overview of findings from the principal studies of external irradiation of the thyroid gland. Observed thyroid cancers and estimates of expected cancers are given. (It should be noted that in estimating expected values, it was not possible to take into account the increases in cancer detection associated with heightened surveillance in several of these populations.) The risk estimates in Table 1 are given in absolute risk form and relative risk form. The absolute risk estimates for juvenile irradiation are reasonably uniform, averaging about $3–4/10^6$ PY-rad, except for the scalp-ringworm studies, which produced a higher estimate. For the relative risk estimates, the values mostly vary from about 0.6% to 1.5% for childhood irradiation, except for the aberrant value from the tinea capitis data. Because there are uncertainties in the dose estimates for the scalp-ringworm studies, the risk estimates derived from them should be treated with caution.

TABLE 1 Thyroid Cancer After External Irradiation

Reference	Series	Number of persons	Type of control[a]	Mean dose (rad)	Observed	Expected	Absolute risk[b]	RR[b] (%)
Wakabayashi et al, 1983; Prentice et al, 1982	A-Bomb, age < 30 (≥ 50 rad)	4377	U	~130	26	2.8	3.4[c]	1.5[c]
Wakabayashi et al, 1983; Prentice et al, 1982	A-Bomb, age ≥ 30 (≥ 50 rad)	2782	U	~130	6	2.6	0.3[c]	—
Shore et al, 1985	Thymus x-ray—Rochester	2652	S,P	140	30	0.7	3.5[c]	0.6[c]
Schneider et al, 1978	Tonsil x-ray—M. Reese	2578	P	780	181	~2	~3.6	~0.6
Maxon et al, 1980	Head/neck x-ray—Cinn.	1266	D	290	16	~0.4	~1.7	~1.3
Ron and Modan, 1984; Shore, 1982	Scalp ringworm x-ray—Israel; New York	13,060	U;S;D	10	29	—	~6.2	~11.8

[a] U, unexposed group; S, siblings; D, same disease control; P, general population control.
[b] Absolute risk = excess cancers/10^6 persons/rad/yr; RR = Relative risk, percent increment/rad.
[c] Estimates based on the dose–response analyses of the original authors. Estimates marked "~" were made by us, based on the original data and, in some cases, our estimates of expected values.

Supported in part by Center Program Grants ES-00260 from the National Institute of Environmental Health Sciences and CA-13343 from the National Cancer Institute to the Institute of Environmental Medicine, New York University Medical Center, and Grant CA-19764 from the National Cancer Institute to the Department of Preventive, Family and Rehabilitation Medicine, University of Rochester School of Medicine and Dentistry.

REFERENCES

Adams W, Harper J, Rittmaster R, Heotis P, Scott W (1984). Medical status of Marshallese accidentally exposed to 1954 Bravo fallout radiation: January 1980 through December 1982. (Technical Report BNL 51761) Upton, NY: Brookhaven National Lab, pp. 51

Albert RE, Omran A (1968) Follow-up study of patients treated by x-ray epilation for tinea capitis. I. Population characteristics, post-treatment illnesses and mortality experience. Arch Environ Health 17:899–918.

Armenian H, Lilienfeld A (1974) The distribution of incubation periods of neoplastic diseases. Am J Epidemiol 99:92–100.

Beebe G, Kato H, Land C (1977) Mortality experience of atomic bomb survivors, 1950–74. In: Life span study, Report 8. Hiroshima: Radiation Effects Research Foundation, Technical report: RERF TR 1–77.

Christov K (1975) Thyroid cell proliferation in rats and induction of tumors by x-rays. Cancer Res 35:1256–1262.

Colman M, Simpson L, Patterson L, Cohen L (1976) Thyroid cancer associated with radiation exposure: Dose-effect relationship. In: Biological and environmental effects of low-level radiation, Vol. II. Vienna: International Atomic Energy Agency, pp. 285–288.

Conard RA (1977) Summary of thyroid findings in Marshallese 22 years after exposure to radioactive fallout. In: DeGroot L, Frohman L, Kaplan E, Refetoff S (eds), Radiation-associated thyroid carcinoma. New York: Grune and Stratton, pp 241–257.

Conard RA, Paglia D, Larsen P, Sutow W, Dobyns B, Robbins J, Krotosky W, Field J, Rall J, Wolff J (1980) Review of medical findings in a Marshallese population twenty-six years after accidental exposure to radioactive fallout. Upton, NY: Brookhaven National Laboratory, pp. 138.

DeGroot L, Paloyan E (1973) Thyroid carcinoma and radiation; A Chicago endemic. J Am Med Assoc 225:487–491.

DeGroot LJ, Frohman L, Kaplan E, Refetoff S (eds) (1977) Radiation-associated thyroid carcinoma. New York: Grune and Stratton, pp 1–539.

Dobyns BM, Sheline G, Workman J, Tompkins E, McConahey W, Becker D (1974) Malignant and benign neoplasms of the thyroid in patients treated for hyperthyroidism: A report of the cooperative thyrotoxicosis therapy follow-up study. J Clin Endocrinol Metab 38:976–98.

Doniach I (1963) Effects including carcinogenesis of I-131 and x-rays on the thyroid of experimental animals: A review. Health Phys 9:1357–1362.

Doniach I (1974) Carcinogenic effect of 100, 250 and 500 rad x-rays on the rat thyroid gland. Br J Cancer 30:487–495.

Duffy BJ, Fitzgerald P (1950) Cancer of the thyroid in children: A report of 28 cases. J Clin Endocrinol Metab 10:1296–1308.

Harley N, Albert R, Shore R, Pasternack B (1976) Follow-up study of patients treated by x-ray epilation for tinea capitis. Estimation of the dose to the thyroid and pituitary glands and other structures of the head and neck. Phys Med Biol 21:631–642.

Hempelmann LH, Pifer J, Burke G, Terry R, Ames W (1967) Neoplasms in persons treated with x-rays in infancy for thymic enlargement. A report of the third follow-up survey. J Natl Cancer Inst 38:317–341.

Hempelmann LH, Hall W, Phillips M, Cooper R, Ames W (1975) Neoplasms in persons treated with x-rays in infancy: Fourth survey in 20 years. J Natl Cancer Inst 55:519–530.

Hempelmann LH, Furth J (1978) Etiology of thyroid cancer. In: Greenfield LD (ed), Thyroid cancer. West Palm Beach, FL: CRC Press, pp 37–49.

Hoffman DA (1934) Late effects of I-131 therapy in the United States. In: J Boice, J Fraumeni (eds.), Radiation carcinogenesis: Epidemiology and biological significance. New York: Raven Press, pp 273–280.

Holm LE, Dahlqvist I, Israelsson A, Lundell G (1980a) Malignant thyroid tumors after Iodine-131 therapy. N Engl J Med 303:188–191.

Holm LE, Lundell G, Walinder G (1980b) Incidence of malignant thyroid tumors in humans after exposure to diagnostic doses of Iodine-131. I. Retrospective cohort study. J Natl Cancer Inst 64:1055–1059.

Holm LE, Eklund G, Lundell Goran (1980c) Incidence of malignant thyroid tumors in humans after exposure to diagnostic doses of Iodine-131. II. Estimation of thyroid gland size, thyroid radiation dose, and predicted versus observed number of malignant thyroid tumors. J Natl Cancer Inst 1980c; 65:1221–1224.

Holm LE (1983) Thyroid cancer after exposure to [131]I. Presented at the Swedish–Japanese Seminar on Radiation and Cancer, Stockholm, Sweden, June 30–July 1.

Lee W, Chiacchierini R, Shleien B, Telles N (1982) Thyroid tumors following I-131 or localized x-irradiation to the thyroid and the pituitary glands in rats. Radiat Res 92:307–319.

Lee W, Youmans H (1970) Doses to the central nervous system of children resulting from x-ray therapy for tinea capitis. Bureau of Radiological Health, FDA, Publication no. BRH/DBE 70–4. Washington, D.C.

Maxon HR, Saenger EL, Thomas S, Buncher R, Kereiakes J, Shafer M, McLaughlin C (1980) Clinically important radiation-associated thyroid disease. J Am Med Assoc 244:1802–1805.

Modan B, Baidatz D, Mart H, Steinitz R, Levin S (1976) Radiation-induced head and neck tumours. Lancet i:277–279.

Modan B, Ron E, Werner A (1977) Thyroid cancer following scalp irradiation. Radiology 123:741–744.

Modan B (1979) Evaluation of risks in medical radiation exposure—The thyroid story. In: Okada S, Imamura M, Terashima T, Yamaguchi H Radiation research: Proceedings of the Sixth International Congress of Radiation Research. Tokyo: Japanese Association for Radiation Research, pp 968–972.

NAS (1980) The effects on populations of exposure to low levels of ionizing radiation: 1980. BEIR III Report. Washington, D.C.

Parker LN, Belsky JL, Yamamoto T, Kawamoto S, Keehn R (1974) Thyroid carcinoma after exposure to atomic radiation: A continuing survey of a fixed population, Hiroshima and Nagasaki, 1958–1971. Ann Int Med 80:600–604.

Prentice R, Kato H, Yoshimoto K, Mason M (1982) Radiation exposure and thyroid cancer incidence among Hiroshima and Nagasaki residents. Monog Natl Cancer Inst 62:207–212.

Rallison ML, Dobyns B, Keating R, Rall J, Tyler F (1974) Thyroid diseases in children. A survey of subjects potentially exposed to fallout radiation. Am J Med 56:457–463.

Rallison ML, Dobyns B, Keating R, Rall J, Tyler F (1975) Thyroid nodularity in children. J Am Med Assoc 233:1069–1072.

Reddy MM, Goh K, Hempelmann L (1976) B and T lymphocytes in man. I. Effects of infant thymic irradiation on the circulating B and T lymphocytes. In: Radiation and the lymphatic system (CONF-740930, ERDA Symposium Series 37). National Technical Information Service Springfield VA 192–196.

Ron E, Modan B (1980) Benign and malignant thyroid neoplasms after childhood irradiation for tinea capitis. J Natl Cancer Inst 65:7–11.

Ron E, Modan B (1980) Thyroid and other neoplasms following childhood scalp irradiation. In: J Boice, and J Fraumeni (eds.), Radiation carcinogenesis: Epidemiology and biological significance. New York: Raven Press, pp 139–151.

Saenger EL, Seltzer A, Sterling T, Kereiakes J (1960) Neoplasia following therapeutic irradiation for benign conditions in childhood. Radiology 74:889–904.

Schneider AB, Favus M, Stachura M, Arnold J, Arnold M, Frohman L (1978) Incidence, prevalence and characteristics of radiation-induced thyroid tumors. Am J Med 64:243–252.

Schneider AB, Pinsky S, Bekerman C, Ryo U (1980) Characteristics of 108 thyroid cancers detected by screening in a population with a history of head and neck irradiation. Cancer 46:1218–1227.

Shore RE, Albert R, Pasternack B (1976) Follow-up study of patients treated by x-ray epilation for tinea capitis—IV. Resurvey of post-treatment illness and mortality experience. Arch Environ Health 31:21–28.

Shore RE, Woodard E, Pasternack B, Hempelmann L (1980) Radiation and host factors in human thyroid tumors following thymus irradiation. Health Phys 38:451–465.

Shore RE (1982) A follow-up study of children given x-ray treatment for ringworm of the scalp (tinea capitis). Doctoral dissertation, Columbia University, pp 1–167.

Shore RE, Woodard E, Hildreth N, Dvoretsky P, Hempelmann L, Pasternack B (1985) Thyroid tumors following thymus irradiation. J Natl Cancer Inst 74:1177–1184, 1985.

Simpson CL, Hempelmann L, Fuller L (1955) Neoplasia in children treated with x-rays in infancy for thymic enlargement. Radiol 64:840–845.

Wakabayashi T, Kato H, Ikeda T, Schull W (1983) Studies of the mortality of A-bomb survivors, Report 7. Part III. Incidence of cancer in 1959–78, based on the tumor registry, Nagasaki. Radiat Res 93:112–146.

Walinder G (1972) Late effects of irradiation on the thyroid gland in mice. I. Irradiation of adult mice. Acta Radiol Ther Phys Biol 2:433–451.

Werner A, Modan B, Davidoff D (1968) Doses to brain, skull and thyroid, following x-ray therapy for tinea capitis. Phys Med Biol 13:247–258.

CARCINOGENIC EFFECTS OF RADIATION ON THE HUMAN SKELETON AND SUPPORTING TISSUES

JANET VAUGHAN, F.R.S., F.R.C.P., D.M.

It is agreed that the bony skeleton and its supporting tissues are resistant to the carcinogenic action of ionizing radiation, compared with the majority of other tissues (UNSCEAR, 1977; BEIR, 1980). Cancer may result in the human skeleton from external radiation and from internal radiation. In the former, both penetrating low-LET radiation, gamma, and x-rays and high-LET from fast neutrons may be involved; in the latter, high-LET radiation from alpha particle-emitting radionuclides. There is at present no evidence in the open literature that beta particle emission from internally deposited radionuclides has resulted in malignancy in humans, though it has in animals.

SUPPORTING TISSUES

The supporting tissues of the human skeleton are the associated muscles, tendons, and synovial membranes of joints. No report has been found of malignancy occurring as a result of radiation in these tissues. A wide variety of natural tumors are described, but they are rare and difficult to classify, especially those arising in muscle (Sissons, 1979).

THE SKELETON

The skeleton is a complex organ. The bones comprise both cartilaginous and bony tissue. Within the bone cavities are the hemopoietic marrow, the osteogenic stroma, the blood vessels, and the nerves. The cells of the hemopoietic marrow originate from the primitive yolk sac, via the embryonic liver, and the cells of the osteogenic stroma from primitive mesenchyme cells, which retain

From the Bone Research Laboratory, Nuffield Orthopaedic Centre, Oxford, England.

their osteogenic and chondrocytic potential (Vaughan, 1981). The osteogenic stroma of the marrow is continuous with the soft connective tissue lining periosteal and endosteal surfaces and Haversian canals (Owen, 1980).

CELLS AT RISK

The cells of the skeleton at risk from ionizing radiation are 1) hemopoietic cells, 2) cells with osteogenic potential, 3) cells with cartilaginous potential, 4) epithelial cells closely applied to bone in the mastoid and other air cells (ICRP 11, 1968), and 5) primitive mesenchyme cells other than osteogenic (Loutit and Vaughan, 1971).

Hemopoietic Cells

The carcinogenic effect of radiation on the hemopoietic cells capable of proliferation results in the induction of leukemia in cells of the granulomonocytic series. For reasons that are not yet understood, chronic lymphatic leukemia is not induced by radiation, whereas, acute lymphoblastic leukemia may occur (Doll, 1981). On the other hand, there is suggestive epidemiologic evidence that myelomatosis, which arises in plasma cells derived from lymphocytes, may be radiation-induced (Mole, 1978; Ichimaru et al, 1980; BEIR, 1980). Brief mention of leukemia is included here because there are interesting differences in its incidence, compared with osteosarcoma, following exposure to external and internal radiation of the skeleton.

Osteogenic Cells

The cells responsible for matrix formation and calcification, both osteoblasts and chondroblasts, are derived from mesenchyme stroma, while the osteoclast is derived from a cell of hemopoietic origin (Owen, 1980). Osteogenic cells of stromal origin are present throughout marrow, but appear in highest concentration near bone surfaces (Ashton et al, 1981).

In young actively growing bone, particularly on the periosteal surface, this layer may be several cells thick, consisting of precursor cells and differentiated osteoblasts. In older bone the layer is often only one cell thick. On endosteal surfaces, therefore, it may often be difficult to distinguish bone cells from closely adjacent hemopoietic cells in sections examined by light microscopy, but electron microscope studies indicate a continuous nonhemopoietic cellular layer (Sissons, 1970; Vaughan, 1970; Luk et al, 1974). The cells involved on the endosteal surface in the adult are now often spoken of as "lining cells," but there is good evidence that some of these cells are capable of mitosis (Vaughan, 1981) and therefore malignant transformation. It has been common practice to calculate radiation dose to cells 0–10 μm from the endosteal bone surface (ICRP, 1968; ICRP, 1977; Marshall and Groer, 1977; Marshall, Groer, and Schlenker, 1978), ignoring the smaller number of osteogenic cells scattered throughout the stroma in the marrow and the lining of Haversian canals. Lloyd (1979–80) suggested that it would be wiser to consider all cells lying within the range of the alpha particle at risk. On examining the endosteal surface of bone

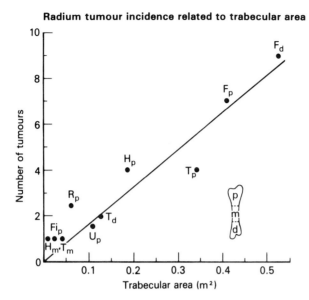

FIGURE 1. Radium data, number of tumors versus measured trabecular area. Note there are points of zero tumor incidence (eight in all) below a trabecular area of 0.03 m². Spiers, King, and Beddoe, 1977; by courtesy of authors and publishers.

from a radium dial painter with a "well differentiated fibrosarcoma," Lloyd and Henning (1978–79) found a fibrotic layer interposed between fibroblast-like cells and the mineral surface, while in a normal control the cells were close to the bone mineral.

The importance of the osteogenic cells on bone surfaces in skeletal radiation carcinogenesis has been analyzed by Spiers et al. (1977; 1983a). Trabecular bone, because of its morphologic character, might be expected to have a greater surface area than cortical bone and, therefore, to have more cells at risk. Indeed, they found that the occurrence of tumors in the long bone of humans shows an approximately linear relationship with the trabecular surface area (Figure 1 (Spiers et al, 1977). This relationship also holds good for the beagle (Spiers et al, 1983) and for 33 human radium cases, 139 naturally occurring cases, and 473 recorded by Dahlin (Thurman et al, 1973).

While accepting the general principle that the osteogenic cells at risk are those on growing bone surfaces, it must be remembered that the number of actively proliferating cells (i.e., those capable of malignant transformation at any site) may vary with a number of factors that are not at present understood. Whereas, in human long bones tumors appear to arise on the endosteum of trabecular bone, trabeculation may not be the only significant factor. Only two of 54 bone sarcomas in radium subjects occurred in the vertebrae (i.e., bones with a high surface to volume ratio) (Mole, 1978). It may be that the initial high radium uptake on the extensive trabecular surfaces in the vertebrae may result in the death, rather than the transformation, of the sensitive endosteal cells. On the other hand, Spiers has reported finding a lower ^{226}Ra content in the verte-brae compared with other bones of a radium worker, which he attributes to greater metabolic activity (Spiers and Burch, 1957).

The Chondroblasts

Chondroblasts appear relatively resistant to radiation-induced malignancy. In the case of children exposed to ^{224}Ra who showed considerable growth retarda-tion, the majority of the proliferating cartilage cells (i.e., the cartilage cells at risk) would lie out of the range of the alpha particles from the radium on the surface of calcifying degenerating cartilage cells in the lower part of the epiph-yseal plate (Kember, 1981). However, they may be affected by ^{224}Ra taken up in the matrix vesicles present in the longitudinal septa adjacent to the proliferat-ing cells (Ali, 1976; Anderson, 1976) and in the mitochondria of the proliferat-ing cells themselves (Martin and Mathews, 1969; Burger and Mathews, 1978). Mitochondria are known to take up calcium, strontium, and barium (Peachey, 1964).

Epithelial Cells in the Sinuses of the Skull

Epithelial cells are closely applied to bone, both in the paranasal and mastoid air sinuses of the skull, and are therefore theoretically at risk from the radionu-clides deposited in the underlying bone. In 1939 Martland postulated that carcinomas of the head occurring in the dial painters arise ". . . in the mucosa . . . as the result of the local effects of radon . . . in the expiratory air." In 1966 Evans reported "very high radon concentrations in the airspaces of the frontal sinuses and mastoid air cells" and noted that "the alpha radiation from this radon and its daughter products augments the alpha radiation from the under-lying bone and the combination appears clearly to be the radiobiological origin of this group of carcinomas." After histologic studies and dose-rate calcula-tions, Schlenker and Harris (1978–79) tentatively concluded that radon and its daughters in the airspace produce a greater dose-rate in the mastoid air cell epithelium than do ^{226}Ra and its daughters in bone. For the paranasal sinuses they suggest that this is also probably the case. Schlenker (1979–1980) has made dose calculations that suggest that ^{228}Ra and ^{226}Ra are of comparable significance for the production of carcinomas in patients exposed to compara-ble levels; further, that ^{224}Ra would also be carcinogenic at the levels used in humans. Indeed, he concludes "one cannot ignore carcinomas of the sinuses and mastoids as a potential risk from all alpha emitting bone seekers," even though they have no gaseous daughter products.

Mesenchyme Cells Other than Osteogenic in Marrow Stroma. The origin of endothelial cells lining the marrow sinuses is still disputed. Vasiform sarco-mas, usually called hemangiosarcoma in humans, are thought to probably arise from such cells or their precursors. They are common in mice exposed to hard beta emitters, such as strontium 90 (Ash and Loutit, 1977; Loutit, 1976). They are not recorded in the populations exposed to ^{226}Ra, ^{228}Ra, or ^{224}Ra. One occurring in the bone marrow is reported in a large series of patients who received thorotrast, a contrast medium containing ^{232}Th (Mole, 1978). Thoro-trast and its daughter products (Jee et al, 1967) may be found in bone marrow as well as on bone surfaces.

INTERNAL RADIATION FROM BONE-SEEKING RADIONUCLIDES

Since Martland published his first reports on the effects of radium deposition in the skeleton of radium dial painters it has been recognized that internal radiation might be a skeletal carcinogenic hazard (Martland, Conlon, and Knef, 1925). The extent of this hazard was extended when Hamilton, in 1947, detailed the number of radionuclides resulting from atomic fission that were bone-seekers.

The different carcinogenic effects of the bone-seeking radionuclides depend on their physical and chemical characteristics, which determine their biological behavior. Hitherto, only the radioisotopes of the radium and thorium series, both alpha emitters, have proved carcinogenic to the skeleton in humans, although animal experiments clearly indicate the potential hazard to other species.

Physical Characteristics

The physical characteristics of the more common bone-seeking radionuclides are shown in Table 1, and the decay chains of the radium and thorium series known to be carcinogenic humans are shown in Tables 2 and 3. These radionuclides vary in the energy and range of their radiations, their half-lives, and their decay products. The injury any radionuclide may do to cells depends not only on the physical character of the initially deposited element but also on the character and biological behavior of the radioactive daughter products. ^{226}Ra decays with a long half-life of 1620 yr, whereas, ^{224}Ra decays with a short half-life of 3.64 days. This suggests that ^{226}Ra will continue to irradiate bone cells as long as it is retained, whereas, ^{224}Ra will decay rapidly and exert its maximum effect on sensitive cells only for a short period (ICRP 20, 1972).

It must be remembered, however, that the radiation dose from ^{224}Ra to sensitive cells on surfaces, for the first 24 hr after injection is appreciable, because 15.5% of an injected dose is present on the surface for the first 24 hr (ICRP 20, 1972). Intravenous injection of 1 μCi of ^{224}Ra to "standard man" (JCRP.20) results in an average dose to the endosteal cells 0–10 μm from bone surfaces of 1.5 rad (Marshall et al, 1978), which is somewhat less than the 1.77 rad originally proposed by Spiess and Mays (1970). Intravenous injection of 1 μC of ^{226}Ra to "standard man" would give a dose of 6.29 rad to the endosteal cells. Marshall et al (1978) have also calculated the dose to endosteal cells and relative distribution factors for ^{224}Ra and ^{239}Uu, compared with ^{226}Ra. This relative distribution factor (RDF) with ^{226}Ra as the standard of reference, they consider, provides a more secure distribution of spatial differences between the dose distribution of alpha emitters than does endosteal dose, itself. The value of RDF for ^{224}Ra/^{226}Ra is 20, and for ^{239}Pu it is about 28 for a surface source of plutonium and 0.96 for a volume source. For dosimetric purposes, as regards limits for intake of radionuclides by workers, ICRP assumes that ^{226}Ra is uniformly distributed throughout the volume of bone matrix at all times after its intake (ICRP 30, 1979), whereas ^{224}Ra is uniformly distributed in an infinitely thin layer over bone surfaces at all times.

A theory of the induction of bone cancer by alpha radiation was developed by Marshall and Groer (1977), largely based on studies of the population ex-

TABLE 1 Physical Characteristics of the More Common Bone-Seeking Radionuclides

	Half-life	Maximum particle energies (MeV)	Gamma ray energies (MeV)	Daughter products	Maximum particle ranges in soft tissue
^{45}Ca	165 days	β-0.254	—	Stable scandium	650 μm
^{89}Sr	51 days	β-1.46	—	Stable yttrium	7 mm
^{90}Sr	28 yr	β-0.54	—	^{90}Y β	2 mm
^{90}Y	64.2 hr	β-2.27	—	Stable zirconium	10 mm
^{224}Ra (Thorium X)	3.64 days	α 5.68 95% α 5.44 4.9%	0.24	^{220}Rn α + β to stable ^{208}Pb	39–88 μm
^{226}Ra (Radium)	1620 yr	α 4.78 94.3% α 4.59 5.7%	0.19	^{222}Rn Half-life 3.8 days α + β to stable ^{206}Pb	31–70 μm
^{228}Ra (Mesothorium I)	5.7 yr	β-0.04	—	^{228}Actinium (Mesothorium II) 6.13 hr α + β to stable ^{208}Pb	39–88 μm
^{228}Th (Radiothorium)	1.91 yr	α 5.42 71% α 5.34 28%	0.084	^{224}Ra	39–88 μm
^{239}Pu	2.4 × 10⁴ yr	α 5.15 72% α 5.13 17% α 5.10 11%	0.013 0.038 0.151	^{235}U (7 × 10⁸ yr)	35 μm
^{241}Am	458 yr	α 5.48 85% α 5.44 13%	0.06 36% 0.03 2.5%	^{237}Np (2.2 × 10⁶ yr)	40 μm
^{32}P	14.3 days	β-1.71	—	Stable sulphur	8 mm

α-particle ranges: Minimum and maximum values for alpha particles in the decay chains.
β-particle ranges: Ranges for maximum energies as given for muscle by Berger and Seltzer, 1966.

TABLE 2 Radioisotopes in the Radium Series

Radioisotope (historical name)	Element	Half-life	Particle energies (MeV)[a]	Gamma-ray energies (MeV)
Radium	^{226}Ra	1620 yr	α, 4.78 (94.3%) α, 4.59 (5.7%)	0.187 (5.7%)
Radon	^{222}Rn	3.82 days	α, 5.49 (99+%) α, 4.98 (< 0.1%)	0.51 (0.07%)
Ra A	^{218}Po	3.05 min	α, 6.00 (99+%)	
Ra B	^{214}Pb	26.8 min	β-, 0.67– 1.03	0.053–0.352
Ra C	^{214}Bi	19.7 min	β-, 0.4–3.18 (99+%) α, 5.51, 5.44 (0.04%)	0.61–2.43
Ra C′ (99+%)	^{214}Po	160 μsec	α, 7.68	
Ra C″ (0.04%)	^{210}Tl	1.32 min	β-, 1.96	0.30–2.36
Ra D	^{210}Pb	21.4 yr	β-, 0.017 (85%) β-, 0.064 (15%)	0.047 (85%)
Ra E	^{210}Bi	5.0 days	β-, 1.16 (99+%)	
Ra F (polonium)	^{210}Po	138.4 days	α, 5.30 (99+%)	
Ra G	^{206}Pb	Stable		

Source: Spiers, 1968; by courtesy of author and publishers

[a] Where the β- or α-spectra contain many lines, only ranges of energy without abundances are given.

posed to radium. They concluded that promotion by division of the irradiated cell is the final required step for bone sarcoma induction. The theory has recently been criticized by Raabe (1984) on the grounds that the importance of dose rate was ignored.

Chemical Characteristics

The avid retention of certain radionuclides in bone is explained in the case of radium isotopes by the fact that radium is an alkaline earth, like calcium, which constitutes the major constituent of the bone mineral. ^{226}Ra that gains access to the blood stream is taken up in high concentration in areas of bone

TABLE 3 Radioisotopes in the Thorium Series

Radioisotope (historical name)	Element	Half-life	Particle energies[a] (MeV)	Ray energies (MeV)
Thorium	^{232}Th	1.4×10^{10} yr	α, 4.01 (76%)	0.059 (24%)
			α, 3.95 (24%)	
Mesothorium 1	^{228}Ra	5.7 yr	β-, 0.02	
Mesothorium 2	^{228}Ac	6.13 hr	β-, 0.45–2.18	0.057–1.64
Radiothorium	^{228}Th	1.91 yr	α, 5.42 (71%)	0.084–0.21
			α, 5.34 (28%)	
Thorium X	^{224}Ra	3.64 days	α, 5.68 (95%)	0.241 (4.9%)
			α, 5.44 (4.9%)	
Thoron	^{220}Rn	55 sec	α, 6.28 (99.7%)	0.54 (0.3%)
			α, 5.75 (0.3%)	
Thorium A	^{216}Po	0.16 sec	α, 6.78	
Thorium B	^{212}Pb	10.6 hr	β-, 0.58 (12%)	0.12–0.41
			β-, 0.34 (84%)	0.24 (84%)
Thorium C	^{212}Bi	60.5 min	β-, 0.08–2.27 (64%)	0.72–2.2
			α, 6.09, 6.05 (36%)	0.04–0.47
Th C′ (64%)	^{212}Po	0.30 μses	α, 8.78	
Th C″ (36%)	^{208}Tl	3.1 min	β, 1.0–2.38	0.04–2.61
Thorium C	^{208}Pb	Stable		

Source: Spiers, 1968; by courtesy of author and publishers.

[a] Where the β- or α-spectra contain many lines, only ranges of energy without abundances are given.

where active mineralization is taking place and also in low concentration throughout the bone mineral. Because of its long half-life (1620 yr) ^{226}Ra so taken up in bone is retained for many years. Figure 2 shows an autoradiograph of a complete tibia in cross section from a case of radium poisoning given ^{226}Ra therapeutically for 1 yr at the age of 46. The estimated body burden was 10 μCi at death, 36 yr later. Both the areas of high concentration and the diffuse pattern are easily seen. Figure 3 shows an autoradiograph left on a section of cortical bone at a much higher magnification. One Haversian system is heavily labeled with alpha tracks, whereas the adjacent system contains none. The labeled osteone was in process of laying down calcium at the time the radium blood level was high, and incorporated radium together with calcium, while the other osteone was either fully calcified at that time or had been formed later. Because of the diffuseness of the final distribution of ^{226}Ra throughout bone mineral, ^{226}Ra is often referred to as a volume-seeker (Marshall, 1969).

Other important alpha-emitting radionuclides, such as plutonium, are referred to as surface-seekers, because they are initially taken up and concentrated by various mechanisms on bone surfaces. They may be removed from bone surfaces by osteoclasts; they may also be buried by the laying down of new bone and will diffuse into the matrix from bone blood vessels (Howells and Green, 1980). There is considerable evidence that one factor involved in their initial surface uptake is their affinity with certain chemical constituents in bone matrix to which they bind (Taylor, 1972).

This division of the bone-seeking radionuclides into volume- and surface-seekers has a certain convenience, but it must be recognized that in some ways it is an oversimplification. This is illustrated by an analysis of the behavior of ^{228}Ra. ^{228}Ra is taken up like calcium and ^{226}Ra throughout bone mineral. It is a weak beta emitter, but the average range of its alpha-emitting daughter products is greater than the range of the alpha emitters of the ^{226}Ra series. Most of the ^{228}Ra daughter products remain in the bone volume, but a small fraction of the daughter ^{228}Th is released from the deposition site of its parent and will deposit on bone surfaces. Rowland et al, have concluded however, that in humans there is no difference in the toxicity of the two isotopes, ^{226}Ra and ^{228}Ra (Rowland, Keane, and Lucas, 1973); but this is not necessarily true of all aspects of tumors induced by ^{228}Ra in dogs (Spiers and Beddoe, 1983).

FIGURE 2. Autoradiograph of a complete tibia cross section from a case of radium poisoning (case 118) given Ra^{226} therapeutically for 1 yr at age 46, estimated body burden 10 μCi at death, 36 yr later. Note hot spots and diffuse distribution throughout bone. Rowland and Marshall, 1959; by courtesy of authors and publishers.

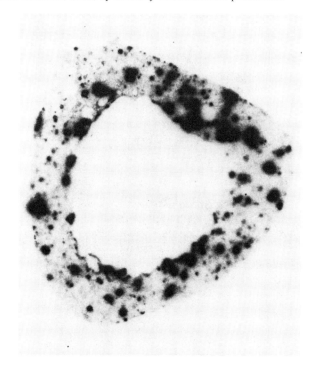

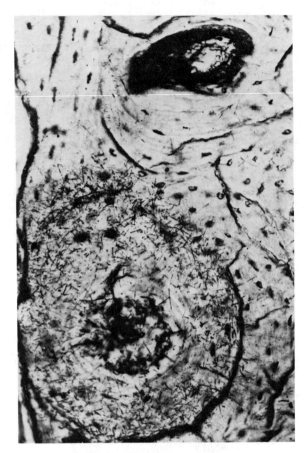

FIGURE 3. Autoradiograph left on section of cortical bone in case of radium poisoning. Note one Haversian system labeled with alpha tracks, whereas adjacent system contains none. × 125. Vaughan, 1962; by courtesy of author and publishers.

RADIUM

Two human populations have been exposed to skeletal alpha radiation from internally deposited radium. First, a population of 3712 persons consisting of dial painters, radium chemists, and individuals given ^{226}Ra, ^{228}Ra therapeutically was collected by the Center for Human Radiobiology (ANL.83.100, 1982–83); second, a group given repeated injections of ^{224}Ra for tuberculosis in childhood and for ankylosing spondylitis in adult life (Spiess, 1969; Mays, Spiess, and Gerspach, 1978) was collected.

^{226}Ra, ^{228}Ra

Bone Tumors. The most recent figures from the Center for Human Radiobiology note 61 bone sarcoma cases among 2312 persons whose body burden of ^{226}Ra and ^{228}Ra is known, and 24 probable or confirmed cases among 1400 persons whose body burden has not been measured (ANL.83.100, 1982–83). The lowest mean dose to bone at death was 888 rad. Some sarcomas have appeared as long as 52 yr after initial ingestion. The shortest recorded appearance time is 6 yr (Keane, 1971). There are interesting age differences in sensitivity to tumor induction, as there appear to be for radiation cancers in other tissues, notably the breast. In the case of bone, the most sensitive individuals were pubertal females aged 12–16 yr; the least sensitive were females age 19–24 yr at the initiation of exposure (Mole, 1979).

Age differences in the anatomical sites of bone sarcoma are shown in Table 4. It is difficult to find any explanation for some of these age differences. Evidence that the cell at risk in the induction of bone cancers by radiation is the proliferating osteogenic cell, the osteoblast, or its precursor present on all bone surfaces, has already been discussed.

The high sarcoma incidence in the proximal limb, knee, and innominate bone of the young may be associated with an increase in cell proliferation associated with growth in these areas; but, will such an increase explain the high tumor incidence in the elbow, not a site of active growth in humans?

Dose–Response Relationship. There are many complicating factors to be taken into account in attempting to analyze the relationship between radiation dose and cancer incidence, such as the fact that the radium paint used by the early dial painters was a mixture of ^{226}Ra and ^{228}Ra, and that there were considerable variations in the age at which contamination occurred, the rate at which the body burden was acquired, and the latent intervals to tumor occurrence.

In 1969, Evans et al, having made an analysis of 496 persons with a skeletal burden of ^{226}Ra and ^{228}Ra, concluded that there was a "practical threshold" of

TABLE 4 Age Differences in Anatomical Sites of Bone Sarcomas (Osteo- and Fibro-) in Radium Subjects*

	Age at start of exposure (yr)	
Anatomical site	12–20	21+
Innominate	9	0
Trunk	3[a]	2
Limbs		
Proximal	10[b]	4
Knee, elbow	12	5
Distal	4	7
Total	36[b]	18
Subjects with average skeletal dose 500 cumulative rads or more		
Female	112	72
Male	4	30

Source: Mole, 1978; by courtesy of author and publishers.

* Data extracted from Center for Human Radiobiology, 1975.
[a] One in the lateral sacrum, one of the only two sarcomas occurring in any vertebra.
[b] Excluding one chondrosarcoma.

dosage below which the required tumor appearance time generally exceeds the life span, hence, radiation-induced tumors appear with negligible frequency (Evans et al, 1969). This view is not entirely supported by a more recent analysis. Following a study of a well defined population of female dial painters, Rowland et al (1978) concluded that the dose–incidence relationship between the quantity of radium acquired in microcuries and the number of bone sarcomas per person-year at risk was best described by a dose-squared exponential function. Recently they have made further assessment of the incidence of bone sarcomas among female dial workers using two methods to evaluate the risk from radium (Rowland et al, 1983). The first utilized all cases who survived at least 5 yr after the start of employment, a cohort based on year of entry into the industry. The second was based on all cases who survived at least 2 yr after first measurement. The mean year of start of follow-up was 1931 for the first method of analysis and 1969 for the second method.

A generalized dose–response function

$$I = (C + \alpha D + \beta D^2)e^{-\gamma D}$$

and simplifications that result when one or two of the coefficients α, β, and γ were set to zero, were fitted to each data set. Here, incidence (I) was expressed as bone sarcomas per person-year, the dose parameter (D) was the quantity (microcuries) of radium that entered the blood during the period of exposure, and C, the natural incidence, in units of bone sarcomas per person-year, was dependent on the composition of each group. Two functions

$$I = (C + \alpha D + \beta D^2)e^{-\gamma D} \text{ and } I = (C + \beta D^2)e^{-\gamma D}$$

fit the cohort based on year of entry into the industry ($p > 0.05$), whereas, both these expressions and $I = (C + \alpha D)$ fit the cohort based on date of first measurement.

The number of bone sarcomas observed as a function of age at first exposure and as a function of time after first exposure matched the predicted numbers quite satisfactorily, indicating no age sensitivity and a constant rate of bone sarcoma induction. There was an indication that bone sarcomas have been missed at early times in other radium groups, most likely in high-dose cases who may have died of their malignancies without awareness of the connection with radium. Further, the results suggest that the risk of bone sarcoma induction is reduced when radium is acquired after the age of 35.

Raabe et al (1983) have proposed a log-normal three-dimensional dose–response relationship, yielding risk as a function of average dose-rate and time after beginning of exposure.

Histology of Radium Tumors. Little is known of the early bone changes in man following radium ingestion. Descriptions of late radiologic and histologic abnormalities are confused by the presence of effects associated with natural aging and with vascular injury induced by radiation (Pool et al, 1983), resulting in a condition described as osteodystrophy, which may terminate in malignancy but does not necessarily do so. It is characterised by the development of large and bizarre resorption cavities, by the production of fibrous and abnormal bone tissue, hypermineralized lacunae, and plugged Haversial canals.

TABLE 5 Primary Malignant Tumors of the Skeleton—Naturally Occurring and Radiation-Induced (BEIR 1980)

Primary malignant tumors of skeleton[a]	Naturally occurring				Radiation-induced							
	U.S.		England and Wales		X-ray literature		X-ray therapy in U.S.		^{226}Ra and ^{228}Ra in bone in U.S.		^{224}Ra in bone in Germany	
	n	%	n	%	n	%	n	%	n	%	n	%
Osteosarcoma	652	43.0	296	60.9	155	59.2	12	44.4	42	70.0	42	84.0
Chondrosarcoma	343	22.6	73	15.0	19	7.3	3	11.1	1	1.7	3	6.0
Ewing's tumor	209	13.8	31	6.4	—	—	—	—	—	—	—	—
Chordoma	122	8.0	25	5.1	—	—	—	—	—	—	—	—
Reticulum-cell sarcoma	101	6.7	10	2.1	—	—	2	7.4	—	—	1	2.0
Fibrosarcoma	82	5.4	49	10.1	66	25.2	8	29.6	17	28.3	1	2.0
Angiosarcoma	7	0.5	2	0.4	—	—	—	—	—	—	—	—
Others	—	—	—	—	22	8.4	2	7.4	—	—	3	6.0
Totals	1516	100	486	100	262	100.1	27	99.9	60	100	50	100

Source: Reproduced from *The Effects on Populations of Exposure to Low Levels of Ionizing Radiation*, Washington, DC: National Academy Press, 1980, by permission.

[a] Excluding leukemia, myeloma, Hodgkin's disease, neuroblastoma, adamantioma, giant-cell tumors, unspecified bone tumors, and soft-tissue tumors invading bone.

Table 5 shows the incidence of primary malignant tumors of the skeleton, both those naturally occurring and those known to be radiation induced in humans (BEIR, 1980).

The majority of skeletal tumors associated with radium are recorded as osteosarcomas, with rather fewer fibrosarcomas (Thurman et al, 1973). In 1967, I had the opportunity to examine all the available pathologic sections from tumors induced by ^{226}Ra and ^{228}Ra (both at the Argonne, by courtesy of Dr. Rowlands, and at M.I.T., by courtesy of Prof. Evans). I was impressed with the number of fibrosarcomas in the series and the amount of fibrous material in the osteosarcomas, compared with a large collection in London of tumors from patients unexposed to radiation (made available by Dr. Sissons). In view of the observation of Lloyd and Henning (1978–79) of a layer of fibrous material between the bone and the osteogenic cells, this impression of the high incidence of fibrosarcoma and fibrous material in the radium patients may be significant.

There is no evidence that internal radiation has induced giant cell tumors (osteoclastomas), Ewing's tumor, angiosarcoma, or any of the rarer types of tumor described in human bone (Sissons, 1979).

Cancer of Cartilage. Only one chondrosarcoma is recorded in the patients with a burden of ^{226}Ra, ^{228}Ra. This may be due to a variation in pathologic nomenclature—chondroosteogenic sarcomas are relatively common in humans.

Sinus and Mastoid Cancers. An analysis of tumor incidence in persons exposed to ^{226}Ra, ^{228}Ra showed 28 sinus or mastoid tumors, compared with 60 bone sarcomas, among 2164 patients whose radium burdens had been measured; 0.8 sinus tumors might have been expected (Schlenker, 1979–80).

In their study of dose–response relationships for female radium dial painters, Rowland et al (1978) concluded that the relationship for head carcinomas was best described by a linear function.

Leukemia. In his early studies, Martland (1931) describes 13 cases of radium poisoning among the early radium dial painters as acute. "These cases showed during life a clinical picture quite different from that in cases which developed later." They had a severe anemia and went on to heal with a patchy fibrosis. Loutit (1970) has since argued that such cases should be classified as examples of leukemia or malignant myelosclerosis.

Spiers et al (1983b) have recently made a fresh analysis of leukemia in the U.S. dial painters. Among a total of 2930 located radium dial workers, 10 cases of leukemia of all types were observed; 9.24 would have been expected on the basis of rates in the general population. The cases included those exposed to low and moderate doses, as well as the highly exposed persons among whom bone and head tumors appeared. In a special subgroup of 1456 persons in whom the mean bone marrow dose in rads varied from 0.088 to 981.8, there were only two cases who developed leukemia. The mean narrow dose in these cases was 18.53 rad and 82.67 rad, a considerably lower figure than the dose received by the ankylosing spondylitics, who received external radiation. The mean marrow dose in the spondylitic patients was 321 rad, although cases of leukemia were recorded at 5.0 rad. It must be concluded that ^{226}Ra and ^{228}Ra deposition in the skeleton is unlikely to result in leukemia.

^{224}Ra

The pattern of radiation dose to sensitive cells in patients receiving ^{224}Ra in repeated injections will differ from that received from ^{226}Ra and ^{228}Ra, because ^{224}Ra will decay rapidly on the bone surface owing to its short half-life, whereas, the ^{226}Ra, ^{228}Ra is present continuously.

Bone Tumors. Bone sarcomas are reported in 54 of 897 patients, of known and unknown dose, with appearance times ranging from 3.5 to 22 yr after the first ^{224}Ra injection. For patients of known dose and injection span bone sarcoma occurred in 35 of 204 juveniles who received an 1110 rad average injection dose of ^{224}Ra and had an 11 mo average injection span. In a group of 612 adults 13 developed osteosarcoma. Their average skeletal dose was 210 rad and their average injection span 6 mo. Mays et al (1978) consider that for equal injection spans the juveniles were only slightly more sensitive per rad to radium-induced bone sarcoma than the adults. Most of the observed sarcomas arose in locations unaffected by tuberculosis or ankylosing spondylitis. The shortest appearance times of 3.5 yr in juveniles and 5 yr in adults agree well with those observed following x-ray therapy of 4 yr in juveniles and 4 yr in adults (Woodard, 1969). The lowest total mean dose to bone associated with a cancer in a ^{224}Ra patient in the original series was 90 rad (Mays, 1978a). In a series of 1000 patients receiving less than 90 rad, two osteosarcomas occurred, the lowest dose being 67 rad (Mays, 1978b), a dose much lower than the lowest dose recorded in an ^{226}Ra patient, of 880 rad.

In the case of ^{224}Ra, the incidence of bone sarcoma increased as the injection span increased, both in juveniles and adults, as shown in Figure 4 (Mays et al,

FIGURE 4. Risk of bone sarcomas in humans versus ^{224}Ra protractions. The risk rises to about 200 bone sarcomas/10^6 person-rad at long protraction. The standard deviation of each point is shown. Mays et al, 1976; by courtesy of authors and publishers.

Bone sarcoma induction vs. protraction of injections

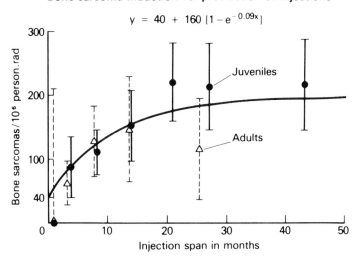

1976). Mole (1979) suggests "that repopulation counterbalancing inactivation in the endosteum would seem to be the most plausible biological mechanism for the protraction effect with Ra^{224}, i.e. the increase in frequency of bone sarcoma induction when multiple injections of Ra^{224} are spread over relatively long periods instead of one short period."

In 1978 Rowland et al considered that a dose-squared exponential function described the dose incidence relationship between ^{224}Ra and the number of bone sarcomas per person-year at risk. Mays, Spiess, and Gerspach (1978) state it is impossible to choose between a variety of dose–response relationships.

Cartilage Pathology. In a group of 217 juveniles and 708 adults reported in 1970 only three chondrosarcomas were noted, compared with 43 osteosarcomas (Speiss and Mays, 1970). Osteochondroma or exostosis occurred in 30 juveniles. Only two would have been expected among 204 juveniles of known dose and injection span who were followed for an average of 20 yr. The younger at the age of injection the higher the exostosis incidence. The majority were present in the region of the metaphyses of the long bones and were often multiple. None have become malignant, though two patients have developed osteosarcoma elsewhere in the skeleton (Mays, Speiss, and Gerspach, 1978). Spiess (1969) has described considerable disturbance, as evidenced by radiology, in the region of the epiphyseal plate and interference in growth of the long bones. The exact pathology of these exostoses merits further study in relation to the site of ^{224}Ra deposition. In nonirradiated individuals an exostosis appears to form in consequence of cartilaginous metaplasia in the periosteum in the neighborhood of the plate. The aberrant cartilage, Sissons suggests, forms the growing cap of the lesion, and as growth proceeds the cartilage becomes replaced by cancellous bone as a result of endochondral ossification (Sissons, 1979). Such cartilaginous metaplasia may arise as the result of ^{224}Ra deposition in the calcifying cartilage of the metaphyseal trabeculae, or in the matrix vesicles of the cartilage and in the mitochondria of the proliferating cartilage cells of the cartilage plate, itself.

Sinus and Mastoid Cancers. No sinus or mastoid tumors are reported in patients receiving ^{224}Ra. This is not surprising, because ^{224}Ra decays rapidly and, therefore, the bone dose will be low and these tumors are characterized by an extremely long latent period.

Leukemia. In the earlier populations treated with ^{224}Ra two cases of leukemia were diagnosed among the injected adults, whereas, about 0.8 would have been expected naturally (Spiess, Gerspach, and Mays, 1978). In addition three cases of "pan myelosis" were noted (Spiess and Mays, 1970). No cases are recorded in children. More recently, a generalized plasmacytoma and a reticulum cell sarcoma of marrow have been recorded in a group of 1531 ankylosing spondylitis patients receiving a skeletal dose less than 90 rad (Wick and Gossner, 1983).

THORIUM-232 (THOROTRAST)

Colloidal thorium dioxide has been used widely, under the trade name Thorotrast, as a contrast medium in diagnostic radiology. It also has important bone-seeking daughter products: ^{224}Ra, ^{228}Ra, and ^{228}Th. Characteristically, the injected Thorotrast tends to become encapsulated in fibrous tissue, especially in the liver, but some of the radioactive daughter products may escape into the blood stream and so reach both bone and marrow. The thorotrast, itself, is taken up by bone marrow macrophages (Jee et al, 1967). Because macrophages are mobile cells, they will move the radiation source in relation to both hemopoietic and endosteal cells. The resulting dosimetry, therefore, is extremely complex (Rundo, 1978; Mays, 1978a; Kaul and Noffz, 1978; Mole, 1979).

Bone Tumors

Subjects receiving Thorotrast at younger ages may have a genuine excess of bone sarcomas, even if subjects receiving Thorotrast at an older age have not. Six cases of bone sarcoma were listed initially in 3772 cases, to which a seventh has since been added (Mole, 1978, 1979). Four of these were histologically confirmed.

Sinus Tumors

Ten cases of neoplasia of the maxillary sinuses after antral injection and incomplete removal of thorotrast have been described (Fabrikant et al, 1964).

Leukemia

Leukemia and related blood dyscrasias have occurred in excess in Thorotrast subjects, as shown in a recent review of 3772 cases (Mole, 1978, 1979). A total of 44 cases of leukemia, excluding chronic lymphatic, are recorded in the same review and 26 cases of myelomatosis.

EXTERNAL IRRADIATION

Humans are exposed to external radiation from various sources, of which the most important are the therapeutic and diagnostic use of x-rays. There is no evidence that background radiation from natural sources in the environment is responsible for skeletal malignancies but, in assessing the importance of any manmade source of radiation, the existence of background radiation, which is usually assessed as 4.7 rem $\pm$ 0.4 to age 60, must not be forgotten (Spiers, 1979).

Exposure to external radiation differs from exposure to internal radiation from alpha-emitting radionuclides already considered by the fact that it involves penetrating radiation which, in the majority of cases, causes approximately uniform tissue irradiation. This means that all the cells in the skeleton are exposed. This uniform tissue irradiation puts the highly cellular hemopoietic bone marrow at far greater risk than occurs with internal irradiation. It is not surprising that leukemia is more common than bone cancer. Some large groups, notably radiologists who, before the risk was recognized, were exposed to continuous low-level radiation, showed an increased leukemia incidence but no excess of bone cancer (Seltser and Sartwell, 1965; Matanoski, 1980; Smith and Doll, 1981). The majority of one group included in the survey could have received an accumulated whole-body dose of between 100 and 500 rad (Smith and Doll, 1981). No excess of bone cancers has been noted in the A-bomb survivors, although there is a high incidence of myeloid leukemia.

Therapeutic Irradiation

The possible carcinogenic effect of external radiation on the skeleton has been analyzed in several studies. Yoshizawa, in an incomplete review, found 262 cases of skeletal neoplasia (Yoshizawa et al, 1977), the site being largely dependent on the condition for which radiation was given. Hutchison (1976) considers the available data to be insufficient to define a dose–response curve. Doll (1981) concludes that an increase in risk of cancer induction is approximately proportional to the dose received, down to doses of the order of 1 rad, the increase being greater in childhood and late middle age than in the young adult. In a group of children irradiated for thymic enlargement, an excess of benign osteochondroma and leukemia are recorded (Hempleman et al, 1967). An excess of leukemia and cancer of the skull bones are noted in large groups of children irradiated for ringworm (Modan et al, 1974).

External irradiation has been used extensively in the treatment of ankylosing spondylitis. The radiation involves only about 40% of the skeleton, including the spine. A follow-up of 14,111 patients who received a *single* course of x-ray treatment records an increased cancer incidence in all heavily irradiated sites except the skin (Smith and Doll, 1982). This included 31 deaths from leukemia, other than chronic lymphatic, when 6.5 cases might have been expected. The ratio of observed deaths from leukemia to expected deaths (4.8 to 1) was considerably greater than that from all other neoplasms combined (1.5 to 1). The estimated mean marrow dose was 321 rad in a group of 903 patients for whom full data on radiation treatment were available. The distribution of the estimated mean bone marrow dose in this group is shown in Figure 5. This is fairly uniform (between 50 and 550 rad), but the number exposed to higher doses then falls off rapidly, and only 2.1% of patients had estimated doses in excess of 650 rad. It is suggested that this may be due to an increasing proportion of cells at risk in the bone marrow having been sterilized with increasing doses of radiation.

The risk of a radiation-induced leukemia or other cancers was dependent on the age of the patient at the time of treatment. Those who were older than 55 when irradiated had an excess death rate from leukemia that was greater than 15 times that in those who were treated when younger than 25 yr. The incidence of osteosarcoma was lower than that of leukemia in the group of 14,111 patients who received a single course of treatment. Three osteosarcomas were noted, when 0.55 were expected. The mean follow-up period was 16.2 yr. The risk of developing a radiation-induced cancer in other heavily irradiated sites was shown to be increased for many years following treatment, so it is not impossible that further osteosarcomas will be noted as follow-up is continued. Patients with ankylosing spondylitis not given x-ray therapy showed no excess of leukemia or osteosarcoma (Radford et al, 1977).

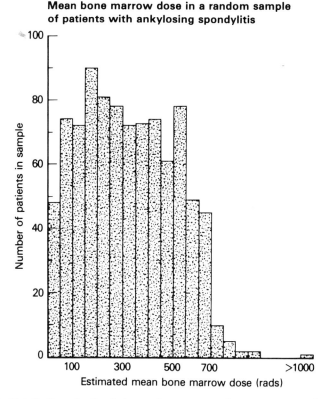

FIGURE 5. Distribution of estimated mean bone marrow doses among a random sample of 903 patients with ankylosing spondylitis. Smith and Doll, 1982; by courtesy of authors and publishers.

Diagnostic Irradiation

The question of the effect of fetal irradiation on cancer incidence has been controversial (MacMahon, 1980), although it is now generally accepted (Mole, 1974; Doll, 1981). It was first reported in 1958 that mothers of children with cancer had more frequently received pelvic x-ray examinations during the relevant pregnancy than mothers of healthy children (Stewart et al, 1958). The cancers included osteosarcomas and leukemias other than chronic lymphatic (Stewart, 1973, 1981). No such relationship has been observed in Japanese A-bomb survivors (Jablon and Kato, 1970). Mole (personal communication to UNSCEAR, 1977), however, suggests that this discrepancy may be explained by the higher fetal doses received by the Japanese, resulting in cell killing effects that may have reduced the subsequent incidence of cancer that would otherwise have been expected (Major and Mole, 1978). UNSCEAR (1977) concludes "that malignancies may be induced in the foetus by exposure in utero at average absorbed doses in the range of 0.2–20 rads from diagnostic X rays."

BONE TUMOR RISK ESTIMATES

Bone tumor risk estimates are given by UNSCEAR (1977) and provisional risk estimates by BEIR (1980). Many of the calculations involved in the BEIR risk estimates are based on animal data. Because there are differences in the human and animal skeletal response to radiation (Spiers and Vaughan, 1976) and in the time factors involved, there must be reservations about accepting the BEIR estimates.

CONCLUSION

Present evidence suggests that ^{226}Ra and ^{228}Ra deposited in the human skeleton may induce cancers of bone, cartilage, and epithelium applied to bone in the cranial air sinuses. ^{224}Ra will induce cancers of bone and cartilage but no radium isotope, at present, is recognized as leukemogenic in humans. ^{232}Th, administered as Thorotrast, may induce osteosarcoma, myeloma, hemangiosarcoma, and a variety of luekemias other than lymphatic. External radiation may induce osteosarcomas and granulocytic-monocytic leukemias in humans, particularly the latter.

I am grateful to Dr. J. F. Loutit, Dr. M. Owen, and Prof. F. W. Spiers who have provided most valuable advice.

REFERENCES

Ali SY (1976) Analysis of matrix vesicles and their role in the calcification of epiphyseal cartilage. Fed Proc 35:135–142.

Anderson HV (1976) Matrix vesicles of cartilage and bone. Fed Proc 35:105–108.

ANL (1982–83) Radiological and environmental research division annual report, Part II.

Ash P, Loutit JF (1977) The ultrastructure of skeletal haemangiosarcomas induced in mice by strontium-90. J Pathol 122:209–218.

Ashton BA, Allen TD, Howlett CR, Eaglesom CC, Hattori A, Owen M (1981) Formation of bone and cartilage by marrow stromal cells in diffusion chambers in vivo. Clin Orthop 151:294–307.

BEIR (1980) The effects on populations of exposure to low levels of ionzing radiation: 1980. Washington, DC: National Academy of Sciences, National Research Council. Committee on the Biological Effects of Ionizing Radiations. National Academy Press.

Burger EH, Mathews JL (1978) Cellular calcium distribution in foetal bones studied with k. pyroantimonate. Calcif Tissue Res 26:181–190.

Doll R (1981) Radiation hazards: 25 Years of collaborative research. Br J Radiol 54:179–186.

Evans RD (1966) The effect of skeletally deposited alpha-ray emitters in man. Br J Radiol 39:881–895.

Keane AT, Kolenkow RJ, Neal WR, Shanahan MM (1969) Radiogenic tumors in the radium and mesothorium cases studied at M.I.T. In: Mays CW, Jee WSS, Lloyd RD, Stover BJ, Dougherty JH, and Taylor GN (Eds.), Delayed effects of bone-seeking radionuclides. Salt Lake City, UT: University of Utah Press.

Fabrikant JI, Dickson RJ, Fetter BF (1964) Mechanisms of radiation carcinogenesis at the clinical level. Br J Cancer 18:458–477.

Hamilton JG (1947) The metabolism of the fission products and the heaviest elements. Radiology 49:325–348.

Hempelmann LH, Pifer JW, Burke GJ, Terry R, Ames WR (1967) Neoplasms in persons treated with x-rays in infancy for thymic enlargement. A report of the 3rd follow-up survey. J Natl Cancer Inst 38:317–341.

Howells GR, Green D (1981) The temporal and spatial distribution of ^{239}Pu within bone In: Bone and bone seeking radionuclides—Physiology, dosimetry and effects. EULEP Symposium, Rotterdam, Aug, EUR-7168-EN. New York: Harwood Academic Publishers, pp 57–71.

Hutchison GB (1976) Late neoplastic changes following medical irradiation. Cancer 37:1102–1107.

Ichimaru T, Ishimaru M, Mikami M, Matsunga A (1980) Incidence of multiple myeloma among atomic bomb survivors. Hiroshima and Nagasaki by dose 1950–76. Quoted BEIR 1980.

ICRP 11 (1968) A review of the radiosensitivity of the tissues in bone. Oxford: Pergamon Press.

ICRP 20 (1972) Alkaline earth metabolism in adult man. Oxford: Pergamon Press.

ICRP 26 (1977) Recommendations of the international commission on radiological protection. Ann ICRP 1:1–47.

ICRP 30 (1979) Limits for intakes of radionucleotides by workers. Ann ICRP 2. 98–99:1979.

Jablon S, Kato H Childhood cancer in relation to prenatal exposure to atomic-bomb radiation. Lancet ii:1000–1003.

Jee WSS, Dockum NL, Mical RS, Arnold JS, Looney WB (1967) Distribution of thorium daughters in bone. Ann NY Acad Sci 145:660–673.

Kaul A, Noffz W (1978) Tissue dose in Thorotrast patients. Health Phys 35:113–121.

Keane AT (1978–71) Skeletal location of primary bone tumors in the radium cases. Argonne National Laboratory Report ANL 7860, Part II, pp 59–66.

Kember NF (1981) Personal communication.

Lloyd EL (1979–80) Radiation dose to the cells at risk for the induction of bone tumours by bone seeking radionuclides, Part II. Radiological and Environmental Research Annual Report, ANL-80-115. Center for Human Biology, pp 29–32.

Lloyd EL, Henning CB (1978–79) Cells at risk for the production of bone tumours in man. An electron microscope study of the endosteal surface of control bone and bone from a human radium case. Part II. Radiological and Environmental Research Division Annual Report, ANL-79-65, pp 39–53.

Loutit JF (1970) Malignancy from radium. Br J Cancer 24:195–207.

Loutit JF (1976) Vasoformative non-osteogenic (angio) sarcomas of bone marrow stroma duet to strontium-90. Intl J Radiat Biol 30:359–383.

Loutit JF, Vaughan JM (1971) The radiosensitive tissues in bone Br J Radiol 44:815.

Luk SC, Nopajaroonsri C, Simon GT (1974) The ultrastructure of endosteum. A topographic study in young adult rabbits. J Ultrastruct Res 46:165–183.

MacMahon R (1980) Childhood cancer and prenatal irradiation. In: Burchenal JF and Oettgen HF (Eds.), Cancer Proceedings 1980, International Symposium on Cancer. New York: Grune and Stratton, pp 223–228.

Major IR, Mole RH (1978) Myeloid leukemia in x ray irradiated CBA mice. Nature (Lond) 272:455–456.

Marshall JH (1969) The retention of radionuclides in bone. In: Mays CW, Jee WS, Lloyd RD, Stover, BJ, Dougherty JH, and Taylor GN (Eds.), Delayed effects of bone-seeking radionuclides. Salt Lake City, UT: University of Utah Press.

Marshall JH, Groer PG (1977) A theory of the induction of bone cancer by alpha radiation. Radiat Res 71:149–192.

Marshall JH, Groer PG, Schlenker RA (1978) Dose to endosteal cells and relative distribution factors for Ra^{224}, Pu^{239} compared to Ra^{226}. Health Phys 35:91–101.

Martin JH, Mathews JL (1969) Mitachondrial granules in chondrocytes. Calc Tissue Res 3:184–193.

Martland HS (1931) The occurrence of malignancy in radioactive persons. Am J Cancer 15:2435–2516.

Martland HS (1939) Occupational tumours, bones. Encyclopaedia of Health and Hygiene. Geneva: International Labour Organization, pp 1–23.

Martland HS, Conlon P, Knef JP (1925) Some unrecognized dangers in the use and handling of radioactive substances; With special reference to the storage of insoluble products of radium and mesothorium in the reticuloendothelial system. J Am Med Assoc 85:1769–1776.

Matanoski GM (1980) Risk of cancer associated with occupational exposure in radiologists and other radiation workers. In: Burchenal JH and Oettgen HF (Eds.), Cancer Proceedings 1980, New York: Grune and Stratton, pp 241–254.

Mays CW (1978a) Endosteal dose to thorotrast patients. Health Phys 35:123–125.

Mays CW (1978b) Risk to bone from present Ra^{224} therapy. In: Muller WA and Ebert HG (Eds.), Biological effects of Ra^{224}, benefit and risk of therapeutic application. The Hague: Nijhoff Medical Division.

Mays CW, Spiess H, Taylor GN, Lloyd RD, Jee WSS, McFarlane SS, Taysom DH, Brammer TW, Brammer D, Pollard TA (1976) Estimated risk to human bone from Pu^{239}. In: Jee WSS (Ed.), The health effects of plutonium and radium. Salt Lake City, UT: The J.W. Press.

Mays CW, Spiess H, Gerspach A (1978) Skeletal effects following Ra^{224} injections into humans. Health Phys 35:83–90.

Mayneord WV, Clarke RH (1975) Carcinogenesis and radiation risk. A biomathematical reconnaissance. Br J Radiol 12 (suppl):1–25.

Modan B, Baidatz D, Mart H, Steinitz R, Levin SG (1974) Radiation Induced head and neck tumours. Lancet i:277–279.

Mole RH (1974) Ante-natal irradiation and childhood cancer. Causation or coincidence?" Br J Cancer 30:199–208.

Mole RH (1978) The radiological significance of the studies with Ra^{224} and Thorotrast. Health Phys 35:167–174.

Mole RH (1979) Carcinogenesis by Thorotrast and other sources of irradiation, especially other emitters. Environ Res 18:192–215.

Owen M (1980) The origin of bone cells in the postnatal organism. Arthrit Rheum 23:1073–1080.

Peachey LD (1964) Electron microscope observations on accumulation of divalent cations in intramitochondrial granules. J Cell Biol 20:95–109.

Pool RR, Morgan JP, Parks NJ, Farnham JE, Littman MS (1983) Comparative pathogenesis of radium-induced intracortical bone lesions in humans and beagles. Health Phys 44 (suppl 1):155–177.

Raabe OG (1984) Comparison of the carcinogenicity of radium and bone seeking actinides. Health Phys 46:1241–1258.

Raabe OG, Book SA, Parks NJ (1983) Life time bone cancer dose response relationships in beagles and people from skeletal burdens of ^{226}Ra and ^{90}Sr. Health Phys 44 (suppl 1):33–48.

Radford EP, Doll R, Smith PG (1977) Mortality among patients with ankylosing spondylitis not given x-ray therapy. N Engl J Med 297:572–576.

Rowland RE, Marshall J (1959) Radium in human bone: The dose in microscopic volumes of bone. Radiat Res 11:299–313.

Rowland RE, Keane AT, Lucas HF (1973) In: Radionuclide carcinogenesis. AEC Symposium Series 20, Conf. 720505, 405-420.

Rowland RE, Stehney AF (1977–78) Radium-induced malignancies, Part II. Argonne National Laboratory Report ANL 78-65, p 259.

Rowland RE, Stehney AF, Lucas HF, Jr. (1978) Dose–response relationship for female radium dial workers. Radiat Res 76:368–383.

Rowland RS, Stehney AF, Lucas HF (1983) Dose–response relationships for radium-induced bone sarcomas. Health Phys 44 (suppl 1):15–31.

Rundo J (1978) The radioactive properties and biological behavior of ^{224}Ra (ThX) and its daughters. Health Phys 35:13–20.

Schlenker RA (1979–80) Dosimetry of paranasal sinus and mastoid epithelia in exposed humans. Radiological and Environmental Research Division Annual Report ANL-80-115, Part II, pp 1–21.

Schlenker RA, Harris MJ (1978–79) Dosimetry of head carcinomas in radium cases. Radiological and Environmental Research Division Annual Report July 1978–June 1979. ANL-79-65, Part II, pp 76–84.

Seltser R, Sartwell PE (1965) The influence of occupational exposure to radiation on the mortality of American radiologists and other medical specialists. Am J Epidemiol 81:2–22.

Sissons HA (1970) Dimensions of cells covering bone surfaces. Medical Research Council, London, Subcommittee on Permissible Levels, PIRC/PL/70/4.

Sissons HA (1979) Bones, diseases of joints, tendon sheath and other soft tissue. In: Symmes W St C (Ed.), Systematic pathology, 2nd Ed. Edinburgh: Churchill Livingstone, pp 2383–2522.

Smith PG, Doll R (1981) Mortality from cancer and all causes. Br J Radiol 54:187–194.

Smith PG (1982) Mortality among patients with ankylosing spondylitis following a single treatment course with x rays. Br Med J 284:449–460.

Spiers FW (1968) Radioisotopes in the human body. New York: Academic Press.

Spiers FW (1979) Background radiation and estimated risks from low dose irradiation. (Health Phys 37:784–789.

Spiers FW, Vaughan (1976) Hazards of plutonium with special reference to the skeleton. Nature 259:531–534.

Spiers FW, King SD, Beddoe AH (1977) Measurement of endosteal surface areas in human long bones: Relationship to sites of occurrence of osteosarcoma. Br J Radiol 50:769–776.

Spiers FW, Beddoe AH (1983a) Sites of incidence of osteosarcoma in the long bones of man and the beagle. Health Phys 44 (suppl 1):49–64.

Spiers FW, Lucas HF, Rundo J, Anast GA (1983b) Leukaemia incidence in the U.S. dial painters. Health Phys 44 (suppl 1):49–64.

Spiers FW, Lucas HF, Rundo J, Anast GA (1983b) Leukaemia incidence in the U.S. dial painters. Health Phys 44 (suppl 1):65–72.

Spiers FW, Burch PRJ (1957) Measurements of body radioactivity in a radium worker. Br J Radiol Suppl 7:81–89.

Spiess H (1969) Ra^{224} induced tumors in children and adults. In: Mays CW, Jee WSS, Lloyd RD, Stover BJ, Dougherty JH, and Taylor GN (Eds.), Delayed effects of bone-seeking radionuclides. Salt Lake City UT: University of Utah Press.

Spiess H, Mays CW (1970) Some cancers induced by Ra^{224} (ThX) in children and adults. Health Phys 19:713–729.

Spiess H, Gerspach A, Mays CW (1978) Soft tissue effects following Ra^{224} injections into humans. Health Phys 35:61–81.

Stewart AM (1973) Cancer as a cause of abortion and still-births: The effect of these early deaths on the recognition of radiogenic leukaemias. Br J Cancer 27:465–472.

Stewart AM (1981) Personal communication.

Stewart AM, Webb J, Hewitt D (1958) A survey of childhood malignancies. Br J Med i:1495–1508.

Taylor DM (1972) Interaction between transuranium elements and the components of cells and tissues. Health Phys 22:575–581.

Thurman GB, Mays CW, Taylor GN, Keane AT, Sissons HA (1973) Skeletal location of radiation-induced and naturally occurring osteosarcomas in man and dog. Cancer Res 33:1604–1607.

UNSCEAR (1977) Sources and effects of ionizing radiation. United Nations Scientific Committee on the Effects of Ionizing Radiation. Annex G. New York: United Nations.

Vaughan J (1962) Bone disease induced by radiation. Intl Rev Exp Pathol 1:244–369.

Vaughn J (1970) Note on the character of cells on trabecular bone surfaces in adult human vertebrae. Medical Research Council, London. Subcommittee on Protection Against Ionizing Radiation PIRC/PL/70/1.

Vaughn J (1981) The physiology of bone, 3rd Ed. Oxford: Clarendon Press.

Wick RR, Gossner W (1983) Follow up study of late effects in ^{224}Ra treated ankylosing spondylitis patients. Health Phys 44 (suppl 1):187–194.

Woodard HO (1969) In: Sikov MR and Mahlum DD (Eds.), Radiation biology of the foetal and juvenile mammal. USAEC Conf 690501. Springfield, VA: National Technical Information Service.

Yoshizawa Y, Kusama T, Morimoto K (1977) Search for the lowest irradiation dose from literature on radiation induced bone tumours. Nippon Acta Radiol 37:377–386.

CARCINOGENIC EFFECTS
OF RADIATION ON THE HUMAN SKIN

ROY E. ALBERT, M.D., AND ROY E. SHORE, Ph.D., D.P.H.

Roentgen discovered x-rays in November 1895; 7 yr later, in Germany, Frieben (1902) reported the first case of cancer of the skin attributable to x-rays, in a technician who had demonstrated x-ray tubes for 4 yr by holding his hands in the beam. He developed a squamous cell carcinoma on the dorsum of one hand with regional lymph node metastases. By 1909, a number of cases of skin cancer in x-ray workers had been reported in both the U.S. and England (Henry, 1950). Skin cancer was also found in radium workers and was regarded an occupational disease in Great Britain in 1924 (Cade, 1948). Radium dermatitis occurs most frequently on the hands; the nails and skin of the fingers become atrophic. Carcinoma of the skin has been described in areas of chronic dermatitis in radium workers most of whom had handled radium for 10 yr or more (Cade, 1948).

There is a very large background of skin cancer in humans against which the effects of ionizing radiation have to be considered. The major cause of skin cancer in humans is chronic exposure to sunlight. In many individuals, exposure to excessive amounts of sunlight over the years results in severe forms of senile atrophy of the skin. The skin becomes thin, sallow, dry, wrinkled, slightly scaling, and inelastic; often freckles, lentigines, and telangiectases are present. Such changes are frequently seen in sailors, farmers, fishermen, and habitual sunbathers, among others, and are more common in blonde or red-headed persons. The frequency of precancerous keratoses and carcinomas in these individuals is very high. A characteristic feature of sunlight-induced cancer is that it occurs in exposed parts of the body. In one series of over 3500 basal cell carcinomas seen at the Dermatology Clinic at New York University Medical Center from 1955 to 1969, 85% occurred on the face, ear, and neck, and 3% on the arm and hand (Kopf, 1979).

From the Institute of Environmental Medicine, New York University Medical Center, New York, New York.

Most of the reports on radiation-induced skin cancer have consisted of cases from medical facilities (Totten et al, 1957; Petersen, 1954; Pack and Davis, 1965; Ridley and Spittle, 1974; Sarkany et al, 1968; Meara, 1968). There are many case reports of skin cancer arising as a consequence of the use and misuse of x-ray for a variety of conditions, including ringworm of the scalp, acne of the face, hypertrichosis, hemangioma, lupus vulgaris, toxic goiter, eczema, and multiple fluoroscopies (Neuman, 1963). Many such cases arise in association with radiodermatitis (Getzrow, 1976). There are few adequate studies of exposed populations because nonmelanotic skin cancers have a low mortality rate and are unreported.

Case-control studies provide supporting evidence about radiation-induced skin cancer but do not permit detailed quantitative evaluations. Martin et al (1970) compared 156 patients with skin cancer of the head or neck with 434 other patients drawn from his private practice, as to the history of radiotherapy of the head and neck, and found a relative risk of 4.4 (19% versus 5%, respectively; $p < 0.0001$). In a series of 368 skin cancer cases following radiotherapy, 25% had been treated for hirsutism and 35% for acne. Of 314 of these irradiation skin cancer cases, 19% showed slight or no skin changes, indicating that chronic radiodermatitis is not a prerequisite for radiation-induced skin cancer.

Takahashi (1964) has reported case-control data indicating that medical radiation is associated with skin cancer among Japanese. Fourteen of 308 (4.5%) cases of skin cancer versus 23 of 4067 (0.6%) controls had a history of previous irradiation. The excess was significant at the lowest dose range, 500–2000 R, and there was a highly significant dose–response relationship (X^2 for trend $= 79.3$, 1 df, $p < 0.0001$). However, the small number of irradiated subjects and the uncertainties of the dose estimates make it impossible to test the shape of this dose–response curve.

Several epidemiologic follow-up studies have shown excessive skin cancer following radiation exposures. These will be reported next, followed by several studies that have not shown radiation-induced skin cancers.

STUDIES FINDING RADIATION-INDUCED SKIN CANCER

It should be noted that in subsequent calculations of excess risk, no account is taken of the amount of skin area irradiated. This is difficult to assess for many studies, and is complicated by uncertainties in carcinogenic susceptibility of the skin according to anatomic location.

In the Rochester study of x-ray therapy for an enlarged thymus gland (Hempelmann et al, 1975), 8 of 2653 persons had a skin cancer in the irradiated area (six basal cell, two malignant melanomas) versus 3 of 4791 in the corresponding skin area among controls (Woodard, 1980). There was no difference between the groups in the incidence of skin cancers outside the irradiated skin area. During years 10–49 postirradiation, the rate in the irradiated area was 4.8 times the rate in the control ($p = 0.01$). Assuming that the skin doses were approximately 20% greater than the air doses (due to backscatter, etc.), the skin doses would range from 40 to about 1500 rad, with a mean of 330 rad. The radiation was given mainly in fractions of approximately 40–400 rad.

Matanoski et al (1975) reported an excess of skin cancer mortality among radiologists, compared with three other groups of medical specialists. The excess was especially pronounced in the earliest cohort (those becoming members of the radiologic society during the 1920s), who presumably had the highest radiation exposures. The average skin doses received by the various cohorts of radiologists were essentially unknown. Estimates for the earlier cohorts range all the way from a low of about 200 rad to a high of 2000 rad (Lewis, 1957; Braestrup, 1957). The NAS Report (1972) used 800 rad as a tentative estimate. With that estimate the absolute risk of skin cancer deaths in the 1920–29 cohort would be $0.5/10^6$ person-year-rad (PYR).

Sevcova et al (1978) found a significantly elevated incidence of skin cancers, primarily basal cell carcinomas of the face, in a large series of uranium miners, who had estimated cumulative alpha radiation doses to the basal cell layer of the skin in the range of 100–200 rad (1000–2000 rem). The observed incidence (per million person-years) over that expected from age-specific population rates was 374 versus 82, or a relative risk of 4.5. The actual numbers of skin cancers and exposed workers were not reported. If an estimate of 150 rad is taken as the average dose, this excess yields an absolute risk value of $1.9/10^6$ PYR. The rate among nonmining uranium workers (with small exposures) was not elevated, suggesting that the elevated rate among miners was not a methodologic artifact of better case detection in the workers than in the general population. However, caution should be taken in assigning the apparent skin cancer excess among miners to radiation alone. Arsenic in the ores may also be a factor, because arsenic is known to produce skin cancer (although mainly on the palms, soles, and trunk).

One of the most extensive follow-up studies of radiation-induced skin cancer involves persons who were treated as children by x-radiation for ringworm of the scalp (tinea capitis) (Albert and Omran, 1968; Shore et al, 1976). The study included a group of 2227 tinea capitis cases who received x-ray epilation and 1387 tinea capitis cases who were treated by other means at the New York University (NYU) Medical Center Skin and Cancer Unit. These cases had been treated between 1940 and 1959; at which time the antifungal agent griseofulvin supplanted the use of x-irradiation. The cases were irradiated with 100 kVp unfiltered x-ray (HVL = 0.85 ml aluminum, equivalent to an effective photon energy of 16 KeV); about 340 R were administered to each of five fields over a 10-min period, in order to distribute the radiation as evenly as possible over the entire surface of the scalp. The average absorbed dose to the scalp was about 450 rad (330–600 rad), the margin of the scalp received 240 rad, and the rest of the face and neck received 10–50 rad (Schultz, 1968). The average age at treatment was about 8 yr, and the average posttreatment elapsed time to follow-up was about 25 yr. In the three surveys to date, a total of 31 cases of skin cancer of the head and neck have been found in the irradiated group and three in the control group. An additional ten cases have been found in a dermatologic clinic evaluation program of 203 irradiated subjects (versus 0 among 90 control subjects); thus, a total of 41 irradiated cases are known to have developed skin cancer. All 41 irradiated cases had basal cell carcinomas. There was a total of 80 skin cancer lesions among the 41 cases. Even though 25% of the irradiated group was black, all 41 skin cancer cases were in whites. If one assumes the average dose to the scalp was about 450 rad, then the skin cancer excess (based on the 31 cases found at survey) was about $2.4/10^6$ PYR.

STUDIES NOT OBSERVING EXCESS SKIN CANCERS

Of the incidence studies of skin cancer in defined irradiated populations, the Japanese atomic bomb study is the largest. As part of its Adult Health Study evaluation program, an extensive dermatologic evaluation was performed on 9646 subjects from Hiroshima or Nagasaki, including 1830 with >90 rad (kerma) doses, and an additional 2081 with 10–89 rad doses (Johnson et al, 1969). These subjects were compared with others in the city at the time of the bombing who had doses <1 rad (2696 subjects). The sample was carefully drawn, and the examinations were conducted 19–21 yr postirradiation, allowing apparently ample time for latent malignant changes to begin to appear. No evidence was found for radiation-induced skin cancer; the only observed skin cancer case received <1 rad.

The A-bomb study is statistically incompatible with other studies that have shown a skin cancer effect at doses under 1000 rad. Using an estimate of 1.0 skin cancer/10^6 PYR as an average of the estimates found in other studies, one would have expected about 5.0 skin cancers in the irradiated group; the probability of finding none by chance is extremely low ($p = 0.007$, Poisson exact test).

A skin examination program was conducted by Sulzberger et al (1952), who evaluated 1000 patients treated 5–23 yr previously with superficial x-rays, 90% of whom had been treated for benign dermatoses and the remainder for skin cancer. For comparison 1000 former patients, treated for similar conditions without irradiation, were evaluated. The bulk (72%) of the irradiated group received between 150 and 1000 rad to one or more localized areas of the skin, and the remainder received larger doses. For the benign conditions the doses were typically given in fractions of 35–85 rad. The patients were reasonably distributed over the full age range at irradiation, with the exception of a deficit under age 20. Six skin cancers were found in the irradiated group, of which only one occurred in an irradiated area, and nine were found in the control group. However, the average interval from irradiation to evaluation was only 9 yr; just 26 irradiated subjects were evaluated at more than 15 yr postirradiation. The methodologic weakness of a short interval since radiotherapy makes it impossible to interpret the negative results.

No skin cancer deaths have been found among the approximately 15,300 patients followed after radiotherapy for ankylosing spondylitis (Court Brown and Doll, 1965) for which the cumulative skin dose in the primary beam was in the region of 1000–1500 rad. Based on the average risk from the studies finding an effect, one would expect about 70 excess skin cancers to have occurred (58,014 PY 9 yr or more postirradiation × 1200 rad × ~1.0 cancers/10^6 PYR = 70 excess skin cancers expected). If one assumes a 1% mortality from skin cancer, (which is probably a high estimate), then about 0.7 deaths would be expected, whereas none was observed, a result compatible with chance ($p = 0.50$). It should be noted that others have reported basal cell carcinomas following such therapy (Sarkany et al, 1968; Meara, 1968).

Boice and Monson (1977) have followed a series of 543 tuberculous women by questionnaire for an average interval of 26 yr since irradiation. These women had a mean cumulative skin dose of about 1300 rad from an average of 102 fluoroscopic examinations (Boice et al, 1978). Three skin cancers were reported in the irradiated group and one among controls, but it was not known if any of the skin cancers was in the primary beam (Boice, 1979). From the average risk estimate of $1.0/10^6$ PYR (for 10 yr or more postirradiation) given above one would expect about 11 excess skin cancers in the irradiated group.

In another multiple fluoroscopy study, Myrden et al (Myrden and Hilz, 1969; Myrden and Quinlan, 1974) have followed 300 irradiated women with questionnaires for up to 32 yr. The average cumulative skin dose was on the order of 1900 rad. An excess of about seven skin cancers would have been expected when in fact none was observed (Myrden, 1977).

Delarue et al (1975) followed 269 tuberculous women for over 20 yr subsequent to multiple fluoroscopies. An average of 142 fluoroscopic examinations was given posteriorly with a skin dose of about 850 rad. Only one skin cancer was observed in the irradiated area of the back (versus none among controls). An excess of about 2.7–3.4 would be expected based on the average risk estimate $(1.0/10^6$ PYR) and the estimated person-years of follow-up. Observing one skin cancer was compatible with expectation ($p = 0.20$ when the expectation is taken as 3.0).

Woodard and Hempelmann (1978) found no excess skin cancer among women given radiotherapy for postpartum mastitis, in which the average skin dose in the primary beam was about 280 rad and the average follow-up was 25 yr. They found six skin cancers among 571 irradiated women and 13 among 993 control women. Considering years 10–34 postirradiation 7.4 skin cancers would be expected in the irradiated group, based on the control group rate, and from the excess risk calculations, one would expect an additional 2.6. Thus, the total expected was about 10.0 versus 6.0 observed.

One of the problems with the studies by Court Brown, Boice, Myrden, Delarue, and Woodard is that skin cancer was not specifically enquired about in the questionnaires or interviews. When asked only a general question, such as, "Any cancers?", skin cancer will probably be underreported. Thus, the negative results cannot be interpreted unambiguously. Modan's study of tinea capitis irradiation did not find an excess of skin cancer (Modan and Ron, 1977). However, he has indicated that he was essentially unable to study skin cancer, because his sources of information were a tumor registry and a death registry—both of which yield gross underreporting of skin cancer incidence.

HUMAN DOSE–RESPONSE CURVES

The study by Takahashi (1964), though showing a trend with dose, is unsuitable for defining the shape of the dose–response curve, because it was not based on a defined population and the doses were all high. The negative skin cancer results of the Japanese A-bomb study and fluoroscopy studies (Johnson et al, 1969; Boice and Monson, 1977; Delarue et al, 1975) make them unusable for defining a dose–response curve.

The high range of skin cancer incidence (10%–35%) among patients with radiodermatitis and the much lower rates among populations with lower doses (negative to 1%) suggests that the power of dose is greater than one. On the other hand, at least at levels under 1000 rad, the data of Woodard and Hempelmann (1978) do not suggest a diminution of effect with lower doses, although the numbers are very small. There was no evidence of a lesser risk at lower doses, when doses <400 versus >400 rad were compared. The absolute risk estimate was numerically (but not significantly) higher in the lower dose group (0.66 versus $0.32/10^6$ PYR, respectively).

DOSE FRACTIONATION EFFECTS

It cannot be concluded from the negative findings in the two multiple fluoroscopy series (Boice and Monson, 1977; Delarue et al, 1975) that dose fractionation reduces skin carcinogenesis. The postpartum mastitis study (Shore et al, 1977), with little fractionation of the radiation doses to the skin of the chest, was also negative. The radiologist study (Matanoski et al, 1975; Matanoski, 1977) indicates a carcinogenic effect to the skin by highly fractionated exposures at both high and lower total dose levels (i.e., early and more recent cohorts). On the other hand, the thymus radiation study does suggest that dose fractionation may reduce the magnitude of the carcinogenic effect (Woodard and Hempelmann, 1978). One of us (RS) examined dose fractionation in this study, according to number of fractions and average dose per fraction. A tabulation by number of fractions gave comparable estimates for subjects with one, two, and three or more fractions, respectively. A course breakdown of the dose-per-fraction data gave estimates of $0.4/10^6$ PYR for 1–199 rad per fraction and 0.5 for 200–400 rad per fraction. However, a finer-grained analysis of these data using the Cox regression model (controlling total skin dose) tentatively suggested that both increased fractionation and smaller dose per fraction decrease the skin cancer yield ($p = 0.05$ for each effect).

AGE AND TEMPORAL FACTORS

No information is available regarding whether or not age at irradiation (AAI) modifies the risk of radiogenic skin cancer. The range of latent intervals for skin cancer following irradiation is extremely variable. Martin et al (1970) reported latencies of 1–64 yr among 357 cases. In only about 6% of the cases was the interval less than 10 yr, whereas, in about 20% it was greater than 30 yr (20% is probably an underestimate because of the skewed distribution of follow-up times since irradiation in the study population). Ridley and Spittle (1974) have reported a mean latency of 45 yr postirradiation for a series of cases.

The temporal pattern of skin cancer induction in the New York tinea capitis study is shown in Figure 1. The cumulative incidence at about 35 yr after irradiation was approximately 5%. The treated population is still young, however, and more cancers will probably occur. When normalized to life span, the temporal pattern of tumor response in the irradiated tinea capitis cases, as shown in Figure 1, is similar to that in rats that received 1100 rad to 24 cm^2 of dorsal skin with 30 KvP x-rays (Albert et al, 1978).

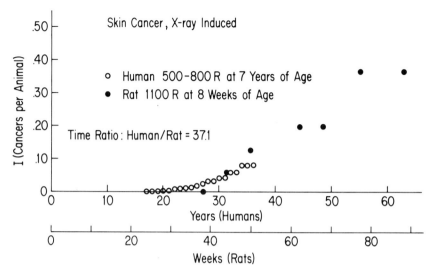

FIGURE 1. The cumulative number of cancers per animal for rats and humans are plotted on linear coordinates. The dose to human skin was about 500–800 rad and the dose to rat skin was 1100 rad. The time scale was shifted by a factor of 37.1 in order to superimpose approximately the two sets of data.

SUSCEPTIBILITY FACTORS AND PATHOGENESIS

The principal classifications of radiation-induced skin cancers are squamous cell and basal cell carcinomas. Anatomic location is one factor determining the relative incidence of the two types: squamous cell (prickle cell) carcinomas have been found most often on the hands; basal cell carcinomas clearly predominate on the head and neck (Traenkle, 1963). An additional factor of dose has been proposed; viz., squamous cell cancers occur primarily following large radiation exposures associated with severe radiodermatitis and ulceration, whereas, basal cell carcinomas predominate at lower exposure levels (Mole, 1972). Fibrosarcomas of dermal origin have also occurred following radiation exposure, but their incidence is an order of magnitude lower than that of squamous or basal cell cancers (Mole, 1972). Additionally, some of the reported fibrosarcomas would be regarded as spindle cell carcinomas today (Martin et al, 1970; Pegum, 1972).

Melanomas and sweat gland tumors have also been reported as occasional radiation sequellae (Traenkle, 1963; Black, 1971; Shore et al, 1976). Austin et al (1981) reported a significant excess of malignant melanoma cases at the Lawrence Livermore National Laboratory (19 observed; approximately 5.3 expected), but it was not found to be associated with radiation exposure. Acquavella et al (1982) attempted to replicate the study at the Los Alamos National Laboratory, but found neither an excess of malignant melanoma nor an association with radiation exposure. The study of cancer incidence among the "Smoky" nuclear test participants initially reported a significant excess of melanomas of the skin (8 observed, 3.5 expected, $p = 0.03$) (Caldwell, 1980). However, further investigation subsequently showed that two of the cases were not melanoma of skin, and the difference then proved to be nonsignificant ($p > 0.10$). In addition, numerous other radiation studies have found no excess of melanomas. Thus, there is no credible evidence for an association of melanomas with ionizing radiation.

The relative sensitivities of various anatomic portions of the skin to radiation-induced cancer are not established, although it is thought that the face and scalp are especially sensitive (Traenkle, 1963). The role of superimposed ultraviolet (UV) radiation by insolation on skin that received ionizing radiation is not defined at this time. UV irradiation is clearly implicated in the genesis of many skin cancers (Emmett, 1973; Anonymous, 1978; Stern et al, 1979), and needs to be taken into account. The carcinogenic effects of UV and ionizing irradiation may be purely additive, but the apparent sensitivity of the face to radiation-induced skin cancers suggests the possibility that UV radiation in some way potentiates ionizing radiation. For instance, the anatomical distribution of tumors on the skin of the head in the tinea capitis study is shown in Figure 2, indicating that about 50% of the lesions were at the nonhair-covered edge of the scalp. This suggests that sunlight has an important cocarcinogenic interaction with the x-rays.

If UV irradiation potentiates the carcinogenic effects of ionizing radiation to the skin, then sensitivity to UV effects would be an important determinant of the magnitude of the ionizing radiation effect. Thus, the well known protection afforded blacks and orientals to the skin-carcinogenic effects of UV irradiation (Segi, 1963; Scotto et al, 1974; Quisenberry, 1963) may also serve to protect them from UV-potentiated effects of ionizing radiation. A lack of UV sensitivity might explain the negative skin cancer effects among blacks in the tinea capitis study, and among the Japanese A-bomb survivors.

FIGURE 2. A scatter diagram showing the location of each of 64 cancers diagnosed and confirmed in the x-irradiated group.

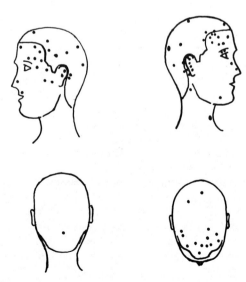

Although chronic radiodermatitis was long thought to be a prerequisite for the induction of skin cancer, ample documentation now exists that basal cell cancers, especially, can occur in skin with little or no gross evidence of radiation skin damage (Ridley and Spittle, 1974; Sarkany et al, 1968; Shore et al, 1976; Albert et al, 1968). It has been suggested that the carcinogenic effect to the skin is much greater if obvious radiodermatitis is present (Traenkle, 1963), with estimates of cumulative incidence ranging from 10% to 35% (versus <1% when there is no radiodermatitis). Calculations on a per-rad basis per unit of irradiated skin area have not been performed to test this difference. Assuming there is a difference, it remains unclear if it results from biological factors having to do with damage in radiodermatitis, or if it is primarily a reflection of similar dose–response relationships for injury and cancer.

Basal cell cancers following radiation exposure are often multiple, either simultaneously or over a period of some years. For instance, Martin et al (1970) reported an average of five lesions per patient when the skin cancer followed irradiation, but 2.5 lesions per patient when there had been no prior irradiation. The comparability of these two groups in length of follow-up after the first lesion was not reported, however, so the comparison may be biased. In the New York series irradiated for tinea capitis, 13 of the 41 basal cell skin cancer cases had multiple lesions. Lesions in cases were developing at the rate of about 0.25/PY (Shore, 1982).

SUMMARY

Ionizing radiation is carcinogenic to the human skin. The character of the dose–response relationships are not well known, nor are the effects of dose fractionation or linear energy transfer. It seems probable that skin on various parts of the body differs in sensitivity to cancer induction by ionizing radiation. There is the possibility that ionizing radiation and UV radiation are cocarcinogenic. What data there are suggest a long period of tumor expression, perhaps of lifetime duration, following irradiation. The rat and human show similar temporal responses when adjustments are made for life span.

REFERENCES

Acquavella J, Tietjen G, Wilkinson G, Key C, Voelz G (1982) Malignant melanoma incidence at the Los Alamos National Laboratory. Lancet i:883–884.

Albert RE, Burns FJ, Shore R (1978) Comparison of the incidence and time patterns of radiation-induced skin cancer in humans and rats. In: Late biological effects of ionizing radiation: Proceedings of A Symposium, Vienna, 13–17 March, Vol. II. Vienna:International Atomic Energy Agency, pp 499–505.

Albert RE, Omran A (1968) Follow-up study of patients treated by x-ray epilation for tinea capitis. I. Population characteristics, post-treatment illnesses, and mortality experience. Arch Environ Health 17:899–918.

Albert R, Omran A, Brauer E, Cohen N, Schmidt H, Dove D, Becker M, Baumring R, Baer R (1968) Follow-up study of patients treated by x-ray epilation for tinea capitis. II. Results of clinical and laboratory examinations. Arch Environ Health 17:919–934.

Anonymous (1978) Ultraviolet radiation and cancer of the skin (Editorial). Lancet i:537–538.

Austin DF, Reynolds P, Snyder M et al (1981) Malignant melanoma among employees of Lawrence Livermore National Laboratory. Lancet ii:712–716.

Black M, Jones E (1971) Dermal cylindroma following x-ray epilation of the scalp. Br J Dermatol 85:70–72.

Boice JD, Land C, Shore R, Norman J, Tokunaga M (1979) Risk of breast cancer following low-dose radiation exposure. Radiology 131:589–597.

Boice J, Monson R (1977) Breast cancer following repeated fluoroscopic examinations of the chest. J Natl Cancer Inst 59:823–832.

Boice J, Rosenstein M, Trout E (1978) Estimation of breast cancer risk and breast doses associated with repeated fluoroscopic examinations of women with tuberculosis. Radiat Res 73:373–390.

Braestrup C (1957) Past and present radiation exposure to radiologists from the point of view of life expectancy. Am J Roentgenol Radium Ther Nucl Med 78:988–992.

Cade S (1948) Malignant disease and its treatment by radium, vol 1. Baltimore:Williams and Wilkins.

Caldwell GG (1981) Cancer incidence and mortality in nuclear test participants—an interim report. In: Quantitative risk in standards setting, proceedings no. 2. National Council on Radiation Protection and Measurements. Washington, D.C.

Court Brown W, Doll R (1965) Mortality from cancer and other causes after radiotherapy for ankylosing spondylitis. Br Med J 2:1327–1332.

Delarue N, Gale G, Ronald A (1975) Multiple fluoroscopy of the chest: Carcinogenicity for the female and implications for breast screening programs: Canadian Med Assoc J 112:1405–1413.

Emmett E (1973) Ultraviolet radiation as a cause of skin tumors. CRC Critical Rev Toxicol 211–255.

Frieben E (1902) Demonstration eines cancroids des rechten handruckens, das sich nach langdauernder einwirkung von roentgenstrahlen entwickelt hatte. Fortsch Roentgenstr 6:106.

Getzrow P (1976) Chronic radiodermatitis and skin cancer. In: Andrade R, Gumport SL, Papkin GL, and Rees TD (eds.), Cancer of the skin. Philadelphia:W. B. Saunders, pp 458–472.

Hempelmann L, Hall W, Phillips M, Cooper R, Ames W (1975) Neoplasms in persons treated with x-rays in infancy: Fourth survey in 20 years. J Natl Cancer Inst 55:519–530.

Henry SA (1950) Cutaneous cancer in relation to occupation. Ann Royal Coll Surg Engl 7:425.

Johnson M, Land C, Gregory P, Taura T, Milton R (1969) Effects of ionizing radiation on the skin, Hiroshima and Nagasaki. Atomic Bomb Casualty Commission, Technical Report no. Hiroshima:Japan 20–69.

Kopf A (1979) Computer analysis of 3531 basal-cell carcinomas of the skin. J Dermatol 6:267–281.

Lewis E (1957) Leukemia and ionizing radiation. Science 125:965–972.

Martin H, Strone E, Spiro R (1970) Radiation-induced skin cancer of the head and neck. Cancer 25:61–71.

Matanoski G (1977) Personal communication.

Matanoski G, Seltser R, Sartwell P, Diamond E, Elliott E (1975) The current mortality rates of radiologists and other physician specialists: Specific causes of death. Am J Epidemiol 101:199–210.

Meara R (1968) Epitheliomata after radiotherapy of the spine. Br J Dermatol 80:620.

Modan B, Ron E (1977) Thyroid neoplasms in a population irradiated for scalp tinea in childhood. In: Radiation-associated thyroid carcinoma. In: DeGroot L, Frohman L, Kaplan E, Refetoff S (eds.), New York:Grune and Stratton.

Mole R (1972) Radiation induced tumors—Human experience. Br J Radiol 45:613.

Myrden J, Hiltz J (1969) Breast cancer following multiple fluoroscopies during artificial pneumothorax treatment of pulmonary tuberculosis. Canadian Med Assoc J 100:1032–1034.

Myrden J, Quinlan J (1974) Breast carcinoma following multiple fluoroscopies with pneumothorax treatment of pulmonary tuberculosis. Ann Royal Coll Physicians Surg Canada 7:45.

Myrden J (1977) Personal communication.

NAS (1972) The effects on populations of exposure to low levels of ionizing radiation, BEIR I Report. Washington, DC:National Academy Press.

Neuman Z, Ben-Hur N, Shulman J (1963) The relationship between radiation injury to the skin and subsequent malignant change. Surg Gynecol Obstet 117–559.

Pack G, Davis J (1965) Radiation cancer of the skin. Radiology 84:436–442.

Pegum J (1972) Radiation induced skin cancer. Br J Radiol 45:613.

Petersen O (1954) Radiation cancer—Report of 21 cases. Acta Radiolog 42:221–236.

Quisenberry W (1963) Ethnic differences in skin cancer in Hawaii. US Natl Cancer Inst Monogr 10:181–189.

Ridley C, Spittle M (1974) Epitheliomas of the scalp after irradiation. Lancet i:509.

Sarkany I, Fountain R, Evans C, Morrison R, Szur L (1968) Multiple basal-cell epitheliomata following radiotherapy of the spine. Br J Dermatol 80:90–96.

Schulz R, Albert R (1968) Dose to organs of the head from the x-ray treatment of tinea capitis. Arch Environ Health 17:935–950.

Scotto J, Kopf A, Urbach F (1974) Non-melanoma skin cancer among caucasians in four areas of the United States. Cancer 34:1333–1338.

Segi M (1963) World incidence and distribution of skin cancer. US Natl Cancer Inst Monogr 10:245–255.

Sevcova M, Sevc J, Thomas J (1978) Alpha irradiation of the skin and the possibility of late effects. Health Phys 35:803–806.

Shore R (1982) A follow-up study of children given x-ray treatment for ringworm of the scalp (tinea capitis). (PhD dissertation, Columbia University.)

Shore R, Albert R, Pasternack B (1976) Follow-up study of patients treated by x-ray epilation for tinea capitis. Arch Environ Health 31:21–28.

Shore R, Hempelmann L, Kowaluk E, Mansur P, Pasternack B, Albert R, Haughic G (1977) Breast neoplasms in women treated with x-rays for acute postpartum mastitis. J Natl Cancer Inst 59:813–822.

Stern R, Thibodeau L, Kleinerman R, Parrish J, Fitzpatrick T (1979) Risk of cutaneous carcinoma in patients treated with oral methoxsalen photochemotherapy for psoriasis. N Engl J Med 300:809–813.

Sulzberger M, Baer R, Borota A (1952) Do Roentgen-ray treatments as given by skin specialists produce cancers or other sequelae? Arch Dermatol Syphil 65:639–655.

Takahashi S (1964) A statistical study on human cancer induced by medical irradiation. Acta Radiolog (Nippon) 23:1510–1530.

Totten R, Antypas P, Dupertuis M, Gaisford J, White W (1957) Pre-existing Roentgen-ray dermatitis in patients with skin cancer. Cancer 10:1024–1030.

Traenkle H (1963) X-ray induced skin cancer in man. US Natl Cancer Inst Monogr 10:423–432.

Woodard E, Hempelmann L (1978) Personal communication.

Woodard E (1980) Personal communication.

CARCINOGENIC EFFECTS OF RADIATION ON THE HUMAN DIGESTIVE TRACT AND OTHER ORGANS

CHARLES E. LAND, Ph.D.

The organs discussed in this chapter are thought to be generally of intermediate to low sensitivity to the carcinogenic effects of ionizing radiation. Little is known about the shapes of the dose–response curves for radiation-induced cancers of the digestive, hepatobiliary, genitourinary, and central nervous systems; rather, the available data suffice merely to establish, or suggest, the existence of a radiation-related excess risk for certain sites. It does not follow, however, that these organs are unimportant in any assessment of the overall cancer risk from exposure to ionizing radiation. They account for a substantial fraction of the usual cancer burden, and a relatively modest proportional increase in risk can account for more excess risk for certain sites. It does not follow, however, that these organs are unimportant in any assessment of the overall cancer risk from exposure to ionizing radiation. They account for a substantial fraction of the usual cancer burden, and a relatively modest proportional increase in risk can account for more excess cancer deaths than a much greater proportional increase in such rare cancers as leukemia or thyroid cancer.

The 1980 report of the National Academy of Sciences Committee on the Biological Effects of Ionizing Radiation (BEIR) includes separate reviews on most of the organ sites of concern here (NAS, 1980). The present review will concentrate on new data published since the BEIR report, including 1) the mortality experience as determined from death certificates of the Life Span Study (LSS) sample of survivors of the Hiroshima and Nagasaki A-bombs for the period 1950–1978 (Kato, 1982), 2) cancer morbidity data for the Nagasaki portion of the LSS sample as determined from the Nagasaki Tumor Registry for 1959–1978 (Wakabayashi, 1983), 3) cancer mortality through 1970 among British ankylosing spondylitis patients following a single course of radiation ther-

---

From the National Cancer Institute, Bethesda, Maryland.

apy (Smith, 1982), 4) a preliminary report of cancer morbidity among 82,000 women treated for invasive cervical cancer by x-ray or intracavity radium, as determined from a multinational study based on tumor registries (Boice, 1983), and 5) the subset of the international study based on the Connecticut Tumor Registry, which has been reported separately (Kleinerman, 1982). The Connecticut data are of particular interest because follow-up was relatively complete and lengthy, relatively few (14%) of the irradiated patients had surgical removal of the ovaries, uterine corpus, or cervix, at least within 4 mo after diagnosis, histologic confirmation was available for 85% of second cancers, and because unpublished site-specific data were available by age at treatment. Relevant data from these five studies are summarized in Tables 1-5, and are referred to as needed in the discussion of the various sites.

METHODS

At the time of this writing, the dosimetric basis for analysis of the LSS sample data is in question (Bond, 1982). A new dosimetry is being developed, a process involving a reassessment of the amount and quality of the radiations released by the two bombs and the attenuation of exposure by distance, shielding materials, and tissue. Eventually new estimates of tissue dose will be calculated on an organ-by-organ basis for almost all sample members. Although drastic changes in linear model risk estimates are not expected, the effects of changing the dosimetry are uncertain. It appears, however, that the importance of the neutron component of dose, which under the current (T65) dosimetry amounts to 19%–27% of tissue kerma in Hiroshima and only 1%–2% in Nagasaki, will be greatly reduced. Accordingly, it no longer seems useful to regard differences in dose response between the two cities as informative with respect to the biological effectiveness of radiations of different qualities, and in this chapter the data from Hiroshima and Nagasaki are treated as the results of replicate studies on two exposed populations with roughly equivalent dosimetry.

Linear model risk estimates are expressed in terms of organ-specific tissue dose in rad, calculated according to the present dosimetry. [For conversion factors from kerma to tissue dose, see Table V-6 of the BEIR report (NAS, 1980).] In these calculations, each rad of neutrons (tissue dose) has been assumed equivalent to 11.3 rad of gamma ray. This conversion is based not on radiobiologic considerations, but on the empirical observation that, under the T65 dosimetry, it brings Hiroshima and Nagasaki into approximate agreement with respect to linear model estimates of leukemia risk (NAS, 1980). The conversion is consistent with the assumptions made by the BEIR Committee to obtain linear estimates for cancer other than leukemia. Because the current dosimetry for Nagasaki is less controversial than that for Hiroshima, the conversion may also produce estimates that will be in better agreement with those eventually obtained from a new dosimetry.

Where feasible, hypothesis tests and risk estimates have been recalculated for the present review, and presented in similar format. In the case of the A-bomb survivor data, the p-values for trend have been recalculated to conform to tissue dose as defined above, and have been adjusted for skewness of the population distribution with respect to dose (Beebe, 1978). Risk estimates were calculated separately, assuming Poisson variability for rates obtained by dividing observed numbers of cancers by person-years (PY) calculated by distributing total PY among dose classes proportionally with respect to expected numbers of cancers; thus, rates were adjusted indirectly, rather than directly, for age at the time of the bombings (ATB), city, and sex. For the most part, risk estimates have been given with their standard errors to facilitate comparison among estimates derived from different studies. Hypothesis tests, and their corresponding p-values, were computed under the null hypothesis of no radiation effect and, thus, with different distributional assumptions from those used to compute risk estimates; therefore, p-values do not generally correspond to normal-theory interpretations of risk estimates and their standard errors.

CANCERS OF THE DIGESTIVE SYSTEM

Cancers of the Digestive Tract and Peritoneum (ICD, 150–159, 1977)*

Although the most important cancer sites in this group are covered separately below, there is some value in discussing the radiation relationship for the entire group. Of 4756 death certificates coded to malignant neoplasms during the period 1950–1978 among members of the LSS sample, 2967 (62%) were attributed to cancers of the digestive organs and peritoneum (Kato, 1982). Statistical evidence of an increasing trend in mortality with increasing radiation dose was strong (Table 1). Proportionally, however, the excess risk was not great, amounting to an estimated 50% excess among survivors with over 200 rad kerma and 3%, or about 85 excess deaths of a total 2967, among exposed sample members generally, whose average exposure level was 27 rad tissue kerma. This excess amounts to about 35% of the estimated radiation-related excess mortality from all cancers, and 55% of that from cancers other than leukemia (Kato, 1982).

For specific cohorts defined in terms of age at the time of the bombings (ATB) inferences are more uncertain, but overall the pattern is consistent with an increased risk following exposure at any age. Linear model estimates of the percent increase in risk per rad kerma are 0.1% overall, and 0.9%, 0.6%, 0.2%, 0.1%, and 0.1% following exposure at ages 0–9, 10–19, 20–34, 35–49, and 50+, respectively (Table 1). The age-specific estimates have large standard errors, particularly those corresponding to the youngest and oldest cohorts, and the general impression of a decrease in relative risk with increasing age at exposure is weakly supported by a two-sided p-value of 0.08 for trend. The absolute risk estimates, on the other hand, increase with increasing age ATB ($p < 0.001$ for trend), a result that may at least in part reflect a general tendency for excess solid tumors to confirm to normal age-specific patterns of temporal distribution of risk (Land, 1978; Kato, 1982; Land, 1984). Absolute risk estimates were closely similar for male and female survivors, but were about twice as high relative to underlying risk among women as among men, reflecting the higher population rates for men.

---

* International Classification of Diseases

TABLE 1 Cancer Mortality Among A-Bomb Survivors, Hiroshima and Nagasaki, 1950–1978

Site	Subgroup	Total deaths	Trend test p-value	Estimated excess risk per rad ± SE	
				Cases/10^{6}PY	(%)
Digestive organs	Total	2967	<0.0001	1.80 ± 0.50	0.12 ± 0.03
and peritoneum	Hiroshima	2393	<0.0001	2.23 ± 0.62	0.14 ± 0.05
	Nagasaki	574	0.0960	1.21 ± 1.04	0.10 ± 0.09
	Males	1690	0.0066	1.90 ± 0.87	0.09 ± 0.04
	Females	1277	0.0004	1.94 ± 0.64	0.18 ± 0.06
	0–9 ATB	28	0.0210	0.51 ± 0.40	0.89 ± 0.80
	10–19 ATB	115	<0.0001	1.24 ± 0.45	0.59 ± 0.24
	20–34 ATB	362	0.0400	1.30 ± 0.74	0.16 ± 0.09
	35–49 ATB	1349	0.0140	2.74 ± 1.41	0.09 ± 0.05
	50+ ATB	1113	0.1200	3.55 ± 3.43	0.06 ± 0.06
Esophagus	Total	156	0.0510	0.21 ± 0.14	0.28 ± 0.20
	Hiroshima	126	0.0076	0.41 ± 0.20	0.52 ± 0.27
	Nagasaki	30	0.8100	—	—
Stomach	Total	1754	0.0031	1.04 ± 0.44	0.12 ± 0.04
	Hiroshima	1443	0.0088	1.16 ± 0.55	0.12 ± 0.06
	Nagasaki	311	0.0860	0.89 ± 0.84	0.14 ± 0.13
	Male	997	0.0660	0.93 ± 0.75	0.07 ± 0.06
	Female	757	0.0056	1.29 ± 0.56	0.20 ± 0.10
	0–9 ATB	21	0.0410	0.30 ± 0.32	0.66 ± 0.81
	10–19 ATB	65	0.0120	0.57 ± 0.35	0.46 ± 0.31
	20–34 ATB	211	0.0670	0.94 ± 0.67	0.20 ± 0.15
	35–49 ATB	779	0.0960	1.36 ± 1.20	0.08 ± 0.08
	50+ ATB	678	0.1800	2.34 ± 3.06	0.06 ± 0.09
Colon	Total	157	0.0010	0.46 ± 0.21	0.62 ± 0.31
	Hiroshima	133	0.0007	0.58 ± 0.26	0.70 ± 0.35
	Nagasaki	24	0.1900	0.21 ± 0.32	0.45 ± 0.75
	Male	77	0.0430	0.48 ± 0.33	0.52 ± 0.38
	Female	80	0.0029	0.46 ± 0.28	0.74 ± 0.50
Rectum	Total	157	0.9000	—	—
Pancreas	Total	148	0.6800	—	—
Other and	Total	595	0.0073	0.53 ± 0.23	0.18 ± 0.08
unspecified	Hiroshima	444	0.0044	0.69 ± 0.30	0.24 ± 0.10
digestive organs	Nagasaki	151	0.2300	0.39 ± 0.54	0.13 ± 0.18
Urinary organs	Total	104	0.0270	0.25 ± 0.14	0.51 ± 0.29
	Hiroshima	90	0.0840	0.23 ± 0.15	0.41 ± 0.28
	Nagasaki	14	0.0610	0.27 ± 0.23	1.20 ± 1.19
	Male	60	0.0700	0.31 ± 0.23	0.44 ± 0.35
	Female	44	0.0720	0.23 ± 0.16	0.69 ± 0.54
Cervix uteri	Total	332	0.3100	0.16 ± 0.41	0.06 ± 0.15
and uterus	Hiroshima	270	0.1400	0.47 ± 0.54	0.16 ± 0.19
	Nagasaki	62	0.7500	—	—
Cervix uteri	Total	72	0.2200	0.14 ± 0.20	0.23 ± 0.33

Source: Kato, 1981.

Salivary Glands

Cancers of the salivary glands normally are rare, and while the excess risk associated with radiation exposure is slight, it can be highly visible against the low background rate in some irradiated populations. The salivary glands were not among the more heavily irradiated sites for the spondylitis or the cervical cancer patients, and because salivary gland cancer is not usually fatal it was not tabulated as a cause of death in the LSS sample mortality series. Only six cases were reported in the Nagasaki Tumor Registry among LSS sample members between 1959 and 1978, and of these five were exposed to less than 10 rad kerma from the A-bomb and one was exposed to between 10 and 99 rad (Table 2). Thus, the evidence of Tables 1–5 for a radiation effect is either negative or nonexistent.

At the time of this writing, the only incidence-level study of salivary gland cancer based on the entire LSS sample covered the period 1950–1970 (Belsky, 1975). Of nine malignant tumors observed, seven were from Hiroshima and two from Nagasaki, a ratio in accord with the 3:1 ratio of Hiroshima to Nagasaki members of the LSS sample. The finding of 20 benign tumors in Hiroshima and only one in Nagasaki, however, suggests strongly that the rate of benign salivary gland tumors, or, more likely, the efficiency of case finding, was much higher in Hiroshima than in Nagasaki ($p = 0.02$). Two of the malignant tumor cases had exposures over 300 rad kerma, whereas, another was in the 50–99

TABLE 2 Cancer Incidence Among A-Bomb Survivors, Nagasaki, 1959–1978

Site	Total cases	Trend test p Value	Estimated excess risk per rad ± SE	
			Cases/10⁶PY	(%)
Esophagus	31	0.6600	—	—
Stomach	404	0.0160	3.07 ± 1.50	0.26 ± 0.13
Colon	45	0.0430	0.95 ± 0.69	0.78 ± 0.64
Rectum	47	0.0850	0.87 ± 0.69	0.67 ± 0.58
Pancreas	36	0.0740	1.15 ± 0.66	1.25 ± 0.86
Liver	55	0.0380	0.70 ± 0.59	0.46 ± 0.41
Gall bladder	36	0.7100	—	—
Salivary glands	6	0.7600	—	—
Urinary tract	32	0.0075	1.22 ± 0.56	1.71 ± 1.00
Prostrate	30[a]	0.0100	2.14 ± 1.27	1.20 ± 0.87
	19[b]	0.0890[c]	1.46 ± 1.29	1.32 ± 1.42
Uterus	132	0.3700	0.38 ± 1.63	0.05 ± 0.23
Ovary	18	0.7400	—	—

Source: Wakabayashi, 1983.

[a] Includes occult cases found at autopsy; autopsy series is known to be biased.

[b] Clinically evident cases only.

[c] Based on tabular data presented in the main reference. Wakabayashi et al (1983) using a more finely divided dose partition, obtained a p-value of 0.20 for trend.

TABLE 3 Cancer Mortality Among British Patients Following a Single Course of X-Ray Treatments for Ankylosing Spondylitis

Site	Dose (rad)	Item	Time since exposure (yr)			p	Excess risk per rad ±SE 9+ yr	
			0–2	3–8	9+		Cases/10⁶ PY	(%)
	—	PY	32,434	43,436	58,004			
Esophagus	306	Obs	0	2	8	0.030	0.25 ± 0.16	0.40 ± 0.26
		Exp	0.67	1.28	3.62			
Stomach	67[a,b]	Obs	6	8	31	0.014	2.81 ± 1.43	0.81 ± 0.41
	89[a,c]	Exp	5.04	9.08	20.10		2.11 ± 1.08	0.61 ± 0.31
	250[d]						0.75 ± 1.21	0.22 ± 0.11
Colon	57	Obs	6	6	16	0.060	1.70 ± 1.21	0.95 ± 0.68
		Exp	2.52	4.39	10.38			
Pancreas	90	Obs	5	3	10	0.110	0.70 ± 0.61	0.64 ± 0.56
		Exp	1.00	2.13	6.35			
Kidney	46[a]	Obs	1	0	7	0.020	1.65 ± 0.99	3.7 ± 2.2
		Exp	0.50	0.98	2.61			
Bladder	31[a]	Obs	0	3	8	0.140	1.63 ± 1.57	1.9 ± 1.8
		Exp	0.84	1.75	5.07			

Spinal cord and nerves	698	Obs	2	2	2	0.050	0.04 ± 0.035	0.63 ± 0.55
		Exp	0.09	0.14	0.37			
Rectum	—[e]	Obs	1	13		0.260		
		Exp	1.86	10.55				
Liver and gall bladder	—[e]	Obs	1	1		0.920		
		Exp	0.69	4.15				
Brain	—[e]	Obs	2	10		0.280		
		Exp	1.66	7.98				
Prostate	—[e]	Obs	3	6		0.610		
		Exp	0.72	6.38				
Uterus	—[e]	Obs	0	4		0.500		
		Exp	0.71	3.68				
Ovaries	—[e]	Obs	0	4		0.330		
		Exp	0.48	2.92				

Source: Smith, 1982.

[a] Estimate from 1980 BEIR report, Table V-7 [NAS, 1980].
[b] Assumes 50% of stomach irradiated, hypersthenic configuration [NAS, 1980].
[c] Assumes 67% of stomach irradiated, asthenic configuration [NAS, 1980].
[d] Estimate from 1972 BEIR Report [NAS, 1972].
[e] Lightly irradiated site, no dose estimate given.

TABLE 4 Cancer Incidence Among Cervical Cancer Patients, International Study

Site	Estimated dose (rad)	Item	Cancer in situ or treated by surgery alone		Radiation therapy	
			<10 yr	10+ yr	<10 yr	10+ yr
Esophagus	50[a]	Obs	3	3	29	13
		Exp	5.8	2.7	16	11
Stomach	90–330	Obs	46	19	115	86
		Exp	49	22	124	86
Small intestine	1000+	Obs	5	2	12	9
		Exp	3.6	1.1	5.7	3.8
Colon	500+	Obs	83	44	167	146
		Exp	83	39	169	133
Rectum	5400–9200	Obs	52	25	69	118
		Exp	44	21	88	69
Liver	250	Obs	7	2	13	10
		Exp	6.3	2.6	13	10
Gall bladder	250[a]	Obs	11	5	22	19
		Exp	12	6.1	28	24
Pancreas	64–300	Obs	28	17	70	51
		Exp	25	12	53	43
Kidney	93–380	Obs	30	15	46	23
		Exp	24	9.2	38	29
Bladder	5400–9200	Obs	32	16	81	112
		Exp	21	9.3	41	33
Brain	3–15	Obs	44	11	36	15
		Exp	42	10	43	25
Uterus	1000+	Obs	38	13	48	78
		Exp	87	36	126	83
Ovary	1400–7210	Obs	87	20	67	70
		Exp	102	31	122	76
Other genital	1000+[a]	Obs	89	23	55	47
		Exp	13	5.4	25	18

Source: Boice, 1983.

[a] No dose given; value in table is an interpolation from nearby organs.

TABLE 5 Cancer Incidence Among Cervical Cancer Patients Following Radiotherapy, Connecticut Tumor Registry Data

Site	Item	Time since radiotherapy		Age at irradiation (cancers 10 yr after irradiation					
		<10 yr	10+ yr	<30	30–39	40–49	50–59	60–69	70+
Esophagus	Obs	4	2						
	Exp	1.0	1.0						
Stomach	Obs	10	9	0	0	2	6	1	0
	Exp	7.9	6.3	0.02	1.8	1.8	2.2	1.6	0.25
Colon	Obs	18	29	0	1	7	10	9	2
	Exp	21.9	23.2	0.9	1.9	7.3	6.9	5.0	0.7
Rectum	Obs	10	20	0	2	10	3	5	0
	Exp	9.5	8.8	0.04	0.9	3.0	2.9	1.7	0.3
Liver	Obs	3	2						
	Exp	3.8	3.5						
Pancreas	Obs	6	4						
	Exp	4.6	4.8						
Kidneys	Obs	4	10	1	2	3	2	2	0
	Exp	2.6	2.6	0.01	0.3	0.9	0.8	0.4	0.05
Bladder	Obs	10	16	0	4	4	5	0	0
	Exp	3.6	4.1	0.01	0.4	1.2	1.4	1.0	0.2
Brain and CNS	Obs	2	1						
	Exp	2.0	1.5						
Uterus	Obs	17	22	0	8	9	4	1	0
	Exp	15.4	12.3	0.1	2.2	5.0	3.5	1.5	0.2
Ovaries	Obs	12	13	0	4	5	2	2	0
	Exp	9.2	6.8	0.1	1.2	2.6	2.0	0.9	0.1

Source: Kleinerman, 1982.

rad range. A contingency table test for increasing linear trend with increasing exposure, using average kerma values and PY from the 1950–1970 LSS mortality study (Jablon, 1972) yielded an approximate, normal-theory p-value less than 0.01 for trend, adjusted for age ATB and city. Assuming the algorithm for conversion of kerma–to–tissue dose to be approximately the same as that for the female breast, a linear regression estimate based on age-city-adjusted rates is 0.10 excess cases, with standard error 0.07, per million PY per rad (0.10 ± 0.07/10^6 PYR), or 3.2% ± 2.8%/rad. Benign tumor risk was only marginally associated with radiation dose, giving a linear model risk estimate of 0.09 ± 0.13/10^6 PYR, or 0.7% ± 1.1%/rad for the Hiroshima survivors. No differences in excess risk were apparent with respect to age ATB.

An independent study based on the so-called "open-city" population of Hiroshima, which is not restricted to the LSS population and includes survivors returning to Hiroshima at various times after 1945, was carried out by Takeichi et al. through a review of records of nearly all private and public hospitals having surgical and anatomic pathology departments in Hiroshima and the nearby city of Kure for the period 1953–1971 (Takeichi, 1976; Ohkita, 1978). Seventeen malignant and 14 benign tumors were identified among persons directly exposed to the A-bomb (within 5000 meters), compared with five malignant and 25 benign tumors in a much larger group of nonexposed residents. In fact, the level of malignant tumors among the nonexposed seems extraordinarily low, $0.1/10^5$ PY, compared with an average of $0.45/10^5$ from four Japanese tumor registries (Waterhouse, 1982) covering, moreover, a generally younger age range. Accordingly, the comparisons considered here have been based solely on the directly exposed population, contrasted by exposure distance. Using numbers of cases, PY and crude rates in the two cited publications [Takeichi, 1976; Ohkita, 1978] it was possible to reconstruct a distribution of cases and PY for exposure distances 0–1500, 1501–2000, and 2001–5000 meters in which the breakdown of PY between the two more distant intervals is approximate (Table 6). Average kerma values for distance intervals were based on the LSS sample (Beebe, 1978). Linear regression estimates were 0.06 ± 0.04 excess malignant and 0.06 ± 0.04 excess benign tumors per 10^6 PYR ($0.7\% \pm 0.6\%$ and $1.1\% \pm 0.9\%$/rad, respectively). Age-specific rates for combined benign and malignant tumors suggested a similar level of effect among survivors 0–19 and 20–49 yr of age ATB whereas, among survivors 50 or older ATB no effect was seen; this difference, however, was statistically nonsignificant.

There is a substantial literature on salivary gland tumors in patient populations after head and neck irradiation, mostly during infancy and childhood. This literature is summarized in Table 7. The studies can be considered in three groups: First, there were five studies of patient populations given X-ray therapy to the head and neck during infancy or childhood (Saenger, 1960; Hempelmann, 1975; Maxon, 1981; Janower, 1971; Schneider, 1978), for which salivary gland doses tended to be greater than 100 rad. Second, children in New York City and Israel were given depilating exposures to the scalp during the treatment of tinea capitis, resulting in salivary gland doses of about 40 rad (Shore, 1976; Modan, 1974). Finally, Hoffman (1982) studied a group of women treated with radioactive iodine, most of them during late middle age; the mean salivary gland dose, based on 10.6 mCi of ^{131}I, was 530 rad (Hoffman, personal communication). In Table 7 the incidence of salivary gland tumors is compared with that in nonexposed control groups or, if there were no cases in an appropriate control group, with the number expected on the basis of population rates. Although the highest risk estimates correspond to the two tinea capitis series, data from the different studies are remarkably consistent. A linear regression using the eight exposed groups and six nonexposed groups from studies following childhood exposure yielded the estimate 0.26 ± 0.06 excess malignant tumors per 10^6 PYR ($6.9\% \pm 5.5\%$/rad, ignoring the first 5 yr after exposure, with a chi-square of 12.7 on 12 df for lack of fit ($p = 0.39$). The analogous regression for benign tumors, using seven exposed and five nonex-

TABLE 6 Incidence of Salivary Gland Tumors Among A-Bomb Survivors, Hiroshima, 1953-1971, Open City Population.

PY	Exposure distance				Trend test, 0–5000m: p-value	Estimated risk per rad	
	<1500m 322,768	1501–2000[a] 366,887[a]	2001–5000[a] 800,486[a]	>5000 4,333,814		Cases/10⁶ PY	(%)
Average kerma[b]	124.3	9.9					
Approximate dose[c]	247.5	18.7					
Malignant	7	4	6	5	0.030	0.056 ± 0.036	0.69 ± 0.57
Benign	7	2	5	25	0.010	0.063 ± 0.035	1.10 ± 0.86
Total	14	6	11	30	0.002	0.120 ± 0.050	0.86 ± 0.49

Source: Takeichi 1976; Ohkita, 1978.
[a] Estimated from numerators and crude population rates.
[b] From Beebe et al (1978) Table 39.
[c] Assuming kerma-to-tissue dose conversion identical to that for the female breast (NAS, 1980), and a neutron quality factor of 11.3 (see text).

posed groups, gave $0.44 \pm 0.11/10^6$ PYR (3.6% $\pm$ 2.1%/rad), and a chi-square of 12.9 on 10 df (p = 0.23).

Overall, the data give no reason to conclude that the risk of salivary gland tumors, malignant or benign, following exposure to ionizing radiation is strongly dependent on age at exposure. The difference between the two A-bomb survivor series and the series abstracted in Table 7 is not easily ignored, but possible explanations include differences in ascertainment criteria and case-reporting procedures, as well as age and population differences.

Esophagus

At the time of the 1980 BEIR report the principal epidemiologic evidence that exposure to ionizing radiation increases the risk of esophageal cancer was from the 1950–1974 LSS sample mortality data for the Hiroshima survivors (Beebe, 1978). The more recent LSS mortality data are similar, with a strong increasing trend with increasing dose in Hiroshima but none in Nagasaki (Table 1), and the greatly expanded Nagasaki tumor registry data continue to be negative (Table 2). The estimated excess mortality for the combined cities is 5.4 deaths out of 156, about $0.2/10^6$ PYR or 0.3%/rad. The data were not tabulated separately by sex or age ATB.

Although no excess mortality from esophageal cancer was observed through 1962 among the sample of spondylitis patients treated by x-ray, follow-up through 1970 of the patients who received only a single series of treatments found 8 deaths versus 3.6 expected 9 yr or more after treatment, compared with 2 deaths versus 2 expected within the first 8 yr (Table 3). The BEIR Committee tentatively estimated the average esophageal dose to be 306 rad (NAS, 1980), from which the average excess per rad after 9 yr must be about 0.4% of normal risk, or $0.25/10^6$ PYR.

Finally, 42 incident esophageal cancers were observed, compared with 27 expected according to population rates, among the cervical cancer patients treated by radiation (Table 4). The esophagus was not considered to be a heavily irradiated organ, however, and the investigators considered that a more important causal factor might be elevated levels of tobacco and alcohol use associated with cervical cancer (Boice, 1983). Also, the excess of esophageal cancer did not increase over time following treatment, as would be expected if the radiation exposure were the cause; 13 cases were observed versus 11 expected more than 10 yr after treatment, compared with 29 observed versus 16 expected within the first 10 yr. On the other hand, no excess risk was seen among the relatively few cervical cancer patients with in situ cancer or with invasive cancer treated surgically. A similar pattern was observed with respect to cases determined from the Connecticut Tumor Registry (Table 5).

Overall, the available evidence concerning the risk of radiation-induced esophageal cancer is about the same as it was at the time of the 1980 BEIR report, and the BEIR estimate of about 0.3 excess incident cases per 10^6 PYR (NAS, 1980) seems reasonable.

Stomach

The first substantial evidence of a dose–response relationship for stomach cancer in an irradiated human population was reported by Court Brown and Doll in their analysis of cancer mortality among spondylitis patients treated by x-ray at some time during 1935–1954 and followed through 1963 (Court Brown, 1965). More recently, the evidence for a stomach cancer effect has been strengthened by the observation of 31 deaths 9 yr or more after treatment versus 20.0 expected among the patients given a single course of x-ray treatment (Table 3), whereas, 14 deaths were observed versus 14.2 expected during the first 8 yr. Estimates of radiation dose to the stomach are extremely tentative, however, ranging from 67 to 250 rad, and correspond to an excess of 0.2–0.8% rad, or $0.8–2.8/10^6$ PYR.

Stomach cancer is a leading cause of death in Japan, contributing 37% of all deaths from malignant neoplasms among members of the LSS sample through 1978. A dose–response relationship was first shown by Nakamura (1977) using death certificate data for the period 1950–1973, and was confirmed by the LSS sample mortality data for 1950–1974 (Beebe, 1978). The effect seemed fairly clear from the Hiroshima data, but in Nagasaki the only evidence of an effect was a high relative risk among survivors with over 400 rad kerma. In the most recent mortality data the evidence for a dose response has strengthened for Hiroshima, and has moved closer to statistical significance for Nagasaki (Table 1). The estimated excess mortality in the combined cities is 42 deaths, or about 2.4% of that expected in the absence of exposure. Linear-model estimates of excess risk are similar for the two cities, corresponding to an increase of about 0.14–0.24% rad, or $0.9–2.3/10^6$ PYR. Risk was (nonsignificantly) higher among women than among men. Estimated risk varied significantly by age ATB, increasing with increasing age in terms of absolute risk ($p < 0.001$) and decreasing in terms of excess risk as a percentage of the risk expected in the absence of exposure ($p < 0.05$).

The Nagasaki tumor registry data for 1959–1978 demonstrate a clear dose–response for stomach cancer incidence, when based on all sources of ascertainment ($p = 0.013$). The estimated excess risk per rad is 0.3%, or $3.1/10^6$ PYR (Table 2).

Given the overall consistency of the LSS and ankylosing spondylitis patient data for cancer of the stomach, it is surprising that the cervical cancer data in Tables 4 and 5 do not suggest an excess risk. Observed and expected numbers of cases agree closely for irradiated and nonirradiated patients, both in the 10 yr immediately after treatment and subsequently. The data are consistent with a relative risk as high as 1.2 for irradiated patients observed beyond 10 yr after treatment. Estimates of the average dose to the stomach range between 90 and 330 rad, from which upper confidence limits can be obtained that are consistent with the estimates obtained from the data of Tables 1–3. Nevertheless, the negative results from the cervical cancer patient studies suggest that the estimates based on the LSS and spondylitis data may be too high, or that other variables, as yet unknown, may affect the sensitivity of stomach tissue to the carcinogenic effects of ionizing radiation.

TABLE 7 Salivary Gland Cancer Incidence In Medically-Irradiated Populations

Reference	Age at exposure	Group	Number of subjects	Average follow-up (yr)	Average dose to salivary glands	Number of cases		Risk estimates: Excess rads/10⁶ PY/rad after 5-yr minimum latent period	
						Malig-nant	Be-nign	Malignant	Benign
Saenger, 1960	<15	Exposed	1644	18.4	200[a]	2	0	0.43 ± 0.32	0
		Control	3777	18.1	0	0	0		
		Pop expect	—	—	—	0.1	0.4		
Hempelmann, 1975	<1	Exp (I)	261	31.0	277[a]	0	2	0	0.37 ± 0.39
		Exp (II)	2611	23.4	135[a]	0	2		
		Control	5055	22.9	0	1	2		
Maxon, 1981	x = 5.1	Exposed	554	21.5	500[b]	3	—	0.65 ± 0.38	—
		Control	958	21.5	500[b]	3	—		
		Pop expect	—	—	—	0.02			
Janower, 1971	x = 5	Exposed	466	30.1	240[a]	0	1	—	0.21 ± 0.37
		Control	2604	27.3	0	0	2		

Study		Group							
Schneider, 1978	x = 5.5	Exposed	1922	29.9	790[c]	8	19	0.21 ± 0.07	0.48 ± 0.12
		Pop expect	—	—	—	0.2	0.7		
Shore, 1976	x = 7.9 s = 2.5	Exposed	2215	20.5	39[d]	1	3	0.67 ± 0.75	1.9 ± 1.3
		Control	1413	20.3	0	0	0		
		Pop expect	—	—	—	0.1	0.4		
Modan, 1974	<15	Exposed	10902	16.8	39[d]	4	3	0.72 ± 0.40	0.47 ± 0.37
		Control	16398	16.8	0	0	1		
		Pop expect	—	—	—	0.4	1.5		
Hoffman, 1982	x = 57	Exposed	1005	15	530[e]	2	—	0.26 ± 0.28	—
		Control	2141	21	0	2	—		

[a] Calculated as 60% of the average air dose in Roeutgens.
[b] As specified by the investigator (Maxon, 1981).
[c] Calculated by Dr. Marilyn Stovall (personal communication) from exposure factors given in the original reference.
[d] (NAS, 1980).
[e] (Hoffman, personal communication).

Small Intestine

Cancer of the small intestine is rare, especially in comparison with cancers of the stomach and colon, and little is known about causal factors (Lightdale, 1982). Cancers of the small intestine and colon often are not tabulated separately in reports of cancer risk in irradiated populations, but it seems safe to assume in such cases that the vast majority of "intestinal cancers" reported are in the colon. Cancer can be induced readily in rats by irradiating temporarily exteriorized intestinal tissue, but until recently the epidemiologic evidence for an effect was limited to the observation of 3 deaths versus 0.4 expected among 2068 women irradiated for the treatment of benign menstrual disease (Smith, 1976). The large sample of cervical cancer patients treated by radiation received very high average doses to the small intestine, and 9 incident cancers were observed more than 10 yr after treatment, compared with 3.8 expected (Table 4). The evidential value of these data is weakened, however, by the 12 cases observed within 10 yr after treatment versus 5.7 expected, and by the observation among nonirradiated patients with invasive or cervical cancer of 5 cases versus 3.6 expected within 10 yr after treatment and 2 cases versus 1.1 expected, subsequently. At this point it seems uncertain whether or not radiation exposure is associated with cancer of the small intestine in man.

Colon

The colon has long been considered an organ of apparent, but uncertain, sensitivity to radiation carcinogenesis, based on studies of patient populations irradiated for benign or malignant pelvic disease, and on the follow-up of the spondylitis patients (ICRP, 1969). Studies of patients treated for benign pelvic disease included a series of 267 patients followed for an average of 16 yr, in which 4 deaths from intestinal cancer were observed versus 1 expected (Brinkley, 1969). In another series of 1893 women treated with radium implants (900 patients) or x-ray (993 patients) for benign gynecologic disorders, 32 colon cancers were found versus 29 expected [Wagoner, 1983]. An incomplete follow-up of women treated with radium for benign uterine hemorrhage found no excess mortality from pelvic cancers (Dickson, 1969). Finally, in a follow-up of patients treated for metropathia haemorrhagica, 21 colon cancer deaths were observed versus 13.5 expected 5 yr or more after treatment, with no excess mortality from colon cancer within 5 yr after treatment (Smith, 1976).

In their reports of cancer mortality among spondylitis patients, Court Brown and Doll (1965) and, later, Smith and Doll (1982) tended to discount their consistent observation of excess colon cancer mortality because of the possibility that the excess might arise from the known associations between spondylitis and ulcerative colitis and between ulcerative colitis and colon cancer. The most recent follow-up of the series demonstrates the reasons for this caution (Table 3). Sixteen colon cancer deaths were observed versus 10.4 expected 9 yr or more after treatment, a nonsignificant excess. Within the first 8 yr there were 12 deaths versus 6.9 expected, a significant excess, and of these, 6 occurred during the first 2 yr after treatment when 2.5 would have been expected. It is difficult to attribute the early excess to radiation, and it seems likely that the later excess might have a similar etiology.

An important development during recent years has been the gradual emergence of colon cancer as a radiation-related cause of death among the Hiroshima members of the LSS sample, although no such relationship is evident from the Nagasaki mortality data (Table 1). The two cities approach statistical inconsistency when compared in terms of the estimated numbers of excess colon cancer deaths per PYR, although the estimates are less different when expressed as percentages of city-specific risks in the absence of exposure. The combined-cities estimate is $0.6/10^6$ PYR, or 0.8%/rad, for all ages at exposure. This estimate corresponds to 16 excess deaths, or 10% of the total colon cancer deaths observed. Estimated risk does not vary by sex. No colon cancer deaths were observed among sample members exposed at ages under 10 yr; for the older cohorts there was wide variation in estimated risk by age ATB, with the extremes at ages 35–49, for which there was an apprent excess, and 50+, for which there was an apparent deficit; both the excess and the deficit were statistically significant when considered in isolation.

The apparent absence of a radiation relationship for colon cancer mortality in Nagasaki is contradicted by a positive relationship with respect to incidence, as determined from the Nagasaki tumor registry (Table 2). Twice as many cases were identified from all sources of ascertainment as from death certificates alone, and the incidence data may well reflect more recent diagnoses than the death certificate data. The Nagasaki portion of the LSS sample is about 5 yr younger on the average than the Hiroshima portion, and the city difference may be a temporal one in which a radiation-related excess risk has been slower to emerge in the generally younger Nagasaki population. The estimated excess incidence is $1.0/10^6$ PYR, a number slightly greater than the estimate derived from the mortality data for the combined cities, and very close to the BEIR report estimate (NAS, 1980).

Although preliminary estimates place the average radiation dose to the colon in excess of 500 rad for the cervical cancer patients treated by radiation, the cancer incidence data in Tables 4 and 5 do not suggest a correspondingly high excess cancer risk. During the first 10 yr after treatment 167 cases were observed versus 169 expected in the international study, while subsequently, 146 were observed versus 133 expected, a nonsignificant excess. A similar pattern was seen among the nonirradiated patients, 83 observed versus 83 expected during the first 10 yr and 44 observed versus 39 expected, subsequently. Assuming the excess to be real in the irradiated population and a random fluctuation in the nonirradiated population, and assuming a 500-rad dose, the excess risk would be about 0.02% rad or $0.1/10^6$ PYR. A 95% upper confidence limit for this excess risk is 0.03% rad or $0.2/10^6$ PYR. The age-specific data from the Connecticut Tumor Registry suggest a greater sensitivity among women irradiated after age 50, contrary to what was seen in the LSS sample data (Tables 1 and 5).

On the strength of the A-bomb survivor data it seems likely that radiation can induce colon cancer in man. The relationship of the excess risk to age at exposure is unclear, however, and the data from irradiated North American and European populations are difficult to interpret. Colon cancer is relatively rare in Japan compared with western countries, and it may be that other risk factors tend to overshadow the radiation effect in western populations.

Rectum

Evidence of a radiation-related excess risk for rectal cancer has been observed in patient populations irradiated for benign pelvic disease (Brinkley, 1969; Smith, 1976; NAS, 1980) and for cervical cancer (Dickson, 1972; Castro, 1973). The A-bomb survivor mortality data do not suggest a dose response (Table 1), although the Nagasaki tumor registry data are somewhat suggestive of an increase in incidence with increasing dose ($p = 0.07$) (Table 2). The estimated risk from the tumor registry data is $0.7/10^6$ PYR, or 0.6%/rad. The rectum was considered to be a lightly irradiated site for spondylitis patients treated by x-ray, and the mortality data in Table 3 do not suggest a radiation effect. The irradiated cervical cancer patients received about 5000 rad to the rectum, however, and the data of Tables 4 and 5 are more than suggestive of an excess risk. These data also suggest that rectal cancer may be somewhat more frequent among cervical cancer patients generally, although not to the extent seen in the irradiated patients more than 10 yr after treatment. The significantly depressed incidence in the international series within 10 yr after treatment may reflect early diagnosis, and subsequent removal from the population at risk, of incipient rectal cancers in conjunction with treatment for cervical cancer (Table 4). The age-specific data from the Connecticut Tumor Registry do not suggest that irradiation at any particular age is more effective than at any other (Table 5).

Overall, the data suggest that the rectum is sensitive to radiation carcinogenesis, but that the effect of doses on the order of a few hundred rad or so may be too small to detect easily.

CANCERS OF THE HEPATOBILIARY SYSTEM

Liver

Liver cancer is most clearly associated with radiation exposure from studies of patient populations who had been injected intravascularly with Thorotrast (colloidal 232 thorium dioxide) as an x-ray contrast medium, usually for the diagnosis of suspected brain disease. About 60% of the injected Thorotrast was deposited in the liver, where it emitted alpha radiation continually at a dose rate to the liver of about 25 rad/yr. Alpha radiation is extremely densely ionizing. Also, it is weakly penetrating and tends to affect only cells very near the emitting material, in contrast to the more uniform irradiation by penetrating x- or gamma rays. The 1980 BEIR report based its review primarily on follow-up studies in Germany, Denmark, and Portugal involving a total of 3046 traced patients who survived at least 10 yr after injection of thorotrast (NAS, 1980). Subsequent to the 10th yr after injection, 301 cases of liver cancer were observed versus 12 expected according to population rates, an enormous excess accounting for about 25% of all deaths in this group. Assuming a minimal induction period of 10 yr, and projecting to the end of life for the population still alive, it was estimated that about 300 liver cancers would be caused per million persons exposed per rad of alpha radiation to the liver. Using a quality factor of 20 for alpha particles with respect to gamma rays, an estimate of 0.7 excess liver cancers per 10^6 PYR was derived for low-LET radiation (NAS, 1980).

One possibility that has not been examined in any detail is that chemical toxicity of Thorotrast, itself, might contribute to the apparent carcinogenic effect from alpha radiation (Mole, 1979).

Liver cancer does not appear to be induced as readily by low-LET radiation as by alpha radiation. In the cervical cancer patient data of Table 4, observed and expected numbers are identical despite an estimated average dose to the liver of 250 rad. The liver is not among the heavily irradiated sites in the spondylitis series, and no excess risk has been observed (Table 3).

Primary liver cancer (PLC) is difficult to study on the basis of death certificates, because the liver is a frequent site for metastasis from primary cancers of other sites, and because it can be difficult to distinguish between primary and secondary liver cancer. Partly for this reason, the LSS mortality reports have not tabulated liver cancer separately, but have included it under the general classification of "other and unspecified digestive cancers." Until the most recent report, no dose–response relationship had been seen for this rubric, but a fairly strong association appears to be present in the material for 1950–1978, reflecting mainly deaths since 1971 (Table 1). The relevance of this trend to PLC is questionable, given that radiation-induced cancers of other sites may have metastasized to the liver, contributing to the observed trend. Asano et al. (1982) reviewed PLC cases obtained from the tumor and tissue registries of Hiroshima and Nagasaki, and from the RERF surgical pathology and autopsy files for 1961–1975, obtaining 128 confirmed cases among LSS sample members, including 77 from Hiroshima and 51 from Nagasaki. The Hiroshima Tumor Registry is known to have been incomplete at the time of the survey, as the ratio 77/51 suggests (the Hiroshima part of the LSS sample is three times as large as the Nagasaki part). No relationship between radiation dose and the incidence of PLC was demonstrated for either city separately or for both cities combined. The Nagasaki Tumor Registry data for 1959–1978 (Table 2) indicate an increasing linear trend with increasing dose, based on 55 cases (p = 0.04). This trend depends on 4 liver cancers observed versus 1.1. expected among survivors with exposures of 400+ rad kerma, whereas, below 400 rad no dose-response is seen. Somewhat surprisingly, the risk estimate in Table 2 is identical to the BEIR report estimate obtained using a quality factor of 20 for alpha particles (NAS, 1980).

Although the existence of a liver cancer effect from high-LET radiation is well documented by the Thorotrast follow-up studies, the available information on liver cancer risk in populations exposed to low-LET radiation permits only the conclusion that an excess risk may someday be established.

Gall Bladder

By any account, the gall bladder would be considered an organ of low sensitivity to the carcinogenic effects of ionizing radiation. Gall bladder cancer is tabulated separately in Tables 2–4, which contain no suggestion of an association between risk and exposure.

Pancreas

ICRP Publication 14 (1969) listed the pancreas among organs of apparent, but uncertain, sensitivity to radiation carcinogenesis. This somewhat ambivalent description still applies after more than a decade during which solid cancers as a group have become well established as important late sequellae of exposure to ionizing radiation.

Pancreatic cancer is the fourth leading cause of death among all sites of cancer in the United States (Fraumeni, 1975). It is, however, an extremely difficult disease to diagnose, and because it is usually diagnosed late in the course of illness, with poor prognosis and poor prospects for successful treatment by surgery, it has a low percentage of histologically proven cases compared with other cancer sites (Mack, 1982). Temporally there has been an increasing trend in pancreatic cancer rates in many countries, a trend which, in the United States, is thought to be due in part to improved accuracy of diagnostic information and in part to a true increase in the disease (Mack, 1982).

Excess mortality from pancreatic cancer was reported among British radiologists who entered the practice of radiology before 1921 (6 deaths versus 1.9 expected through 1976) but not among those who began practice later and who, possibly because of improved safety practices, also had less risk of other cancers that have been linked to radiation (Smith, 1981). A study of American radiologists reported no excess risk of pancreatic cancer among cohorts beginning practice in 1920–29, 1930–39, or 1940–49 (Matanoski, 1975).

The strongest evidence for a causal role of radiation exposure comes from studies of patient populations given radiation therapy for benign or malignant disease. A significant excess mortality was found in the initial study of irradiated spondylitis patients (Court Brown, 1965). In the more recent study summarized in Table 3, there were 18 deaths from pancreatic cancer versus 9.5 expected, but 5 deaths were within 2 yr of first treatment compared with 1.0 expected, while 13 occurred after 3 yr compared with 8.5 expected. Thus, the early excess, which seems unlikely to correspond to a radiation etiology at least in terms of initiation, complicates the interpretation of the later (and statistically nonsignificant) excess.

Excess pancreatic cancer mortality has been reported among patients treated by radiation for lymphoma (Jochimsen, 1976) and for cervical cancer (Dickson, 1972). By far the largest series is that summarized in Table 4. In that series the greatest elevation in risk among the irradiated women occurred within 1–4 yr after exposure, with a decreasing trend over time since exposure that was of marginal statistical significance ($p = 0.06$) (Boice, 1983). No excess risk was seen in the Connecticut series (Table 5).

Mortality from pancreatic cancer as reported on death certificates for members of the LSS sample of Japanese A-bomb survivors has been homogeneous with respect to radiation dose (Table 1). Incidence data from the Nagasaki Tumor Registry for 1959–1978 might be better described as nonhomogeneous with respect to dose, rather than suggestive of an increase in risk with increasing dose (Table 2). The usual test for nonhomogeneity with dose was highly significant (p < 0.001) while a trend test gave a marginal result (p = 0.07). About 50% of the cases were histologically confirmed, and these were less suggestive of a dose response. Data from the (then incomplete) Hiroshima Tumor Registry for 1959–1970 suggested no dose relationship (Beebe, 1978).

A report of a dose-related excess of deaths from pancreatic cancer among radiation monitored workers at the Hanford Plutonium Works, which was controversial because it was seen at radiation doses far below any associated with excess risk in any other study (Mancuso, 1977; Marks, 1978; Kneale, 1978; Gilbert, 1979; Hutchison, 1979), was not confirmed by more recent follow-up data on that population, for which the variation by dose was unremarkable (Tolley, 1983).

Overall, the evidence linking pancreatic cancer risk to radiation exposure seems less clearcut than it seemed in 1969. Closer examination of the variation of observed risk by radiation dose and time following exposure to radiation raises more questions than it answers. In the absence of a compelling need for precise estimates of the risk of radiation-induced pancreatic cancer, the best course of action may be simply to consider the pancreas as an organ possibly susceptible to radiation carcinogenesis, and when making risk estimates, to group it with cancers of other organs like the stomach, with which it may be associated in exposure but also confused in diagnosis.

CANCERS OF THE GENITOURINARY SYSTEM

Ovary, Uterine Corpus, and Cervix Uteri

The induction by ionizing radiation of ovarian tumors in mice is an established experimental result, and provides a useful experimental model for investigations of the effects of changes in dose, dose rate, and radiation quality on risk (Ullrich, 1979a, 1979b). No similar experimental findings are available with respect to uterine cancer. The human evidence for radiation induction of ovarian and uterine cancer rests almost entirely on studies of patients treated for benign or malignant disease, and is complicated by aspects of treatment other than radiation that influence the risk of subsequent cancer.

For none of the sites considered in this section has cancer emerged as a radiation effect from the A-bomb survivor data, in terms of either mortality or incidence (Tables 1 and 2). The apparent high-dose excesses seen in the Hiroshima Tumor Registry data for 1959–1970 (Beebe, 1978) should be interpreted cautiously because of the incompleteness of the series. No significant excess risk has been seen in the relatively small number of women in the British ankylosing spondylitis patient series (Table 3).

Palmer and Spratt (1956) found 8 cases of ovarian cancer versus 2.6 expected (p < 0.001), in a retrospective study of 731 women treated with intracavity radium or external x-ray for benign pelvic disorders. Average tissue dose from x-ray was about 700 rad, but the dose from radium exposure could not be estimated. The study also found 29 cancers of the uterine corpus versus 4.9 expected (p < 0.001), and 11 cervical cancers versus 6.5 expected (p = 0.06). In the metropathia haemorrhagica series of Doll and Smith, 8 deaths from ovarian cancer were observed 5 yr or more after treatment compared with 7.66 expected from population rates (Smith, 1976). They also observed 16 uterine cancer deaths versus 10.34 expected (p = 0.06). Given 2068 women with an average of 19 yr follow-up (range, 10–31), and ovarian doses between 500 and 1000 rad, the excess mortality from uterine cancer was on the order of $0.3/10^6$ PYR 5 yr or more after treatment.

Brinkley and Haybittle (1969) reported 3 deaths from cancer of the uterine corpus versus 1.1 expected, and 1 death from ovarian cancer versus 1.0 expected in 277 women induced for artificial menopause by x-irradiation, more than 5 yr after treatment. Dickson (1969) identified 50 cancers of the uterine corpus and 33 of the cervix among 4010 women treated by radium for benign uterine hemorrhage between 1926 and 1966; 16 of the cervical cancers and 23 of the cancers of the uterine corpus were diagnosed more than 10 yr after radiation treatment. The number of cancers found seems excessive, but expected frequencies for the periods 1–10 and 10+ yr after treatment were not given, making it difficult to discern whether the later excess was due to radiation or was associated with the treated disease. In another study, 199 deaths from cancer of the uterine corpus were reported in 923 women surviving more than 5 yr after radium treatment for cancer of the cervix; nearly 50% of these deaths occurred within 10 yr after treatment and the excess may be disease-related, rather than treatment-related (Dickson, 1972). Only 5 deaths from ovarian cancer were observed, versus 3.44 expected.

Wagoner (1984) studied 1893 Connecticut women who had been treated by radiation for benign gynecologic disease during the period 1935–1964. He reported 107 cancers of the female genital organs compared with 54.9 expected according to Connecticut Tumor Registry rates during that period. This highly significant excess (p < 0.001) pertained mainly to cancers of the ovary and uterine corpus; there was no excess risk of cervical cancer, possibly because the cervix had been amputated in 12% of the population. Of particular interest was the observation of 12 uterine sarcomas versus 1.5 expected; most were mesodermal carcinosarcomas, in contrast to the general population ratio of three leiomyosarcomas for every carcinosarcoma seen in the Connecticut Tumor Registry. A fourfold excess of uterine sarcoma was also seen in a group of Connecticut patients given radiation therapy for cervical cancer.

In the large international series of women treated by radiation for cervical cancer there have been statistically significant *deficits* of ovarian and uterine cancer among women treated by radiation or by surgery, but not among women with cancer in situ (Table 4). A likely explanation is that, to an extent that has yet to be determined (John Boice, personal communication), radiation therapy was sometimes combined with surgical removal of the ovaries or the uterine corpus, or both. It is interesting that there were statistically significant increases over time in the incidence of cancers of the ovary and the uterine corpus, from marked deficits compared with population rates within 15 yr after treatment to marked excesses after 30 yr (Boice, 1983).

More to the point, in the Connecticut Tumor Registry data reported separately (Table 5), in which 86% of the patients did not have surgical removal of pelvic organs prior to 4 mo after diagnosis, 12 ovarian cancers were observed versus 9.2 expected (p = 0.22) in the first 9 yr after treatment, but subsequently

13 were observed versus 6.8 expected (p = 0.02). Similarly, 17 cancers of the uterine corpus were seen versus 11.7 expected within 9 yr (p = 0.09),. whereas, 22 were observed versus 11.7 expected, subsequently (p = 0.005). The increase in relative risk with time since treatment is marginally significant for cancer of the uterine corpus (p = 0.089), but not for ovarian cancer (p = 0.22). The later excess in cancers of the uterine corpus was observed in women who were under age 50 at treatment (17 observed versus 7.2 expected), whereas, there was no particular age dependence for ovarian cancer risk.

Although cancer does not appear to be induced readily in either the ovary or the uterus by exposure to ionizing radiation in doses of a few hundred rad or less, there is some evidence that an increased risk obtains after partial-body exposure to very high levels of radiation. This evidence is not particularly strong, and many uncertainties remain, including the extent to which the effect, if any, has been masked by surgical removal of the ovaries or uterus in some members of the irradiated populations under observation. Examination of the data from the large international study of cervical cancer patients is just beginning, and it is reasonable to expect that many of the uncertainties mentioned will be resolved in due course. Similarly, a more nearly complete case finding among members of the Hiroshima portion of the LSS sample, similar to that already undertaken for the Nagasaki portion, can be expected to resolve uncertainties about the apparent ovarian cancer excess in the Hiroshima tumor registry material.

Prostate Gland

Until very recently, the prostate gland was considered to be remarkably insensitive to the carcinogenic effects of ionizing radiation (Beebe, 1982). Prostate cancer is chiefly a disease of old men, increasing with age through the most advanced ages for which data are available (Greenwald, 1982). Its geographic variation is great, with a difference between US blacks, who have the highest rates, and Japanese, who have the lowest, of more than 20-fold (Waterhouse, 1982).

The prostate was a "lightly irradiated" site for the British spondylitis patients treated by x-ray, and no excess mortality has been observed (Table 3). At the death certificate level, no dose response has ever been observed among members of the LSS sample nor, indeed, have tabulations been published for this site in any of the periodic reports of mortality. No dose response was detected in either the Nagasaki or the (incomplete) Hiroshima tumor registry data for 1959–1970 with the LSS mortality survey data for 1950–1974 (Beebe, 1978).

It is of some interest, therefore, that the Nagasaki Tumor Registry data for the period 1959–1978 suggest that prostate cancer has been more frequent among the more heavily irradiated survivors of the Nagasaki A-bomb (Table 2). The investigators point out, however, that 11 of 30 prostate cancer cases recorded in the registry were discovered only at autopsy, and that of those LSS sample members dying during the interval 1961–1975, a (nonsignificantly) higher proportion were autopsied if their estimated exposures were to 100+ rad kerma (114 of 324, or 36%) than if their exposures were under 1 rad (188 of 619, or

30%) (Wakabayashi, 1983). Overall, the test for linear trend is statistically significant (p = 0.01), and yields a linear model risk estimate for all ages ATB, of $2.1/10^6$ PYR or 1.2%/rad. When restricted to the clinically evident cases, however, the trend is only suggestive (p = 0.09) and the corresponding estimate is $1.5/10^6$ PYR or 1.4%/rad.

It is surely too soon to conclude that the prostate gland is a sensitive site for radiation carcinogenesis, given the marginal nature of the evidence from the Nagasaki tumor registry and the absence, so far, of supporting evidence from other irradiated populations. It is not unreasonable, however, that a positive dose response should appear in an irradiated Japanese population and not in one of the European or North American populations under study. An excess risk sufficient to be seen against the low population rate among Japanese men might well be invisible against the more than tenfold greater population rates seen elsewhere. For the present, the prostate gland can be classified as a possibly sensitive site for radiation carcinogenesis, probably of low sensitivity both absolutely and relative to population rates.

Kidney and Urinary Bladder

The 1980 BEIR report concluded that the kidney and the urinary bladder seemed susceptible to radiogenic cancer in both human beings and experimental animals, but that the degree of susceptibility was probably low in comparison with other organs (NAS, 1980). Kidney cancer has been observed to be in excess among patients in whom Thorotrast used as an x-ray contrast medium was introduced directly into the urinary tract by catheterization of the ureter; 26 of 124 cancers attributed to Thorotrast were of the kidney (Wenz, 1967). The average time from exposure to onset or diagnosis of kidney cancer was 28 yr. Except for the possibility that the chemical properties of Thorotrast might be carcinogenic (Mole, 1979), the Thorotrast data suggest that alpha particles can cause kidney cancer, but provide little information about exposure levels.

Smith and Doll's study (1976) of women treated by radiation for metropathia haemorrhagica found only 3 deaths from bladder cancer 5 yr or more after treatment versus 2.15 expected. Wagoner (1984) observed 7 cases of kidney cancer versus 3.4 expected (p = 0.046), and 10 cases of bladder cancer versus 5.1 expected (p = 0.026), among women receiving radiotherapy for benign gynecologic disorders in Connecticut during the period 1935–1966. Based on estimated ovarian doses of 500–1000 rad to the metropathia patients, kidney and bladder doses were probably of similar magnitude in both studies.

A dose response for cancers of the urinary tract has been suggested by the two most recent LSS sample mortality surveys (Beebe, 1978; Kato, 1982). The data summarized in Table 1 indicate a significantly increasing trend for the two cities combined (p = 0.03). Although 90 deaths were coded to urinary cancer among exposed LSS sample members in Hiroshima and only 14 among those in Nagasaki, the test for trend approaches statistical significance in each city considered separately. The LSS sample data were not tabulated by age ATB. For all ages combined, the overall regression estimate is $0.27/10^6$ PYR or 0.5%/rad. This estimate may be too low, however, because the detection rate by death certificate for urinary cancers, as determined from autopsy findings, has been low (Steer, 1976).

Sanefuji and Ishimaru (1979) studied bladder cancer incidence in the LSS sample for the period 1961–1972, reviewing diagnoses from the mortality and pathology series and the tumor registries of Hiroshima and Nagasaki. Additional efforts were made in collaboration with urologists of the larger hospitals of the two cities to ascertain urinary bladder tumors not reported to the tumor registries. In all, 112 cases were identified, including only five based on death certificate diagnosis alone. There was only a marginally significant increasing trend with increasing dose ($p = 0.09$), and no significant variation by city or sex. All but 8 cases occurred among persons over 35 yr of age ATB; in this group the estimated excess risk was $1.6 \pm 1.1/10^6$ PYR or $0.6 \pm 0.4\%$/rad.

The Nagasaki tumor registry data in Table 2 include 32 cases of urinary tract cancer based on all sources of ascertainment. The overall test for linear trend is highly significant statistically, and the linear estimate of absolute risk is $1.2/10^6$ PYR or a 1.7%/rad increase over population rates. According to Wakabayashi et al (1983), the trend test is no less significant when applied to the somewhat smaller number of histologically confirmed cases in the registry.

Urinary tract cancers also appear to be in excess in the follow-up data on spondylitis patients given one course of x-ray treatment (Table 3), even though the estimated radiation doses, 46 rad to the kidneys and 31 rad to the bladder, are not particularly high. For the kidney, 7 deaths occurred more than 9 yr after beginning treatment compared with 2.6 expected ($p = 0.02$), whereas, 8 bladder cancer deaths were seen versus 5.1 expected ($p = 0.14$). During the first 9 yr, the corresponding numbers were 1 kidney cancer death versus 1.5 expected and 3 bladder cancer deaths versus 2.6 expected. The observed and expected values more than 9 yr after beginning treatment correspond to 1.7 excess kidney cancer deaths, and 1.6 excess bladder cancer deaths, per 10^6 PYR or, in relative terms, 3.7% and 1.9%/rad, respectively.

Given the generally positive findings from the spondylitis study, it is somewhat surprising that despite an average dose to the kidneys of about 250 rad, there should be no unequivocal evidence of a radiation-related excess risk among the cervical cancer patients treated by irradiation in either the large international study or among the subset covered by the Connecticut Tumor Registry (Tables 4 and 5). Both sets of data indicate an excess risk within the first 10 yr after treatment, which seems too soon; the Connecticut data suggest an excess after 10 yr that is highly significant statistically when viewed in isolation ($p < 0.001$) but only suggestive in comparison with the earlier excess ($p = 0.09$), whereas, the data for the entire study indicate a deficit after 10 yr. Boice and Day (1983) note that the pattern of risk over time following treatment was complex, with a large excess (not shown in Table 4) within 4 yr after treatment, followed by a decline and then a subsequent increase after 20 yr. Possibly, early detection produced an early excess of cases and a subsequent deficit which was gradually overcome by an excess due to radiation exposure.

The experience of the smaller number of patients with invasive cancer not treated by radiation offers little support to the radiation hypothesis: 18 kidney cancers were observed versus 8.4 expected, a statistically significant ($p = 0.001$) but unexplained excess which, moreover, showed no variation by the time since treatment (Boice, 1983). For patients with cervical cancer in situ the numbers of observed and expected kidney cancers agreed closely.

For bladder cancer the Connecticut Tumor Registry data are equivocal, with highly significant excesses over expected numbers both within the first 10 yr after treatment and subsequently, but with only a marginal increase in relative risk between the two periods ($p = 0.26$). In the larger study, however, relative risk increased from 2.0 (81 observed versus 41 expected) in the first 10 yr to 3.4 (112 observed versus 33 expected) subsequently, a highly significant increase ($p < 0.001$). For the patients with invasive cancer treated surgically or with cancer in situ the relative risk increased only slightly, from 1.5 to 1.7 ($p = 0.40$). The investigators suggest that radiation did, in fact, increase risk of bladder cancer, but that some other risk factor, such as smoking, may be associated with cervical cancer causing the radiation-related excess to operate on an already elevated level of risk. Radiation doses were estimated to be approximately 5000–9000 rad to the bladder.

The weight of the evidence would seem to be that radiation exposure can cause bladder cancer in man, and that the effect can occur at doses of a few hundred rad or less. The evidence regarding kidney cancer is considerably weaker, and the only quantitative estimate available is that calculated from the spondylitis data. To the extent that the excess risks in Table 5 represent a radiation effect, that effect seems to be fairly independent of age at exposure, at least after age 30 or so.

BRAIN AND CENTRAL NERVOUS SYSTEM

Both benign and malignant brain tumors can have serious consequences for the patient; furthermore, the malignancy of certain brain tumors (e.g., astrocytomas) is not well established. For these reasons, primary attention in this section is paid to brain tumors as a group, rather than to malignant or benign forms in particular.

Studies of central nervous system (CNS) cancer risk following atenatal irradiation reviewed in the 1980 BEIR report included a comparison by Bithell and Stewart (1975) of the histories of irradiation in utero for 1332 British children who died of malignant CNS tumors before the age of 15 and 8513 children without tumors. A significantly greater frequency of exposure in utero was found among the cancer cases, leading to an estimate of 6.1 excess deaths per 10^6 PYR (80% confidence limits 3.9 and 8.6) based on an unmatched comparison, and $4.4/10^6$ PYR based on a comparison with matched controls. MacMahon (1962), working from a base of 734,000 children born in selected hospitals during 1947–1954, searched death certificate lists for the years 1947–1959 and, for all cancer deaths and for a 1% sample of the total population, searched obstetrical records for evidence of prenatal x-ray exposure. Estimates of excess CNS cancer mortality associated with irradiation were $11.2/10^6$ PYR (80% confidence limits 2.0 and 23.6) based on a crude risk ratio and $6.3/10^6$ PYR (-1.1 and 17.2) after adjustment for birth order, religion, maternal age, sex, and whether the pay status was that of a private or clinic patient. Two negative cohort studies of populations with antenatal exposure to medical x-ray (Diamond, 1973) or the Hiroshima and Nagasaki A-bombs (Jablon, 1970) because of the relatively small numbers of exposed persons studied were nonetheless consistent with the risk estimates obtained in the two positive studies.

Studies of postnatal CNS irradiation included the New York tinea capitis study, in which 8 incident brain tumors (3 malignant) were observed among 2215 persons treated by x-ray as children for tinea capitis and followed an average of 25 yr versus none in 1413 controls (Shore, 1976; NAS, 1980). More recently, Shore (1982) has calculated that 1.4 brain tumors would have been expected in the exposed group according to population rates, from which, given an average brain dose of 140 rad, the estimated excess risk is $1.0 \pm 0.4/10^6$ PYR or $3.4\% \pm 1.5\%$/rad. No brain tumors were observed within 5 yr after irradiation, and 4 of the 8 occurred more than 25 yr after irradiation.

An updated report on the Israeli tinea capitis series through 1978 identified 21 brain tumors (10 malignant) among 10,842 persons irradiated as children versus only 6 (4 malignant) among an equal number of population controls and 5400 sibling controls, after a mean follow-up of 22.6 yr (Ron, 1984). Nine other CNS tumors (2 malignant) were found among the exposed versus none in the controls. For both malignant and benign CNS tumors (brain and other), the relative risk increased with the number of x-ray treatments. Brain dose at the surface was estimated to range between 121 and 139 rad, depending on filtration, whereas, irradiation at 2.5 cm below the surface ranged between 95 and 121 rad. If we take 125 rad as the mean dose to the tissue at risk, and ignore the first 5 yr of follow-up, the estimated excess risk per 10^6 PY per rad to the brain is 1.09 ± 0.24 for all CNS tumors, and 0.71 ± 0.20 for the brain, itself. There was no significant variation in relative risk by age at exposure, based on a comparison among age intervals 0–5, 6–8, and 9–15 yr. Although the study population was almost evenly divided by sex, 21 out of 30 CNS tumor cases among the exposed, and all six among the controls, were male. There was no significant variation in excess risk by country of origin for these mostly immigrant subjects.

Colman et al. (1978) reported 14 intracranial tumors (six malignant) among 3108 patients given x-ray treatment to the head and neck during childhood and followed for an average of 22 yr since irradiation. Based on an average 790 rad dose to the midplane of the neck, Stovall has calculated an average 80 rad to the midbrain on the basis of exposure information given by Colman et al. Stovall, personal communication). Given about 1.6 expected cases (Shore, 1982), the corresponding risk estimate, ignoring the first 5 yr of follow-up, is $2.9 \pm 0.9/10^6$ PYR or $9.7\% \pm 2.9\%$/rad.

Sandler et al (1982) found three brain tumors in 904 patients treated with radium implants in the nasopharynx and none in 2021 patients treated by other means. Given an average follow-up of 25 yr, an average brain dose in the range 15–40 rad, and 0.57 expected brain tumors in the irradiated patients (Shore, 1982), the estimated excess risk is between 3.4 ± 2.4 (for 40 rad) and 9.0 ± 6.4 (for 15 rad) cases per 10^6 PYR.

Brain cancer was nearly three times as frequent as a cause of death among American radiologists beginning practice during the decade 1920–1929, compared with other medical specialists (Matanoski, 1975). While this finding is generally confirmatory of other findings, it is difficult to evaluate further, as neither numbers of deaths nor average radiation doses were given.

A case-control study of intracranial meningiomas among women in Los Angeles County, California, found, among other things, an apparent association with exposure to medical and dental diagnostic x-rays to the head (Preston-Martin, 1980). The strongest association was to exposure to full-mouth dental x-ray series, especially before age 20 (RR = 4.0, p < 0.01) or before 1945 (RR = 2.1, p = 0.03). The investigators speculated that neural tissue could be more sensitive to radiation carcinogenesis at young ages or, alternatively, older dental x-ray machines in use during the 1940s, 1950s, and earlier may have delivered high doses to the brain. The series was based on intracranial meningiomas diagnosed during 1972–1975, and over 50% of the cases were over 50 yr old at diagnosis. No dose estimates were given.

The major sources of information represented by Tables 1–5 contain little that is relevant to the risk of brain tumors following exposure to ionzing radiation. Seyama et al (1979) studied incident brain tumors in the LSS sample during 1961–1975. Of 45 cases identified, 29 were among nonexposed sample members and survivors with less than 10 rad kerma, nine were in the 10–99 rad range, three had kerma estimates of 100 or more rad, and four were among those survivors whose exposures, while known to be high, were associated with such complicated shielding that numerical estimates of kerma could not be calculated. Curiously, all three cases in the 100+ rad range were among Nagasaki males, while the four unknown-dose cases were evenly distributed by city and sex. The data for survivors with estimated kerma do not support a dose relationship for brain tumors, but if the unknown-dose class is assumed to have the same average kerma as the 100+ rad class, the estimated excess risk is 0.16 $\pm$ 0.11/10^6 PYR (0.6% $\pm$ 0.4%/rad), kerma. Brain tumor prevalence at autopsy was also evaluated in the ABCC-RERF autopsy series, but no association with dose was found.

The spinal cord and nerves were heavily irradiated during x-ray therapy for ankylosing spondylitis, but the evidence for a radiation effect from the British series is equivocal. Although the observation of two deaths more than 9 yr after treatment is a statistically significant excess over expectation, even more stiking excesses were observed during years 0–2 and 3–8 following treatment (Table 3).

Although the risk of brain and other CNS tumors appear to be associated with exposure to ionizing radiation, many details of this risk remain unclear. The data are consistent with a tendency for risk to decline with increasing age at exposure, but uncertainties about comparability of case reporting and diagnostic criteria are reasons for caution. Exposures from therapeutic irradiation, in particular, often result in markedly nonuniform doses to different parts of the brain, and it would seem desirable for this important factor to be taken into account in any study attempting to synthesize existing data rigorously.

SUMMARY

The organ sites discussed in this chapter vary in their normal risks of cancer and in their susceptibility to radiation carcinogenesis. As a group, they may contribute half or more of the overall burden of radiation-induced cancer in many irradiated populations. Nevertheless, because of high background levels of risk or paucity of cases, much less is known about dose–response relationships, age dependence, and induction period than is known for such cancers as leukemia and breast cancer. Another reason for relative ignorance about many of these cancers is that information about radiation carcinogenesis is fragmented among many different studies, and has been integrated only at the necessarily superficial level of reviews. This is particularly true for salivary gland and CNS tumors, for which the relationship of risk to radiation dose seems well established, based on many separate studies. A more thorough synthesis, involving parallel analysis of basic data from the original studies and, perhaps, a more detailed dosimetry, would seem to be a promising expenditure of scientific resources.

REFERENCES

Asano M, Kato H, Yoshimoto K, Seyama S, Itakura H, Hamada T, Iijima S (1982) Primary liver carcinoma and liver cirrhosis in atomic bomb survivors, Hiroshima and Nagasaki, 1961–75, with special reference to HBs surface antigen. J Natl Cancer Inst 69:1221–1227.

Beebe GW. 1982. Ionizing radiation and health. Am Scientist 70:35–44.

Beebe GW, Kato H, Land CE (1978) Studies of the mortality of A-bomb survivors. 6. Mortality and radiation dose, 1950–1974. Radiat Res 75:138–201.

Belsky JL, Takeichi N, Yamamoto T, Cihak RW, Hirose F, Ezaki H, Inoue S, Blot WJ (1975) Salivary gland neoplasms following atomic radiation: Additional cases and reanalysis of combined data in a fixed population, 1957–1970. Cancer 35:555–559.

Bithell JF, Stewart AM (1975) Pre-natal irradiation and childhood malignancy: A review of British data from the Oxford survey. Br J Cancer 31:271–287.

Boice JD, Jr., Day NE (1983) Cancer risk following radiotherapy of cervical cancer. Preliminary report. In: Boice JD, Jr., and Fraumeni JF, Jr. (eds.), Radiation carcinogenesis: Epidemiology and biological significance. New York: Raven Press.

Bond VP, Thiessen JW (eds) (1982) Reevaluation of dosimetric factors, Hiroshima and Nagasaki. DOE Symposium Series; 55 CONF-810928 (DE81026279). Springfield, VA: National Technical Information Service, US Department of Commerce.

Brinkley D, Haybittle JL (1969) The late effects of artificial menopause by x-radiation. Br J Radiol 42:519–521.

Castro EB, Rosen PP, Quan SHQ (1973) Carcinoma of large intestine in patients irradiated for carcinoma of cervix and uterus. Cancer 31:45–52.

Colman M, Kirsch M, Creditor M (1978) Radiation induced tumors. In: Late biological effects of ionizing radiation, Vol. 1. Vienna: International Atomic Energy Agency, pp 167–180.

Court Brown WM, Doll R (1965) Mortality from cancer and other causes after radiotherapy for ankylosing spondylitis. Br Med J 2:1327–1332.

Diamond EL, Schmerler H, and Lilienfeld AM (1973) The relationship of intrauterine radiation to subsequent mortality and development of leukemia in children. Am J Epidemiol 97:283–313.

Dickson RJ (1969) The late results of radium treatment for benign uterine haemorrhage. Br J Radiol 42:582–594.

Dickson RJ (1972) Late results of radium treatment of carcinoma of the cervix. Clin Radiol 23:528–535.

Fraumeni JF, Jr. (1975) Cancers of the pancreas and biliary tract. Epidemiological considerations. Cancer Res 35:3437–3446.

Gilbert ES, Marks S (1979) An analysis of the mortality of workers in a nuclear facility. Radiat Res 79:122–148.

Greenwald P (1982) Prostate. In: Schottenfeld D and Fraumeni JF, Jr. (eds.), Cancer epidemiology and prevention. Philadelphia: WB Saunders.

Hempelmann LH, Hall WJ, Phillips M, Cooper RA, Ames WR (1975) Neoplasms in persons treated with x-rays in infancy: Fourth survey in 20 years. J Natl Cancer Inst 55:519–530.

Hoffman DA, McConahey WM, Kurland LT. 1982. Cancer incidence following treatment for hyperthyroidism. Int J Epid 11:218–224.

Hutchison GB, MacMahon B, Jablon S, Land CE (1979) Review of report by Mancuso, Stewart, and Kneale of radiation exposure of Hanford workers. Health Phys 37:207–220.

ICRP (1969) Radiosensitivity and spatial distribution of dose. Reports prepared by two task groups of ICRP committee 1, Publication 14. Oxford: Pergamon Press.

Jablon S, Kato H (1970) Childhood cancer in relation to prenatal exposure to atomic-bomb radiation. Lancet II:1000–1003.

Jablon SD, Kato H (1972) Studies of the mortality of A-bomb survivors. 5. Radiation dose and mortality, 1950–1970. Radiat Res 50:649–698.

Janower ML, Miettinen OS (1971) Neoplasms after childhood irradiation of the thymus gland. J Am Med Assoc 215:753–756.

Jochimsen PR, Pearlman NW, Lawton RL (1976) Pancreatic carcinoma as a sequel to therapy of lymphoma. J Surg Oncol 8:461–464.

Kato H, Schull WJ (1981) Life span study report 9, 1950–78. Supplementary tables. Hiroshima: Radiation Effects Research Foundation.

Kato H, Schull WJ (1982) Studies of the mortality of A-bomb survivors. 7. Mortality, 1950–1978: Part 1. Cancer mortality. Radiat Res 90:395–432.

Kleinerman RA, Curtis RE, Boice JD, Jr., Flannery JT, Fraumeni JF, Jr. (1982) Second cancers following radiotherapy for cervical cancer. J Natl Cancer Inst 69:1027–1033.

Kneale GW, Stewart AM, Mancuso TF (1978) Re-analysis of data relating to the Hanford study of the cancer risks of radiation workers. In: Late biological effects of ionizing radiation, Vol. I. Vienna: International Atomic Energy Agency, pp 386–412.

Land CE, Norman JE (1978) Latent periods of radiogenic cancers occurring among Japanese a-bomb survivors. In: Late biological effects of ionizing radiation, Vol I. Vienna: International Atomic Energy Agency, pp 29–47.

Land CE, Tokunaga M (1984) Induction period. In: Boice JD, Jr. and Fraumeni JF, Jr. (eds.), Radiation carcinogenesis: Epidemiology and biology significance. New York: Raven Press.

Lightdale CJ, Koepsell TD, Sherlock P (1982) Small intestine. In: Schottenfeld D and Fraumeni JF, Jr. (eds.), Cancer epidemiology and prevention. Philadelphia: WB Saunders.

Mack TM (1982) Pancreas. In: Schottenfeld D and Fraumeni JF, Jr. (eds.), Cancer epidemiology and prevention. Philadelphia: WB Saunders.

MacMahon B (1962) Prenatal x-ray exposure and childhood cancer. J Natl Cancer Inst 28:1173–1191.

Mancuso TF, Stewart A, Kneale G (1977) Radiation exposures of Hanford workers dying from cancer and other causes. Health Phys 33:369–385.

Marks S, Gilbert ES, Breitenstein BD (1978) Cancer mortality in Hanford workers. In: Late biological effects of ionizing radiation, Vol I. Vienna: International Atomic Energy Agency, pp 369–386.

Matanoski GM (1975) The current mortality rates of radiologists and other physician specialists: Specific causes of death. Am J Epidemiol 101:199–210.

Maxon HR, Saenger EL, Buncher CR, Kereiakes JG, Thomas SR, Shafer ML, McLaughlin CA (1981) Radiation-associated carcinoma of the salivary glands. A controlled study. Ann Otol 90:107–108.

Modan B, Baidatz D, Mart H, Steinitz R, Levin SG (1974) Radiation-induced head and neck tumours. Lancet i:277–279.

Mole RH (1979) Carcinogenesis by Thorotrast and other sources of irradiation, especially other alpha-emitters. Environ Res 18:192–215.

Nakamura K (1977) Stomach cancer in atomic-bomb survivors. Lancet ii:866–867.

National Academy of Sciences, Committee on the Biological Effects of Ionizing Radiation (1980). The effects on populations of exposure to low levels of ionizing radiation. Washington, DC: National Academy of Sciences

Ohkita T, Takehashi H, Takeichi N, Hirose F (1978) Prevalence of leukemia and salivary gland tumors among Hiroshima Atomic Bomb Survivors. In: Late biological effects of ionizing radiation, Vol. 1, Vienna: International Atomic Energy Agency, pp 71–81.

Palmer JP, Spratt DW (1956) Pelvic carcinoma following irradiation for benign gynecological diseases. Am J Obstet Gynecol 72:497–505.

Preston-Martin S, Paganini-Hill A, Henderson BE, Pike MC, Wood C (1980) Case-control study of intracranial meningiomas in women in Los Angeles County, California. J Natl Cancer Inst 65:67–73.

Ron E, Modan B (1984) Thyroid and other neoplasms following childhood scalp irradiation. In: Boice JD, Jr., Fraumeni JF, Jr. (eds.) Radiation Carcinogenesis: Epidemiology and Biological Significance. New York: Raven Press.

Saenger EL, Silverman FN, Sterling TD, Turner ME (1960) Neoplasia following therapeutic irradiation for benign conditions in childhood. Radiology 74:889–904.

Sandler DP, Cornstock GW, Matanoski GM (1982) Neoplasms following childhood irradiation of the nasopharynx. J Natl Cancer Inst 68:3–8.

Sanefuji H, Ishimaru T (1979) Urinary bladder tumors among atomic bomb survivors, Hiroshima and Nagasaki, 1961–72. RERF TR 18–79. Hiroshima: Radiation Effects Research Foundation.

Schneider AB, Favus MJ, Stachura ME, Arnold MJ, Frohman LA (1978) Salivary gland neoplasms as a late consequence of head and neck irradiation. Ann Int Med 87:160–164.

Seyama S, Ishimaru T, Iiyima S, Mori K (1979) Primary intracranial tumors among atomic bomb survivors and controls, Hiroshima and Nagasaki, 1961–75. RERF TR 15-79. Hiroshima: Radiation Effects Research Foundation.

Shore RE (1982) A follow-up study of children given x-ray treatment for ringworm of the scale (tinea capitis). (Unpublished doctoral thesis, Columbia University Faculty of Medicine.)

Shore RE, Albert RE, Pasternack BS (1976) Follow-up study of patients treated by x-ray epilation for tinea capitis: Resurvey of post-treatment illness and mortality experience. Arch Environ Health 31:17–24.

Smith PG, Doll R (1976) Late effects of x irradiation in patients treated for metropathia haemorrhagica. Br J Radiol 49:224–232.

Smith PG, Doll R (1981) Mortality from cancer and all causes among British radiologists. Br J Radiol 54:187–194.

Smith PG, Doll R (1982) Mortality among patients with ankylosing spondylitis after a single treatment course with x-rays. Br Med J 284:449–460.

Steer A, Land CE, Moriyama IM, Yamamoto T, Asano M, Sanefuji H (1976) Accuracy of diagnosis of cancer among autopsy cases: JNIH-ABCC population for Hiroshima and Nagasaki. Gann 67:625–632.

Takeichi N, Hirose F, Yamamoto H (1976) Salivary gland tumors in atomic bomb survivors, Hiroshima, Japan. I. Epidemiologic observations. Cancer 38:2462–2468.

Tolley HD, Marks S, Buchanan J, Gilbert ES (1983) A further update of the analysis of mortality of workers in a nuclear facility. Radiat Res 95:211–213.

Ullrich RL, Storer JB (1979) Influence of irradiation on the development of neoplastic disease in mice. II. Solid tumors. Radiat Res 80:317–324.

Ullrich RL, Storer JB (1979) Influence of irradiation on the development of neoplastic disease in mice. III. Dose-rate effects. Radiat Res 80:325–342.

Wagoner JK (1984) Leukemia and other malignancies following radiation therapy for benign gynecological disorders. In: Boice JD Jr., Fraumeni JF, Jr. (eds.) Radiation Carcinogenesis: Epidemiology and Biological Significance.

Wakabayashi T, Kato H, Ikeda T, Schull WJ (1983) Studies of the mortality of A-bomb survivors, Report 7. Part 3. Incidence of cancer in 1959–1978, based on the tumor registry, Nagasaki. Radiat Res 93:112–146.

Waterhouse J, Muir C, Shanmugaratnam K, Powell J (Eds.) (1982) Cancer incidence in five continents, Vol IV, Lyon: International Agency for Research on Cancer.

Wenz W (1967) Tumors of the kidney following retrograde pyelography with colloidal thorium dioxide. Ann NY Acad Sci 145:806–810.

RADIOGENIC CANCER AFTER PRENATAL OR CHILDHOOD EXPOSURE

ROBERT W. MILLER, M.D., AND JOHN D. BOICE, Jr., Sc.D.

Exposures to ionizing radiation during prenatal life or childhood may induce cancers within the pediatric years or far beyond. We now know, for example, that a single exposure to ionizing radiation at any time during the first 10 yr of life may induce breast cancer in females 30 yr later (Tokunaga et al, 1984).

The first case-reports of cancer following childhood exposure to radiotherapy appeared in 1922 and concerned osteosarcoma (reviewed by Cahan et al, 1948). Then, in 1950, relatively low doses of radiotherapy for thymic enlargement were first linked with ten cases of thyroid carcinoma by Duffy and Fitzgerald (1950) from a review of the clinical information on 28 patients with the neoplasm.

LEUKEMIA

Leukemia was known to occur excessively in early radiation workers, and children were expected to be as susceptible to radiogenic leukemia or perhaps even more so (Miller, 1953). The first clear evidence for radiation-induced leukemia during childhood was reported in 1956 by Miller, who noted 17 cases in the 10 yr following exposure within 1500 meters of the hypocenter in Hiroshima. The number of child-years at risk was a few thousand, so essentially no cases were expected. In 1962, Brill et al reported on the relation between the type of leukemia and age, and noted a "markedly increased incidence in acute leukemia in the younger age group [0–19 years at the time of the bomb (ATB)], as well as the unusual finding of five chronic granulocytic leukemia cases in the age range of zero to nine years." Among survivors over 19 yr of age at irradiation (AAI) and within 1500 meters of the hypocenter, none developed acute lymphocytic leukemia, but granulocytic leukemia developed in 41 (15

From the Clinical Epidemiology Branch and the Environmental Epidemiology Branch, National Cancer Institute, Bethesda, Maryland.

acute and 26 chronic). Japanese adults seldom develop chronic lymphocytic leukemia, a disease that is rare, if not absent, among children throughout the world.

The most recent analyses of data on A-bomb survivors show that in persons under 15 yr AAI, the excess in leukemia ran its course faster and reached an earlier, higher peak than was seen in older age groups (BEIR, 1980). Boys were affected more than girls, to the same extent that they are among children with leukemia not due to radiation exposure. A small excess in the frequency of leukemia has been reported in patients given radiotherapy for Wilms' tumor (Schwartz et al, 1975).

Fallout from nuclear weapons tests over southern and eastern Utah in the 1950s reportedly increased the mortality from leukemia among children, according to Lyon et al (1979). The rates, however, rose from below those for the nation to the national level, and then fell back again. The rates for all other childhood cancer moved in the opposite direction. This inconsistency suggested to Land (1979) that the observations were due to random fluctuation. Further studies are planned. For additional problems in ascribing the rise in leukemia rates to radiation, see the chapter on leukemia (p 249).

A much heightened susceptibility to cancers in childhood after intrauterine exposures to diagnostic radiation was first suggested by Stewart et al in 1956, and a fuller report was published in 1958. Similar findings were made by a different epidemiologic approach (MacMahon, 1962). Although Stewart seemed to strengthen the evidence for a causal relationship (reviewed by Bithell and Stewart, 1975), doubts about the interpretation of the results began to arise. Graham et al (1966) reported similar results when exposure of either parent occurred before conception. Other studies failed to replicate Stewart's findings. Diamond et al (1973) reported that the rates for all causes of death among prenatally exposed white children were 100% higher than in a nonexposed comparison group, except for cancers other than leukemia and two causes other than cancer, for which no increases were found. Among their sample of black children Diamond et al found no difference between cases and controls.

None of the Japanese children exposed in utero to the A-bomb developed leukemia and only one child died of another form of cancer (Jablon and Kato, 1970), contrary to the number (at least five) predicted by Stewart and Kneale (1970).

MacMahon's series has been extended in number and time. The original risk ratio (1.5) for leukemia remained unchanged, but the 1.5–fold increase in mortality from other cancers was no longer present (Monson and MacMahon, 1984). In still another study, a relative risk of only 1.1 was found for leukemia and for other cancer among children who died of cancer and whose births were in military hospitals (Robinette and Jablon, 1976). Children in the comparison group were born in the same hospitals, and their mothers had the same access to diagnostic procedures as the case-mothers did.

In an extensive series of animal studies, Brent (1979) was unable to show an oncogenic effect of prenatal exposure to ionizing radiation. Overall, the question of whether diagnostic x-rays increase the risk of the fetus to leukemia and other cancers, is as yet uncertain, and may never be resolved (MacMahon, 1981; Monson and MacMahon, 1984).

LYMPHOMA

The epidemiology of lymphoma is different from that of nonlymphocytic leukemias, and there is at present no convincing evidence that ionizing radiation induces lymphoma in the human (Kato and Schull, 1982; Miller and Beebe, 1986).

THYROID TUMORS

The radiation-induction of thyroid tumors, first observed in a retrospective study (Duffy and Fitzgerald, 1950), was evaluated in a prospective study by Hempelmann et al (1975). In their most recent resurvey of 2872 persons treated with radiation in infancy for enlargement of the thymus, 24 thyroid cancers were found, compared with 0.29 expected. No thyroid cancers occurred among 5055 untreated siblings. The average dose to the thyroid was estimated to be 119 rad, and the risk was 2.5 cases per million person-year-rad (PYR). Female subjects were more frequently affected than male. Benign tumors of the thyroid also occurred excessively. This and other studies (e.g., Becker et al, 1975) have found that the increase begins in adolescence and continues unabated through mid-life, the longest interval of follow-up yet possible. The cell-type is usually papillary, and can be effectively treated. An analysis of data from the Connecticut Tumor Registry has revealed that the incidence of thyroid cancer decreased among persons born in the 1960s, after radiotherapy was discouraged for benign diseases of the head, neck, or chest (Pottern et al, 1980). No change in mortality has occurred (McKay et al, 1982) because radiogenic thyroid cancer is usually curable, and presumably the more malignant nonradiogenic thyroid cancers have not diminished in frequency.

Among Japanese A-bomb survivors, thyroid cancer was more common in persons who received 50+ rad and were under 20 yr AAI, than in those who were older. The age group that was 0–19 AAI contained four of the five male subjects affected and nine of the 30 female (Parker et al, 1974).

The frequency of thyroid cancer was also increased among 10,842 Israeli children given radiotherapy for tinea capitis (Ron and Modan, 1980). Twenty-three thyroid cancers developed, compared with five expected. The estimated dose to the thyroid was low, only 9 rad on the average. An alignment error may have greatly increased the exposures, however. The affected group contained a disproportionate number of persons from North Africa (Ron and Modan, 1984). Moroccan immigrants to Israel had a high frequency of ataxia-telangiectasia (Levin and Perlov, 1971), an autosomal recessive disorder with unusual sensitivity to the acute effects of ionizing radiation (Pritchard et al, 1982). Possibly the numerous heterozygotes among Moroccan immigrants have an increased susceptibility to radiation-induced thyroid carcinoma. If so, tumors among this group might be due to a host–environment interaction.

Radioactive iodine is 1) used in medicine, 2) a major release product from nuclear reactors, and 3) a major component in fallout from nuclear weapons tests. Studies of Marshallese children heavily exposed to fallout from a weapons test in Bikini in 1954 revealed that two who were infants at the time of exposure suffered ablation of the thyroid. Among the other 20 who were under 10 yr of AAI, 17 developed benign tumors of the thyroid (including two of three exposed in utero), and one developed thyroid carcinoma (Sutow et al, 1982). The dose to the thyroids of these children from several radioisotopes of iodine plus external radiation was estimated to be 810–1800 rad.

Weapons tests in Nevada in the 1950s have raised concern about radiogenic cancers of the thyroid and other sites among persons in the area of fallout. In 1965–1971 clinical examinations were made of 5179 persons 11–18 yr of age, some of whom lived in selected communities in Utah and Nevada that received fallout, and comparison was made with others who subsequently moved into the area or who lived in Arizona where they were not in the path of fallout (Rallison et al, 1975). Thyroid carcinoma was not found in the exposed group, as contrasted with two cases among the Arizona children. Benign nodules were equally frequent among the three groups. The estimated dose to the thyroid of exposed children was about 100 rad. An excess of 73–100 children with radiogenic thyroid nodules was expected, according to risk estimates then current, assuming no latent period. Failure to find the excess, according to Boice and Land (1982), may be due to insufficient time elapsed since exposure, to less biological effectiveness of radioactive iodine than for external radiation, or to overestimation of the thyroid dose. A reexamination of the exposed and unexposed groups will soon begin, to determine the frequency of thyroid disease since 1971.

BREAST CANCER

About 9300 female subjects under 10 yr of age were exposed to the A-bomb in Japan. When last studied they were 35–45 yr old, and eight had developed breast cancer, compared with two expected (Tokunaga et al, 1984). The cases were evenly distributed throughout the age-interval at exposure. This observation indicates that a single exposure at any time in childhood can induce breast cancer decades hence, in contrast to leukemia, which runs its course of increased frequency in about 20 yr. The risk of breast cancer was higher in female victims exposed at 10–19 yr of age than in those who were exposed at older ages (Land et al, 1980). Those who were 0–9 yr AAI may ultimately be at still higher risk of radiogenic breast cancer.

An excess of breast cancer has also been observed after children were given radiotherapy. Hildreth et al (1983) described 5 such cases versus 0.5 expected after exposure to 50–199 rad as treatment for thymic enlargement in infancy. The earliest diagnosis of breast cancer was at 29 yr. Li et al (1983a, 1983b) described four children, including two males, who developed breast cancer in the field of therapeutic radiation for cancer under 10 yr of age. The patients developed breast cancer at 31–38 yr.

Adolescents who had multiple chest fluoroscopies for tuberculosis did not begin to develop an excess of breast cancers until 15 yr later, and the increased risk still persists 45 yr later (Boice and Monson, 1977).

BONE SARCOMA

External radiation induces osteosarcoma, as indicated, for example, in patients given radiotherapy for bilateral retinoblastoma (Sagerman et al, 1969). Beginning just after World War II, several hundred children were given radium-224 intravenously as empirical therapy for tuberculosis of bone. Among 218 children who were traced, 35 developed osteosarcoma or chondrosarcoma, and 29 developed benign tumors of bone (Mays and Spiess, 1984). The average skeletal dose was 1100 rad. The shortest latent period was 4 yr, the peak was at 6–8 yr, and the last bone cancer developed in 1974, 25 yr after treatment. The radioactivity of ^{224}Ra diminishes rapidly, thus, accounting perhaps for the fade-out of its carcinogenic effect on bone, according to Mays and Spiess. The finding is remarkable, and reflects a neoplastic process seemingly like that for leukemia and unlike that for breast cancer.

Thorotrast (thorium dioxide) is a radioactive compound given years ago to thousands of people as a radiologic contrast medium. In studies in various countries (reviewed by BEIR, 1980) excesses of hemangioendothelioma of the liver and, to a lesser extent, leukemia have occurred in these patients. Bone sarcoma has developed in persons given Thorotrast early in life (van Kaick, 1978; Sindelar et al, 1978).

Women who worked as radium-dial painters in the 1920s have developed great excesses of bone sarcomas and carcinomas of the endothelial lining of the mastoid sinuses (from radon gas trapped there). These women gave birth to an estimated 3000 children, who were exposed to radium in utero. Rowland and Lucas (1984) calculated that the fetal doses were 1–10 rem to the bone marrow during gestation, with additional exposure from radium deposited in the bones until it was eventually excreted. No radioactivity has been found in the few adults who were exposed in utero and were available for whole-body counts (Rowland, personal communication). The health status of this group has not been evaluated.

BRAIN TUMORS

Apparently, brain tumors have been induced among Israeli children treated with x-rays for tinea capitis. The diagnosis of definite or probable tumors was made in four persons with glioma and four with meningioma, compared with one case expected (Modan et al, 1974). The estimated dose to the brain was 140 rad. In a study of New York children similarly treated, three developed glial tumors and two developed meningioma, compared with none in the comparison group (Shore et al, 1976). An excess of brain tumors has not been reported among Japanese A-bomb survivors.

SOFT-TISSUE TUMORS

Radiotherapy for childhood cancer may induce soft-tissue tumors (mesenchymoma, fibrosarcoma, rhabdomyosarcoma) (e.g., Sagerman et al, 1969). Infants irradiated for enlargement of the thymus developed an excess of benign tumors of bone, breast, skin, and nerve in the field of radiation (Hempelmann et al, 1975).

COLON CANCER

Three children who received heavy doses of radiotherapy for Wilms' tumor developed colon cancer at ages 12, 24, and 27 yr (reviewed by Li, 1980). Although only three cases have been reported to date, the early age at diagnosis of colon cancer, in the absence of genetic predisposition as in polyposis coli, strongly suggests that the cancers were radiogenic.

PAROTID TUMORS

In each of the two studies of children given radiotherapy for tinea capitis, four developed parotid tumors, compared with none in the comparison groups (Modan et al, 1974; Shore et al, 1976). Among Japanese survivors of the A-bomb exposed within 1500 meters of the hypocenter, 14 cases of salivary gland tumors were observed compared with three expected (Takeichi et al, 1976). Among persons under age 20 yr AAI, the crude incidence of salivary gland tumors was similar to that for persons 20–49 yr AAI. Hence, no special susceptibility in children was evident.

HOST–RADIATION INTERACTION

Perhaps the best evidence of an interaction between the host and radiation in carcinogenesis is seen when children with the gene for multiple basal cell nevus syndrome receive radiotherapy to the chest. Several instances have been described in which radiation, given for medulloblastoma (occasionally an early feature of the syndrome), has been followed by basal cell nevi in the field of radiation much sooner than they usually appear (Stong, 1977). The most dramatic example of this interaction was described in 1949 by Scharnagel and Pack. They published a photograph of a 5 year old boy who developed a myriad of nevi on both the front and back of his chest following radiotherapy for thymic enlargement 4 yr earlier.

Strong (1977) has reported that second primary tumors occur earlier and more often after radiotherapy for heritable retinoblastoma than in children given radiotherapy for other cancers not known to be inherited. This observation also suggests the interaction of host susceptibility and exposure to ionizing radiation.

OVERVIEW

Studies of radiation exposures of children have revealed that they tend to be more susceptible than adults to certain cancers, that cancer may occur almost half a century after a single exposure, and that an interaction between radiation and host susceptibility can be demonstrated in certain genetic disorders.

REFERENCES

Becker FO, Economou SG, Southwick HW, Eisenstein R (1975) Adult thyroid cancer after head and neck irradiation in infancy and childhood. An Int Med 83:347–351.

Biological Effects of Ionizing Radiations (1980) The effects on populations of exposure to low levels of ionizing radiation: 1980. Washington, DC: National Academy Press.

Bithell JF, Stewart AM (1975) Pre-natal irradiation and childhood malignancy: A review of British data from the Oxford survey. Br J Cancer 31:271–287.

Boice JD, Jr., Land CE (1982) Ionizing radiation. In: Schottenfeld D and Fraumeni JF, Jr. (eds.), Cancer epidemiology and prevention. Philadelphia: W.B. Saunders, pp 231–253.

Boice JD, Jr., Monson RR (1977) Breast cancer in women after repeated fluoroscopic examinations of the chest. J Natl Cancer Inst 59:823–832.

Brent RL (1979) Effects of ionizing radiation on growth and development. Contr Epidemiol Biostat 1:147–183.

Brill AB, Tomonaga M, Heyssel RM (1962) Leukemia in man following exposure to ionizing radiation. A summary of the findings in Hiroshima and Nagasaki, and comparison with other human experience. Ann Int Med 56:590–609.

Cahan WG, Woodard H, Higinbotham NL, Stewart FW, Coley BL (1948) Sarcoma arising in irradiated bone: Report of eleven cases. Cancer 1:3–29.

Diamond EL, Schmerler H, Lilienfeld AM (1973) The relationship of intra-uterine radiation to subsequent mortality and development of leukemia in children: A prospective study. Am J Epidemiol 97:283–313.

Duffy BJ, Fitzgerald PJ (1950) Thyroid cancer in childhood and adolescence: A report on twenty-eight cases. Cancer 3:1018–1032.

Graham S, Levin ML, Lilienfeld AM, Schuman LM, Gibson R, Dowd JE, Hempelmann L (1966) Preconception, intrauterine, and postnatal irradiation as related to leukemia. Natl Cancer Inst Monogr 19:347–371.

Hempelmann LH, Hall WJ, Phillips M, Cooper RA, Ames WR (1975) Neoplasms in persons treated with x-rays in infancy: Fourth survey in 20 years. J Natl Cancer Inst 55:519–530.

Hildreth NG, Shore RE, Hempelmann LH (1983) Risk of breast cancer among women receiving radiation treatment in infancy for thymic enlargement. Lancet ii:273.

Jablon S, Kato H (1970) Childhood cancer in relation to prenatal exposure to atomic-bomb radiation. Lancet ii:1000–1003.

Kato H, Schull WJ (1982) Studies of the mortality of A-bomb survivors. 7. Mortality, 1950–1978: Part 1. Cancer mortality. Radiat Res 90:395–432.

Land CE (1979) the hazards of fallout or of epidemiologic research? N Engl J Med 300:431–432.

Land CE, Boice JD, Jr., Shore RE, Norman CE, Tokunaga M (1980) Breast risk from low-dose exposures to ionizing radiation: Results of parallel analysis of three exposed populations of women. J Natl Cancer Inst 65:353–376.

Levin S, Perlov S (1971) Ataxia-telangiectasia in Israel: With observations on its relationship to malignant disease. Israeli J Med Sci 7:1535–1541.

Li FP (1980) Colon cancer after Wilms tumor. J Pediatr 96:954–955.

Li FP, Roser E (1983) Radiotherapy for childhood tumours followed by breast cancer. Lancet ii:738–739.

Lyon JL, Klauber MR, Gardner JW, Udall KS (1979) Childhood leukemias associated with fallout from nuclear testing. N Engl J Med 300:397–402.

MacMahon B (1962) Prenatal x-ray exposure and childhood cancer. J Natl Cancer Inst 28:1173–1191.

MacMahon B (1981) Childhood cancer and prenatal irradiation. In: Burchenal, JH and Oettgen HF (eds.), Cancer achievements, challenges, and prospects for the 1980s, Vol 1. New York: Grune and Stratton, pp 223–228.

Mays CW, Spiess H (1984) Bone sarcomas in patients given radium-224. In: Boice JD, Jr. and Fraumeni JF, Jr. (eds.), Radiation carcinogenesis: Epidemiology and biological significance. New York: Raven Press, pp 241–252.

McKay FW, Hanson MR, Miller RW (1982) U.S. Cancer Mortality 1950–1977. Natl Cancer Inst Monogr 59:

Miller RW (1953) Some potential hazards of the use of roentgen rays in pediatrics. Pediatrics 11:294–303.

Miller RW (1956) Delayed effects occurring within the first decade after exposure of young individuals to the Hiroshima atomic bomb. Pediatrics 18:1–18.

Monson RR, MacMahon B (1984) Prenatal x-ray exposure and cancers in children. In:

Boice JD, Jr. and Fraumeni JF, Jr. (eds.), Radiation carcinogenesis: Epidemiology and biological significance. New York: Raven Press, pp 97–105.

Parker LN, Belsky JL, Yamamoto T, Kawamoto S, Keehn RJ (1974) Thyroid carcinoma after exposure to atomic radiation. A continuing survey of a fixed population, Hiroshima and Nagasaki, 1958–1971. Ann Int Med 80:600–604.

Pottern LM, Stone BJ, Day NE, Pickle LW, Fraumeni JF, Jr. (1980) Thyroid cancer in Connecticut, 1935–1975: An analysis by cell type. Am J Epidemiol 112:764–774.

Pritchard J, Sandland MR, Bretnach FB, Pincott JR, Cox R, Husband P (1982) The effects of radiation therapy for Hodgkin's disease in a child with ataxia telangiectasia. Cancer 50:877–886.

Rallison ML, Dobyns BM, Keating, FR, Jr., Rall JE, Tyler FH (1975) Thyroid nodularity in children. J Am Med Assoc 233:1069–1072.

Robinette CD, Jablon S (1976) Childhood cancer and fetal x-ray exposure in children born in military hospitals. Radiat Res 67 (abstr):627.

Ron E, Modan B (1980) Benign and malignant thyroid neoplasms after childhood irradiation for tinea capitis. J Natl Cancer Inst 65:7–11.

Ron E, Modan B (1984) Thyroid and other neoplasms following childhood scalp irradiation. In: Boice JD, Jr. and Fraumeni JF, Jr. (eds.), Radiation carcinogenesis: Epidemiology and biological significance. New York: Raven Press, pp. 139–151.

Rowland RE, Lucas HF, Jr. (1984) Radium-dial workers. In: Boice JD, Jr. and Fraumeni JF, Jr. (eds.), Radiation carcinogenesis: Epidemiology and biological significance. New York: Raven Press, pp 231–240.

Sagerman RH, Cassady JR, Tretter P, Ellsworth RM (1969) Radiation induced neoplasia following external beam therapy for children with retinoblastoma. Am J Roentgenol Radium Ther Nucl Med 105:529–535.

Scharnagel IM, Pack GT (1949) Multiple basal cell epitheliomas in a five year old child. Am J Dis Child 77:647.

Schwartz AD, Lee H, Baum ES (1975) Leukemia in children with Wilms tumor. J Pediatr 87:374–376.

Shore RE, Albert RE, Pasternack BS (1976) Follow-up study of patients treated by x-ray epilation for tinea capitis: Resurvey of post-treatment illness and mortality experience. Arch Environ Health 31:21–28.

Sindelar WF, Costa J, Ketcham AS (1978) Osteosarcoma associated with Thorotrast administration: Report of two cases and literature review. Cancer 42:2604–2609.

Stewart A, Webb J, Giles DD, Hewitt D (1956) Malignant disease in childhood and diagnostic irradiation in utero: Preliminary communication. Lancet ii:447.

Stewart A, Webb J, Hewitt D (1958) A survey of childhood malignancies. Br Med J 1:1495–1508.

Stewart AM, Kneale GW (1970) Radiation dose effects in relation to obstetric x-rays and childhood cancers. Lancet i:1185–1188.

Strong LC (1977) Theories of pathogenesis: Mutation and cancer. In: Mulvihill JJ, Miller RW, Fraumeni JF, Jr. (eds.), Genetics of Human cancer. New York, Raven Press, pp 401–414.

Sutow WW, Conard RA, Thompson KH (1982) Thyroid injury and effects on growth and development in Marshallese children accidentally exposed to radioactive fallout. Cancer Bull 34:90–96.

Takeichi N, Hirose F, Yamamoto H (1976) Salivary gland tumors in atomic bomb survivors, Hiroshima, Japan. I. Epidemiologic observations. Cancer 38:2462–2468.

Tokunaga M, Land CE, Yamamoto T, Asano M, Tokuoka S, Ezaki H, Nishimori I, Fujikura T (1984) Breast cancer among atomic bomb survivors. In: Boice JD, Jr. and Fraumeni JF Jr. (eds.), Radiation carcinogenesis: Epidemiology and biological significance. New York: Raven Press, pp 45–56.

van Kaick G, Lorenz D, Muth H, Kaul A (1978) Malignancies in German Thorotrast patients and estimated tissue dose. Health Phys 35:127–136.

CARCINOGENIC EFFECTS OF OCCUPATIONAL RADIATION EXPOSURE

PHILIP E. SARTWELL, M.D., AND
ROY E. SHORE, Ph.D., D.P.H.

Although an industrial hazard from exposure to ionizing radiation (to be termed simply "radiation" in this chapter) has existed for centuries in the mining industry, interest in the topic has arisen largely since the end of World War II and the beginning of the "atomic age." It would seem that study of occupational exposures would provide one of the best ways to learn the hazards, because exposure can be measured and employees kept under observation. In fact, more information has come from other sources, especially studies of the A-bomb survivors and the medical use of x-rays. This is mainly due to the fortunate fact that occupational exposures have usually, with exceptions to be noted, been low-level. The only occupational groups that have provided clear-cut positive information as to hazards are uranium miners, radiologists, and radium-dial painters. The present most important challenge is to learn what effects, if any, result from continued exposures such as those sustained by workers in the repair of nuclear-powered ships, in the range of 1–5 rad accumulated over years—in other words, to acquire information about the lower end of the dose–response curve. This may provide further insight into mechanisms of carcinogenesis and permit the setting of sounder maximum permissible limits.

Animal studies cannot be substituted for human experience, and there is inevitably a long lag time in the acquisition of human experience. The usual latent period of leukemia after brief intensive exposure is 5–10 yr, although the maximum range may be as much as 2–20 yr. For solid tumors, the latent period is generally more than 10 yr, and some excess risk may persist throughout the remainder of life. Furthermore, the time at which cancer is initiated in occupational situations is presumably not at first exposure but after several, perhaps

From the Institute of Environmental Medicine, New York University Medical Center, New York.

many, years of cumulative small exposures. Exposures beginning in 1982 and continuing for 20 yr, if carcinogenic, might first detectably increase the observed incidence of solid tumors only after the termination of exposure.

The problem of following workers over long periods is formidable. It is important that industries in which exposure is incurred keep full records of each individual's exposures and information relevant to other carcinogenic hazards, such as chemical exposures and smoking practices, and that they do what they can to make possible follow-up after termination of employment.

Because of the time-lag problem, the chief method of epidemiologic study is the historical prospective, or cohort, method. Rosters of employees at risk, going back as far as possible, are secured and their experience is followed up to the last available year, so as to determine mortality from, and if possible incidence of, disease, as well as the numbers lost to observation, year by year. This information will provide person-years at risk of the events of interest, and permit calculation of rates. Similar information is secured from an unexposed body of personnel within the same industry for purposes of comparison, if possible; if not, rates for the nation or appropriate demographic subdivision may have to be substituted. It is usual to compare directly the observed deaths or cases with the expected number obtained by multiplying person-years of the study group by rates of the comparison group, specific for age, time, and other variables. Dividing the observed by the expected number yields the standardized mortality or morbidity ratio (SMR).

The case-control method (Schlesselman, 1982) would not be very useful for studying occupational radiation exposures in a general population, because such exposures are incurred by only a small percentage of the population. (Case-control studies are mainly useful for studying common exposures.) However, the case-control method is useful in some situations. In particular, a variant of this method that has been termed the "nested case-control study" has proved valuable. This is a study that draws on a prospective study in progress. Cases of the disease under investigation that have arisen during the course of the prospective study constitute the case series, and a sample of persons in that study who have not developed the disease constitute the controls. It is often possible to obtain more and better information from this limited number of subjects than would be practicable from the whole study population, and there are other advantages, including more confident selection of controls.

Accumulative intensity and duration of exposures are of course important; a dose–response relationship strengthens the evidence that the suspected agent is causative, although it does not establish it.

In general, the three principal issues to be dealt with are: choice of a control group, dealing with possible biases in determining exposure and disease status, and taking into account confounding factors, of which smoking will serve as an example. Age, sex, race, calendar time, and follow-up time, plus other variables need to be considered. The "healthy worker effect" must be taken into consideration, particularly if the comparison group is the whole population. This is an expression for the familiar observation that employed workers characteristically have lower mortality from all causes combined than does the general population of similar demographic structure, owing to selective factors for employment.

A study of confounding factors in occupational mortality (Gilbert, 1982) illustrates some pitfalls in the use of industrial mortality rates. Analyses of 323,000 person-years of experience over 30 yr at the Hanford nuclear plant, compared with U.S. mortality experience, showed the expected large "healthy worker" effect. An internal comparison of groups of workers at the plant, by categories, was then made. The endpoints were deaths from cancer and from all other causes, respectively. The categories were: length of time since entering the industry; employment status (years since termination of employment); length of employment; job category; and calendar year of initial employment, each divided in several subclasses. In examining the effect of each category, adjustment was made for all the others, and of course for age. There were found differences in SMR between subclasses of each category, several of which were statistically significant. A reduced risk of death characterized the early years of employment; and increased risk was found for those with less than 2 yr of employment at Hanford, and was particularly striking for those whose employment had terminated. After adjustment for all these factors, exposure to radiation had no detectable influence on all cancers or other causes of death. There were, as previous analyses of the same data had shown, significant excesses of cancer of the pancreas and multiple myeloma, based on quite small numbers.

Of the studies cited in this chapter, few if any have examined and adjusted for all these factors, partly because of the unavailability of the needed data, or too small numbers. While this should lead to caution in their interpretation, it by no means nullifies them.

There have been a few industrial accidents involving the exposure of small numbers of persons to very large doses of radiation, with or without acute symptoms occurring within hours or days after exposure. In survivors of such accidents, the occurrence of cancer years later has sometimes been recorded. Where acute myelogenous leukemia arises a decade later, it is a reasonable inference that it was probably a result of the exposure; yet in the individual case this can never be known with assurance. Therefore, incidents of this nature, which really do not contribute to the knowledge of radiation carcinogenesis, will not be further discussed.

Before considering those industries having a clear or postulated radiation hazard, it will be well to identify the industries in which some exposure exists, with the numbers of personnel exposed and the annual average dose in millirems. These estimates for the United States are taken from the 1980 report on the effects on populations of exposure to low levels of ionizing radiation, produced by a committee of the National Research Council (1980), and commonly known as the BEIR III report, as it will be termed in the remainder of this chapter (Table 1). It will be noted that the estimates of average dose do not vary greatly between industries, and that the number of workers in the medical and related fields constitute the largest groups.

WORKERS IN MEDICAL RADIOLOGY

Some of the pioneer radiologists in the early years of the century sustained severe x-ray burns and skin cancers. Later, several investigators in the U.S. noted that the proportionate mortality from leukemia among radiologists was higher than in the general population. This information was commonly

TABLE 1 Estimate of Whole-Body Dose of Radiation in U.S. to Workers from Industrial Sources

| Source of exposure | Number of workers exposed | Average dose rate (mrems/yr) | |
		Exposed group	Prorated over total population
Medical x-rays			
Medical personnel	195,000	300–350[a]	0.30
Dental personnel	171,000	50–125[a]	0.05
Radiopharmaceuticals			
Medical personnel	100,000	260–350	0.10
Nuclear Industry			
Commercial nuclear power plants	67,000	400[b]	0.10
Industrial radiography	11,250	320	0.02
Fuel processing and fabrication	11,250	160	0.01
Handling byproduct materials	3,500	350	0.01
Federal contractors	88,500	~250	0.01
Naval nuclear propulson program	36,000	220	0.04
Research activities			
Particle accelerators	10,000	Unknown	<<1
X-ray diffraction units	10–20,000	Unknown	<<1
Electron microscopes	4,400	50–200	0.003
Neutron generators	1–2,000	Unknown	<<1
Airlines			
Crew members (cosmic radiation)	40,000	160	0.03
Natural background, for comparison	220×10^6	54[c]	54

Source: Adapted from BEIR III.

[a] Based on personal dosimeter readings; because of relatively low energy of medical x-rays, actual whole-body doses are probably less.

[b] Average dose rate to the ~40,000 workers who received measurable exposures was 600–800 mrems/yr.

[c] Includes cosmic and terrestrial radiation, but no internal sources.

gleaned from obituary notices in medical journals giving the cause of death. Warren (1956) called attention to the earlier age at death of radiologists than other professionals. In Britain (Court Brown, 1958) and in the United States (Seltser, 1965), cancer mortality in radiologists was studied more systematically by the historical prospective method.

The British report showed an excess mortality from cancer among men who entered the practice of radiology before 1921, but no clear excess of leukemia, as contrasted with all members of the upper socioeconomic classes. The American study indicated a substantial risk not only of leukemia but also of several solid-tissue cancers. The comparison groups were members of other medical specialty bodies. Both studies have been recently updated.

The British follow-up study (Smith, 1981) found the final mortality rate from cancer among 339 radiologists who entered the study before 1921 to be 75% higher than that of other medical practitioners. Cancer of the pancreas, lung, and skin, and leukemia were significantly raised. Among 999 men entering the study after 1920 there was little evidence of an excess risk, and that little was confined to those entering in the earlier period, 1921–1935. In the latter group, for no single neoplasm was there a significant excess over other medical practitioners.

The U.S. workers (Matanoski, 1975, 1981) had a larger number of subjects available for study (6524 male radiologists contributing 104,483 man-years); the comparisons were with several other specialty societies presumed to have a gradient of diminishing exposure, due to the nature of their practice. These included internists, pathologists and bacteriologists, otorhinolaryngologists, and ophthalmologists. They were arrayed by 10-yr cohorts of entry. Cancer mortality was higher for members of the radiologic societies than the others. In the particular entry period shown, with observations terminating in 1969, the following malignancies as coded from the death certificates showed statistically significant differences: all cancer, oral cancer, skin cancer, and leukemia. For an earlier cohort contrasted with pathologists and bacteriologists, the excess of leukemia was 15-fold, the difference being significant for acute and myeloid forms. Radiologists entering in 1940–1969 had no excess of leukemia, and only a slight excess in a few forms of cancer, but a significant doubling in SMR for multiple myeloma.

There was no dosimetry in these studies, because film badges were not worn during the period when the heavy exposures presumably occurred, but there can be little doubt that prior to 1950 exposures were high. It was not possible to evaluate the members' exposures to other risk factors for cancer, or to determine if health-related factors influenced their choice of specialty. The quantitative difference between the British and U.S. studies may be partly due to the comparative study sizes and the choice of comparison groups. Differences in protective equipment and in adherence to protective practices may also have been involved.

Clearly, however, there was an excess risk of cancer overall, estimated at 1.5–2 times the expected, and at certain specific sites, among the earlier radiologists (Matanoski, 1981). Leukemia was especially increased. These excesses have greatly diminished, and perhaps disappeared entirely, in recent experience. Too little time has passed since the most recent generations of radiologists entered the field to be wholly confident of this, because they have not yet entered the age-classes with the highest risks.

A registry of American radiologists and pathologists was established in 1962 to advance understanding of this problem. Questionnaires were sent to the members of the American College of Radiology and the College of American Pathologists, first in that year and periodically, thereafter, to new members (Silverman, 1971). To date, the only findings reported have concerned the use of x-rays by members of the two societies and their families. Both diagnostic and therapeutic uses by the male members, their spouses, and their children were more frequent than such uses by families of the pathologists. Therapeutic procedures were used by 19% of radiologists and 8% of pathologists; thus, the radiologists' exposures include a component of personal use (Jessup, 1981).

Long-term follow-up of x-ray technicians is far more difficult than for physicians, owing to the effort required to trace them. However, deaths of U.S. veterans with war service are reported to the Veterans Administration. Army personnel who served as radiologic technicians during World War II, numbering 6560, and a comparison group of 6828 other medical technologists, were followed up for 29 yr, 1946–1974 (Jablon, 1978). Follow-up consisted of ascertaining the deaths, obtaining death certificates, and coding the causes. The total number of deaths in the two groups was identical; malignant neoplasms were assigned as the cause in 145 former x-ray technicians and 158 other technicians, and leukemia in 12 and seven, respectively. The x-ray technicians served in that capacity for an average of less than 3 yr in the Army, and only an estimated 19% continued in similar work afterward. This study is essentially negative to date, but its limitations include the presumably low exposures of the technicians and the restricted time that has elapsed.

It is estimated from film badge data that in 1975 96% of U.S. dental personnel received less than 100 mrem of radiation annually (BEIR III); thus, their dosage is unlikely to lead to perceptible effects. The corresponding value for hospital radiological personnel was 69%; 95% of these workers were exposed to less than 1 rem/yr.

WORKERS AT NUCLEAR FACILITIES AND POWER PLANTS

The Hanford, Washington, plant has processed plutonium, conducted nuclear research, and served as a nuclear power station; records of employees have been kept since 1944. Several reports on the health of workers, including the one cited earlier in this chapter, have appeared. Several by Mancuso, Stewart and Kneale (e.g., Mancuso, 1977; Neale, 1981) have reported elevated cancer risks and have generated considerable controversy. Exposures were said not to be excessive by existing standards. The first analysis contrasted the exposures of men dying of cancer with those dying of other causes, and found higher mean radiation doses, and a higher proportion of exposed men, among those dying of lymphomas, myelomas, myeloid leukemias, and all solid tumors as a class, particularly cancers of the pancreas and lung.

Hutchison et al (1979) were asked by the Department of Energy to review this report. The abstract of their review reads, in part, "There is no suggestion of a radiation relationship for lymphatic and hemopoietic cancers other than myeloma, or for solid tumors of sites other than the pancreas, with the possible, and very weak, exception of the kidney . . . Radiobiologic considerations, including the results of other studies, suggest that the excess proportional mortality at doses above 10 rem for cancer of pancreas and multiple myeloma is likely to be explainable in terms of a correlate of dose rather than in terms of radiation . . ." The data have also been analyzed by Sanders (1978), and Gofman (1979), Darby and Reissland (1981), and several others.

Gilbert and Marks (1979, 1980) also studied the Hanford mortality experience by the prospective method. They first compared it with the U.S. death rates and showed the anticipated healthy worker effect; deaths from all causes were 75% of the expected, and for malignant neoplasms, 85%. (It seems reasonable to suppose that cancer is less affected by the healthy worker effect than conditions such as cardiovascular disease). An internal, within-plant comparison showed no correlation between dosage and either all cancers, or all causes. A trend with dosage was shown for multiple myeloma and cancer of the pancreas, but not for other forms of cancer, including leukemia. The most recent analysis has shown that with further accrual of person-years cancer of the pancreas no longer has a significant association with radiation dose.

Thus, the one consistent positive finding in all of the analyses of the Hanford data has been for radiation and multiple myeloma. It should be noted that this finding is essentially based on three cases who had doses in the range of 15–50 rem. In retrospect, had these sparse data not been used to generate estimates of the "doubling dose" for cancer, which were one to two orders of magnitude lower than conventional estimates, probably no controversy would have erupted over them.

Two studies from laboratories dealing with nuclear physics have produced contradictory findings with respect to the occurrence of malignant melanoma. The first (Austin, 1981) found an excess number of cases among employees of the Lawrence Livermore National Laboratory in California, U.S. (19 observed, 6.4 expected at the rates of the local area). The second, conducted at the Lost Alamos National Laboratory in New Mexico (Aquavella, 1982), failed to find an excess; there were 6 cases observed and 5 expected. In neither study was there evidence that the cases had experienced heavier radiation exposure than other employees.

The only positive finding in the nuclear industry that has not been challenged and that is consistent with similar findings in other exposed occupations appears to be the excess of multiple myeloma. Such an excess was seen among Windscale (England) nuclear energy workers, American radiologists, and radium-dial painters (Cusick, 1981). In several nonoccupational groups, such as diagnostically or therapeutically irradiated subjects, an excess was also seen.

URANIUM AND HARD-ROCK MINING

The longest-existing industrial exposure to radiation, as stated earlier, is inhalation of radon daughters in mining operations, leading to lung cancer. This topic is dealt with in Chapter 18; here, only the epidemiologic evidence will be discussed.

The activity that chiefly gives rise to this hazard is underground mining in which there is exposure to dust from hard rock in areas where the rock contains some uranium, but uranium milling operations may also entail some risk. Even in the 16th C. it was known that a fatal lung disease occurred among miners in the Erz Mountains of central Europe. Alpha radiation, given off by radon daughters inhaled into the lungs, is mainly responsible. Epidemiologic studies did not begin until after World War II. A "working level" of 100 pCi/L of air from ^{222}Rn in decay equilibrium with its daughters has been adopted. Working level months (WLM) are defined as number of working levels multiplied by the length of underground exposure in "working months" of 170 hr.

In the U.S. the studies have been done in the four-state Colorado Plateau region, where mining of uranium on a large scale began in 1948. In these mines, measurements for radon show levels approximating those in the Erz Mountains.

The most detailed report of this experience is that by Lundin et al (1971). An excess of respiratory cancer was found in white uranium miners with cumulative exposures upwards of 120 WLM. The excess over the numbers expected at general population rates became evident after 10 yr of exposure. Although the SMR was higher in cigarette smokers, it was fully apparent in nonsmokers. For small-cell undifferentiated tumors, which are the most characteristic radiation-induced type, there was a suggestion that excess risk might appear at an even lower level. Improved underground ventilation and other measures are said to have reduced exposures to an average of about 1.3 WLM/yr, or 60 in a working lifetime (Cohen, 1982).

Studies of Czechoslovakian miners (Sěvc, 1976; Kunz, 1978), done in similar fashion, led to generally similar results. The lowest level at which distinct evidence of carcinogenicity was observed was in the 100–200 WLM range. The SMR continued to rise to above eight for exposure above 400 WLM.

Several other types of mining have been found to lead to lung cancer. Fluorspar miners in Nova Scotia, working in mines with exposure above usual limits, had a high risk (de Villiers, 1964). Iron ore miners in Cumberland, England (Boyd, 1970) showed a small excess risk, which was considered due either to the radon concentration or to a carcinogenic effect of iron oxide. Cornish underground tin miners, who also had exposure to raised levels of radiation, had a twofold excess of lung cancer (Fox, 1981). Gastric cancer, and all cancers combined, also showed an excess. Surface miners were not affected.

There can be no doubt of the carcinogenicity of underground mining in certain rock formations. Soft-coal miners apparently escape this risk. Along with respiratory cancer, other serious hazards including pulmonary silicosis may occur. The remedy is better ventilation of the work areas.

RADIUM-DIAL PAINTERS

The biological effects of ingestion of radium are discussed in Chapter 20; here we shall present the epidemiologic findings that relate to the occupational disease incidence and mortality.

Several publications from the Argonne National Laboratory in the past few years have dealt with this topic. Radium-dial painters were young women, exposed between 1915 and 1930 to large quantities of alpha-emitting radionuclides, partly through pointing their brushes between their lips. These compounds are bone-seeking and gave rise to many cases of bone cancer. The latency period of this disease is prolonged, from a few years to more than 40 yr after the first exposure; because the radionuclides are deposited in bone, they continue to emit internal radiation for long periods. When the intake dose is high, the latent period is shortened (Polednak, 1977). Mortality rates of 634 women employed in this industry were higher than those for U.S. white females (adjusted for age and time), the mortality ratio being 1.3. Substantial excesses were recorded for all malignant neoplasms collectively, bone cancer (with a mortality rate more than 80 times the expectation), external causes, and "other unspecified sites." A possible relation to colon cancer and blood and blood-forming organs was also noted, but no mention was made of breast cancer (Polednak, 1978).

Life tables based on all 1235 women who could be followed (including the above 634) were presented in another paper (Stehney, 1978). Mortality was tabulated for intervals following first exposure and observed deaths were compared with those expected for all white females, adjusted for age and time.

Over the first 25 yr since entering this employment, observed deaths from all causes exceeded expected deaths by an average SMR of 1.5; thereafter, they were scarcely above the expected level. When the deaths involving tumor types that are known to be related to radium exposure (bone sarcoma, and carcinomas originating in the paranasal sinuses and mastoid cells) were removed from consideration, the observed deaths exceeded the expected appreciably only in the first decade after exposure. Although the healthy worker effect would be expected to lower general mortality rates somewhat, especially in the first years of employment, it is evident that the excess was not of great magnitude, was operative chiefly during the first 25 yr, and was due almost entirely to the two cancers.

An excess incidence and mortality from breast cancer, seen only among the women whose body burden was unmeasured and those with intake dose of 50 μCi or more (the latter comprising 9 observed and 2.7 expected cases) has been reported (Adams, 1980). A suggestively increased mortality for this cancer site has also been found in British workers who were exposed between 1939 and 1961, whose body content of radium was small, but who also had exposure to external gamma rays (Baverstock et al, 1981).

WORKERS EXPOSED IN REPAIR OF NUCLEAR-POWERED SHIPS

An investigation of workers at the Portsmouth, New Hampshire Naval Shipyard (Najarian, 1978) yielded suggestive evidence of a cancer and leukemia risk among the men who carry out repairs of nuclear-powered submarines and whose exposures are to pure gamma radiation. In this industry radiation exposures have been carefully monitored and found to be nearly always low. The procedure was to screen over 100,000 death certificates filed in the geographic area in order to locate the 1722 that mentioned employment at the shipyard. Of these, the ones mentioning cancer were identified, and the next-of-kin of 33% of the deceased workers were queried by telephone as to whether or not the workers were thought to have been exposed to radiation, and as to the cause of death. Proportionate mortality from cancer was estimated using U.S. 1973 rates to derive the expected values. The observed proportionate mortality for all cancer, and especially leukemia, was somewhat higher than expected; for non-nuclear workers this was not the case.

This study was followed by a Federal investigation (Rinsky, 1981) of the same shipyard, done by the historical prospective method, and employing official records of radiation dosage. Comparisons were with expected mortaltiy based on U.S. rates, for three groups; 7615 men who received cumulative exposures of 1 mrem or more; 15,585 never assigned to work in the radiation area; and 1345 qualified for radiation work but receiving no exposure. Fewer than 5% of the men were lost to follow-up. No excess mortality from all causes or from cancer, including leukemia, was found in any of the subgroups. Analysis according to dose received also showed, in general, no relationship. The difference between these findings and the former ones was attributed to the more complete ascertainment of the study population and more accurate classification of workers as to their exposure in this study. It may be added that proportionate mortality is a less reliable measure of mortality rate from a disease than the cause-specific mortality rate itself (MacMahon, 1970). Further study of all workers in this industry is in progress.

PROSPECTS FOR FUTURE ADVANCES IN KNOWLEDGE

For a number of years, a major concern of workers in health physics has been to quantify the effects of low-dose radiation. For a variety of reasons, especially the great number of subjects required in order to detect the expected small effects, there has been pessimism as to whether it was possible to do this without an inordinate expenditure of resources. Considering the widespread fear of radiation, others have pointed out that political and social purposes should perhaps have priority in this area.

Whatever the merit and feasibility of the goal, clearly one of the best opportunities for its achievement lies in study of industries with known and measured exposures. The U.S. Government recently contracted with a private agency to study the feasibility of epidemiologic investigations of the health effects of low-level radiation. A large number of population groups that might be suitable were identified and rated according to their promise (Dreyer, 1980, 1981). Those receiving the highest "feasibility scores" included: the Japanese A-bomb survivors; seven different patient groups who received radiation therapy; three receiving diagnostic procedures; and six occupational groups. These last included radiologists, radium-dial painters, radionuclide workers, power reactor workers, workers in DOE facilities, and uranium miners. Occupational groups were considered the most promising, but even these were not regarded as outstanding in the sense of giving a good prospect of a useful answer. The three final tentatively proposed occupational groups for prospective study in the U.S. were nuclear plant workers, workers in DOE facilities, and radiologic and nuclear medical technologists. This chapter has cited studies already done in several of these fields.

In addition to the studies already mentioned, a number of other epidemiologic studies of radiation workers are ongoing. Summaries of several were presented at a recent Department of Energy workship (Goldsmith, 1982) and a recent Health Physics Society conference (1983). These include studies at Oak Ridge of about 140,000 radiation workers at six DOE facilities and of 3200 workers who received 5+ rems of exposure in any single year; a nationwide study based at Los Alamos of plutonium workers; a study by the Centers for Disease Control of participants in nuclear tests; and a study at Johns Hopkins University of radiation workers in the U.S. Naval shipyards. Large occupational radiation surveillance programs are also being conducted in other countries, including ones in Canada (Newcombe, 1980) and Britain (Reissland, 1982).

SUMMARY

Some idea of the relative importance of all exposure to radiation, and of occupational exposures, in the fatal cancer burden can be gained from a publication by Jablon and Bailar (1980). They estimated the annual person-rems of exposure from all sources of ionizing radiation to the U.S. population, and from this the number of fatal cancers. (A person-rem is defined in BEIR III as a unit of population exposure obtained by summing individual dose-equivalent values for all people in a population. Thus, the number of person-rems contributed by 100,000 people exposed to one millirem is equal to that contributed by one person exposed to 100 rems.) They assumed that one cancer death would result from each 4000 person-rems of exposure. From all sources of radiation, out of 365,000 annual cancer deaths in 1975, slightly less than 10,000 (2.7%), might be attributed to radiation. For these estimates they used some data provided by the Interagency Task Force on the Health Effects of Ionizing Radiation (1979). They assumed a linear model for extrapolation purposes; a sublinear model would, of course, give a lower estimate. Their figures (Table 2) suggest that 50–60 deaths per year out of the total 10,000 radiation-associated cancer deaths might be attributable to industrial exposures to radiation, inclusive of the healing arts. The various elements in these calculations are necessarily subject to considerable uncertainty.

TABLE 2 Estimates of U.S. Occupational Exposures, and Lifetime Burden of Fatal Cancer

Source	Annual person-rems (thousands)[a]	Number of persons exposed annually[a]	Lifetime cancer mortality commitment[b]
Healing arts	40–80	500,000	10–20
Manufacturing and industrial	50	7,000,000	12.5
Nuclear energy (fuel cycle)	52	62,000	13
Research	12	100,000	3
Naval reactors	8	36,000	2
Nuclear weapons development and production	0.8	?	0.2
Other occupations	50	?	12.5
Total			52–62

Source: Adapted from Jablon and Bailar, 1980.

[a] From Interagency Task Force on the Health Effects of Ionzing Radiations "Final Report," Washington, DC 1979 (the Libassi report).
[b] Estimated, using a risk factor of 250 deaths/10^6 person-rems.

TABLE 3 Types of Malignant Disease Found in Excess in Occupational Groups

	Occupational group			
Type of cancer	Radium-dial painters	Uranium miners	Radiologists	Nuclear workers
Leukemia			++	?
Lung		++		?
Bone	++			
Lymphoma			+	?
Sinuses-head	+			
Skin		+	+	
Pancreas				?
Colon	?			
Multiple myeloma	+		+	+

Source: Adapted from Upton, 1982.

++, Substantial hazard, confirmed; +, small hazard; ?, small hazard, reported but unconfirmed.

Table 3 is a rough summary of the evidence with regard to radiation carcinogenesis in broad occupational groups (adapted from a report by Upton, 1982). Four such groups are listed, of whom three have clearly suffered an excessive incidence of cancer at one or another site. It is of interest that two of the groups—radium-dial painters and uranium miners—have been exposed to alpha radiation in doses long known to be excessive. These two groups have primarily experienced cancer of a single organ, bones and lungs respectively. The third group, radiologists, had external exposures, of unknown but presumably large amount. They experienced excesses of leukemia, lymphoma, skin cancer, and recently, myelomatosis, but the present exposures are presumably much lower.

The nuclear workers comprise mainly two groups: employees in the nuclear power industry, and those in shipyards engaged in the repair of atomic-powered vessels. Both groups afford the opportunity to examine risks in relation to careful and consistent dosimetry over many past years.

The questions of carcinogenicity of prolonged low-level radiation and the shape of the lower end of the dose–response curve may never be firmly settled, owing to the size, complexity and cost of the epidemiologic studies entailed, and the presence of confounding factors such as smoking and asbestos. We can, however, if the presently ongoing studies prove essentially negative, be reassured that the risks are too small to be of consequence compared to those of other larger and unavoidable exposures.

REFERENCES

Acquavella JF, Tietjen GL, Wilkinson GS et al (1982) Malignant melanoma incidence at the Los Alamos National Laboratory. Lancet i:883–884.

Adams EE, Brues AM (1980) Breast cancer in female radium dial workers first employed before 1930. J Occup Med 22:583–587.

Austin DF, Reynolds PJ, Snyder MA et al (1981) Malignant melanoma among employees of the Lawrence Livermore National Laboratory. Lancet ii:712–716.

Baverstock KF, Papworth D, Vennart D (1981) Risks of radiation at low dose rates. Lancet i:430–433.

Boyd JT, Doll R, Faulds JS et al (1970) Cancer of the lungs in iron ore (haematite) miners. Br J Indust Med 27:97–105.

Cohen BL (1982) Radon daughter exposure to uranium miners. Health Phys 42:449–457.

Court Brown WM, Doll R (1958) Expectation of life and mortality from cancer among British radiologists. Br Med J ii:181–187.

Cusick J (1981) Radiation-induced myelomatosis. N Engl J Med 304:204–210.

Darby SC, Reissland J (1981) Low levels of ionising radiation and cancer—Are we under-estimating the risk? J Roy Statist Soc A 144:298–331.

de Villiers AJ, Windish JP (1964) Lung cancer in a fluorspar mining community. Br J Indust Med 21:94–109.

Dreyer NA, Kohn HI, Clapp RW et al (1980) The feasibility of epidemiologic investigations of the health effects of low-level ionizing radiation: Final report. Prepared for U.S. Nuclear Regulatory Commission. NUREG/CR-1728.

Dreyer NA, Loughlin JE, Friedlander ER et al (1981) Choosing populations to study the health effects of low-dose ionizing radiation. Am J Publ Health 71:1247–1252.

Fox AJ, Goldblatt P, Kinlen LJ (1981) A study of the mortality of Cornish tin miners. Br J Indust Med 38:378–380.

Gilbert ES (1982) Some confounding factors in the study of mortality and occupational exposures. Am J Epidemiol 116:177–188.

Gilbert ES, Marks S (1979) An analysis of the mortality of workers in a nuclear facility. Radiat Res 79:122–148.

Gofman JW (1979) The question of radiation causation of cancer in Hanford workers. Health Phys 37:617–639.

Goldsmith R (1982) DOE radiation epidemiology contractors workshop, April 13–14, Program and working papers. Washington, DC: Department of Energy.

Health Physics Society: Epidemiology applied to health physics. Sixteenth Midyear Topical Meeting of the Health Physics Society, January 10–13, 1983. Proceedings (in press)

Hutchison GB, MacMahon G, Jablon S et al (1979) Review of report by Mancuso, Stewart and Kneale of radiation exposure of Hanford workers. Health Phys 37:207–220.

Interagency Task Force on the Health Effects of Ionizing Radiation (1979) F Libassi, Chairman. Final Report. Washington, DC: Department of Health, Education and Welfare.

Jablon S, Bailar JC, III (1980) The contribution of ionizing radiation to cancer mortality in the U.S. Prev Med 9:219–226.

Jablon S, Miller RW (1978) Army technologists: 29-year follow up for cause of death. Radiology 126:677–679.

Jessup GL, Silverman C (1981) Personal usage of medical radiological procedures by radiologists, pathologists, and their families. Am J Epidemiol 114:53–62.

Kneale GW, Mancuso TF, Stewart AM (1981) Hanford radiation study III: A cohort study of the cancer risks from radiation to workers at Hanford (1944-77 deaths) by the method of regression models in life tables. Br J Indust Med 38:156–166.

Kunz E, Sěvc J, Plaček V (1978) Lung cancer mortality in uranium miners (methodological aspects). Health Phys 35:579–580.

Lundin FE, Wagoner JK, Archer VE (1971) Radon daughter exposure and respiratory cancer: Quantitative aspects. Joint monograph no. 1, National Institute for Occupational Safety and Health, National Institute of Environmental Health Sciences. Washington, DC: U.S. Department of Health, Education and Welfare.

MacMahon B, Pugh TF (1970) Epidemiology: Principles and methods. Boston: Little, Brown and Co, pp 59–60.

Mancuso TF, Stewart AM, Kneale GW (1977) Radiation exposures of Hanford workers dying from cancer and other causes. Health Phys 33:369–385.

Matanoski GM, Seltser R, Sartwell PE et al (1975) The current mortality rates of radiologists and other physician specialists: Deaths from all causes and from cancer. Am J Epidemiol 101:188–198.

Matanoski GM, Seltser R Sartwell PE et al (1975) The current mortality rates of radiologists and other physician specialists: Specific causes of death. Am J Epidemiol 101:199–210.

Matanoski GM (1981) Risk of cancer associated with occupational exposure in radiologists and other radiation workers. 1980 International Symposium on Cancer. New York: Grune and Stratton.

Najarian T, Colton T (1978) Mortality from leukemia and cancer in shipyard nuclear workers. Lancet i:1018–1020.

Newcombe HB (1980) Design and future uses of national dose registers for regulatory control and epidemiology. Health Phys 39:783–796.

National Research Council, Committee on the Biological Effects of Ionizing Radiation, BEIR III (1980) The effects on populations of exposure to low levels of ionizing radiation. Washington, DC: National Academy Press.

Polednak AP (1977) Bone cancer among female radium dial workers. Latency periods and incidence rates by time after exposure. J Natl Cancer Inst 60:77–82.

Polednak AP (1977) Bone cancer among female radium dial workers. Latency periods and incidence rates by time after exposure. J Natl Cancer Inst 60:77–82.

Polednak AP, Stehney AF, Rowland RE (1978) Mortality among women first employed before 1930 in the U.S. radium dial-painting industry: a group ascertained from employment lists. Am J Epidemiol 107:179–195.

Reissland JA (1982) Epidemiological methods of assessing risks from low level occupational exposure to ionising radiation. Radiat Protect Dosimet 2:199–207.

Rinsky RA, Zumwalde RD, Waxweiler RJ et al (1981) Cancer mortality at a Naval nuclear shipyard. Lancet i:231–235.

Sanders BS (1978) Low level radiation and cancer deaths. Health Phys 34:521–588.

Schlesselman JJ (1982) Case-control studies: Design, conduct, analysis. New York: Oxford University Press.

Seltser R, Sartwell PE (1965) The effect of occupational exposure to radiation on the mortality of physicians. Am J Epidemiol 81:2–22.

Sěvc J, Junz E, Plaček V (1976) Lung cancer in uranium miners and long-term exposure to radon daughter products. Health Phys 30:433–437.

Sliverman C, Seltser R (1971) Radiation registry of physicians. Radiology 99:559–568.

Smith PG, Doll R (1981) Mortality from cancer and all causes among British radiologists. Br J Radiol 54:187–194.

Stehney AF, Lucas HF, Rowland RE (1978) Survival times of women radium dial workers first exposed before 1930. Vienna: International Atomic Energy Agency.

Upton AC (1982) The biological effects of low-level ionizing radiation. Sci Am 246:41–49.

Warren S (1956) Longevity and causes of death from irradiation in physicians. J Am Med Assoc 162:464–468.

SECTION V
MODIFYING FACTORS AND RISK ASSESSMENT

INHERITED INFLUENCES ON SUSCEPTIBILITY TO RADIATION CARCINOGENESIS

ALFRED G. KNUDSON, Jr., M.D., Ph.D., AND
SURESH H. MOOLGAVKAR, M.D., Ph.D.

Carcinogenesis is the complex interplay of heredity and environment. It is now clear that there are single gene defects, both dominant and recessive, that predispose to radiation-induced cancer. In addition, there may be other more diffuse host factors that are at least partially genetically determined, which modify the response to irradiation. In order to incorporate these facts into a general framework for carcinogenesis, we discuss the interaction of heredity and irradiation within the context of a specific model for the pathogenesis of cancer. This is the only model that has been shown to be consistent with the main body of epidemiologic and experimental data on carcinogenesis (Moolgavkar and Knudson, 1981).

A MODEL FOR CARCINOGENESIS

Evidence from diverse sources suggests that both mutation and the dynamics of tissue growth and differentiation play important roles in carcinogenesis. A genetic regulatory schema proposed by Comings (1973) has been incorporated into a model that recognizes the importance of tissue kinetics and mutations in carcinogenesis and that is consistent with data from human epidemiology and animal experiments (Moolgavkar and Knudson, 1981). Specifically, Comings postulated that all cells contain genes capable of coding for transforming factors that can release the cell from normal growth constraints. These genes, which correspond to viral-like host oncogenes, would be expressed during histogenesis and tissue renewal, their expression controlled by diploid pairs of regulatory genes. Malignant transformation of a cell would occur when the oncogenes are turned on to inappropriately high levels. This could happen in

From the Fox Chase Cancer Center, Philadelphia, Pennsylvania.

one of two ways: 1) by direct activation of oncogenes, or 2) by inactivation of regulatory genes (antioncogenes).

Recent investigations on model tumor viruses suggest various ways in which the oncogenes could be activated directly. Chromosomal rearrangement might bring a host oncogene adjacent to a "promoter" site, or a viral "promoter" sequence might be inserted next to an oncogene. Both these circumstances would lead to an abrogation of normal cellular control of the oncogene. Indeed, the latter mechanism has been shown to be responsible for some virally induced avian tumors (Hayward et al, 1982), and the possibility that some human tumors arise by direct activation of oncogenes must be recognized. Candidates for such tumors are the lymphomas and leukemias in which specific chromosomal rearrangements are a characterizing feature.

We have argued in a previous publication (Moolgavkar and Knudson, 1981) that human tumors most commonly arise by mutations of the regulatory genes, because complex controls have probably evolved to prevent disastrous one-step mutations in or around oncogenes. Thus, the model we have developed to describe most human cancers requires the occurrence of two rare and irreversible events (mutation of each of the two homologous regulatory genes). There is evidence that, at least in some tissues, mutations at one of several gene loci may be involved in carcinogenesis. For example, in the colon as many as four distinct genes may predispose to malignancy. Then, in an extension of the Comings scheme, homozygous mutations at any one of these loci would lead to malignancy.

Figure 1 represents a model for carcinogenesis by mutation of antioncogenes and incorporates two features: 1) transition of target stem cells into cancer cells, via an intermediate stage, in two irreversible steps, and 2) growth and differentiation of normal target and intermediate cells. The first step is called the initiating step, and cells that have sustained the first event are called initiated or intermediate cells. The second step is called the completing step, and cells that have sustained both events are malignant or transformed cells. Within the framework of this model, mutagens act by affecting transition rates, whereas, promoters influence the kinetics of growth, especially of initiated cells. The model provides a good description of the age-specific incidence curves of childhood and adult cancers, and is consistent with much of the data on human and animal carcinogenesis (Moolgavkar and Knudson, 1981). Note that this model does not explicitly assume that the two events confer homozygosity at a gene locus.

Environmental agents and genetic predisposition to cancer could facilitate two-step carcinogenesis by increasing one or both transition rates above spontaneous background levels or by increasing the proliferation of normal or intermediate cells. Further, in some genetic conditions the first step could be inherited. There may be genetic conditions in humans that predispose to cancer in each of these ways. Perhaps the most important examples of genetic predisposition in humans are provided by those cancers that, on segregation analysis, are inherited in an autosomal dominant fashion. Examples are hereditary retinoblastoma and carcinoma of the colon in familial polyposis. However, even though every cell in the susceptible tissue carries the cancer gene, only a few of the cells go on to become malignant, indicating that inheritance of the gene is

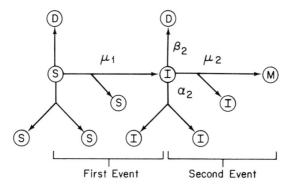

FIGURE 1. Two-stage model for carcinogenesis. S, normal stem cell; I, intermediate or initiated cell; D, differentiated or dead cell; M, malignant cell. μ_1, rate at which first event occurs; μ_2, rate at which second event occurs; α_2, rate of division of intermediate cells; β_2, rate of differentiation or death of intermediate cells.

In a small time interval, a given stem cell may divide with a certain probability to give rise to two daughter stem cells, or it may differentiate (or die) and, thus, leave the pool of susceptible cells, or it may divide (with a small probability) into two cells, one of which is normal and the other of which has suffered the first event to become an intermediate (initiated) cell. The intermediate cell may in turn give rise to two intermediate daughters, die or differentiate, or give rise to one intermediate cell and one malignant cell. The important parameters of the model are the two transition rates μ_1 and μ_2 and the difference $\alpha_2 - \beta_2$. Mutagens increase μ_1 and μ_2, whereas, the most important effect of promoters is to increase $\alpha_2 - \beta_2$.

not sufficient (at the cellular level) for malignant transformation and that at least one other event is necessary. The two-stage model accounts for the dominantly inherited forms of cancer by postulating that the first event—probably a mutation—occurred in an ancestral germ cell. This mutant gene would then act as a cancer gene in affected families. The second event is postulated to occur in a somatic cell. Both events would be rare at the cellular level in healthy persons. However, in individuals who carry the gene, there would be numerous cells in which a single event (the second) could give rise to malignant transformation. Thus, the probability that at least one cell would undergo malignant change is very high, and segregation analysis would be consistent with autosomal dominant inheritance with high penetrance. In tissues with relatively small numbers of target cells, the penetrance would be low.

Two recessive conditions, xeroderma pigmentosum (XP) and Bloom's syndrome, both seem to affect transition rates but possibly in different ways. In XP, defective DNA repair (Cleaver, 1968) leads to an increase in the mutation rates (i.e., to an increase in both the transition rates). The possible mechanism in Bloom's syndrome is more interesting. If malignancy were the result of genomic change at homologous sites, then such change could be brought about by mutations (including deletion and chromosomal loss) at both sites or by mutation at one site followed by mitotic recombination. In this regard it is interesting to note that in Bloom's syndrome there is greatly increased frequency of sister chromatid and homologous chromosome exchanges (Chaganti et al,

1974) in addition to elevated mutation rates (Warren et al, 1981). Thus, Bloom's syndrome may preferentially increase the *second* transition rate. Predisposition to cancer would be general. There is no good example of a genetic condition that predisposes to malignancy because of a profound disturbance in tissue kinetics. A possible candidate for such a condition is Fanconi's anemia (FA).

To summarize, and to relate the above discussion to the schema proposed by Comings, most cancers in humans may derive from mutations at a pair of regulatory genes, thus, abrogating cellular control of oncogenes. If a mutant nonfunctional regulatory gene is inhereited, the cancer would appear, on segregation analysis, to occur in a dominant fashion. Some recessive conditions such as XP may increase the mutation rate at the regulatory genes in tissues exposed to specific carcinogens. At least one recessive condition, Bloom's syndrome, may facilitate homozygosity for mutant regulatory genes by mitotic recombination.

Ionizing and ultraviolet (UV) radiation are strongly mutagenic and, thus, would increase the transition rates. The consequences of this mode of action within the context of the model proposed here are discussed in a recent publication (Moolgavkar and Knudson, 1981). The interaction of radiation with genetic conditions predisposing to malignancy could occur in one of two ways. In a recessive condition such as XP, UV-B radiation would simply increase both transition rates. However, in dominantly inherited conditions in which the risk of radiation-induced cancer is increased, the mechanism of action would be somewhat different. According to the model, the first mutation has already occurred in such individuals, and radiation effects the second event in some of the cells in the target tissue, leading to malignant transformation of these cells. Examples of such conditions are the B-K mole, or dysplastic nevus syndrome, and the nevoid basal cell carcinoma syndrome. Both these genetic conditions segregate in an autosomal dominant fashion. In the former, affected individuals are at greatly elevated risk for malignant melanoma. We have suggested that the dysplastic nevi in these individuals represent identifiable clusters of cells in the intermediate stage (Moolgavkar and Knudson, 1981). Exposure to UV-B radiation may cause a few of these cells to become malignant. In the nevoid basal cell carcinoma syndrome, affected individuals are at greatly increased risk of developing multiple basal cell carcinomas. Some of these individuals also develop medulloblastomas, which are treated with radiation. Individuals so treated develop large numbers of basal cell carcinomas in the field of irradiation, with a very short latent period (Strong, 1977). Again, according to the model, radiation has effected the second event in cells that had inherited the first.

GENETIC CONDITIONS PREDISPOSING TO RADIATION CARCINOGENESIS

The idea that some persons are inherently more susceptible to radiation carcinogenesis is best illustrated by the vast differences in susceptibility to sunlight-induced skin cancer shown by members of different racial groups. Whites as a group are more susceptible, and within them, those who are of fair complexion are still more so. The susceptibility is obviously genetic, but not attributable to a single Mendelian gene. On the other hand, albinos of all races are homozygous for a single recessive mutation and very susceptible to skin cancer. In albinos the radiation is simply not absorbed by pigment cells. The relationship of pigmentation of the skin to susceptibility to skin cancer in normal persons is based on a complex genetic polymorphism and in albinos on a Mendelian gene. We should assume that there is a similar basis for differential susceptibility to radiation carcinogenesis generally. However, the differences in sunlight sensitivity among races correlate with their geographic circumstances, whereas, susceptibility to ionizing radiation probably does not. Just as with sunlight sensitivity, however, there should be individuals with single Mendelian gene abnormalities that render them more or less discontinuous from the range of variation among normals. For both UV and ionizing radiation it is the mendelian disorder from which we can learn most, because it is much easier to identify and characterize. Here we discuss some Mendelian conditions that predispose to radiation carcinogenesis.

Xeroderma Pigmentosum

There are a few recessively inherited disorders that impart an increased risk of one or more cancers and also show an altered response to radiation. The paradigm of these conditions is xeroderma pigmentosum, in which skin cancer is inevitable and UV light damage to DNA is not repaired normally.

The skin cancers are not specific, as basal and squamous cell carcinomas and melanomas are all increased in frequency. Carcinomas appear frequently in the first two decades of life (Kraemer et al, 1982). Melanoma is much less common. The relationship of these cancers to sun exposure is well illustrated by twins who were protected from sunlight from earliest childhood. For two decades neither had any cancers, although one, through relaxation of vigilance, developed a carcinoma and a melanoma at 21 yr (Lynch et al, 1981).

It is generally thought that these are the only cancers to which such persons are at increased risk. A recent report, however, suggests that this may not be the case (Kraemer, 1980). The most common other cancers involve the oral cavity, but internal cancers, including leukemia and brain tumors, have been reported at early ages. Because these are unlikely to be induced by radiation, it may be that XP also predisposes to chemical or spontaneous carcinogenesis at sites other than the skin.

The most dramatic laboratory finding related to XP has been the discovery that cultivated fibroblasts are deficient in the repair of UV-induced damage to DNA (Cleaver, 1968). UV light induces thymine dimers in DNA and there ensues a repair process, defective in most cases of XP, that begins with excision of the dimers. Seven different complementation groups for excision defectiveness have been recorded since then (Keijzer et al, 1979), but the fundamental defect has not been characterized for any. There are additional cases, called XP variants, in which cell survival and excisional repair are normal, but postreplication repair is not. Cleaver (1982) has proposed that the different XP mutations produce defects at different sites in a repair enzyme complex of molecular weight around 10^6 daltons. Progress in defining the defects in XP may come from gene cloning. XP and its pathogenic mechanisms are discussed by Cleaver elsewhere in this volume (pp 43–55).

The means by which DNA damage leads to cancer in XP is not known, but sensitivity to UV light cannot account for the internal cancers or for the severe neurologic symptoms, dementia, small brain size, and general diminution in numbers of neurones found in some XP patients (Robbins et al, 1974). Because certain carcinogenic chemicals, such as N-acetoxyacetylaminofluorene, produce DNA damage that is not repaired in XP cells (Regan and Setlow, 1974), these internal effects may be produced by commonly encountered metabolites. If somatic mutations account for the occurrence of cancer, then one would expect that XP cells would show higher than normal rates of induced locus-specific mutation and of transformation in vitro. Indeed, both of these phenomena have been observed (Maher et al, 1976; Maher et al, 1982).

Ataxia Telangiectasia

Ataxia telangiectasia (AT) is another recessively inherited disorder that enhances the prospect of cancer and also imparts a sensitivity to radiation. The cancers are particularly in the lymphoid system, although other kinds have been reported at a frequency that is difficult to evaluate. Both the patients and their cells manifest a marked sensitivity to ionizing radiation. The patients do not have excessive skin cancer, so they are apparently not unduly sensitive to UV light. There is thought to be some defect in the normal mechanism for dealing with radiation damage, because AT cells do not show the normal delay in the reinitiation of DNA synthesis that follows x-irradiation (Painter and Young, 1980). AT cells also show increased chromosomal breakage, both single- and double-strand breaks, occurring spontaneously and following x-irradiation. There is considerable heterogeneity in AT, at least some of which is attributable to different mutations. To Murnane and Painter (1982) the five complementation groups suggest a complex system for initiating DNA synthesis after damage. As with XP there may be many sites in which the system can be defective.

Much needs to be learned about the AT mutation in relation to radiation carcinogenesis. The lymphoid neoplasms that have been recorded did not follow ionizing radiation. The immune deficiencies and the severe loss of Purkinje cells from the cerebellum that characterize the disease also suggest that cellular damage can occur through other means. Some chemicals, including N-methyl-N'-nitro-N-nitrosoguanidine, mimic the effects of ionizing radiation on AT cells (Regan and Setlow, 1974), so it may be that both the cancers and the other effects are produced by metabolites of exogenous, or even endogenous, origin. Radiation, chemicals, and apparently even "spontaneous" changes to which AT cells are susceptible all cause unrepaired chromosomal damage that can lead to cancer. This process is possibly mediated by chromosomal translocation, particularly involving the long arm of chromosome #14. Translocations at this site have been repeatedly observed in the lymphocytes of AT patients and may be responsible for the lymphoid neoplasms to which AT pateints are predisposed (McCaw et al, 1975; Oxford et al, 1975). They may also be responsible for the immune deficiencies so often seen. The somatic genetic changes that underlie carcinogenesis in AT apparently belong to some subclass of all genetic changes that cause mutations as measured in locus-specific in vitro tests, because the specific locus mutation rate is not elevated in AT cells, in contrast with XP cells (Arlett and Lehmann, 1978). It is possible that the translocation leads directly to activation of an oncogene and that cancer in these patients is a one-step process. It may be possible to improve our understanding of pathogenic mechanisms in AT now that a mouse model of the disease has been discovered (Shultz et al, 1982).

The significance of AT for human cancer may be considerable, because persons *heterozygous* for the AT mutation are also at an increased risk of cancer. Swife et al (1976) have estimated that this increase is approximately fivefold for persons under age 45 yr. Such persons may be rather frequent in the population. For example, if the incidence of AT were 1 of 40,000 persons, then 1% of the population would be heterozygous, and approximately 5% of cancer in persons under age 45 would be occurring in AT heterozygotes.

Bloom's Syndrome

In BS there is a predisposition to a variety of cancers. The patients are small at birth and growth is impaired after birth. There is a sensitivity to sunlight, but apparently not to skin cancer. Cells from patients with BS are sensitive to killing by ethyl methanesulphonate (Arlett and Lehmann, 1978), and it may be that some endogenous chemicals are responsible for the elevated mutation rate observed in vitro (Warren et al, 1981) and for the increased cancer incidence. Associated with the chromosomal quadriradials are the phenomena of sister chromatid exchange and homologous chromosome exchange in somatic cells (Chaganti et al, 1974). This has the important implication that cells heterozygous for a somatic cancer mutation could become homozygous by mitotic recombination (Passarge and Bartram, 1976; Festa et al, 1979). If, as suggested in the discussion of the two-step model for carcinogenesis, the second step entails the development of homozygosity, then the BS gene would be a consitutive "second-step" disorder.

Retinoblastoma

The retinoblastoma gene is an example of a tumor-specific gene that can impart susceptibility to radiation carcinogenesis. Patients with the hereditary form of retinoblastoma develop retinoblastoma with a 95% or greater probability. They also have an approximately 10% incidence of osteosarcomas. The hereditary cases of retinoblastoma are usually bilateral, and it is in these cases that radiation is sometimes employed to preserve one eye. When radiation therapy was primarily of the orthovoltage type, significant absorption by surrounding bone occurred, and the incidence of osteosarcoma of orbital bone rose to as high as 30% of cases (Sagerman et al, 1969), whereas that site was virtually never affected in persons not receiving radiation. This gene seems to be an example of susceptibility to radiation carcinogenesis at a specific site, viz, bone. Radiation has the effect of increasing gene penetrance for osteosarcoma.

There is evidence that the inherited mutation in retinoblastoma is an intiating step that is identical to the one that results from somatic mutation in the nonhereditary form of the disease. Transition rates are presumably normal and locus-specific mutation rates also should be. Radiogenic osteosarcoma seems to result more readily than otherwise because the first step on the path to ostero-sarcoma is present in all cells at birth. We know from the incidence of re-tinoblastoma that the germinal mutation is not *sufficient* to produce that tumor and that some further event must occur. That further event is the second step in the model, and is the one we believe to be effected by radiation.

The evidence supporting the idea that the inherited mutation acts as an initiating event stems from the study of a small set of genetic cases in which there is heterozygosity for a constitutional deletion within band 14 of the long arm of chromosome #13 (13q14) (Yunis and Ramsay, 1978). Such individuals are hemizygous for the enzyme esterase D, showing that the genes for re-tinoblastoma and esterase D are near each other. Advantage of this fact has been taken to study linkage in those cases that do not show a deletion. This is made possible because of the existence of heterozygotes for an electrophoretic variant of esterase D. In those families where this variant is segregating with the retinoblastoma gene, linkage can be tested. Indeed, there is very close linkage in those cases that are genetic but do not show constitutional deletion (Sparkes et al, 1983). Deletion at this same site is also found in some cases of tumor occurring in individuals who do not show a constitutional deletion (Balaban et al, 1982; Gardner et al, 1982). It is suggested, therefore, that genetic change at a particular site initiates tumorigenesis in all cases of retinoblastoma, whether hereditary or not; in the former the change is germinal, in the latter, somatic. It would seem that mutation or deletion at this site is a *necessary* condition for formation of retinoblastoma. The gene also predisposes to osteosarcoma, an event whose probability is increased by ionizing radiation. We assume that in hereditary retinoblastoma an initiating mutation is inherited by all cells and that a tumor, either retinoblastoma or osteosarcoma, develops following some second event. For retinoblastoma this gene it the major, perhaps the only, one that so predisposes. For osteosarcoma it may prove to be just one of several, because many hereditary cases of osteosarcoma are not associated with re-tinoblastoma. In at least one case the second event for the retinoblastoma was a loss of the other chromosome #13, so the tumor cell contained no copy of the critical segment of band 13q14 (Benedict et al, 1983).

Nevoid Basal Cell Carcinoma Syndrome

Another dominantly heritable condition that predisposes to radiation-induced cancer is the nevoid basal cell carcinoma syndrome. In this condition basal cell carcinomas appear in the skin, usually during the second decade of life. There is apparently sensitivity to UV-induced cancer, because the carcinomas most often appear in sun-exposed areas. This sensitivity also seems to extend to ionizing radiation. Some subjects with this syndrome develop a brain tumor, medulloblastoma, which is often treated by craniospinal irradiation. There are now several cases in which basal cell carcinomas appear in large numbers, as early as 6 mo after exposure, at the edges of the field of irradiation (Strong, 1977). It may be that cells in the central part of the irradiation field are killed rather than mutated to survive to produce cancer. The study of cells from these individuals has not revealed mutagen sensitivity or a defect in DNA repair. The best interpretation is that, whereas, radiation induces an initiating event in normal persons, it produces a second event in these subjects. As for osteogenic sarcoma in retinoblastoma, the patients with the nevoid basal cell carcinoma syndrome may have inherited an event that is initiating, and irradiation produces the genetic change(s) necessary to accomplish a second event that completes the process of carcinogenesis, hence, greatly compressing the usual latent period of radiation carcinogenesis.

Neurofibromatosis

In neurofibromatosis (NF) a benign lesion, the neurofibroma, can give rise to neurofibrosarcoma. There is also an increased probability of other sarcomas in NF, and these latter, as well as neurofibrosarcoma, have been found in previously irradiated areas (Meadows et al, 1977). NF is also a noteworthy disease because the intermediate premalignant lesions and the corresponding malignant tumor have both been studied for the clonality of their origin. Fialkow et al (1971; Friedman et al, 1983) have demonstrated in female patients with NF, and who are also heterozygous for electrophoretic variants of an X-linked enzyme, glucose-6-phosphate dehydrogenase, that neurofibromas are multicellular in origin, whereas neurofibrosarcoma is clonal. The neurofibromas are apparently formed from multiple cells that were initiated by a germinal mutation and the malignant tumor follows a second, somatic mutation. When radiation induces a tumor in NF subjects, it probably causes a second event.

CONCLUDING REMARKS

Our discussion, in this chapter, of hereditary factors in susceptibility to radiation-induced carcinogenesis has been limited to mendelian conditions, and has been conducted within the framework of a model for which there is some circumstantial evidence. The details of the model are largely speculative. From the viewpoint of the model, mendelizing conditions that predispose to carcinogenesis may be classified into two principal groups: 1) those, such as XP, in which event (mutation) rates are increased in the presence of specific carcinogens; 2) those in which a nonfunctional "antioncogene" is inherited from a parent, such as the BK mole syndrome. In addition there is at least one condition, Bloom's syndrome, in which the second event rate may be increased due to mitotic recombination.

Despite the abundant evidence that susceptibility to specific cancers can be inherited as single-gene defects, very little is known about the location or function of these genes. The retinoblastoma gene is an exception in that it has been localized to a particular band on the long arm of chromosome #13 (13q14). More recently, this gene has been shown to be closely linked with the gene for esterase D. Moreover, as discussed above, there is some evidence that genetic change at the same chromosomal location is involved in the nonhereditary cases of retinoblastoma as well, thus, supporting the argument that the mutation is initiating in the sense of the model.

One of the implicit theses in our discussion in this chapter and elsewhere is that fundamental pathogenetic mechanisms are identical in hereditary and nonhereditary forms of the same cancer. Thus, although hereditary cancer forms only a small part of the total cancer burden, it provides a prototype for the study of cancer in general. Whether or not this viewpoint is correct will be known only after the genes that predispose to cancer have been thoroughly investigated. A promising beginning has been made with XP and retinoblastoma, and here there is hope of progress.

This work was supported in part by Public Health Service Grants CA06927 (a CORE grant), CA30671 and CA22780 awarded by the National Cancer Institute, DHHS, and by an appropriation from the Commonwealth of Pennsylvania.

REFERENCES

Arlett CF, Lehmann AR (1978) Human disorders showing increased sensitivity to the induction of genetic damage. Ann Rev Genet 12:95–115.

Balaban G, Gilbert F, Nichols W, Meadows, AT, Shields J (1982) Abnormalities of chromosome #13 in retinoblastomas from individuals with normal constitutional karyotypes. Cancer Genet Cytogenet 6:213–221.

Benedict WF, Murphree AL, Banerjee A, Spina CA, Sparkes MC, Sparkes RS (1983) Patient with 13 chromsome deletion: Evidence that the retinoblastoma gene is a recessive cancer gene. Science 219:973–975.

Chaganti RS, Schonberg S, German J (1974) A manyfold increase in sister chromatid exchanges in Bloom's syndromes lymphocytes. Proc Natl Acad Sci USA 71:4508–4512.

Cleaver JE (1968) Defective repair replication of DNA in xeroderma pigmentosum. Nature 218:652–656.

Cleaver JE (1982) Inactivation of ultraviolet repair in normal and xeroderma pigmentosum cells by methyl methanesulfonate. Cancer Res 42:860–863.

Comings DE (1973) A general theory of carcinogenesis. Proc Natl Acad Sci USA 70:3324–3328.

Festa RS, Meadows AT, Boshes RA (1979) Leukemia in a black child with Bloom's syndrome: Somatic recombination as a possible mechanism for neoplasia. Cancer 44:1507–1510.

Fialkow PJ, Sagebiel RW, Gartler SM, Rimoin DL (1971) Multiple cell origin of hereditary neurofibromas. N Engl J Med 284:298–300.

Friedman JM, Fialkow PJ, Greene CL, Weinberg MN (1983) Probable clonal origin of neurofibrosarcoma in a patient with hereditary neurofibromatosis. J Natl Cancer Inst 69:1289–1292.

Gardner HA, Gallie BL, Knight LA, Phillips RA (1982) Multiple karyotypic changes in retinoblastoma tumor cells: Presence of normal chromosome no. 13 in most tumors. Cancer Genet Cytogenet 6:201–211.

Hayward WS, Neel BG, Astrin SM (1982) Avian leukosis viruses: Activation of cellular "oncogenes." In: Klein G (ed.), Advances in viral oncology. New York: Raven Press, pp 207–233.

Keijzer E, Jaspers NGJ, Abrahams PJ, Taylor AMR, Arlett CF, Zelle B, Takebe H, Kinmont PDS, Bootsma D (1979) A seventh complementation group in excision-deficient xeroderma pigmentosum. Mutat Res 62:183–190.

Kraemer KH (1980) Oculo-cutaneous and internal neoplasms in xeroderma pigmentosum: implications for theories of carcinogenesis. In: Pullman B, Ts'o POP, Gelboin H (eds.), Carcinogenesis: Fundamental mechanisms and environmental effects. Holland: D. Reidel Publishing, pp 503–507.

Kraemer KH, Lee MM, Scotto J (1982) Early onset of skin and oral cavity neoplasms in xeroderma pigmentosum. Lancet i:56–57.

Lynch HT, Fusaro R, Edlund J, Albano W, Lynch J (1981) Skin cancer developing in xeroderma pigmentosum patient relaxing sunlight avoidance. Lancet ii:1230.

McCaw BK, Hecht F, Harnden DG, Teplitz RL (1975) Somatic rearrangement of chromosome 14 in human lymphocytes. Proc Natl Acad Sci USA 72:2071–2075.

Maher VM, Ouellette LM, Curren RD, McCormick JJ (1976) Frequency of ultraviolet light-induced mutation is higher in xeroderma pigmentosum variant cells than in normal human cells. Nature 261:593–595.

Maher VM, Rowan LA, Silinskas KC, Kateley SA, McCormick JJ (1982) Frequency of UV-induced neoplastic transformation of diploid human fibroblasts is higher in xeroderma pigmentosum cells than in normal cells. Proc Natl Acad Sci USA 79:2613–2617.

Meadows AT, D'Angio GJ, Miké V, Banfi A, Harris C, Jenkin RDT, Schwartz A (1977) Patterns of second malignant neoplasms in children. Cancer 40:1903–1911.

Moolgavkar SH, Knudson AG (1981) Mutation and cancer: A model for human carcinogenesis. J Natl Cancer Inst 66:1037–1052.

Murnane JP, Painter RB (1982) Complementation of the defects in DNA synthesis in irradiated and unirradiated ataxia-telangiectasia cells. Proc Natl Acad Sci USA 79:1960–1963.

Oxford JM, Harnden DG, Parrington JM, Delhanty JD (1975) Specific chromosome aberrations in ataxia telangiectasia. J Med Genet 3:251–262.

Painter RB, Young BR (1980) Radiosensitivity in ataxia-telangiectasia: A new explanation. Proc Natl Acad Sci USA 77:7315–7317.

Passarge E, Bartram CR (1976) Somatic recombination as possible prelude to malignant transformation. In: Bergsma D (ed.), Cancer and genetics. New York: March of Dimes, Alan R. Liss, 12:177–180.

Regan JD, Setlow RB (1974) Two forms of repair in the DNA of human cells damaged by chemical carcinogens and mutagens. Cancer Res 34:3318–3325.

Robbins JH, Kraemer KH, Lutzner MA, Festoff BW, Coon HG (1974) Xeroderma pigmentosum. An inherited disease with sun sensitivity, multiple cutaneous neoplasms and abnormal DNA repair. Ann Int Med 80:221–248.

Sagerman RH, Cassady JR, Tretter P, Ellsworth RM (1969) Radiation induced neoplasia following external beam therapy for children with retinoblastoma. Am J Roentgenol Radium Ther Nucl Med 105:529–535.

Shultz LD, Sweet HO, Davisson MT, Coman DR (1982) 'Wasted,' a new mutant of the mouse with abnormalities characteristic of ataxia telangiectasia. Nature 297:402–404.

Sparkes RS, Murphree AL, Lingua RW, Sparkes MC, Field LL, Funderburk SJ, Benedict WF (1983) Gene for hereditary retinoblastoma assigned to human chromosome 13 by linkage to esterase D. Science 219:971–973.

Strong LC (1977) Theories of pathogenesis: Mutation and cancer. In: Mulvihill JJ, Miller RW, Fraumeni JF (eds.), Genetics of human cancer. New York: Raven Press, pp 401–415.

Swift M, Sholman L, Perry M, Chase C (1976) Malignant neoplasms in the families of patients with ataxia-telangiectasia. Cancer Res 36:209–215.

Warren ST, Schultz RA, Chang CC, Wade MH, Trosko JE (1981) Elevated spontaneous mutation rate in Bloom syndrome fibroblasts. Proc Natl Acad Sci USA 78:3133–3137.

Yunis JJ, Ramsay N (1978) Retinoblastoma and subband deletion of chromosome 13. Am J Dis Child 132:161–163.

INFLUENCE OF DOSE RATE AND LET IN RADIATION CARCINOGENESIS: THEORY AND OBSERVATIONS

V. P. BOND, M.D.

This chapter will explore, using modified hit theory-microdosimetric approaches, the shape and the influence of radiation quality and dose rate on the dose–response functions for quantal cell responses. Responses expected are explored first in "simple" autonomous cell systems, followed by increasingly complex systems. The approaches used appear to account well for most experimental findings in autonomous cell systems. Complications seen with increasingly complex systems appear to be confined largely to the higher dose and dose rate changes. The low-level radiation* (LLR) exposure range is emphasized because it is in this range that the response of cells to single energy-depositing events is linear and can be evaluated at present.

The term quantal cell response†, as used here (Finney, 1964), denotes responses not usually reversible spontaneously, such as some chromosome abnormalities, mutations, neoplastic cell transformation in vitro or in vivo, and cell death. Such responses are scored either by noting their presence in the individual cell, or by scoring abnormalities (e.g., tumors) presumably derived

---

* Low-level radiation (LLR) exposure refers to the initial linear portion of the absorbed dose-cell response curve for any quality radiation, or to the (linear) curve for higher doses of low-LET radiation delivered at very low average dose-rates. High-level radiation (HLR) refers to higher doses of any quality, and specifically to the quadratic portion of the low-LET dose–response curve, seen only with larger doses delivered at high dose rates. The "high" and "low," as will be seen, refer to the risk of exposure, and not to cell doses. For LLR and HLR, respectively, the fraction of exposed cells hit at all is low.

† The term is appropriate because all such cell responses are caused by stochastic (random), quantal physical processes. The ICRP (1977) uses the term "stochastic effects" to refer exclusively to the two quantal cell responses known to be serious or lethal in humans, mutagenic or oncogenic transformation. However, other stochastic effects (responses) are seen in cells, and stochastic quantal responses are also seen in organs as a result of macro stochastic physical events, or accidents.

From Brookhaven National Laboratory, Associated Universities, Inc., Upton, New York.

from a single quantally altered cell. Although the response is scored only as present or absent (all-or-none), it represents a specific threshold level of cell injury, which separates the "no response possible" range of severity from the "response possible" range. Not considered as quantal are all forms of "subeffective" cell injury—for example, single-strand breaks in DNA—because they are not directly observable in individual cells and are usually reparable.

LIMITATIONS OF ABSORBED DOSE: BIOPHYSICAL CONSIDERATIONS

To explain the shapes of the curves for cell responses and the influences of LET and dose rate, it is pointed out that for LLR exposure the quantity "absorbed dose" is neither 1) the fundamental quantity for measurement of the amount of radiation involved when a population of cells is exposed, nor 2) the appropriate quantity for measurement of the amount of energy that may be deposited stochastically in any given cell.*

With regard to absorbed dose, it is mathematically calculable but conceptually misleading. To expose a cell to any radiation means to place the cell(s) for an exposure time t_E in a radiation field of either primary or secondary charged particles, the strength of which is characterized by the fluence rate (flux). Injury to any relevant cell can result only if energy is deposited in a critical volume (CV)† within that cell, which happens only if a stochastic collison occurs between a charged particle and the CV. The probability of a stochastic collision depends solely on the number of charged particles per centimeter squared in the *environment* of and hence, seen by, the relevant cell. Therefore, it is the charged particle fluence that is the fundamental physical quantity for measurement of the amount of radiation involved in an exposure of the cell, and that must serve as the *primary independent* variable. Any quantity that measures the number of hit cells, or the average amount of energy deposition or dose absorbed in the relevant cells or the supporting medium, is then a dependent function of the fluence.

With respect to the absorbed dose, with LLR, it cannot provide accurate information on either the average energy absorbed in the hit cells, or the amount of energy deposited in a given cell.‡ Thus, microdosimetric concepts

---

* This fact is evident from microdosimetric considerations, and is widely stated or implied (Rossi and Kellerer, 1972; Kellerer, 1976; Rossi, 1979; Bond, 1981; Bond et al, 1965). To quote directly from Kellerer (1976), "absorbed dose is a meaningful concept only if it is sufficiently high in value," and "microdosimetry is the extension of classic dosimetry to those situations (i.e., small absorbed doses) for which the concept of absorbed dose is not applicable." The same ideas are expressed by Rossi (1979).

† The CV is a volume within the cell, the diameter or "cross section" σ of which can be calculated, and within which the macromolecular target(s) must reside. The tissue content of the CV must be "hit" by a charged particle in order for the chance of an all-or-none effect on the target(s) to be other than zero. Thus, a single hit is on the CV and not necessarily on the molecular target(s). The terms single and multiple track are avoided, because the implied assumptions as to target multiplicity are not required with the approach used here.

‡ The concept of dose, reserved in pharmacology and toxicology for use in connection with (multicellular) organ effects, becomes acceptable as the primary variable only as the absorbed dose increases into the HLR region. This is because all cells are then hit at least once, and most have several hits. Thus, the mean value of the multiple-hit energy depositing event sizes ("cell doses") approaches the absorbed dose to the organ, which is nonstochastic. The biological response of interest must then shift from single cell quantal responses to the result of cell population depletion in the organ [i.e., to organ quantal responses (Bond et al, 1965)].

and measurements must be employed. However, the need for fluence has not been similarly recognized. Thus, although "absorbed dose" will often of necessity be employed here because radiobiologic data are now usually presented in terms of this quantity only, the term will be placed in quotation marks to designate that with LLR it is used as an inappropriate surrogate for fluence (i.e., as the charged particle fluence multiplied by a constant k, equal to the mean energy per particle).

Expression of the amount of radiation in terms of charged particle fluence permits the formulation of three conditional probabilities that must be evaluated in order to predict, in a cell population exposed to a given "absorbed dose" of radiation of any quality, the *incidence* of cells showing the quantal response in the exposed cell population (incidence is in terms of exposed, or hit plus unhit, cells; fraction refers to hit cells only). These probabilities, for a given LLR "absorbed dose," are as follows:

p_1. The probability that a given relevant (i.e., mutable or transformable) exposed cell will be hit by (will undergo a stochastic collision with) a charged particle, with a consequent energy deposit in the CV of the cell.

p_2. The probability that the hit on the cell will be of a given size*, measured in terms of the amount of energy deposited in the CV.

p_3. The probability that a hit of that size and the consequent amount of injury to the relevant molecular target(s) will, in fact, result in the given quantal response.

The risk to a cell, of being hit and developing a quantal response, in the population exposed to the given "absorbed dose" of LLR is equal to the product of p_1 and p_2, and p_3. The expected excess incidence in the population is equal to the sum of the products of the three probabilities.

Neither the number nor the size of the charged particle-cell CV collisions from which p_1 and p_2 are evaluated can be measured in living cells. However, the techniques of microdosimetry (Rossi and Kellerer, 1972; Kellerer, 1976; Rossi 1979; Bond, 1981; Bond et al, 1965) do permit such measurements to be made. The basic instrument of microdosimetry is a proportional counter filled with tissue equivalent gas and operated at reduced pressure. It can be viewed conceptually as simply a scaled-up physical surrogate for a single cell or part of a cell (e.g., cell CV, cell nucleus), or as a cell CV phantom, in which the occurrence rate and magnitude of single-hit events that would be expected to take place in similarly exposed living cell(s) can be measured. This physical information on phantom cells exposed in a given radiation field can then be correlated with the observed incidence of quantal cell responses in a population of living cells exposed in the same field. However, the cellular radiobiologic data used for this purpose must also be confined at present to the linear (or LLR) range in order to ensure that the responses are in singly hit cells only.

---

* The size of hit on a cell CV can be expressed in terms of any of the microdosimetric quantities, energy deposit ϵ; lineal energy, y; or the specific energy, z (ICRU, 1980). The energy deposit ϵ is used here, because it is simply the energy transferred in a single hit and thus least committal with respect to which impact parameter may be the most relevant.

THE NEED FOR A HIT SIZE EFFECTIVENESS FUNCTION

Schematic and not-to-scale microdosimetric spectra, for both a relatively low and a relatively high LET radiation, are shown in Figure 1a, each for the same (small) fractional number of cells hit. The area under each of the curves in Figure 1a equals the number of actual hits on the scaled-up phantom cell. When this number is scaled down to the subcellular dimensions of the CV, by a factor as large as 10^6 or more, the resulting value provides the number of hit cells per centimeter squared expressed as the fraction of singly hit cells* in the exposed population, without regard to the amount of energy deposited or the hit size. The incidence of hit cells provides p_1 above.

The hit size spectra in Figure 1a also provide the distribution of the total incidence of hit cells, grouped on the basis of equal hit size. Thus the fraction of the total incidence for a given hit size, equal to p_2 above, is readily determined from the spectra in Figure 1a. Obviously needed, then, is a curve showing the fraction of hit cells responding quantally as a function of hit size, for hit cells also grouped according to hit size (i.e., a hit size-cell response, or hit size-effectiveness function). The needed curve, the derivation of which is given below, is shown as curve A (Figure 1b). The fraction showing the quantal response for any given hit size, obtained from this curve, provides p_3 above. The fraction of the total incidence of hit cells for a given hit size in Figure 1a, when multiplied by the fraction of responding hit cells given by curve A in Figure 1b for that hit size, yields the fraction of the total incidence of quantally responding cells shown in Figure 1c or Figure 1d for that hit size. The total incidence of quantally responding cells, for the given absorbed dose, is equal to the sum of the fractional incidence values so obtained for all hit sizes (i.e., to the area under the curves in Figure 1c. or d). The sum also equals the risk of a quantal response in an average cell.

The ratio of each of the areas in Figures 1c and d, to the corresponding area in Figure 1a (i.e., the fraction of hit cells showing the quantal response) must remain constant in the linear range because, although the incidences of hit and responding cells increase proportionally, the shapes of the spectra in Figure 1a, c, or d do not change with "absorbed dose."

Because of the central role of the previously undescribed hit size-cell-response function shown as curve A, Figure 1, the function is shown in more detail in Figure 2. The hatched area is the region of some form of cellular injury, such as DNA strand breaks. The average amount of injury per hit cell would be expected to increase monotonically with hit size, and the curve for this graded response should not saturate below quite large hit sizes. Above some level of cell injury (type unspecified), the fraction of cells showing a quantal response would be expected to increase monotonically. The curve for this quantal response should saturate at 1.0 (i.e., curve A). It is only curve A, termed the "hit size-cell response function," that is dealt with in this report.

Curve A represents the analogue for hit cells (i.e., the classic pharmaco-

---

* Because a single phantom cell CV is used to record the number of singly hit cells, the value obtained is equal to the number of hit cells per exposed cells. Thus, for example, if the scaled-down number of hit cells per cell CV is 10^{-2}, the incidence of hit cells in the exposed population of relevant cells is 1 in 100.

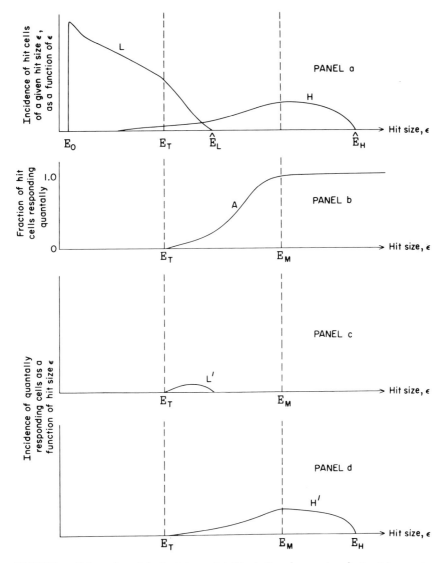

FIGURE 1. Schematic plots (not to scale) illustrating how microdosimetric spectra (panel *a*), which give the incidence of hit cells per hit size for a given "absorbed dose" (panel *a*), if folded with the hit-size-cell response function showing the fraction of hit cells with the quantal response as a function of hit size (panel *b*), yield the incidence of quantally responding cells per hit size (panels *c* and *d*) for that "absorbed dose." The area under spectra in panels *c* and *d* yields the total incidence of quantally responding cells, for the given "absorbed dose." L and H, low and high LET radiations, respectively; ε, energy deposit size; ε_O, ionization potential; ε_L and ε_H, upper limit energy deposit sizes for the radiations of different LET; ε_T, threshold energy deposit size; ε_M, value of ε at which curve A saturates.

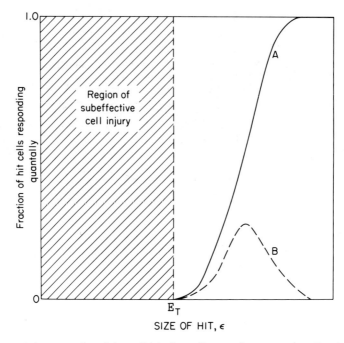

FIGURE 2. Schematic plot of the cell hit size-cell quantal response function (curve A). The shaded region refers to subeffective and usually-reparable types of cell injury, such as DNA stand breaks. Curve A is the integral of the distribution of individual cell sensitivities ascribed to normal biological variation, shown schematically as curve B.

logic–toxicologic organ dose–response curve for dosed animal organs), which gives the fraction of equally dosed animals (organs) responding quantally as a function of dose size, for dosed animals grouped according to dose size. Each curve is the integral of the distribution of organ (cell) sensitivities, due to biological variation, as a function of dose (hit) size. However, the energy is generally less uniformly distributed if delivered in a stochastic versus a non-stochastic mode. Consequently, the slope (variance) of the stochastic cell hit size-quantal response curve could be relatively shallow.

The area under the curves in panel Figure 1a, used to determine the number of hit cells/cm^2, also provides the charged particle fluence (i.e., the particles per CV cross section area is a measure of the fluence). There is no need to measure absorbed dose in order to obtain fluence.

DETERMINATION OF THE HIT SIZE-CELL RESPONSE FUNCTION

The necessarily broad range of single-hit CV hit sizes cannot be obtained with only one quality of radiation, because holding the radiation quality constant and varying the "absorbed dose" cannot alter the spectrum of cell hit sizes other than by changing the number of hits per cell. Thus, the desired cell function for single hits alone can be obtained only by holding the "absorbed dose" constant at a given value in the L R linear range and varying the hit size spectrum by varying the quality of the radiation. The slope ratio (relative biological effectiveness, RBE) values thus obtained provide the relative incidences for the same "absorbed dose," for the entire hit size distribution for the different radiation qualities. Also provided is multiple input information, where the spectra overlap, on the fraction of cells responding to each common value of hit size. With a different spectrum for each of the several different qualities, the corresponding incidence spectra for quantally responding cells, an assumed σ, and a computer program, the curve for the cell hit-cell response function can be approximated by means of successive iterations. The procedure is described elsewhere in detail (Varma and Bond, 1982).

Adjustments are made with each successive iteration using a physics "cross section", or "hit theory" formulation, modified from

$$N_H(\varepsilon) = N_E \Phi \sigma_H(\varepsilon),\tag{1}$$

to

$$N_H(\varepsilon)f(\varepsilon)/N_E = I(\varepsilon) = \Phi \sigma_H(\varepsilon)f(\varepsilon),\tag{2}$$

where N_H is the number per cm^2 of hit cells between hit size ϵ and $(\epsilon + \Delta\epsilon)$; I is the incidence of quantally-responding cells; σ_H is the average probability of a hit and interpretable as the average cross section of the CV; and $f(\epsilon)$ is the hit size weighting function, and N_E is the number/cm^2 of exposed cells. The total incidence is obtained by summing over all values of ϵ. With the incidence of quantally responding cells serving as the "detector" for the incidence of physical events of interest, the cross section for that interaction can thus be determined.

Although several functions have been proposed previously to describe an increasing cell response, using various parameters to represent the *average* energy deposited in groups of cells receiving widely disparate energy deposit event sizes (Rossi and Kellerer, 1972; Kellerer, 1976; Rosi, 1979; Barendsen, 1964), only recently (Bond, 1981; Bond and Varma, 1981; Varma and Bond, 1982) has the approach described here been suggested for determination of P_3—the hit size-cell response function. Preliminary evaluation (Bond and Varma, 1981; Varma and Bond, 1982) suggests that the fraction of quantally reponding cells does rise monotonically above a threshold hit size, as shown in Figure 1b, and reaches unity at some large value of hit size.

"ABSORBED DOSE"—CELL RESPONSE FUNCTIONS EXPECTED IN AUTONOMOUS CELLS

It was shown that the incidence of quantally responding cells and, thus, the risk to the individual cell, in principle can be determined without reference to "absorbed dose"-cell response functions. Thus, there is no need in principle for such functions in the LLR range. However, there is a continuing need to deal with the transitional zone between LLR, in which cell transformation in the single cell is the prime focus and where absorbed dose is inapplicable, and the HLR region, in which depletion of a cell population from cell death (in an organ) is of primary interest and absorbed dose does apply. Hence "absorbed dose"-cell response curves are now considered.

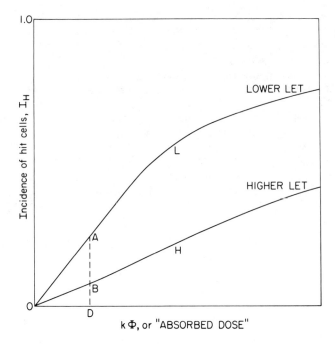

FIGURE 3. Schematic plot for the incidence of hit cells as a function of "absorbed dose," for radiations of low (L) and high (H) LET. The curves bend because of physical saturation due to the decrease in the fraction of unhit cells with increasing exposure.

Figure 3 shows the functions from which p_1 is derived, namely $k\Phi$ or "absorbed dose," versus the accumulated incidence of hit cells per unit $k\Phi$ (p_1 is the slope). The plot is trivial in the LLR range since the two clearly are derived from the same measurement and are proportional. However, it does show that the no-threshold function can result from purely physical processes involving a charged particle and a physical surrogate for a living cell. The curves for the different qualities of radiation have different slopes because the number of charged particles per rad changes with radiation quality (decreases with increasing LET). Were fluence alone used instead of "absorbed dose," curves L and H in Figure 3 would superimpose, and the slpe would be 45°.

Figure 4 shows (schematically, not to scale) "absorbed dose"-living cell response curves for a low- and a high-LET radiation (based on actual curves in Figures 5, 6, and 7). The initial portion of these curves, for any LET, is also linear and without threshold.

Thus, the initial "linear, no-threshold" relationships observed in Figure 4 when the (proportional) incidence of quantally responding living cells is substituted for incidence of hit phantom cells, has its origin in purely physical processes. Hence the no-threshold relationship for the quantal cell response can have little or no bearing on whether or not cells require a threshold amount of energy deposit in order to cause a quantal, or any other cell response or injury. Nor can the slope of the linear curve provide direct information on the

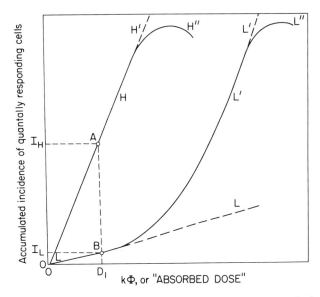

FIGURE 4. "Absorbed dose" - excess incidence curves, for a low (L) and a high (H) LET radiation. Note that the relative positions of curves H and L are reversed over those in Figure 3 (see text). Curve L is for low "absorbed doses," or for larger "absorbed doses" given at very low average "dose rates." Both curves saturate at about the same incidence, due mainly to cell killing.

absolute or relative sensitivity of cells, as measured by the fraction of cells responding quantally to the amount of cell energy deposited.

Note that although the initial portion of all of the curves remains linear, the relative positions of the low- and high-LET curves are reversed (Figures 3 and 9). This reversal emphasizes what is shown schematically in Figure 1a; namely, that a very large fraction of hit sizes from a low LET radiation is effectively below a threshold and, therefore, of vanishingly small effectiveness. Additional support for this explanation is obtained from microdosimetric measurements, which show that at CV diameters of 1 micron and larger and for low LET radiation, a large fraction of the exposed cell CV can have more than one hit at absorbed doses of 1 rad or less. Nonetheless, the curve for living cells (Figure 7) does not bend accordingly, but remains effectively linear up to at least 7–8 rads or more and then rises. This indicates also that the vast bulk of low-LET hit sizes are so small that even two hits on the same cell CV cannot induce a quantal response* (i.e., most hit sizes must be less than half of the

---

* Additional evidence for a threshold amount of energy deposit for a quantal response (marked ϵT in Figure 1) can also be deduced from Figure 7. The curve for low-LET radiation remains linear well above the region of essentially single hits, as shown by microdosimetric measurements. This suggests that the energy deposited by three or more small hits is required to enhance the number of all-or-none effects from single hits. Thus, in the context of LLR, any cell CV with a hit size less than half of the threshold value (ϵT, Figure 1) should be considered unhit.

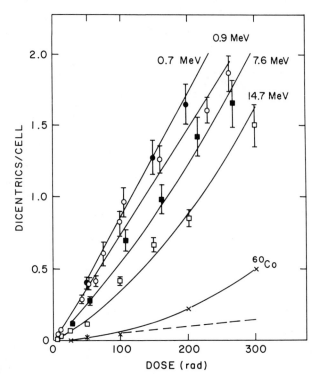

FIGURE 5. Yield of dicentric chromosome abnormalities in human lymphocytes after external exposures to neutrons of four different radiation energies (from Lloyd et al, 1975).

threshold value and, thus, even doubly hit cells are effectively unhit). Thus, with LLR any cell with a hit size less than half of the threshold value could be regarded as unhit.

With respect to the "quadratic" or HLR portion of the low-LET curve shown in Figure 2a, many hits cause only subeffective cell (CV) injury, incapable of causing a quantal response, alone. However, if additional "absorbed doses" are then delivered within a time interval short with respect to that required for repair of the injury to take place, by means of multiple hits additional cells will acquire a hit size large enough to cause, through the cumulative action of the combined subeffective cell injury from each smaller hit, a quantal cell response. It is this multihit, cumulative, or "positive enhancement" phenomenon that leads to the higher order component(s) of the well known formulation

$$I_A = \alpha D + \beta D^2 + - - - \tag{1}$$

in which I_A is the excess incidence of the all-or-none effect in the exposed cell population, D is the "absorbed dose," and α and β are constants.

The higher order exponents in **(1)** would not necessarily be expected to be integers, because D in the equation is conceptually Φ or the number of hit cells N_H, and because of the small-hit phenomenon just described. With the biologi-

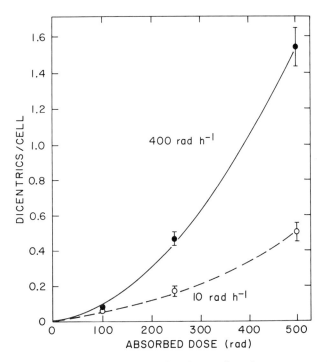

FIGURE 6. Frequency of dicentrics induced in human lymphocytes exposed to ^{137}Ce gamma radiation delivered at 400 rad/hr (—) and 10 rad/hr (- - - -). At dose magnitudes of 250 and 500 rad, the low-dose rate yield of dicentrics is approximately 33% that observed at the high-dose rate (from Purrot and Reeder, 1976, by permission).

cal system shown in Figure 7, the βD^2 exponent does not rise above about 1.6 even at very high dose-rates, over the relatively small "absorbed dose" range in which it can be measured.

It is apparent from the above that there will be a continuum of changes in curve slope and shape as the LET changes (Figure 5). At very high LET, a large fraction of hits on cells will be of a size large enough to produce a quantal response. Hence, the αD term will dominate and it will be difficult to see or demonstrate a βD^2 component (Brusted, 1962). However, its existence has been demonstrated with combined effects experiments (Ngo et al, 1981), in which the effect of "absorbed doses" of high- and low-LET radiations, given in close time juxtaposition is greater than the sum of each individually. This is due to the added cumulative action of the small amount of subeffective injury in the cells exposed to high-LET radiation, and the large amount in the cells exposed to low-LET radiation. With very low-LET radiation, on the other hand, the overall curve will be dominated by the βD^2 component, such that, at low doses, the linear component can be demonstrated only in very large populations of exposed cells. Between these extremes, the overwhelmingly linear response for very high-LET radiation gradually gives way to increasing curvilinearity as the LET is decreased.

424

VP BOND

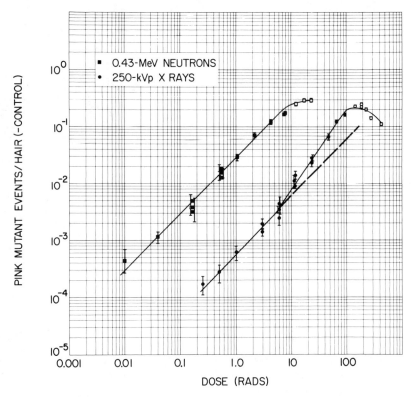

FIGURE 7. Neutron and x-ray dose–response curves for pink mutant events in stamen hairs of *Tradescantia* clone 02. The points represent average values obtained by dividing the total number of mutant events by the total number of stamen hairs scored from day 11 through day 15 after irradiation, when the mutation frequency is highest. The open symbols are saturation points and were not used in computing the true slopes (from Underbrink and Sparrow, 1974).

The continuum of changes in curve slope and shape is shown for living cells in Figure 5. The linear curve extending into the HLR region for most systems is due to the relative unimportance of cell killing for this quantal response (chromosome abnormalities), because early scoring is possible, and because there are multiple targets per cell for what is scored as the same type of abnormality.

CELL RADIOSENSITIVITY; RBE

Curves A and B in Figure 2 are the *cell analoges* of the curves of classical pharmacology for the distribution of *organ* sensitivities as a function of organ dose (curve B), and the integral of this distribution (curve A). Thus, quantitative comparisons of the relative radiation sensitivities of cells of different types should be made in terms of parameters of the cell hit size-cell quantal response, or cell sensitivity functions shown in Figure 2. The absolute or relative hit sizes (cell "doses") at the median response level, or ED_{50} value, and the slopes

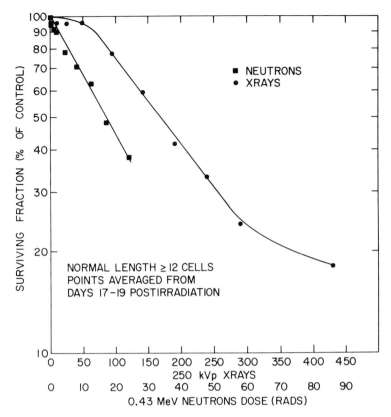

FIGURE 8. Survival curves for stamen hairs exposed to nuetron or x-irradiation. The surviving fraction is the percentage of normal length hairs as a percentage of the control value for the terminal third of the filament. The surviving fraction consists of hairs both with and without abberations (from Underbrink and Sparrow, 1974).

(variance of the integral curves) should be compared for this purpose, as is done in classical pharmacologic toxicology in order to compare the sensitivities of different organ types. Similarly, if the relative potency of radiation and another radiomimetic chemical or physical agent are to be assessed quantitatively, this should be done in terms of parmeters of the curve(s) shown in Figure 2.

In sharp contrast to the cell hit size-cell quantal response functions shown in Figure 2, none of the "$k\Phi$, or absorbed dose"-cell quantal response functions shown in Figures 4–9, in the LLR region of interest for single cell responses, can be construed to represent the integral of a spectrum of cell sensitivities. On the contrary, the slope of the differential curve is constant, indicating that changes in cell sensitivity are not involved. This simply confirms what has been demonstrated above; namely, that with any quality of radiation, an increase in "absorbed dose" or $k\Phi$ and, thus, in the *incidence* of responding cells, means only that one is dealing with a *larger number of hit ("dosed") cells*, with

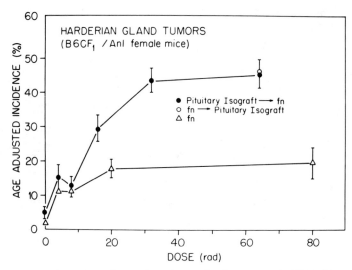

FIGURE 9. Age-adjusted incidence of Harderian gland tumors in B6CF$_1$/Anl female mice as a function of the dose of neutrons from the JANUS reactor (from Fry et al, 1982, by permission).

no change in the distribution of hit sizes, amounts of cell injury, and probability of response in accordance with cell sensitivity. The increase in absorbed "dose" or kΦ does not mean what an increase in "dose" means in pharmacology; namely, that each cell in a group has been given the identical dose of planned size, and that an increase in dose can then mean only an increase in both the dose per cell and the amount of injury in each cell involved and, thus, an increased probability of a quantal response reflecting differences in cell sensitivity.

It follows then, that the ratio of the slopes of different "linear, no threshold" curves shown in Figures 4, 5, and 7 do not represent potency ratios in the pharmacologic sense. In fact, no analog of the potency ratio is involved when cells respond to radiations of different LET. This is because cells responding to hits of any size from any quality of radiation are all responding to "doses" of a single agent, transferred energy. The effectiveness of an energy deposition in a cell CV, in the ranges of overlap, appears to be independent of the quality of radiation from which that amount of energy was derived.

Accordingly, the RBE, rather than being a potency ratio, is merely the ratio of the incidences of the quantal response per rad, for radiations of different LET, or different spectra of transferred energy or hit sizes. Values for those ratios involve complex and differing mixtures of numbers of hit cells, spectra of hit sizes, and ranges of cell sensitivity. Even if normalized to the same number of cells hit, by using fluence instead of "absorbed dose," what is observed and compared is still the normal responses of cells within different but normal ranges of sensitivity responding to different preparations of the same agent with different distributions of hit sizes or cell "doses," and not responses to the same hit size or "dose" of different agents. Thus, RBE is not a single fundamental quantity or parameter, rather it is an empirical ratio involv-

Although no
cell lethality cor
ceivably be cau:
such multiple a
shape of the in
significant or de

From Eq. 4 it
depending on tl
tors, and the va
knowledge of tl
effects, includin;
but should becc
approached.

NONAUTONOM

Although radiog
tissue culture, r
play a large role.
systems to chan
factors (e.g., horr
tion of tissues (ce
of genetic damaş
altered offspring.
or at most a few (
by influences ext
multi- and intra
present or of radi
or supplied fron
drugs). Also invc
1977; Storer et a.
Han and Elkind,
in vivo (Fry and
hancement of tur
Bond et al, 1962)
has been observe

If such enhanc
system to promoi
whatever agent, tl
mations radiogen
LLR) affect each
initial linear curv
substantially and
tumors).

On the other hi
cally altered, qua
that is difficult to
dose" levels wher
or dominate.

ing a complex and varying mixture of quantities, which is inherent in the way energy transfers are packaged by nature.

INFLUENCE OF "DOSE RATE" (FLUENCE RATE), AUTONOMOUS CELLS

The excess incidence per rad in the initial linear (LLR) portion of the curve, in populations of autonomous cells of invariant composition during the exposure, cannot be influenced by "dose rate" if the linearity is in fact due to single hits. This is because the successive single hits are delivered instantaneously and essentially exclusively on previously unhit cells. Because these independently hit cells by definition do not interact, the incidence cannot vary with the fluence ("dose") rate.

Thus, "dose-rate effects" can play a role only if the total amount of cell injury responsible for the quantal response is caused by more than one hit on the same cell, and if those hits are separated in time. In other words, "dose rate" can affect only the βD^2 part of the relationship: those quantal responses due to the cumulative and positively enhancing effects of more than one increment of subeffect injury, neither capable individually of causing a quantal response. A decrease in "dose rate" (i.e., an increase in the time interval between successive hits on the same cells) can alter the incidence of all-or-none effects only if increments of subeffective cell injury effectively disappear (i.e., are reversed, by repair or otherwise) in the time interval between hits, a process by which the total "absorbed dose" is also in effect decreased by the increment responsible for the first hit on the cell.

Thus, the degree to which "dose rate" has an influence is highly dependent on the time constant for repair of subeffect cell injury. If repair can take place, and if sufficient time is allowed for complete repair (half-time frequently in the range of hours or less), then the βD^2 term becomes zero. Thus, in Figure 4, a large "absorbed dose" of low-LET radiation that would yield a relatively high incidence if given rapidly in one large dose (i.e., lie on the βD^2 portion of curve L), if delivered in small, well-separated fractions, would yield a much smaller incidence [i.e., lie essentially on the extended linear portion (L) of the initial curve]. Thus, by the use of large doses delivered at very low dose rates, one can in principle obtain the slope of the linear curve at very low doses (Bond, 1979; Bond, 1980; NCRP, 1980). An advantage of this "high-dose, low-dose rate" approach is that the curve remains linear up to larger absorbed doses, thus, increasing the observed incidence and improving the confidence limits.

It is apparent that "dose rate" is a misnomer, because it is a weighted average of the time intervals between successive hits on individual cells that determines the magnitude of a "dose-rate" effect.

A relatively unexplored area is the degree to which the subeffective but comparatively severe cell injury from the large hit sizes produced by high-LET radiation can be repaired. Such studies are difficult to do because of the large proportion of hit cells that do show the quantal response. There is some evidence that such large cell injuries are poorly repaired. Thus, the survival curve for fast neutrons in the C3H/10T$\frac{1}{2}$ system shows curvilinearity at high doses for both low- and high-LET radiations, consistent with multihit effects (Bond, 1979; Bond, 1980; NCRP, 1980; Han et al, 1980). However, the sparing effect of fractionation is seen only with low-LET radiation (NCRP, 1980), and is mini-

mal or absei
probable ex]
increments (
relatively lai

MODIFYIN(

In autonomo
initial linear
unit "absorb
either to mu
and response
same or a dif
can be writte

I = αD +

where [βD² +
cell quantal
algebraic sur
able modifyi

1. *Physic*
   purely
   Figure
   increas
   numbe
   tinues
   sorbed
   in curv
   be calc
   phenor
   curve,
2. *The cu*
   tor yiel
   that le
   princip
   saturat
   fected
   numbe
3. *Small l*
   tive hit
4. *Cell ki*
   preven
   dent or
   Thus, t
   mulati\
   radiatic
   This ef:
   large d

The critical question then is not can such complicating factors play a role, because they can drastically affect expression. Rather, it is at what "absorbed dose" level are they radiogenically altered, and is this low enough to affect the initial linear *shape* of the curve and, thus, the slope. Even in autonomous cell systems, enhancing factors can change the shape of the initial linear part of the curve at "absorbed doses" of 10 rad or lower, of either low- or high-LET radiation (Figure 9). It may be of little or no value to invoke data above approximately 10 rad, in complex or even in autonomous systems, in an effort to shed light on the shape or slope of the initial part of the curve.

The considerations just mentioned emphasize the need to differentiate clearly between the questions: What is the actual shape and slope of the curve at the low doses encountered in radiation protection and general population exposure (i.e., lifetime "absorbed doses" of less than 5 rad of high-LET radiation, and less than 10 to generally 20–30 rad for low-LET radiation); and, What is the shape of the overall curve for purposes of "extrapolation" (largely academic unless it is from actual HLR data *in humans*, to the LLR region). It is only the shape and slope of the initial curve that is of primary importance in developing the theoretical basis for single-cell radiobiologic responses and in developing theory on which to base radiation protection practice (the question addressed here).

Data in complex systems are now legion, showing positive and then negative enhancement with low-LET radiation, but only negative enhancement with high-LET radiation. Negative enhancement with high-LET radiation may appear at surprisingly low doses in tissue culture (Han and Elkind, 1979) and in animal tumorigenesis experiments (Fry and Ainsworth, 1977). However, there are reasons why such low "absorbed dose" enhancement may be essentially unique to the systems studied. Departure from linearity at the lower "absorbed doses" of high-LET radiation, and even a threshold in some cases, is evident in rodent carcinogenesis (NCRP, 1980; Bond et al, 1962). The marked and perhaps unique radiosensitivity of the mouse ovary is well known, as is the marked role of hormones in the promotion of many rodent tumors (Fry and Ainsworth, 1977; Storer et al, 1982; Bond et al, 1962). Such high sensitivity appears to be absent, however, in the human ovary. Such a departure from linearity may also be seen in neoplastic transformation in vitro, particularly in the C3H/10T½ mouse embryo-derived cell line (Hall, 1981), and "reverse dose-rate" effects may be seen at moderate "absorbed doses." This system is difficult to work with, however, and results are inconsistent [e.g., a "reverse dose-rate" effect" for low-LET radiation is reported by one group (Hall, 1981) but not by another (Han et al, 1980). The system involves long culture times and contact inhibition at confluence. Humoral factors may be present in larger concentration than would be present in vitro. Most striking are the recent data indicating a "reverse dose-rate" effect for neutrons, down to "absorbed doses" of 10 rad (Hill et al, 1982).

Although the explanation for the above unexpected phenomena seen with neoplastic cell transformation in vitro, and their possible relevance to animal and human carcinogenesis, are unclear at present, there are indications that the phenomena are absent or at least much less marked in systems in vivo. Exposure of *Tradescantia* to 0.55 rad of 0.43 MeV neutrons resulted in the same incidence of pink cell mutations, whether exposed at 60 or 0.2 rad/hr (Underbrink and Sparrow, 1974). Studies to date on the influence of dose rate on the high-LET tumorigenesis response in animals (Ullrich et al, 1977), though limited, fail to give consistent evidence of the "reverse dose-rate" effect, and the dose–response curve for neutrons is linear for some tumors up to as much as 20 rad (Ullrich et al, 1977), which would argue against a reverse dose-rate effect. Also, high-LET irradiation from radium in human beings (Evans, 1966) fails to show other than a vanishingly small, if any, tumorigenic effect at very low rates of dose delivery.

Although studies with rat mammary gland tumors (Shellabarger et al, 1980) may show a linear response to low doses, and perhaps even a reverse "dose-rate" effect (Vogel, 1981), the data and analyses are complex and the scoring may include a nonstochastic component. At any rate, the results to date indicate only a possible change in curve slope below 10 rad, and not a departure from the linearity predicted by biophysical-"microdosimetric" theory.

Cell killing can also play a substantial role if moderate doses are delivered at an insufficiently low "dose rate." For instance, the bone marrow stem cell pool size can be significantly reduced under these circumstances, because the time constant for population restitution is measured in days or weeks (compared with hours for subeffective intracellular damage).

Another well known potential complication is "partial synchronization of cells," due to differences in cell sensitivity as a function of stage of cell cycle and the selective removal of those in the more sensitive phase(s). This effect plays a role only with multiple doses spaced in time, and is detectable only with large doses.

The single cell origin of radiogenic tumors is of obvious significance in relation to a linear, no-threshold cell induction function. Many, if not most, human tumors are of monoclonal origin (Gould, 1982), and there appear to be no data to rule out a single-cell orgin of the monoclonicity. Although it has been argued from certain biophysical considerations that radiogenic cancer is most likely multicellular in origin (Rossi and Kellerer, 1972), reasons have been given to explain why this interpretation does not necessarily follow from the data used (Bond, 1981).

EXPERIMENTAL "ABSORBED DOSE"-CELL RESPONSE CURVES

Figure 5 shows dose–response curves for chromosome abnormalities, for which multiple abnormalities due to different charged particle-cell target(s) interactions within the same cell can be scored separately, and in which cell death is not a major complicating factor, because the endpoints are scored even in lethally injured cells (before death removes cells from the population) (Lloyd et al, 1975). Note first that the high-LET curves have the steepest slopes (i.e., the largest RBE), as predicted above, and that these curves remain linear in this system up to at least the 100- to 200-rad region. The lack of either positive or negative enhancement is due to the overwhelming predominance of single-hit all-or-none effects from the spectrum of very large hit sizes, from the fact that many abnormalities are scored before cell death can be a large complication, and because there are multiple targets per cell for similar chromosome breaks. As the LET is reduced, a definite but shorter initial linear portion of the curve remains. That the expected "dose-rate" effect occurs is shown in Figure 6 (Purrst and Reeder, 1976). At still lower dose rates, the curve for "10 rad hr^{-1}" would be expected to be linear.

The competing influence of cell killing is illustrated in Figure 7 for pink cell mutations in the stamen hairs of the plant *Tradescantia* (Bond, 1979; Bond, 1980; NCRP, 1980; Underbrink and Sparrow, 1974). Because there were approximately two mutable cells per stamen hair, the incidence of mutated cells is about half of that shown on the ordinate. Note that the pattern for both high- and low-LET radiation is identical to that for chromosome abnormalities, except that the slope of both curves begins to decrease sharply at a mutation frequency of about 20% corresponding to neutron and gamma doses of about 10 and 100 rad, respectively. A physical saturation effect at these relatively low doses and response frequencies would not be expected. However, from Figure 8, it is clear that the sharp bends in the curves in Figure 7 concide with the dose levels at which cell killing becomes quite significant, and above which the survival rate decreases exponentially. Thus, cells in which the initial radiogenic alteration necessary for the quantal response has been induced die before the mutation can be expressed. From the cell lethality curves shown in Figure 8 it is evident that this function is responsible for most, if not all, of the marked departure from linearity.

An example of the complicating effect of radiogenic hormonal imbalance at very low "absorbed doses" is shown in the fast neutron dose–response curves for mouse Harderian gland tumors (Figure 9). The fact that the curve for data obtained with the use of a pituitary isograft is different from (i.e., above) that for neutrons alone, indicates that a pituitary hormone plays a positively enhancing role in the promotion or the expression of induced cancer cells (i.e., that all "induced" tumors are not expressed in the absence of the isograft). This effect is marked only at high doses, however, and is of questionable significance at low doses. Although the apparent discontinuity at about 5 rad may or may not be significant, there is no question that the initial apparent linearity is compromised at "absorbed doses" of 10 rad or less.

DISCUSSION

The hit size effectiveness theory puts to the test a major basic assumption inherent in "microdosimetry"—that it is the energy transferred to the individual cell, and not the type or energy content of the original source from which the energy was transferred (charged particle), that is the physical quantity primarily responsible for the extent of injury to, and the probability of a quantal response in, the individual cell. Results to date indicate that the assumption is true, in that the hit-size cell response function appears to apply across those qualities of radiation for which the hit size spectra overlap.

Results to date also indicate that the problem of determining the incidence of quantally responding cells with a given size CV involves at least four separate factors: 1) the number of agent sources in the vicinity of the cell CV; 2) the number of hit cell CV; 3) the amount of energy transferred (hit sizes); and 4) the hit size-quantal response function. Classical hit or target theory, in treating the problem as essentially purely physics, focused on the use of 1) to obtain 2), and gave little or no attention to 3) and 4). Microdosimetry, which in essence treats the problem as toxicologic in focusing on the amount of physical insult to the individual cell CV (hit size, "dose"), has focused mainly on 3), and has paid little or no attention to 2), other than to use it to determine the average hit size, or to 4). The approach here contributes 4), and uses all of the factors employed in both hit theory and microdosimetry. Thus, the hit size effectiveness theory unifies and adds to the two earlier approaches, and appears to provide a complete method for determining the expected excess incidence of quantally responding cells for any given amount of radiation of any type or quality.

The hit size effectiveness theory provides a basis for appreciation of the close analogy that exists between the risks to cells (CV) exposed to microagent sources (charged particles) in the environment of the cells, and risks to individuals (organs) exposed to macroagent sources (gross objects in the environment of an individual), in motion relative to the individual, from which the agent (energy) can be transferred in the event of an accidental encounter or collision. Under both of these circumstances there is no real need to characterize or quantify the exposure field. With macroaccidents there is no requirement to consider even the amount of energy ("dose" of energy) transferred to and received by the individual organ, because the number of victims and the severity of injury in each individual, are determinable at once from the observed biological responses. With LLR, however, both the number of hit individuals and a function relating hit size to severity of injury are necessary because of 1) the inability to identify any hit with any cell, 2) the long latent period between a cell transformational event and the visible manifestation of that transformation, for those quantal responses of most practical interest (genetic and malignant cell transformations), 3) the lack of knowledge for carcinogenesis of the fraction of transformed cells that develop into a cancer and 4) the inability to identify the visible manifestations of a cell transformation because of the baseline or normal incidence. Under these circumstances it is only with the approaches outlined above that it is possible to determine, at the time of exposure, both the expected number of casualties and the spectrum of severities, even though the visible manifestations will be seen much later.

The analogy with macroaccidents also makes it clear that the lack of a threshold with a linear (single-event) relationship means simply that it is quite possible to be severely or lethally injured in a single, accidental physical event or collision, whether the event is a severe or lethal injury to an organ, as the result of a macrostochastic event (e.g., auto crash, lightning strike), or to a relevant cell, as the result of a microevent (i.e., a charged particle-cell CV collision in the course of LLR exposure). The shallow slope of the curve indicates the extreme rarity of collisions that are large enough to have the potential for, and which actually will result in, severe or lethal injury.

The initial linearity of the "absorbed dose"-cell response curve, in even the simplest autonomous eukaryotic cell systems, may be overridden by additional mechanisms at "absorbed doses" as low as 10 rad or less, for either low- or high-LET radiation. Thus, inferences as to the shape or slope of the curve in these very low "absorbed dose" ranges are highly questionable in the absence of actual data for those ranges. At present, there appear to be no data in any system that indicate nonlinearity for cellular initiating events below about 5–10 rad. However, it is possible that for some types of carcinogenesis in animals and in some tissue culture systems normally present radiogenic inhibitors of expression may reduce the slope, perhaps even to zero, for the expression of cell transformational events.

Extrapolation of human carcinogenesis data obtained with low-LET radiation in the nonlinear, high-dose, high dose rate portions of the curve to the low-dose region is well justified to obtain an upper bound risk coefficient for LLR. Because no human data for the carcinogenic effects of external high-LET radiation are currently available, the question of extrapolation is academic (as is extrapolation of high-LET tissue culture or animal data, in terms of shedding light on the shape or slope of the initial part of the curve for humans). It is most unlikely that even if external neutron data on human carcinogenesis were to become available, extrapolation from doses above 10–20 rad would be necessary in light of the expected steepness of the slope. Thus, at doses of interest in radiation protection of workers and the general public (i.e., cumulative lifetime doses of less than 5 rad of high-LET radiation, and generally less than 10–30 rad of low-LET radiation, delivered at low dose-rates), there is more than adequate scientific justification for use of a linear, no threshold relationship, with a slope obtained by "extrapolation" of human data, for use as an upper limit value for the initial slope.

The risk associated with LLR exposure is very low because it is the product of three or more (low) probabilities. This differs from classical toxicology and (multicellular) quantal organ responses seen with HLR, for which, because p_1 and p_2 are both 1.0, dose becomes the appropriate independent physical variable on which p_3 depends. Thus, the simple probability of a quantal organ response can be high or low, depending on the dose planned and given.

It is suggested that fluence be introduced to replace "absorbed dose" in the LLR range only. This would serve to emphasize that the risk of a cell being hit and showing a stochastic quantal effect is to be sharply distinguished from the simple probability, above a threshold of nonstochastically delivered dose, of a stochastic quantal response in toxicology. The latter probability is purely biological, and reflects the rate of change of biological sensitivity as the dose increases. The former includes two additional probabilities that are of physical origin and, thus, provide no direct information on biological sensitivity. The use of fluence would serve also to emphasize that the risk of LLR exposure belongs in the same category as the risks from exposure in a field of macro agent sources with the potential for macrostochastic events or accidents, for which the curve for the proportion of individuals "singly hit" in all accidents of a given type and without regard to "hit size" versus the number or incidence of those hit individuals who are lethally injured to the stochastic event, is also characteristically linear and without threshold.

REFERENCES

Barendsen GW (1964) Impairment of the proliferative capacity of human cells in culture by alpha particles with differing LET. Intl J Radiat Biol 8:453.

Becker FF (Ed) (1975) Cancer, a comprehensive treatise, Part I. New York: Plenum.

Bond VP, Cronkite EP, Shellabarger CJ, and Aponte G (1962) Radiation-induced mammary gland neoplasia in the rat. In: Mammalian cytogenetics and related problems in radiobiology. Symposium. New York: Pergamon. pp. 361–82

Bond VP, Archambeau J, Fliedner TM (1965) Radiation lethality, a disturbance in cellular kinetics. New York: Academic Press.

Bond VP (1979) Quantitative risk in radiation protection standards. Radiat Environ Biophys 17:1–28.

Bond VP (1980) A basis for estimating the risks of low-level radiation. In: Fullerton GD (ed), Biological risks of medical irradiation, Medical Physics Monogr no. 5. New York: American Institute of Physics.

Bond VP (1981) The conceptual basis for evaluating risk from low-level radiation exposure. In: Critical issues in setting radiation protection dose limits. Proceedings of the 17th Annual Meeting, NCRP, April 8–9.

Bond VP, Varma MN (1981) The threshold-microdosimetric approach in radiation. Abstract presented at Radiation Research Meeting, Minneapolis, MN, June 1981.

Brusted T (1962) Heavy ions and some aspects of their use in molecular and cellular radiobiology. Adv Biol Med Phys 8:161.

Evans RD (1966) The effect of skeletally-deposited alpha emitters. Br J Radiol 39:881–895.

Feinendegen LE, Mühulensiepen H, Proschen W, Booz J (1981) Acute non-stochastic effect of very low dose whole-body exposure, a thymidine equivalent serum factor. Intl J Radiat Biol 41:139–150.

Finney DJ (1964) Probit analysis, 2nd Ed. Cambridge: Cambridge University Press.

Fry M, Ainsworth EJ (1977) Radiation injury: Some aspects of the oncogenic effects. Proc 36:1703–1707.

Fry RJM, Ley RD, Grube D, Staffeldt E (1982) Studies on the multistage nature of radiation carcinogenesis. In: Hecker E et al (eds.), Carcinogenesis, Vol. 7. New York, Raven Press, pp 155–165.

Gould MN (1982) Radiation initiation of carcinogenesis in vivo: A rare or common event. In: Proceedings of symposium, Radiation Carcinogenesis, Epidemiology and Biological Significance, May 24–26, Bethesda, MD.

Hall EG (1981) The role of in vitro cell studies in low dose extrapolations. In: Critical Issues in Setting Radiation Dose Limits, Proceedings of NCRP Annual Meeting, April, 1981. Washington, DC: NCRP and Measurements.

Han A, Elkind MM (1974) Transformation of mouse C3H10T½ cells by single and fractionated doses of x-rays and fission-spectrum neutrons. Cancer Res 39:123–130.

Han A, Hill CK, Elkind MM (1980) Repair of cell killing and neoplastic transformation at reduced dose rates of ^{60}Co γ-rays. Cancer Res 40:3328–3332.

Hill CK, Buonaguro MF, Myers CP, Han A, Elkind MM (1982) Fission-spectrum neutrons at reduced rates enhance neoplastic transformation. Nature Vol 298, pp 67–69 (July 1, 1982)

ICRP (1977) Publication 26: Recommendations of the International Commission on Radiological Protection. Annals of the ICRP, Vol 3.

International Commission on Radiation Units and Measurements, Washington, D.C. (1980) Report 33: Radiation Quantities and Units.

Kellerer AM (1976) Microdosimetry and its implication for the primary processes in radiation carcinogenesis. In: Yuhas JM, Tennant RW, and Regan JD (eds.), Biology of radiation carcinogenesis. New York: Raven Press.

Kennedy AR, Fox M, Murphy G, Little JB (1980) Relationship between x-ray exposure and malignant transformation in C3H/10T½ cells. Proc Nat'l Acad Sci USA 77:7262–7266.

Lloyd DC, Purrott RJ, Dolphin GW, Bolton D, Edwards AA, Cork MJ (1975) The relationship between chromosome aberrations and low-LET radiation dose to human lymphocytes. Intl J Radiat Biol 28:75.

NCRP (1980) Report 64: Influence of dose and its distribution in time on dose–response relationships for low-LET radiations. Washington, DC: National Council on Radiation Protection and Measurements.

Ngo FQH, Blakeley EA, Tobias CA (1981) Sequential exposures of mammalian cells to low and high LET radiations. Radiat Res 87:59–78.

Purrot RJ, Reeder E (1976) The effects of changes in dose rate on the yield of chromosome aberrations in human lymphocytes exposed to gamma radiation. Mutat Res 35:437.

Richter KH, Jepsen H, Marks F (1984) A system for the study of epidermal G1-chalone in cell culture. Exp Cell Res 150:68–76.

Rossi HH, Kellerer AM (1972) Radiation carcinogenesis at low doses. Science 175:200–202.

Rossi HH (1979) The role of microdosimetry in radiobiology. radiat Environ Phys 17:29–40.

Shellabarger CJ, Chmelevsky D, Kellerer AM (1980) Induction of mammary neoplasms in the Sprague–Dawley rat by 430 keV neutrons and x-rays. J Natl Cancer Inst 64:821–833.

Storer JB, Mitchell TJ, Ullrich RL (1982) Causes of death and their contribution to radiation-induced life shortening in intact and ovariectomized mice. Radiat Res 89:618–643.

Ullrich RL, Jernigan MC, Storer JB (1977) Neutron carcinogenesis: Dose and dose rate effects in BALB/c mice. Radiat Res 72:487–498.

Underbrink AG, Sparrow AH (1976) The influence of experimental endpoints, dose, dose rate, neutron energy, nitrogen ions, hypoxia, chromosome volume and ploidy level on RBE in Tradescantia stamen hairs and pollen. IAEA Symposium on Biological Effects of Neutron Irradiation, Vienna, 1974.

Varma MN, Bond VP (1982) Empirical evaluation of a cell critical volume dose vs cell response function for pink mutation in Tradescantia. Proceedings of the Eighth Symposium in Microdosimetry, Jülich, West Germany, EUR 8395, Sept 27–Oct 1, pp 439–450.

Vogel HH (1981) Mammary neoplasia following acute and protracted irradiation with fission neutrons and ^{60}Co gamma rays. Radiat Res 87(abstr):453–454.

COMBINED EFFECTS OF RADIATION AND OTHER AGENTS

R. J. M. FRY, M.D., AND R. L. ULLRICH, Ph.D.

We are exposed to a gallimaufry of physical and chemical agents ranging from sunlight to synthetic chemical compounds, all of which may have biological effects. In order to establish risk estimates of cancer resulting from exposure to a specific agent it is important to know what the effect may be when there is a combination of agents. For example, smokers exposed to asbestos are at greater risk for lung cancer than smokers, or than nonsmokers exposed to asbestos (Hammond et al, 1979). Such combined effects may be restricted to cancer of a particular organ, although the agents may cause or influence cancer incidence at other sites.

The risk and nature of the effects of exposure to combinations of radiation and other agents are being revealed by epidemiological and experimental investigations. Persons exposed occupationally to radiation are likely to be exposed to other carcinogenic agents, if only sunlight. Patients undergoing therapy for cancer may receive a combination of radiation and chemotherapy. These populations are just two examples of the need to understand combined effects of radiation and other agents.

Investigations of combined effects are usually designed to establish if the interaction between effects is synergistic, additive, or antagonistic. Unfortunately, these three simple terms have not been adequate for some investigators who have used augmentation, potentiation, enhancement, and inhibition to describe the effects of combinations of agents. The currently popular division of agents into complete carcinogens, initiators, and promoters, has also increased the lexicon used to describe combined effects.

Radiation is a good example of a complete carcinogen of which a single dose may induce cancer. It has also been shown that some exposures to radiation may initiate cells that have a low probability of expression as an overt cancer

From the Biology Division, Oak Ridge National Laboratory, Oak Ridge, Tennessee.

but may express their malignant phenotype following exposure to a second agent. On the other hand, irradiation after exposure to a chemical carcinogen may increase the response. The effect of the combination of radiation and other agents depends among other things on the sequence, timing, frequency, and total duration of exposure to the agents.

The use of various chemical agents in combination with radiation has proved useful in probing the mechanisms of the biological, including carcinogenic, effects of radiation. This chapter is restricted to the carcinogenic effects of combinations of ionizing radiation and various physical and chemical agents.

ASSESSMENT OF COMBINED EFFECTS

A combination of agents may result in additive, synergistic, or antagonistic interactive effects. Additivity suggests that the agents act independently. Although it may be important to establish that the action of some specific combination of agents is additive, such effects provide little help in elucidating mechanisms. On the other hand, synergistic and antagonistic effects offer potential for investigating one or more aspects of carcinogenesis.

When the individual responses for both radiation and the second agent are linear, the analysis of interaction should be simple. In this case, the dose–effect relationship for each agent can be described by

$$I = Ic + \alpha D \tag{1}$$

where I is the incidence of tumors in the treated group, Ic is the natural incidence of the specific type of tumor, D is the radiation dose, and α is a constant.

If the response to the two agents is independent, the additivity may be described as follows:

$$\Sigma I = 1 - [(1 - (Ic + \alpha_1 D_1) \times (1 - (Ic + \alpha_2 D_2)] \tag{2}$$

$$\Sigma I = Ic + \alpha_1 D_1 + \alpha_2 D_2$$

A linear response, of course, indicates that the effect per increment of dose is additive, and it is simple to show whether or not the combined effect is greater or less than additive (Figure 1, panel I). Most, if not all, dose–response curves for radiation induction of cancer are nonlinear, however, indicating that increments of dose are not additive. In the case of two agents with curvilinear dose–responses that are dissimilar, the delineation of additivity becomes complex. In pharmacology, the problem of analyzing and depicting the combined effects of varying dose levels of two drugs was tackled by devising isobolograms (Figure 1, panel II). The concepts of isobolograms, developed in particular by Loewe (1953), have been applied to the description of the combined effects of radiotherapy and chemotherapy by Steel and Peckam (1979). The problems of analyzing interactions between agents has been reviewed by Berenbaum (1981). A full discussion of the use of isobolograms can also be found in UNSCEAR's 1982 report of the effects of atomic radiation. This method for delineating the bounds of additivity between agents has recently been applied to studies of carcinogenesis (Reif, 1984). When the responses of the two agents

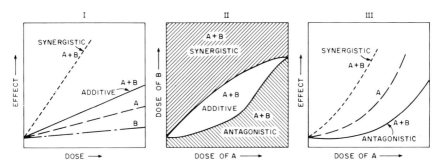

FIGURE 1. *Panel I.* The individual effects of radiation (A): ———, and a second agent (B): —·—, as a function of dose and the combined effects of (A) + (B): Additive, ———, and synergistic ----. When the dose–response relationship for each agent is linear. *Panel II.* A schematic isobologram which delineates the interaction of radiation and a second agent when the shapes of the dose–response for the induction of cancer by radiation and the second agent are dissimilar. *Panel III.* A schematic illustration of the carcinogenic response to radiation: ——— (A) alone and two of the possible responses to a noncarcinogenic agent: ———, and ----. Any response significantly greater or less than the response for radiation would be considered synergistic and antagonistic respectively.

under study are dissimilar, the isobologram makes it possible to define the response to the combination of agents that can be considered additive. If the response lies above the envelope delineating additivity the response can be considered synergistic, and if the response lies below the envelope the combined effect is antagonistic (Figure 1, panel II). If the second agent is not carcinogenic, the demonstration of either a synergistic or enhancing effect, or an antagonism, will depend on confidence limits for the radiation dose–response curves and the curve for the combined effects (Figure 1, panel III).

THERAPEUTIC AGENTS: HUMAN EXPERIENCE

In recent years, more patients with certain types of cancer are surviving because of improved therapy. Lymphomas and cancers of childhood are two classes of cancer that have been treated with radiotherapy, chemotherapy, and combinations of both. Because of the increased survival time in these patients it has become possible and important to study the risks of a second cancer and its association with the specific treatment (Canellos et al, 1975; Nelson et al, 1981; Coleman, 1982). The doses of the agents used in therapy in these patients are known precisely. Patients with Hodgkin's disease have been followed, to determine the risk of cancer in relation to therapy. Although there are a number of confounding factors in such studies, it appears that the risk of a secondary acute leukemia (as a result of treatment) is significantly greater in cases treated with combined chemotherapy and radiotherapy than with radiotherapy alone (Coleman, 1982).

With Wilm's tumor, on the other hand, the risk of secondary cancer after combined treatment with radiation and actinomycin D is smaller than after radiation alone (D'Angio et al, 1976). It is not known why actinomycin D reduces the risk of radiation-induced cancer, but such an effect also has been noted with a cell transformation system in vitro (Little, 1981).

A third population of humans that appears to illustrate interactions between ionizing radiation and other therapeutic modality is the group of psoriasis patients treated with the photosensitizer 8-methoxypsoralen (8-MOP) and ultraviolet (UV) radiation, usually called PUVA (Parrish et al, 1974). Assessments of the risk of skin cancer in patients treated with PUVA have been reported by Stern et al (1979, 1984). Many of the psoriasis patients had received one or another treatment before they entered the PUVA trial, and those that had received previous treatment with x-rays showed an excess incidence of squamous cell carcinomas, which appeared in a surprisingly short time after the exposure to PUVA. Although exposure to either ionizing radiation or PUVA alone presents a risk of skin cancer, an interaction between the two seems likely as the explanation of the increased incidence and rapid appearance of cancer after combined treatments.

EXPERIMENTAL STUDIES

There have been surprisingly few studies of the effect of combinations of radiation and chemotherapeutic agents. Arseneau et al (1977) studied the combined effect of the chemotherapeutic agent procarbazine (PCB) followed by x-irradiation and vice versa. After the treatments mice were observed for 12 wk. PCB is a known carcinogen in experimental animals and in this experiment PCB alone increased the incidence of lung tumors, though radiation alone did not. The incidence of tumors in the combined treatment groups was significantly greater than additive. The multiplicity of tumors was also greater when the interval between administration of the two agents was 3 days rather than 3 wk. Despite the shortness of the experimental period, thymic lymphomas were also found in each of the combined treatment groups.

The combined effect of myleran and radiation on the induction of thymic lymphoma in mice was investigated by Upton et al (1961). The combined effect was synergistic and greatest when myleran was given 15 days before irradiation.

TOBACCO SMOKE

Human Experience

Uranium miners exposed to radon and its daughters are at risk for lung cancer (Lundin et al, 1969). An increase in lung cancer incidence has been attributed to radiation and it has been suggested that there is a synergistic effect between radiation and tobacco smoke. The results of the recent analysis of the data from uranium miners by Whittemore and McMillan (1983) suggests that miners that smoked a pack or more of cigarettes daily for 20 yr had a lung cancer rate of about five times that of their nonsmoking colleagues. On the other hand, in atomic bomb survivors that developed lung cancer the interaction of radiation and smoking appeared to be additive (Prentice et al, 1983). A number of differences between uranium miners and A-bomb survivors come to mind as potential explanations for the discrepancy, including the dose distribution in the lung.

Experimental Animals

Experimental studies of the interaction of tobacco smoke and radiation have attempted to simulate the human experience. In a major study (Chameaud et al, 1979, 1980) rats were exposed to radon with 40-fold range in total doses. In the year after the radiation regime the rats had multiple exposures (over 2000) to tobacco smoke. The radon daughters caused lung tumors, but the tobacco smoke did not. Exposure to the combination was markedly more effective than irradiation alone. When the exposure to tobacco smoke was reversed there was no interaction. This finding supports the contention that tobacco acts as a promoter (Lafuma, quoted in UNSCEAR 1982).

Different experimental conditions in dogs that involved high doses of irradiation indicated an antagonistic effect of tobacco smoke on radiation-induced lung tumors (Cross et al, 1982).

CHEMICAL CARCINOGENS

Experimental Animals

Skin. The early experimental investigations of interactions between ionizing radiation and chemical carcinogens were carried out on the skin (Cramer, 1932; Mottram, 1937). Although these early experiments demonstrated interactions, interpretations were complicated by high doses, which caused marked cell killing and a lack of adequate dose–response curves for both agents. Cloudman et al (1955) reported additive effects when treatments with methylcholanthrene (MCA) followed beta radiation. Argus et al (1962) reported that exposure to x-rays, either before or after exposures to dimethylbenzanthracene (DMBA), reduced the incidence of skin tumors. The reason for the apparent antagonism is not clear and is in conflict with the finding of Burns et al (1977) who found x-irradiation and DMBA acted additively in the production of tumors in rat skin.

McGregor (1976, 1982) noted that the incidence of skin tumors induced by beta radiation was increased by subsequent topical treatment with cigarette smoke condensate although the condensate was not carcinogenic, itself. Myers and McGregor (1982) found that 2-anthramine had a synergistic effect when applied to skin that had been exposed to 16 Gy from a ^{90}Sr-^{90}Y source.

These results appear to be examples of radiation initiated skin tumors that can be brought to expression by chemical agents. There is convincing evidence that radiation can initiate cells in various tissues, which persist for considerable periods. These cells may be stimulated subsequently by various agents to express malignancy. Shubik et al (1953) reported promotion by croton oil of skin initiated by exposure to beta radiation. Hoshino and Tanooka (1975) showed that treatment with 4-nitroquinoline 1-oxide (4NQO) promoted beta-irradiated skin even up to 1 yr after the irradiation. When caffeine was painted on the skin on alternate days of the 4NQO treatment the combined effect of 4NQO and radiation was enhanced.

Less is known about how irradiation influences the expression of epidermal cells initiated with other agents, but Epstein (1972) showed that Grenz irradiation 4 wk after topical application of DMBA advanced the time of appearance compared to irradiation alone. Furthermore, the combined treatment caused more invasive tumors than either of the agents alone. Bock and Moore (1959) found that local irradiation increased the susceptibility of distant areas of skin to the induction of tumors by cigarette-smoke condensate.

Other Tissues

Vogel and Zaldivar (1971) investigated the carcinogenic effect of combinations and sequences of exposures to fission neutron radiation and N,N'-2-7-fluoranylenebisacetamide. The interpretation of the results was that there was a synergistic effect for the induction of hepatic tumors, which was not influenced by the sequence of exposures to the two agents. In the case of gastric carcinoma, a synergism was also noted but only when the chemical was given prior to irradiation.

Cole and Foley (1969) reported that x-irradiation and urethan acted additively in the production of lung tumors of mice. High doses of irradiation in combination with urethan reduced the number of tumors induced by urethan alone.

McGandy et al (1974) and Little et al (1978) examined the effect of intratracheal instillations of benzo(a)pyrene B(a)P and ^{210}Po an alpha radiation emitter on the incidence of lung tumors in hamsters and found it to be additive.

The dangers in the interpretation of combined effects in complex tissues such as the lung are underlined by the finding of Little's group that saline instillations into the lungs of hamsters following a single intratracheal instillation of ^{210}Po increased manyfold the yield of lung tumors (Little, 1981). The only hint of a possible mechanism is that the saline instillations stimulate, temporarily, cell proliferation in the terminal bronchioles.

Shellabarger et al (1967, 1972), using Sprague–Dawley rats, found that the carcinogenic effects of high doses of both to MCA and x- or neutron irradiation were additive, whether the radiation preceded or followed MCA administration.

Armuth and Berenblum (1967) found that DMBA-induced mammary cancer in Wistar rats could be promoted by phorbol, but Shellabarger et al (1979) could not demonstrate any promotion by phorbol when x-rays, DMBA, or procarbazine was used as the initiator in Sprague–Dawley rats, and attributed the differences in the results to a strain-dependent susceptibility to phorbol promotion.

A synergistic effect on the induction of mammary tumors in BALB/c mice was found when a low dose of DMBA was administered prior to gamma radiation. The effect was only additive with a higher dose of DMBA. However, with a higher DMBA dose reversing the sequence gave a synergistic effect (Ullrich and Ethier, 1983).

These results reinforce the concern of statements about interactions that are based on studies that do not cover a wide dose range, different sequences and intervals, as well as dose-rates of the exposures. The value of experiments carried out with low doses consist not only in the decreased likelihood of confounding effects, such as cell killing, but because the exposures of concern in human populations occur either with low doses or low dose-rates.

The sequence in which the agents are administered has been shown to be important, and in the case of promoters, of course, it is all important. With some combinations of radiation and chemical agents the influence of the sequence is quantitative, rather than qualitative. For example, Cole and Nowell (1964) found that CCL_4 administered either before or after neutron irradiation had a synergistic effect. However, the effect was greater when CCL_4 was administered 1 day prior to irradiation than 1 mo after exposure to neutrons. Habs et al (1983) confirmed that CCL_4 administered after neutron radiation enhanced the incidence of liver tumors, but only of carcinomas and not of benign tumors.

The effects of combining x-irradiation and urethan have been studied by several groups. Vesselinovitch et al (1972) administered urethan to mice on the 3rd, 6th and 12th days of life and exposed them to x-rays when the mice were 42 days old and found an additive effect on leukemogenesis. This finding is in contrast to the less than additive effect in adult mice reported by Berenblum and Trainin (1960) when urethan was first in the sequence of treatments. When urethan was given concurrently or followed the x-irradiation a greater than additive effect was found. Myers (1976) gave urethan concurrently with multiple exposures of x-rays to three strains of rats. Both the cumulative mortality and incidence of specific tumors suggested additivity.

The interaction of radiation and chemical agents in the production of lueke-mia, especially thymic lymphoma, has been studied by a number of workers (Furth and Boon, 1943; Berenblum and Trainin, 1960; Upton et al, 1961). The mechanism of induction of thymic lymphoma is complex, and damage to the hematopoietic and lymphoid tissues appears to be important. Therefore, it is perhaps not surprising that cytotoxic agents have been found to enhance radiation induction of thymic lymphoma.

Berenblum and Trainin (1960) interpreted their results with radiation and urethan in terms of promotion by urethan of radiation-initiated cells. There are too many variables in the experimental induction of thymic lymphoma to be able to interpret unequivocally results of the effect of exposure to two agents when one does not know the mechanism by which either agent produces lymphomas. Presumably agents such as MCA (Furth and Boon, 1943) and urethan (Berenblum and Trainin, 1960) that enhance the leukemogenic effect of radiation when administered after exposure to radiation influence expression of the initiated cells. Whereas, the less common effect that depends on exposure to the chemical agent prior to irradiation alters the susceptibility of the target cells.

The influence of dose level and fractionation has been studied, in particular with DMBA and low-LET radiation in hamster cheek pouch. Lurie used multiple exposures of 20 R x-rays and found that greater-than-additive effects occurred when irradiation was concurrent or after DMBA administration but not when radiation was the first treatment (Lurie, 1977, 1982).

RADIATION PROTECTORS AND SENSITIZERS

There are various agents that are antagonistic to radiation effects, including the thiol compounds described collectively as radioprotectors (Thomson, 1962). Such compounds must be present in the cells at the time of radiation exposure to be effective. The mechanism of action is the scavenging of free radicals. Although there have been a number of studies of the effects of radioprotectors on the radiation-induction of tumors (Maisin et al, 1978, 1980; Davis et al, 1970; Mewissen and Brucer, 1957; Shellabarger and Schmidt, 1967; Upton et al, 1959) no clear-cut pattern emerges. The induction of thymic lymphoma appears to involve cell killing as part of the mechanism, and the antagonistic or protective effect of radioprotectors, either singly or more frequently in combination, in this type of tumor is clear (Maisin et al, 1978; Cosgrove et al, 1964; Upton et al, 1959). Maisin et al (1978) also found a combination of radioprotectors reduced the incidence of lung tumors in BALB/c mice. However, the antagonistic effect of some of the more effective radioprotectors on the induction of carcinomas has not been investigated sufficiently (Yuhas and Walker, 1973), and we know of no studies that examine critically the influence of the level of thiol compounds on radiation induced-malignant transformation in vitro. Many aspects of radioprotectors and sensitizers have been reviewed recently (Nygaard and Simic, 1983).

The study of the use of chemical agents for preventing cancer induced by chemical carcinogens has blossomed, and the term chemoprevention is now accepted. Retinoids have been shown to protect against chemical carcinogens in animal studies (Sporn, 1976), and the indications from an experiment in progress is that retinyl acetate inhibits either the induction or the time of appearance of mammary tumors in x-irradiated Sprague–Dawley rats (Stone et al, 1984). Retinoids have been shown to inhibit x-ray–induced transformation of cells in vitro (Harisiadis et al, 1978; Miller et al, 1981).

A number of roles have been proposed for proteases in carcinogenesis (Troll, 1976; Kennedy, 1983). Troll et al (1980) reported a reduction in the incidence of mammary tumors in both unirradiated control and x-irradiated Sprague–Dawley rats that were fed a diet rich in protease inhibitors.

Protection against in vitro malignant transformation with the protease inhibitor antipain is now well documented (Kennedy and Little, 1978; Borek et al, 1979; Geard et al, 1981; Kennedy, 1983). Different protease inhibitors appear to influence different phases of transformation in vitro that have been called fixation, expression, and promotion (Kennedy, 1983). Antipain appears to inhibit all three phases.

A number of other compounds have been found to inhibit radiation-induced cell transformation in vitro, for example selenium, which has been suggested to interfere with free radicals (Borek, 1982). The importance of free radicals is once again receiving considerable attention. Because promoters, such as TPA, appear to be free radical generators (Goldstein, 1981) it is thought that free radicals could be involved in promotion. Certainly the addition of superoxide dismutase (SOD) and catalase inhibits both the induction of transformation by x-rays and the enhancement by TPA (Borek and Troll, 1983).

Hypoxic cell sensitizers are being developed and tested for use in radiotherapy. Hall et al (1978) found that misonidazole, a nitroimidazole malignantly transformed C3H 10T$\frac{1}{2}$ cells in vitro. The combined effect of misonidazole and x-rays was greater but not significantly different from additive (Miller and Hall, 1978).

Mian et al (1982) found no interaction between radiation and misonidazole on the induction of lung tumors in strain A mouse, however, the radiation dose may have been too high to demonstrate an interaction.

RADIATION AND CHEMICAL AGENTS

Studies In Vitro

Cell systems in vitro offer opportunities to study various interactions between radiation and other agents, including prevention of malignant transformation; these subject areas have been reviewed recently (Kennedy, 1983). By and large, the results from studies in vitro have been consistent with comparable studies in vivo.

DiPaolo et al (1971, 1976) reported that pretreatment x-rays enhanced cell transformation induced by B(a)P and that no enhancement was found when the x-irradiation followed exposure to B(a)P. The importance of the sequence and the timing of the exposures has been noted with other agents and the explanation is not always apparent.

Phorbol ester (TPA) appears to enhance transformation of cells in vitro after an initial exposure to ionizing radiation (Kennedy et al, 1978; Kennedy and Little, 1980; Miller et al, 1981; Han and Elkind, 1982). It is difficult to distinguish between a weak carcinogen and a promoter with no carcinogenic properties. In the C3H 10T$\frac{1}{2}$ cell system, Han and Elkind (1982) considered the combined effect of TPA with either x-rays or fission neutrons was synergistic rather than promotion because they found TPA alone to increase malignant transformation.

RADIATION AND HORMONES

Studies In Vivo

The influence of hormones in carcinogenesis is well documented Furth (1975) and interactions between radiation and hormones can occur in a number of ways. Hormones that stimulate cell proliferation may increase the number of cells at risk, especially if there is a cell stage specificity for transformation. In such cases interactions should occur when hormone administration precedes irradiation. It is clear that certain hormones increase the expression of radiation-initiated cells in specific tissues (Clifton et al, 1976), but it is not clear that the mechanisms involve only increased cell proliferation. Some investigators have considered the action of certain hormones to be analogous to promotion. Obviously, hormones required for tissue growth and cell proliferation must at least influence the time of appearance of radiation-induced tumors if not susceptibility of cells to induction.

In Figure 2, the effect of pituitary isograft, which raises the prolactin blood level, can be seen on both the naturally occurring Harderian gland tumors in

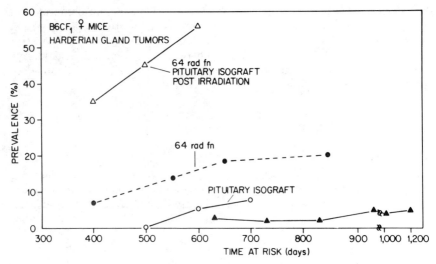

FIGURE 2. The prevalence of Harderian gland tumors after pituitary isograft only (O-O); after a single exposure to 64 rad fission neutrons (fn) only (■-■); and to 64 rad fn followed by pituitary isograft (△-△). Reproduced from Fry et al, 1982, by permission.

mice and the radiation-induced tumors. It can be seen that the raised hormone level advances the time of appearance of the naturally occurring tumors but does not increase the cumulative incidence. When the prolactin levels are raised by pituitary isografts after exposure to radiation the incidence is increased above that induced by radiation alone (Fry et al, 1982). In this example the altered hormone level appears to increase the expression of radiation-initiated cells.

The interaction of radiation and hormones has been studied extensively in radiation-induced breast cancer in rats. Synergism between both estrogens and diethylstilbestrol (DES) and radiation has been demonstrated (Segaloff and Maxfield, 1971; Bekkum et al, 1979; Shellabarger et al, 1976, 1982, 1983; Stone et al, 1980; Holtzman et al, 1979, 1981). These hormones do not necessarily act directly, since both estrogen and DES increase the blood level of prolactin, which has been shown to evoke the expression of the radiation-transformed mammary cells (Yokoro et al, 1977, 1980). Yokoro et al (1977) showed that elevated prolactin levels revealed the persistence of radiation-transformed mammary cells that had remained dormant for months. Implantation of estradiol pellets shortened the latent period, and increased both the incidence of mammary tumors and the proportion of tumors that were malignant (Bekkum et al, 1979).

Tamoxifen, an estrogen antagonist, has been shown to inhibit radiation-induced mammary carcinomas but not benign tumors in Sprague–Dawley rats (Welsch et al, 1981). Since tamoxifen did not affect serum prolactin levels the antiestrogen effect appears to be direct. The lack of inhibition of fibroadenoma induction by tamoxifen underlies the difference in the factors involved in the genesis of benign and malignant tumors. Synergistic effects between diethyl-stilbestrol and radiation have also been found for liver and pituitary tumors (Sumi et al, 1980).

The complexity of the influence of hormones in tumorigenesis is also evident from the in vitro cell transformation studies. Borek et al (Guernsey et al, 1980, 1981) found that thyroid hormones had little effect on cell survival or the growth characteristics after x-irradiation but had profound effect on the radiation-induced transformation rate in both Chinese hamster embryo cells and C3H 10T$\frac{1}{2}$ cells. No transformations were found when the culture medium lacked thyroid hormone for a few days before irradiation. The effect was considered a direct one because addition of the hormone to the medium just prior to irradiation restored the expected frequency. It was found that the critical period for the presence of thyroid hormone was during the 12 hr before irradiation. Somewhat surprisingly, the hormone effect appears to be associated with initial radiation-induced lesions rather than their expression. Based on experiments with cyclohexamide it was suggested that thyroid hormone induces the synthesis of a host protein that is required for the radiation-induced transformation (Guernsey et al, 1981).

Kennedy and Weichselbaum (1981a) found that 17-β estradiol and x-irradiation were additive in transforming C3H 10T$\frac{1}{2}$ cells and that cortisone and radiation acted synergistically (Kennedy and Weichselbaum, 1981b). The same investigators also found that the glucocorticoid dexamethasone acted at least additively with radiation. This finding was of interest, because dexamethasone suppressed TPA-enhanced DMBA-induced skin tumors (Troll, 1976), thus, raising the question of the difference between promotion caused by TPA and the changes in carcinogenesis that occur with a complete carcinogen and which, presumably, correspond to those changes described by the term promotion (Scribner and Suss, 1978). The effect of hormones is not limited to systemic hormones; Fisher et al (1981) showed that the polypeptide epidermal growth factor, which alone does not induce transformation, increases the transformation frequency induced by x-irradiation about fourfold, which is comparable with the increase with TPA.

IONIZING RADIATION AND OTHER PHYSICAL AGENTS

Ionizing Radiation and UVR

Human Studies. Although there has been no unequivocal demonstration of interaction between UV radiation and ionizing radiation the evidence suggests that UV radiation can act as a promoter.

Between 1940 and 1959, 2215 children with tinea capitis (ringworm) were treated with x-rays. This population has been followed carefully and compared with 1300 controls who also had tinea capitis but were not treated with x-irradiation (Albert et al, 1968; Shore et al, 1984).

The doses of x-rays to various parts of the head and neck ranged from 0.2 to 8.5 Gy but it has not been possible to determine the shape of the dose–response curve. The suggestion that skin cancer in this irradiated population is due to the interaction of UV radiation and x-rays is based on the fact that 24% of the patients were black and skin cancer has occurred only in the white patients and in areas exposed to sunlight. The difference in the incidence of skin cancer between white and black patients is significant at the 5% level. The evidence suggests that UV radiation may have caused changes that allowed the expression of the cells initiated by the x-rays.

Uranium miners in Czechoslovakia are a second population in which an interaction between UV radiation and alpha radiation may be involved in the observed increase in skin cancer. Ševcová et al (1978) found an incidence of skin cancer of 104 cases per 10,000 workers compared with the expected 13 cases (O/E = 8). The cancers occurred predominantly on the face.

Asbestos

The effects of the interaction between asbestos and radiation in humans has not been assessed quantitatively. In rats, asbestos and $^{239}PuO^2$ particles were found to induce mesothelioma of the peritoneum in an additive fashion (Sanders, 1973) but less than additively in the induction of lung tumors (Sanders, 1975). A combination of multiple exposures to ^{222}Ra and intrapleural injections of chrysotile fibers induced mesotheliomas and the effect was considered synergistic (Lafuma et al, 1980). Hei et al (1984) found exposure to crocidolite and amosite fibers to be cocarcinogenic with radiation. Pretreatment with asbestos fibers and subsequent irradiation of C3H 10T$\frac{1}{2}$ cells in vitro caused higher transformation frequencies than either agent alone. No interaction was found when asbestos was added 3 days after irradiation.

CONCLUSION

The studies that have examined interactions in the strict sense are those in which both agents were present concurrently at known dose levels. The effects of radiation protectors and radiation sensitizers in combination with radiation are examples of effects resulting from interactions.

Studies of such interactions with radiation protectors, for example, should be useful for probing facets of carcinogenesis in tissues, and further studies could be fruitful.

Many of the studies of the effects of combinations of radiation with other agents are not chemical interactions, but biological interactions in which time becomes an important factor. The sequence, the interval between exposure to the agents, and the number of exposures to either or both agents are of importance. The sequence is of importance because the first agent may alter the susceptibility to a second agent.

There are not many studies of radiation based on the initiation–promotion paradigm. Nevertheless, it is clear that ionizing radiation initiates cells which may express their neoplastic characteristics at a later time in response to a second agent. Whether the second agent, such as a hormone, alters the environment of the initiated cell and allows the expression of the altered phenotype or induces an additional change in the initiated cell itself is not yet clear.

Most of the studies of combined effects have reported results from a limited number of dose levels. Furthermore, because of the expense of experiments required to determine low-dose effects, the experiments have been carried out with relatively high doses which may not be optimal for revealing synergistic effects.

It is clear that there is a need for experiments in which the dose–responses for both radiation and the second agent are adequately defined, and that include the lowest possible dose levels.

Exposure of human populations to carcinogenic agents is usually intermittent or protracted and at a low dose-rate. Such exposures may initiate cells that have little or no probability of expression as overt cancers unless a second agent, which might be either endogenous or exogenous, arouses the potential cancer cell. We have little or no quantitative data on this type of risk. Information is needed on the induction and persistence of potentially malignant cells and the factors that influence their fate.

One hopes that the next generation of experiments on the combined effects of radiation and other agents will be designed to answer such specific questions and will help to unravel mechanisms and to define risks.

Research sponsored by the Office of Health and Environmental Research, U.S. Department of Energy under contract DE-AC05-840R21400 with the Martin Marietta Energy Systems, Inc.

The authors are grateful to J. F. Young for her help in the preparation of this paper.

REFERENCES

Albert RE, Omran AR, Brauner EE, Cohen NC, Schmidt H, Dove DC, Becker M, Baumring R, Baer RL (1968) Follow-up study of patients treated by x-ray epilation for tinea capitis. II. Results of clinical and laboratory examinations. Arch Environ Health 17:919–934.

Argus MF, Kane JF, Sakuntala M, Ray FF (1962) Effect of ionizing radiation on 9,10-dimethyl-1,2 benzanthracene tumorigenesis. Radiat Res 16:37–43.

Armuth V, Berenblum I (1967) Promotion of mammary carcinogenesis and leukemogenic action by phorbol in virgin female Wistar rats. Cancer Res 34:2704–2707.

Arseneau JC, Fowler E, Bakemeier RF (1977) Synergistic tumorigenic effect of procarbazine and ionizing radiation in (BALB/c × DBA/2)F_1 mice. J Natl Cancer Inst 59:423–425.

van Bekkum DW, Broerse JJ, van Zwieten MJ, Hollander CF, Blankenstein MA (1979) Radiation-induced mammary cancer in the rat. In: Okada S, Imamura M, Teresima T, and Yamaguchi H (eds.), Proceeding of the 6th International Congress of Radiation Research, New York: Academic Press, pp 743–752.

Berenbaum MC (1981) Criteria for analyzing interactions between biologically active agents. In: Klein G and Weinhouse S (eds.), Advances in cancer research, vol 35. New York: Academic Press, pp 269–335.

Berenblum I, Trainin N (1960) Possible two-stage mechanism in experimental leukemogenesis. Science 132:40–41.

Bock FG, Moore GE (1959) Carcinogenic activity of cigarette-smoke condensate. I. Effect of trauma and remote x-irradiation. J Natl Cancer Inst 22:401–411.

Borek C (1982) Vitamins and micronutrients modify carcinogenesis and tumor promotion in vitro. In: Arnott MS, van Eys J, and Wang YM (eds.), Molecular interrelations of nutrition and cancer. New York: Raven Press, pp 337–350.

Borek C, Miller R, Pan C, Troll W (1979) Conditions for inhibiting and enhancing effects of the protease inhibitors antipain on x-ray induced neoplastic transformation in hamster and mouse cells. Proc Natl Acad Sci USA 76:1800–1804.

Borek C, Troll W (1983) Modifiers of free radicals inhibit in vitro the oncogenic actions of x-rays, bleomycin, and the tumor promoter 12-0-tetradecanoylphorbol 13-acetate. Proc Natl Acad Sci USA 80:1304–1307.

Burns FJ, Strickland P, Albert RE (1977) The combined carcinogenic action of ionizing radiation and DMBA on rat skin. Radiat Res 70(abstr):607.

Canellos GP, Arseneau JC, DeVita VT, Whang-Peng J, Johnson REC (1975) Second malignancies complicating Hodgkin's disease in remission. Lancet i:947–949.

Chameaud J, Perraud R, Chretien J, Masse R, Lafuma J (1979) Etude experimentale de action combinee de la fumee de cigarettes et du depot actif du radon-222. In: Late effects of ionizing radiation, Vienna: IAEA, pp 429–435. (IAEA-SM-224-805).

Chameaud J, Perraud R, Chretien J, Masse R, Lafuma J (1980) Combined effects of inhalation of radon daughter products and tobacco smoke. In: Sanders CL, Cross FT, Dagle GE, Mahaffey JA (eds.), Pulmonary toxicology of respirable particles. Proceedings of the 19th Annual Hanford Life Sciences Symposium, Richlands, WA, 1979, pp 551–557.

Clifton KH, Douple EB, Sridharan BN (1976) Effects of grafts of single anterior pituitary glands on the incidence and type of mammary neoplasms in neutron- or γ-irradiated Fischer female rats. Cancer Res 36:3732–3735.

Cloudman AM, Hamilton KA, Clayton RS, Brues AM (1955) Effects of combined local treatment with radioactive and chemical carcinogens. J Natl Cancer Inst 15:1077–1083.

Cole LJ, Foley WA (1969) Modification of urethan-lung tumor incidence by low x-radiation doses of cortisone and transfusion of isogenic lymphocytes. Radiat Res 39:391–399.

Cole LJ, Nowell PC (1964) Carcinogenesis by fast neutrons relative to X-rays in mice. In: Biological effects of neutron and proteon irradiations, Vol. II. Vienna: IAEA, pp 129–141. STI/PUB/80.

Coleman CN (1982) Secondary neoplasms in patients treated for cancer: Etiology and perspective. Radiat Res 92:188–200.

Cosgrove GE, Upton AC, Congdon CC, Doherty DG, Christenberry KW, Gosslee DG (1964) Late somatic effects of x-irradiation in mice treated with AET and isologous bone marrow. Radiat Res 21:550–574.

Cramer W (1932) Experimental observations on the effects of radium on a precancerous skin area. Br J Radol 5:618–630.

Cross FT, Palmer RF, Filipy RE, Dagle GE, Stuart BO (1982) Carcinogenic effects of radon daughters, uranium ore dust and cigarette smoke in beagle dogs. Health Phys 42:33–52.

D'Angio GJ, Meadows A, Mike V, Harris C, Evans A, Jaffe N, Newton W, Schweisguth O, Sutow W, Morris-Jones P (1976) Decreased risk of radiation-associated second malignant neoplasms in actinomycin-D treated patients. Cancer 37:1177–1185.

Davis WE, Cole LJ, Nowell PC (1970) Late effects of x-irradiation in chemicaly protected mice, alteration of tumor incidence after AET treatment. Radiat Res 41:400–408.

DiPaola JA, Donovan PJ, Nelson RL (1971) Irradiation enhancement of transformation by benzo(a)pyrene in hamster embryo cells. Proc Natl Acad Sci USA 68:1734–1737.

DiPaolo JA, Donovan PJ, Popescu NC (1976) Kinetics of Syrian hamster cells during x-irradiation enhancement of tranformation in vitro by chemical carcinogens. Radiat Res 66:310–325.

Epstein JH (1972) Examination of the carcinogenic and cocarcinogenic effects of Grenz radiation. Cancer Res 32:2625–2629.

Fisher PB, Mufson RA, Weinstein IB, Little JB (1981) Epidermal growth factor, like tumor promoters enhances viral and radiation-induced cell transformation. Carcinogenesis 2:183–187.

Fry RJM, Ley RD, Grube D, Staffeldt E (1982) Studies on the multistage nature of radiation carcinogenesis. In: Hecker E et al (eds.), Carcinogenesis, Vol. 7. New York: Raven Press, pp 155–165.

Furth J (1975) Hormones as etiologic agents in neoplasia. In: Becker FF (ed.), Cancer: A comprehensive treatise, Vol. 1. New York: Plenum Press, pp 75–120.

Furth J, Boon MC (1943) Enhancement of leukemogenic action of methyl-cholanthrene by pre-irradiation with x-rays. Science 98:138–139.

Geard CR, Rutledge-Freeman M, Miller RC, Borek C (1981) Antipain and radiation effects on oncogenic transformation and sister chromatid exchanges in Syrian hamster embryo and mouse C3H 10T$\frac{1}{2}$ cells. Carcinogenesis 2:1229–1233.

Goldstein BD, Witz G, Amoruso M, Stone DS, Troll W (1981) Stimulation of human polymorphonuclear leukocyte superoxide anion radical production by tumor promoters. Cancer Lett 11:257–262.

Guernsey DL, Ong A, Borek C (1980) Thyroid hormone modulation of x-ray-induced in vitro neoplastic transformation. Nature 288:591–592.

Guernsey DL, Borek C, Edelman IS (1981) Crucial role of thyroid hormone in x-ray induced neoplastic transformation in cell culture. Proc Natl Acad Sci 78:5708–5711.

Habs H, Kunstler K, Schmahl D, Tomatis L (1983) Combined effects of fast-neutron irradiation and subcutaneiously applied carbon tetrachloride or chloroform in C57BL6 mice. Cancer Lett 20:13–20.

Hall EJ, Miller R, Astor M, Rini F (1978) The nitroimidazoles as radiosensitizers and cytotoxic agents. Br J Cancer 37:120–123.

Hammond EC, Selikoff IJ, Seidman M (1979) Asbestos exposures, cigarette smoking and death rates. Ann NY Acad Sci 330:473–490.

Han A, Elkind MM (1982) Enhanced transformation of mouse 10T$\frac{1}{2}$ cells by 12-0-tetradecanoyl-13-acetate following exposure to x rays or to fission-spectrum neutrons. Cancer Res 42:477–483.

Harisiadis L, Miller RC, Hall EJ, Borek C (1978) A vitamin A analogue inhibits radiation-induced oncogenic transformation. Nature 276:825–826.

Hei TK, Hall EJ, Osmak RS (1984) Asbestos, radiation and oncogene transformation. Br J Cancer 50:717–720.

Holtzman S, Stone JP, Shellabarger CJ (1979) Synergism of diethylstilbestrol and radiation in mammary carcinogenesis in female F344 rats. J Natl Cancer Inst 63:1071–1074.

Holtzman S, Stone JP, Shellabarger CJ (1981) Synergism of estrogens and x rays in mammary carcinogenesis female ACI rats. J Natl Cancer Inst 67:455–459.

Hoshino H, Tanooka H (1975) Internal effect of β-irradiation and subsequent 4-nitroquinoline 1-oxide painting on skin tumor induction in mice. Cancer Res 35:3661–3666.

Kennedy AR (1983) Promotion and other interactions between agents in the induction of transformation in vitro in fibroblast. In: Slaga TJ (ed.), Mechanisms of tumor promotion, Vol. III, Tumor promotion and cocarcinogenesis in vitro. Boca Raton, FL: CRC Press, pp 13–55.

Kennedy AR, Little JB (1978) Protease inhibitors suppress radiation-induced malignant transformation in vitro. Nature(London) 276:825–826.

Kennedy AR, Little JB (1980) Investigation of the mechanism for enhancement of radiation transformation in vitro by 12-0-tetradecanoyl-phorbol-13-acetate. Carcinogenesis 1:1039–1047.

Kennedy AR, Mondal S, Heidelberger C, Little JB (1978) Enhancement of x-ray transformation by 12-0-tetradeconoylphrobol-13-acetate in a cloned line of C3H mouse embryo cells. Cancer Res 38:439–443.

Kennedy AR, Weichselbaum RR (1981) Effects of dexamethasone and cortisone with x-ray irradiation on transformation of C3H 10T$\frac{1}{2}$ cells. Nature 294:97–98.

Kennedy AR, Weischselbaum RR (1981) Effects of 17 β-estradiol on radiation transformation in vitro: Inhibition of effects by protease inhibitors. Carcinogenesis 2:67–69.

Lafuma J, Morin M, Poncy JL, Masse R, Hirsch A, Bignon J, Monchaux G (1980) Mesothelioma induced by intrapleural injection of different types of fibers in rats: Synergistic effect of other carcinogens. In: Biological effects of mineral fibres, Vol. 1. Lyon, France: IARC Scientific Publication 30, pp 311–320.

Little JB (1981) Influence of noncarcinogenic secondary factors on radiation carcinogenesis. Radiat Res 87:240–250.

Little JB, McGandy RB, Kennedy AR (1978) Interactions between polonium-210 α-radiation, benzo(a)pyrene, and 0.9% NaCl solution instillations in the induction of experimental lung cancer. Cancer Res 38:1929–1935.

Loewe S (1953) The problem of synergism and antagonism of combined drugs. Arzneimittelforschung 3:285–290.

Lundin FE, Lloyd JW, Smith EM, Archer VE, Holaday DA (1969) Mortality of uranium miners in relation to radiation exposure, hard-rock mining and cigarette smoking—1950 through September 1967. Health Phys 16:571–578.

Lurie AG (1977) Enhancement of DMBA tumorigenesis in hamster cheek pouch epithelium by repeated exposures to low level x-radiation. Radiat Res 72:499–511.

Lurie AG (1982) Interactions between 7,12-dimethylbenz(a)anthracene (DMBA) and repeated low-level x radiation in hamster cheek pouch carcinogenesis: Dependence on the relative timing of DMBA and radiation treatments. Radiat Res 90:155–164.

Maisin JR, Decleve A, Gerber GB, Mattelin G, Lambiet-Collier M (1978) Chemical protection against the long-term effects of a single whole-body exposure to mice to ionizing radiation. II Causes of death. Radiat Res 74:415–435.

Maisin JR, Gerber GB, Lambiet-Collier M, Mattelin G (1980) Chemical protection against long-term effects of whole-body exposure of mice to ionizing radiation. Radiat Res 82:487–497.

McGandy RB, Kennedy AR, Terzaghi M, Little JB (1974) Experimental carcinogenesis: Interaction between alpha radiation and benzo(a)-pyrene in the hamster. In: Karbe E and Park JF (eds.), Experimental lung cancer, carcinogenesis and bioassays. New York: Springer Verlag, pp 485–491.

McGregor JF (1976) Brief communication: Tumor-promoting activity of cigarette tar in rat skin exposed to irradiation. J Natl Cancer Inst 56:429–430.

McGregor JF (1982) Enhancement of skin tumorigenesis by cigarette smoke condensate following β-irradiation in rats. J Natl Cancer Inst 68:605–611.

Mewissen DJ, Brucer M (1957) Late effects of gamma irradiation on mice protection with cysteamine or cystamine. Nature 179:201–202.

Mian TA, Theiss JC, Grdina DJ (1982) Lung tumorigenic response of strain A mice exposed to hypoxic cell sensitizers alone and in combination with γ-radiation. Cancer Res 43:146–149.

Miller RC, Geard CR, Osmak RS, Rutledge-Freeman M, Ong A, Mason H, Napholtz A, Perez N, Harisiadis L, Borek C (1981) Modification of sister chromatid exchanges and radiation-induced transformation in rodent cells by the tumor promoter 12-0-tetradecanoyl-phorbol-13-acetate and two retinoids. Cancer Res 41:655–659.

Miller RC, Hall EJ (1978) Oncogenic transformation in vitro by the hypoxic cell sensitizer misonidazole. Br J Cancer 38:411–417.

Mottram JC (1937) Production of epithelial tumors by irradiation of a precancerous skin lesion. Am J Cancer 30:746–748.

Myers DK (1976) Effects of x-radiation and urethane on survival and tumor induction in three strains of rats. Radiat Res 65:292–303.

Myers DK, McGregor JF (1982) Interaction of β radiation and 2-anthramine for induction of skin tumors in rats. Radiat Res 90:228–231.

National Research Council, Committee on the Biological Effects Ionizing Radiations (BEIR) (1980) The effects of populations of exposure to low levels of ionizing radiation. Washington, DC: National Academy Press.

Nelson DF, Cooper S, Weston MG, Rubin P (1981) Second malignant neoplasms treated for Hodgkin's disease with radiotherapy or radiotherapy and chemotherapy. Cancer 48:2386–2393.

Nygaard OF, Simic M (eds) (1983) Radioprotectors and anticarcinogens. New York: Academic Press.

Parrish JA, Fitzpatrick TB, Tanenbaum L, Pathak MA (1974) Photochemotherapy of psoriasis with oral methoxsalen and longwave ultraviolet light. N Engl J Med 291:1207–1211.

Prentice RL, Yoshimoto Y, Mason MW (1983) Relationships of cigarette smoking and radiation exposure to cancer mortality in Hiroshima and Nagasaki. J Natl Cancer Inst 70:611–622.

Reif AE (1984) Synergism in carcinogenesis. J Natl Cancer Inst 73:25–39.

Sanders CL (1973) Radionuclide carcinogenesis. In: Sanders CL, Busch RH, Ballou JE (eds.), AEC Conf-720505, Springfield, VA: NTIS, p 119.

Sanders CL (1975) Dose distribution and neoplasia in the lung following intratracheal instillation of ^{239}PuO2 and asbestos. Health Phys 28:383–386.

Scribner JD, Suss R (1978) Tumor initiation and promotion. In: Richter GW and Epstein MA (eds.), International review of experimental pathology. New York: Academic press, pp 138–198.

Segaloff A, Maxfield WS (1971) The synergism between radiation and estrogen in the production of mammary cancer in the rat. Cancer Res 31:166–168.

Ševcová M, Sevc J, Thomas J (1978) Alpha irradiation of the skin and the possibility of late effects. Health Phys 35:803–806.

Shellabarger CJ (1967) Effect of 3-methylcholanthrene and x-irradiation given singly or combined on rat mammary carcinogenesis. J Natl Cancer Inst 38:73–77.

Shellabarger CJ, Schmidt RW (1967) Mammary neoplasia in partial-body-irradiated rats treated with AET. Radiat Res 30:507–514.

Shellabarger CJ, Straub RF (1972) Effect of 3-methycholantrene and fission neutron irradiation given singly or combined on rat mammary carcinogenesis. J Natl Cancer Inst 48:185–187.

Shellabarger CJ, Stone JP, Holtzman S (1976) Synergism between neutron radiation and diethylstilestrol in the production of mammary adenocarcinomas in the rat. Cancer Res 36:1019–1022.

Shellabarger CJ, Holtzman S, Stone JP (1979) Apparent rat strain-related sensitivity to phorbol promotion of mammary carcinogenesis. Cancer Res 39:3345–3348.

Shellabarger CJ, Chmelevsky D, Kellerer AM, Stone JP, Holtzman S (1982) Induction of mammary neoplasms in the AC1 rat by 430-keV neutrons, x-rays and diethylstilbestrol. J Natl Cancer Inst 69:1135–1146.

Shellabarger CJ, Stone JP, Holtzman S (1983) Effect of interval between neutron radiation and diethylstilbestrol on mammary carcinogenesis in female AC1 rats. Environ Health Persp 50:227–232.

Shore RE, Albert RE, Reed M, Harley N, Pasternack BS (1984) Skin cancer incidence among children irradiated for ringworm of the scalp. Radiat Res 100:192–204.

Shubik P, Goldfarb AR, Ritchie AC, Lisco H (1953) Latent carcinogenic action of beta-irradiation on mouse epidermis. Nature 171:934–935.

Sporn MB, Dunlop NM, Newton DL, Henderson WR (1976) Relationships between structure and activity of retinoids. Nature 263:110–113.

Steel GG, Peckham MJ (1979) Exploitable mechanisms in combined radiotherapy-chemotherapy: The concept of additivity. Intl J Radiat Oncol Biol Phys 5:85–91.

Stern RS, Thibodeau LA, Kleinerman RA, Parrish JA, Fitzpatrick TB (1979) Risk of cutaneous carcinoma in patients treated with oral methoxsalen photochemotherapy for psoriasis. N Engl J Med 300:809–813.

Stern RS, Laird N, Melski J, Parrish JA, Fitzpatrick TB, Bleich HL (1984) Cutaneous squamous-cell carcinoma in patients treated with PUVA. N Engl J Med 310:1156–1161.

Stone JP, Holtzman S, Shellabarger CJ (1980) Synergistic interactions of various doses of diethylstilbestrol and x-irradiation on mammary neoplasia in female AC1 rats. Cancer Res 40:3966–3972.

Stone JP, Shellabarger CJ, Holtzman S (1984) The long-term inhibition of induced and spontaneous rat breast carcinogenesis by retinyl acetate: Interim results In: Proceedings of American Association for Cancer Research, Vol. 25, p 126.

Sumi C, Yokoro K, Kajitani T, Ito A (1980) Synergism of diethyl-stilbestrol and other carcinogens in concurrent development of hepatic mammary and pituitary tumors in castrated male mice. J Natl Cancer Inst 65:169–175.

Thomson JF (1962) Radiation protection in mammals. New York: Reinhold Publishing.

Troll W (1976) Blocking tumor promotion by protease inhibitors. In: Magee PN (ed.), Fundamentals in cancer prevention. Maryland: University Park Press, pp 41–55.

Troll W, Weisner R, Shellabarger CJ, Holtzman S, Stone JP (1980) Soybean diet lowers breast tumor incidence in irradiated rats. Carcinogenesis 1:469–472.

Ullrich R, Ethier S (1983) Mammary tumorigenesis after exposure to radiation and 7,12-dimethylbanzantracene. In: Broerse JJ, Barendsen GW, Kal HB, and van der Kogel AJ (eds.), Proceedings of 7th International Congress of Radiation Research. C6–17.

UNSCEAR (1982) Ionizing radiation: Sources and biological effects, Annex L. New York: United Nations.

Upton AC, Doherty DG, Melville GS, Jr. (1959) Chemical protection of the mouse against leukemia induction by roentgen rays. Acta Radiol 51:379–384.

Upton AC, Wolff FF, Sniffen EP (1961) Leukemogenic effect of myleran on the mouse thymus. Proc Soc Exp Biol Med 108:464–467.

Vesselinovitch SD, Simmons EL, Mihailovich N, Lombard LS, Rao KVN (1972) Additive leukemogenicity of urethan and x-irradiation in infant and young adult mice. Cancer Res 32:222–225.

Vogel HH, Zaldivar R (1971) Cocarcinogenesis: The interaction of chemical and physical agents. Radiat Res 47:644–659.

Welsch CW, Goodrich-Smith M, Brown CK, Miglorie N, Clifton HK (1981) Effect of estrogen antagonist (Temoxifen) on the initiation and progression of γ-irradiation-induced mammary tumors in female Sprague–Dawley rats. Eur J Clin Oncol 17:1255–1258.

Whittemore A, McMillan A (1983) Lung cancer mortality among US uranium miners. J Natl Cancer Inst 71:489–499.

Yokoro K, Nakano M, Ito A, Nagao K, Kodama Y, Hamada K (1977) Role of prolactin in rat mammary carcinogenesis: Detection of carcinogenicity of low-dose carcinogens and of persisting dormant cancer cells. J Natl Cancer Inst 58:1777–1783.

Yokoro K, Sumi C, Ho A, Hamada K, Kanda K, Kobayashi T (1980) Mammary carcinogenic effect of low-dose fission radiation in Wistar/Furth rats and its dependency on prolactin. J Natl Cancer Inst 64:1459–1465.

Yuhas JM, Walker AE (1973) Exposure-response curve for radiation-induced lung tumors in the mouse. Radiat Res 54:271–273.

Index